AF668433

Aesthetic Dermatology
Current Perspectives

Get Video Contents Online at *emedicine360.com*

Video 1: Botulinum Toxin Reconstitution
Chapter 11: Patient Selection, Dilution, and Storage

Video 2: Botulinum Toxin for Frown Lines
Chapter 13: Upper Face Indications

Video 3: Botulinum Toxin for Forehead Lines
Chapter 13: Upper Face Indications

Video 4: Botulinum Toxin for Crow's Feet
Chapter 13: Upper Face Indications

Video 5: Botulinum Toxin for Bunny's Lines
Chapter 14: Mid Face Indications

Video 6: Botulinum Toxin for Gummy Smile
Chapter 14: Mid Face Indications

Video 7: Botulinum Toxin for Depressor Anguli Oris
Chapter 15: Lower Face and Neck Indications

Video 8: Botulinum Toxin for Mentalis
Chapter 15: Lower Face and Neck Indications

Video 9: Botulinum Toxin for Platysma
Chapter 15: Lower Face and Neck Indications

Video 10: Botulinum Toxin for Masseter
Chapter 15: Lower Face and Neck Indications

Video 11: Hyaluronic Acid Fillers for Tear Trough and Midface
Chapter 24: Soft Tissue Augmentation of the Midface

Video 12: Fillers for Lower Face
Chapter 25: Dermal Fillers in Lower Face Rejuvenation

Video 13: Soft Tissue Augmentation of Chin with Hyaluronic Acid Fillers
Chapter 25: Dermal Fillers in Lower Face Rejuvenation

Video 14: Lip Augmentation with Fillers
Chapter 26: Hyaluronic Acid Fillers for Lip Rejuvenation

Aesthetic Dermatology
Current Perspectives

Editor-in-Chief

Jaishree Sharad MBBS DDV FAAD

International Mentor, American Society of Dermatologic Surgery
Board of Directors, International Society of Dermatologic and Aesthetic Surgery
Medical Director, Skinfiniti Aesthetic and Laser Clinic
Mumbai, Maharashtra, India

Co-Editor

Maya Vedamurthy MDDD FRCP (Edin and Glasg) MAMS

Consultant Dermatologist and Aesthetic Physician
RSV Skin and Laser Center
Apollo Hospitals
Chennai, Tamil Nadu, India

Foreword

Stephen H Mandy

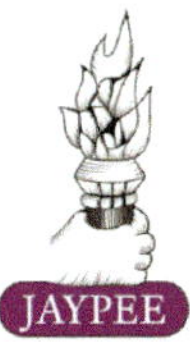

JAYPEE BROTHERS MEDICAL PUBLISHERS

The Health Sciences Publisher

New Delhi | London

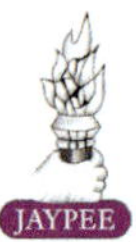

Jaypee Brothers Medical Publishers (P) Ltd

Headquarters
EMCA House
23/23-B, Ansari Road, Daryaganj
New Delhi 110 002, India
Landline: +91-11-23272143, +91-11-23272703
+91-11-23282021, +91-11-23245672
E-mail: jaypee@jaypeebrothers.com

Corporate Office
4838/24, Ansari Road, Daryaganj
New Delhi 110 002, India
Phone: +91-11-43574357
Fax: +91-11-43574314
E-mail: jaypee@jaypeebrothers.com

Overseas Office
J.P. Medical Ltd
83 Victoria Street, London
SW1H 0HW (UK)
Phone: +44 20 3170 8910
E-mail: info@jpmedpub.com

EU GPSR Authorised Representative
Logos Europe, 9 rue Nicolas Poussin
17000, La Rochelle, France
Phone: +33 (0) 6 67 93 73 78
E-mail: contact@logoseurope.eu

Website: www.jaypeebrothers.com
Website: www.jaypeedigital.com

© 2019, Jaypee Brothers Medical Publishers

The views and opinions expressed in this book are solely those of the original contributor(s)/author(s) and do not necessarily represent those of editor(s) of the book.

All rights reserved. No part of this publication may be reproduced, stored or transmitted in any form or by any means, electronic, mechanical, photocopying, recording or otherwise, without the prior permission in writing of the publishers.

All brand names and product names used in this book are trade names, service marks, trademarks or registered trademarks of their respective owners. The publisher is not associated with any product or vendor mentioned in this book.

Medical knowledge and practice change constantly. This book is designed to provide accurate, authoritative information about the subject matter in question. However, readers are advised to check the most current information available on procedures included and check information from the manufacturer of each product to be administered, to verify the recommended dose, formula, method and duration of administration, adverse effects and contraindications. It is the responsibility of the practitioner to take all appropriate safety precautions. Neither the publisher nor the author(s)/editor(s) assume any liability for any injury and/or damage to persons or property arising from or related to use of material in this book.

This book is sold on the understanding that the publisher is not engaged in providing professional medical services. If such advice or services are required, the services of a competent medical professional should be sought.

Every effort has been made where necessary to contact holders of copyright to obtain permission to reproduce copyright material. If any have been inadvertently overlooked, the publisher will be pleased to make the necessary arrangements at the first opportunity. The **CD/DVD-ROM** (if any) provided in the sealed envelope with this book is complimentary and free of cost. **Not meant for sale.**

Inquiries for bulk sales may be solicited at: jaypee@jaypeebrothers.com

Aesthetic Dermatology: Current Perspectives / *Jaishree Sharad*

First Edition: 2019
Reprint: **2026**

ISBN: 978-93-5270-347-0

Printed in India

Dedications

This book is dedicated to my mom and dad who have taught me to believe in my passion and pursue my dreams.

Jaishree Sharad

I dedicate this book to my parents who were visionaries, my husband and children for being my greatest strength and support in my life, and above all my patients who have inspired me throughout my career.

Maya Vedamurthy

Contributors

EDITOR-IN-CHIEF

Jaishree Sharad MBBS DDV FAAD
International Mentor, American Society of Dermatologic Surgery
Board of Directors, International Society of Dermatologic and Aesthetic Surgery
Medical Director, Skinfiniti Aesthetic and Laser Clinic
Mumbai, Maharashtra, India

CO-EDITOR

Maya Vedamurthy MDDD FRCP (Edin and Glasg) MAMS
Consultant Dermatologist and Aesthetic Physician
RSV Skin and Laser Center
Apollo Hospitals
Chennai, Tamil Nadu, India

CONTRIBUTING AUTHORS

Madhuri Agarwal MD
Medical Director
Yavana Aesthetic Clinic
Mumbai, Maharashtra, India

Shehnaz Z Arsiwala MD DDV
Founder and Director
Renewderm Skin, Hair, Laser Aesthetics Centre
Consultant
Saifee Hospital, Prince Aly Khan Hospital
Mumbai, Maharashtra, India

Aditi Bhagat-Patil MD
Dermatologist
Private Practise
Mumbai, Maharashtra, India

Kshama G Bingewar DDV DVD
Consulting Cosmetic Dermatologist
Skin World Clinic
Mumbai, Maharashtra, India

Sebastian Cotofana MD PhD
Associate Professor
Department of Medical Education
Albany Medical College
Albany, New York, USA

Rasya Dixit MD
Medical Director
Dr Dixit Cosmetic Clinic
Bengaluru, Karnataka, India

Zoe D Draelos MD
President
Dermatology Consulting Services
High Point, North Carolina, USA

Jason J Emer MD
Cosmetic Dermatologist
Department of Cosmetic Dermatology and Body Contouring
Spalding Drive Plastic Surgery and Dermatology
Beverly Hills, California, USA

Neetu Gehi MD
Director and Consultant Cosmetic Dermatologist
Skinhance Skin, Hair and Laser Clinic
Mumbai, Maharashtra, India

Jasmine M Gandhi DDVL
Associate Dermatologist
Skinfiniti Aesthetic and Laser Clinic
Mumbai, Maharashtra, India

Harish Kasetty MD
Consultant Dermatologist and Hair Transplant Surgeon
Neoderm Skin Clinic
Hyderabad,Telangana, India

Renita Lourdhurajan MD DNB
Chief Consultant and Director
Department of Cosmetic Dermatology
RENDER Skin and Hair
Chennai, Tamil Nadu, India

Amit Luthra DNB
Cosmetic Dermatologist and
Medical Director, Ishira Skin Clinic
New Delhi, India

Stephen H Mandy MD
Volunteer Professor
Department of Dermatology
Miller School of Medicine
University of Miami
Miami, Florida, USA

Mansi S Mukherjee MD
Head Medical and Service
Innovation
Department of Dermatology
Kaya Skin Clinic
Dubai, UAE

Venkatram Mysore MD DNB DVD
DipRCPath FRCP FISHRS
Director
Department of Dermatology
Venkat Charmalaya Centre for
Advanced Dermatology and
Post Graduate Training
Bengaluru, Karnataka, India

Keyvan Nouri MD
Director
Department of Dermatology and
Cutaneous Surgery
Miller School of Medicine
University of Miami
Miami, Florida, USA

Anuj Pall MD PhD FISD
Chief Director
Department of Dermatology and
Aesthetic Medicine
Escallent Institute of Lasers and
Aesthetic Medicine
Gurugram, Haryana, India

Vrushali Rane DNB FCPS DDVL
Consultant Dermatologist
Private Practise
Mumbai, Maharashtra, India

Rekha A Sheth MD DVD
Consulting Dermatologist
Yuva Skin and Hair Clinic
Mumbai, Maharashtra, India

Neha Sud MD DNB
Consultant Dermatologist
Yuva Skin and Hair Clinic
Mumbai, Maharashtra, India

Abhay Talathi DNB MD FCPS DDVL
Dermatologist
SkinSpace Clinic
Mumbai, Maharashtra, India

Salim Thurakkal MD DNB MNAMS
Medical Director and
Clinical Head
Cutis Institute of Advanced
Dermatology and Aesthetic
Sciences
Calicut, Kerala, India

Anurag Tiwari DVD DNB
Director and Consultant
Dermatologist
Center For Skin Disease and Laser
Treatment
Bhopal, Madhya Pradesh, India

Elizabeth George MD
Fellow Aesthetic Dermatolgy
Venkat Charmalaya Centre for
Advanced Dermatology and Post
Graduate Training
Bengaluru, Karnataka, India

Heidi Waldorf MD
Associate Clinical Professor
Department of Dermatology
Micah School of Medicine of
Mount Sinai
Nanuet, New York, USA

Foreword

It is with great pleasure that I introduce you to this textbook *"Aesthetic Dermatology: Current Perspective"* by Dr Jaishree Sharad and Dr Maya Vedamurthy.

In 2011, I had the delight of mentoring Dr Jaishree Sharad in Miami, Florida. She has been one of the most enthusiastic, well-informed, and skilled physicians I have had the pleasure of teaching over the past 40 years. She has led a distinguished career, lecturing with distinction in the United States, Europe, and South-East Asia. I wish her all the best.

This text is the compilation of the state-of-the-art knowledge in the world of cosmetic treatments written by some of the most experienced dermatologists. This comprehensive text covers all aspects of aesthetic treatments from patient assessment to topical cosmetics, injectables, and energy-based therapies. Each of these areas requires expertise in the anatomy, the structure, and the function of the body's largest organ. This is an ever changing and advancing field of endeavor and it is essential that its practitioners stay informed, invest in the latest technologies, and share their expertise in teaching forums. They advise their patients in the prevention of age and sun related damage, and the maintenance of healthy attractive skin. Surveys of patients who have benefited from skilled aesthetic physicians reveal that they feel and appear 4–7 years younger than their chronological age. For the consumer it is wise to seek the best trained and equipped physician to receive the most natural and pleasing results. The art of aesthetic dermatology is to make your patient look "good," but not "done." Aesthetic dermatology will provide the reader with an in-depth understanding of the art and the science of the specialty at the current time and in the foreseeable future.

Stephen H Mandy MD FAAD
Founding Member and Past President
American Society for Dermatologic Surgery and
the Florida Society of Dermatologic Surgeons
Volunteer Professor, Department of Dermatology
Miller School of Medicine, University of Miami
Miami, Florida, United States

Preface

The great aim of education is not knowledge but action

–Herbert Spencer

When Jaypee Brothers Medical Publishers (P) Ltd. approached me in 2013, to write a textbook on Aesthetic Dermatology, I accepted their invite with great enthusiasm, not realizing what a daunting task it would be. I approached some of my seniors and colleagues to contribute chapters. Few months down the line, I had only three authors who wrote back and my heart sank. It struck me that I was probably too junior to edit an entire book. However, the publisher did not lose hope, they kept pursuing me till the point of my embarrassment. Finally, at the ACSICON 2016 in Mahabaleshwar, two stalwarts and my mentors, Dr Venkataram Mysore and Dr Maya Vedamurthy, encouraged me to complete the book. I took the opportunity and requested Dr Maya to be co-editor. She was extremely kind to accept my request. This gave me confidence to restart the process of editing the book. Our esteemed authors have contributed to this journey to make the book one of a kind.

This book is a comprehensive compilation of various aspects of aesthetic dermatology.

It comprises four sections, the first being on cosmeceuticals. With the market being flooded with cosmeceuticals, it is our duty to guide our patients to choose the right cosmeceutical for themselves. The authors have thrown light on all the newer molecules too.

The second section comprises botulinum toxin. We have discussed anatomy, techniques, and complications in order to help all beginners inject with a clear understanding of neuromodulators.

The third section is on soft tissue augmentation with fillers. The upper face, midface, lower face, and complications have been discussed at length.

The last section is about lasers and miscellaneous procedures like microneedling, thread lifts, body contouring, and platelet-rich plasma, giving an insight to every procedure in depth.

Together with Dr Maya Vedamurthy, I hope that this book benefits postgraduates, dermatologists, and all the physicians who practice aesthetic dermatology. So, here's to reading and getting into action.

Jaishree Sharad

Acknowledgement

I would like to express my deepest gratitude towards:

- Dr Maya Vedamurthy for encouraging me to take up this challenge and helping me sail through this task
- All the amazing authors of this book for their valuable contribution
- My mentors Dr Stephen Mandy, Dr Gerhard Sattler, Dr Zoe Draelos, Dr Rebecca Fitzgerald, Dr Niwat Polnikorn, Dr Satish Savant, Dr Venkataram Mysore, and Dr Rekha Sheth for inspiring me and instilling the confidence in me to look beyond the horizon
- Dr Anuj Pall, Dr M Kumaresan, Dr Chandan Ashokan, Dr Ginni Chhabria, Dr Aarthi Senthil, Dr Jasmine Gandhi, and Dr Snehal Shende for helping us with editing and proofreading
- Senior Acquisition Editor, Dr Neeraj Choudhary; Editorial Coordinator, Ms Barkha Arora; and the entire team at Jaypee Brothers Medical Publishers (P) Ltd. who worked towards the making of this book
- All my patients who have been my biggest supporters
- My associate doctors for being my backbone and my staff for tolerating my idiosyncrasies along the journey of this book
- Allergan for providing injectables for the training videos that come along with this book
- My little angels Aarav and Giana for being my reviving bundles of joy every time I felt this book was impossible
- Last but not the least, my husband, Dr Sharad Sharma for being my rock of Gibraltar.

Jaishree Sharad

Contents

SECTION 1: COSMECEUTICALS

SECTION 2: BOTULINUM TOXIN

SECTION 3: SOFT TISSUE AUGMENTATION

SECTION 4: ADJUNCTIVE TREATMENTS

1

SECTION

COSMECEUTICALS

1

CHAPTER

Cleansers

Jaishree Sharad, Neha Sud

INTRODUCTION

Cleansers can be defined as products used to clean a surface of dirt and grime. Our skin has a plethora of products that collect on the surface and need to be removed on a regular basis to maintain a basic standard of hygiene. The skin surface produces sebum which attracts and attaches dust to the skin surface as dirt. Cosmetics, creams and makeup can also increase this greasy feel and compound the above effect attracting dirt and clogging pores. Over this is added the external pollutants and bacteria. Bacterial action on the sweat with the excreted urea and different salts can produce repugnant body odor. In addition the stratum corneum also sheds or desquamates its cells. Cleansers help remove all the above to maintain personal hygiene and health.

HOW DO CLEANSERS WORK?[1,2]

Cleansers can employ a physical or chemical method to clean the skin. Physical cleansing is primarily by the use of friction, like wiping the skin with a cotton ball or tissue. The friction helps to dislodge the soils from the stratum corneum. Whereas for chemical cleansing, this act of loosening can be by emulsification or dissolving, depending on the composition of the cleanser, primarily its surfactant component and solution properties. Surfactants or "surface active agents" help to loosen the dirt from the sebum and grease and aid its removal by rinsing or wiping thereafter. It is their amphiphilic nature, i.e., surfactants have a polar and a nonpolar end, that aids in removing dirt by reducing the surface tension between the dirt and water. Surfactants position themselves at the oil-water interface. Here they emulsify dirt and grease by forming micelles or surfactant spheres holding the oil phase in the center. Their hydrophobic nonpolar ends point in and the hydrophilic polar ends point out in the water phase. For micelles to form, the concentration of the surfactant should be above a critical value, that is called the critical micellar concentration for that surfactant. There are multitude of surfactants, from those in soaps which are the most basic, sodium stearate or sodium tallowate and are anionic, to those in syndets which can be silicone containing[3] or depending on the surface charge can be (Table 1):

- Anionic
- Cationic
- Amphoteric, or
- Nonionic.

Silicone surfactants (e.g., dimethicone) serve two purposes as they are able to penetrate into follicular orifices and surface grooves; they enhance removal of grime therein and also form an effective barrier for TEWL (trans epidermal water loss) as a result of the smooth surface film that they form on the skin. Hence, these surfactants are noncomedogenic and have a low irritation potential with hypoallergenicity.[7]

From these multitudes of surfactants primarily two are used in manufacturing bar cleansers—alkyl carboxylate (for soaps) and acyl isethionate (for syndets).

Liquid cleansers or personal care products use a combination of different surfactants for optimal and desired end results.

Cleansing by dissolving involves the basic principle of "like dissolves like", and this is in reference to the solvent phase of the cleanser. Surface dirt and body secretions, solids and other liquids get suspended in a homogeneous solution as a result of solvent use. Greasy residue or oil-based makeup would best be cleared by an oil-based nonpolar solvent and would work well in dry aged skin as

TABLE 1: Surfactants types based on surface charge with examples and salient properties[4-6]

Surfactant type	Example	Properties
Anionic (negatively charged)	• Sodium lauryl sulfate • Sodium laureth sulfate • Cocoylisethionate • Sodium stearate • Sodium tallowate	• Good detergents • Good lathering properties • Alkyl sulfates: Poor skin tolerance • Sodium cocoyl isethionate: Excellent skin compatibility
Cationic (positively charged)	• Sodium triethanolamine	• Poorly tolerated alone
Amphoteric (both positive and negative charge)	• Betaines, like cocamidopropylbetaine • Alkylamino acids	• Lather well • Well tolerated
Nonionic (uncharged)	• Polyglucosides • Polysorbates • Propylene glycol	• Lather poorly • Well tolerated

they have a tendency to leave an oil film. On the other hand polar cleansers, which are alcohol based, would work well in oily acne-prone young skin. They may simply be wiped by a cotton ball or swab and do not require water for the same.

Cleansers and Stratum Corneum Interaction

Product and stratum corneum interaction depends on chemical attributes of individual ingredients in a preparation and change in properties and behavior as a result of intraformulation interactions. The collective response determines if a cleanser or a moisturizer is a mild one or not.[8]

Ingredients of skin cleansers:[2]

- Water
- Surfactants
- Moisturizers
- Stabilizers
- Hardeners
- Foam enhancers
- Preservatives
- Fragrance
- Dyes and pigments.

Factors governing skin interaction and result with cleanser use:

- Surfactant: Type, chemical structure, and concentration
- Hydrophobically modified polymers
- Moisturizing agents
- pH of the cleansers
- Fragrances and preservatives
- Rinsabilty factor.

In the process of skin cleansing, some surfactants do bind to the skin lipids and get left over on the skin surface too after rinsing. This distorts and disrupts the intercellular lipid barrier. The surfactant may bind to the proteins and make them swell and become more permeable with the resultant loss of NMFs and TEWL, thus making the skin dry, dull, flaky, red, and itchy with an after wash tightness.

The ability of different surfactants for this skin irritation potential follows the following order:

Cationic = anionic > amphoteric > nonionic.[9,10] Even though anionic and cationic surfactants lead the order for skin irritation, their lather forming properties and antimicrobial properties make them an important part of cleansers in general and antimicrobial washes, respectively.

To reduce their overall irritation potential incorporation in lower concentrations in combination with amphoteric and nonionic surfactants can help.[11-13]

Hydrophobically modified polymers reduce the surfactant skin interaction by forming surfactant polymer complexes, hence reducing skin irritation.

Many products have the ability to deposit moisturizing factors, emollients, occlusive or humectants, on the skin to counteract the dryness caused by the action of surfactants. However, due to the short skin-cleanser contact time, this ability for barrier restoration and skin hydration is guarded.[14]

Even though the skin has an inherent buffering capacity, another factor that on repeated exposure can alter moisture content, bacterial flora, and skin pH and result in skin irritation is the pH of the cleanser.[15] Cleansers with pH close to 5.5 are considered the most compatible with SC integrity causing minimal lipid alteration. Neutral and acidic cleansers are preferable over alkaline ones.[9]

Fragrances and preservatives are the other major irritants present in cleansers and surfactant effect on the skin can pave a pathway for deeper skin entry of these molecules also. Formaldehyde or formaldehyde releasers, like quaternium 15 or diazolidinyl urea or imidazolidinyl urea, followed by methylchloroisothiazolinone/methylisothiazolinone mixture with diazolidinyl urea have been implicated as the most common nonfragrance allergens in cosmetics and personal care products.[16,17] All these are commonly used as preservatives in cleansers.

The skin-cleanser contact time should be minimal to reduce the irritation potential of the cleanser. This property varies for different molecules and this rinsability factor is high for liquid lipid free cleansers.[18]

TYPES OF SKIN CLEANSERS

- Cleansing bars
    - Routine or basic bars
    - Moisturizing or beauty bars
        - Superfatted bars
        - Transparent bars
        - Syndet bars
    - Antibacterial or medicated or deodorant bars
- Liquid washes
    - Body washes
        - Regular body washes
        - Moisturizing body washes
        - Speciality body washes
    - Facial cleansers
        - Lathering cleansers
        - Nonlathering cleansers
            - Lipid-free cleansers
            - Cleansing creams
            - Cleansing milk/lotions
            - Astringents/toners
            - Waterless cleansers
            - Scrubs
    - Antibacterial washes—face/body
- Cleansing cloths
    - Dry
    - Wet.

Cleansing Bars[19]

The basic active ingredient in cleansing bars is the surfactant. Primarily two surfactants are used—alkyl carboxylate and acyl istheonate. Cleansing bars that use the former are called soaps and the ones using the latter are called synthetic detergent bars or syndets.

Basic Bars or Soaps

These are the simplest and most basic type of bars. Soaps are formed by a process called saponification wherein alkalis are made to react with fats and oils, hence making them simply sodium salts of fatty acids. The source of the fatty acids can be animal (e.g., tallow or lard)) or plant/vegetable (e.g., coconut oil, olive oil, palm oil). They can be used in different combinations, mostly animal to plant fatty acid ratio 4:1. Qualities of the final soap bar depend on the type of fatty acids used: longer carbon chain lengths, less soluble and remain solid whereas shorter lengths, lather easily. Basic soaps have a high pH and are irritating to the skin as a result of damaging effects of the surfactant on the skin barrier.

Moisturizing or Beauty Bars

These bars have skin moisturizing properties because of the presence of skin benefit agents and hence are less irritating to the skin.

Superfatted Soaps

In the process of soap making if excess fat/oil is left in the soap after saponification is complete, it results in superfatted soaps. The excess fats could be lanolin, paraffin, shea butter, cocoa butter, etc. and as a common effect reduce the drying effect of the soap on the skin.

Transparent Soaps

These are common bar soaps where glycerine (most commonly), a polyhydric alcohol, is added as a moisturizer, making it less irritating for the skin. Other polyhydric alcohols are polyethylene glycol and propylene glycol. Polyhydric alcohols are solvents that render the bar transparent.

Syndet Bars

Syndets are synthetic detergent-based cleansers. They have a pH, 5.5–7, close to the skin acid mantle with less than 10% soap content, hence less skin dryness and better skin compatibility.[9,20] The surfactant here is most commonly acyl isethionate which renders it less damaging to the stratum corneum lipids. They do not form a soap scum layer.

Medicated Bars

These have added antibacterial agents like triclosan, carbanilide and trichlocarbon. These antibacterial agents inhibit bacterial growth and indirectly help in reducing body odor too. Some antibacterial bars are also marketed as deodorant bars, which in addition have added fragrances to mask the body odor. Their primary beneficial effect would be to suppress the harmful bacteria but in the process they also disrupt or harm the natural skin flora and cause skin dryness and irritation. Antiacne bars

TABLE 2: Highlighting differences in different types of cleansing bars[15,21]

	Basic bars	Superfatted bars	Transparent bars	Syndet bars	Antibacterial bars
Surfactant	Soap based*	Soap based*	Soap based*	Nonsoap based*	Soap based*
pH#	9–11	8–10	8–9	5.5–7	9–11
Added ingredients	None	Excess fatty acids	Glycerine or polyhydric alcohols	Creams	Triclosan, carbanilide, trichlocarbon
Drying effects on skin	+++	++	++/+	+/–	+++

Note: *Soap-based, having alkyl carboxylate as the surfactant, nonsoap based, having acyl isethionate as the surfactant.
#pH varies from bar to bar within the given categories also, this is a rough guide.[15]

too have some antibacterial agent, e.g., triclosan, azelaic acid, zinc oxide, benzoyl peroxide, tea tree oil, neem extract, clove oil, etc. to control the activity of *Propionibacterium acnes* or some active agents like α- or β-hydroxy acids like glycolic and salicylic acid, respectively. They help to reduce the sebaceous activity and help in exfoliation. Table 2 highlights the differences in different types of cleansing bars.

Liquid Cleansers[5,22]

Like bars liquid cleansers are also based on soap or nonsoap surfactants, albeit at a lower concentration, but with a higher water percentage than bars.

There can be a diverse combination of syndets which lather well with hard water but can irritate. To mitigate the irritation potential of surfactants, surfactants with different properties can be combined, e.g., alkyl sulphates (anionic surfactants) while having relatively poor skin compatibility, lather well. So combining an alkyl sulphate with an amphoteric surfactant such as cocamidopropyl betaine can improve both lather and skin compatibility. This lends an aesthetic appeal and better acceptability to liquid cleansers. Facial cleansers have a high percentage of amphoteric surfactants as they lather well and are tolerated well. They have a high rinsability factor too.

Liquid cleansers have a higher percentage of water that offers advantage of form and possibility to add a number of skin benefit agents but risk contamination, hence need preservatives, and increased molecular interactions challenging chemical stability. They contain antioxidants, chelating agents and are formulated around specific pH. Additives like shea butter, olive oil, glycerine, silicones, petrolatum, pulverized fruit seeds, and beads in liquid cleansers help to provide skin benefits ranging from moisturization to soft post rinse feel and exfoliation. Though due to a short contact time of cleansers on the skin, these changes may not be as evident. Dyes and fragrances in addition help to increase the consumer appeal of the product by stimulating visual and olfactory senses. Liquid cleansers can be categorized as those used primarily for the body, face, or hands. Division is guided by surfactant/solvent choices and combinations and delivery systems in addition to specific benefits designed for different body areas and needs.

Discussing a few nuances about the different liquid cleansers below.

Body Washes[1,22]

Regular Body Washes

They primarily serve the purpose of skin cleansing though added fragrances may help win over consumers' olfactory senses.

Moisturizing Body Washes

These body washes help deposit a skin benefit agent, moisturizing factors in this case, on use in addition to the primary action of skin cleansing and this ameliorates their inherent irritancy. Moisturizing ingredients are diverse: lanolin, olive oil, bees wax, paraffin, shea butter, cocoa butter, glycerine, urea, petrolatum, vegetable oils like sunflower and soybean oil, ceramides, cholesterol, etc. Coacervation of molecules like petrolatum in body washes can effectively help moisturize the skin along with cleansing.[1]

Speciality Body Washes[23]

These cleansing systems have ingredients apart from the above that benefit the skin.

As mentioned earlier they may have beads, e.g., polyethylene, aluminum oxide, sodium tetra borate decahydrate; or pulverized or ground fruit seeds, e.g., apricot seeds; or oatmeal that help in mechanical skin exfoliation and provide a dry skin benefit by removing dead skin cells in the scales. Of these, aluminum oxide and fruit pits have the most abrasive action because of their sharp edged surfaces and may lead to skin irritation in sensitive skins. Polyethylene microspheres on the other hand have a smooth surface and provide a gentle and effective exfoliation. They have been cited as an environmental hazard though, because of their nonbiodegradable nature after they were found as contaminants in the water in the Great lakes of North America.[24] There are others like sodium decahydrate granules that dissolve during use. Sugar granules mixed with detergents also melt away during use.

Menthol, another ingredient, in body washes helps provide a cooling and relaxing sensation on use.

Facial Cleansers[5,23,25]

Lathering Cleansers

Lathering cleansers produce a good amount of lather as a result of high concentration, above the critical micelle concentration, of mostly anionic or amphoteric surfactants. To minimize the lipid stripping effect on skin lipids, syndets are primarily incorporated in these systems along with the addition of skin-benefitting moisturizing agents.

Nonfoaming/low Foaming Cleansers[25]

This group is specially formulated for care of the facial skin. They comprise the cleansing creams, cleansing milks and lotions, lipid-free cleansers and waterless cleansers. These "gentle" cleansing systems have "gentler acting" surfactants like sarcosinates and betaines, e.g., cocamidopropyl betaine. Incorporation of humectants, like glycerine, butylene glycol or propylene glycol, in addition helps to attract water to the skin. Some skin care product ranges also introduce hyaluronic acid for its amazing water-retaining properties. Another way to make a product less irritating to the skin is to reduce the levels of irritants like fragrances and preservatives.

Lipid-free cleansers

They do not contain any naturally derived fats or lipids and are also called as "soap-free" cleansers. Fatty alcohols evaporate not leaving any film behind. So, these cleansers offer high rinsibility.[18] They work well as cleansers for dry to normal skin. They are rubbed to produce lather on dry skin and thereafter wiped away so do not need water for cleansing. Their main constituents are water, glycerine, cetyl alcohol and propylene glycol.

Cleansing creams

As the name defines they cleanse and moisturize, so are suited more for dry skin. They work on solvent action of the oil component; mineral oil or wax. Borax lends the detergent action. Heavy, longlasting oil-based makeup can be effectively removed with these cleansers.

Cleansing milk or lotions

They are water-based counterparts of cleansing creams. Their primary mode of action is through emulsification/dissolving in contrast as the external phase here is water. They can be effectively used to remove water-based makeup with a cotton ball or wipe or can be easily rinsed away with water, though generally water is not used.

Astringent or toners

Astringent/tonic/refresher—the nomenclature can vary depending on the concentration of the alcohol component, which imparts the toner with its solvency or dissolving properties. Toners are best suited for oily acne-prone skin or skin areas producing excess of sebum, the T zone especially the nose, and for removing makeup. They can be directly applied to a cotton ball or tissue wipe and used over the target area. This action in addition helps to dislodge the soil or dirt by physical means or friction. The alcohol as it evaporates in addition provides a cooling sensation as do added menthol and camphor in some.

Waterless cleansers

These cleansers are alcoholic preparations, mostly containing isopropyl alcohol, that dissolve oils and sebum. Surfactants if present are in minimal amounts.

Scrubs

Scrubs help to remove lodged dirt by a physical abrasive action imparted by particulate ingredients—natural or synthetic. Natural particles include seeds of fruits (e.g., peach, apricot, or apple), nut shells (e.g., walnut, almond), grains (oats, wheat), sandlewood or sugar. Synthetic particles include polyethylene or polypropylene beads or aluminum oxide or sodium tetraborate decahydrate granules. They help to exfoliate and control excess sebum production suiting oily flaky skin. Sensitive skin types may not be able to tolerate the abrasive action of the beads on the skin and may become red and inflamed. They are best used on intact skin.

Antibacterial Washes[26,27]

These can be called the liquid counterparts of medicated bar cleansers. Their primary indications are as cleansers for acne prone or seborrheic skin and as antiseptic hand cleansers. Antiacne cleansers with antibacterial agents, like benzoyl peroxide, sodium sulfacetamide, sulfur or natural extracts like neem extract or tea tree oil extract, quite similar to their bar counterparts, can be used as a part of a comprehensive treatment plan for acne. They have a bacteriostatic action on the *P. acnes* population and other skin pathogens too. But most of these ingredients irritate the skin. Added emollients can help to mitigate this dryness. Variation in mode of formulation delivery, like in foam form (property because of the added aerosols), can make it less messy and easy to use, especially for large areas, without residue and can enhance cosmetic acceptability and compliance. Salicylic acid, benzoyl peroxide and sodium sulphacetamide-sulfur combination are available as foam-based cleansers. The latter combination has been used for the treatment of rosacea and seborrheic dermatitis in addition to acne.[26]

Cleansing Cloths or Substrate Cleansers

These are the most recent addition to the armamentarium of skin cleansers. Here, the chemical ingredients are absorbed on a nonwoven cloth. They are a double-edged sword; having a dual, physical (imparted by the friction of the cloth with the skin), and a chemical action (role donned by the surfactants and solvents either by emulsifying or dissolving). The cloth can be a natural material, like cotton or synthetic, like rayon, polypropylene or a blend of the two. Because of parallel mechanisms acting at the same time the concentration and type of surfactants used can be skin friendly, i.e., milder surfactants at lower concentrations can be incorporated without worrying about the degree of skin cleansing. Surfactants with one-fourth the concentrations of that in regular liquid cleansers can suffice for substrate cleansers. With the benefit of better cleansing, they prevent overcleansing on part of the consumer as the dirt and soils removed are visible on the cloth as an evidence of effectiveness.

Dry Cleansing Cloths

Here, the cleansing chemicals are directly applied to a cleansing cloth. The cloth needs to be wet before use and needs to be rubbed to produce lather. Petrolatum as an additive hydrates the skin and serves as a barrier to TEWL.[5]

Wet Cleansing Cloths

They are another product range that works well in people with dry skin as they leave a film of humectants and lipids on the skin after use. They are packaged in the wet state, much like baby wipes for the diaper area, and are use and throw products alike.

The most recent are the cleansing brushes. Companies with patent technologies, like the Clarisonic, have innovated cleansing heads with circumferential rows of grouped bristles oscillating at sonic frequencies (300 movements per second), which they claim works with the skin elasticity resulting in flexion action that loosens deeply impregnated impurities from skin pores too (claims of up to six times better cleansing action than the hands used alone). Heads of this handy equipment can be replaced depending on the body area and skin type to be treated.

CLEANSERS IN USE

Expectations from a good cleanser:

- Lather easily and in good amount
- Good smell or fragrance
- Remove all dirt and makeup
- Good post rinse feel to skin
- Does not excessively dry the skin
- Remove body odor
- Does not become mushy in humid surroundings and keeps its shape (for bars)
- Does not dry up and break in between use (for bars).

Primary goals of good cleansing:

- To remove soils (dirt, grease, makeup) from the skin surface effectively
- To remove skin contaminant bacteria effectively
- To exfoliate or remove the dead skin cells
- To cause minimal harm to the skin lipid barrier.

Adverse effects of cleansers:[9]

- After wash tightness is due to enhanced rate of water loss from the skin surface and is the sensation perceived after washing with a soap
- Skin dryness, scaling and roughness can be due to alcohol-based solvents, surfactants, over usage, vigorous cleansing which is further aggravated in dry and cold weather
- Skin irritation, erythema, and itching as a result of damage to the skin barrier
- Allergic contact dermatitis; sensitivity to preservatives, fragrances, and dyes.

HOW TO CHOOSE A CLEANSER

One can choose a cleanser depending on answers to the following questions:

- What is the skin type?

- What is the cleanser form preference—soap/liquid/substrate?
- Any associated problem skin/diseased skin states?

The following table outlines properties of facial and skin cleansers suited in special case scenarios (Table 3).

TABLE 3: Selection based on accompanying skin condition or specific needs[28-35]

Skin condition	Type of cleanser
Newborn skin	• Bars or liquid cleansers with neutral pH (5.5–7.0) • Mild surfactants • Emollients • Preservative-free • Fragrance-free • Nonirritating to the eyes
Oily skin	• Lathering cleansers • Substrate-based cleansers • Toners • Scrubs
Acne-prone skin	• Nonionic bar or liquid cleanser • Antibacterial cleansers/bars • Good rinsability • Fragrance-free
Dry xerotic skin	• Cleansers containing humectants, emollients or ceramides • Coacervated petroleum body washes
Atopic skin	• Liquid cleansers or syndets with pH 5.5–6 • Hypoallergenic • Fragrance-free • Preservative-free
Rosacea skin	• Syndet cleansers and lipid-free cleansers • Neutral to slightly acidic pH • With emollients and humectants • Without irritants and allergens • Avoid alcohol-based cleansers
Photoaged skin	• Lipid-free cleansing agents • Containing humectants and emollients
Makeup-loaded skin	• Heavy oil-based makeup • Substrate, lathering cleansers or toners or cream-based cleansers • Light water-based makeup—cleansing lotions work well

CONCLUSION

There has been a gradual evolution from the traditional soap bars to synthetic detergents to speciality skin cleansers with a major boom at the turn of the century. Consumer demands, habits, and acceptability have been a major catalyst or driving force for technological progress in making more satisfactory cleansers, which respect the skin barrier function at the root level. From merely cleansing, cleansers have come a long way in providing moisturizing benefits too to the skin but cannot surpass the effects of a moisturizer per se on the skin.

REFERENCES

1. Mukhopadhyay P. Cleansers and their role in various dermatological disorders. Indian J Dermatol. 2011;56(1): 2-6.
2. Corazza M, Lauriola MM, Zappaterra M, et al. Surfactants skin cleansing protagonists. J Eur Acad Dermatol Venereol. 2010:24(1):1-6.
3. Hasenoehrl E. Facial cleansers and cleansing cloths. In: Draelos ZD (Ed). Cosmetic Dermatology: Products and Procedures, 1st edition. London: Wiley-Blackwell; 2010. pp. 95-101.
4. Kaimal S. Cosmetics in children. In: Thappa DM (Ed). Clinical Pediatric Dermatology, 1st edition. Noida: Elseiver; 2009. pp. 181-91.
5. Kirsner RS, Froelich CW. Soaps and detergents: understanding their composition and effect. Ostomy Wound Manage. 1998;44(Suppl 3A):62S-70S.
6. Loden M. Role of topical emollients and moisturizers in the treatment of dry skin barrier disorders. Am J Clin Dermatol. 2003;4(11):771-8.
7. Ananthapadmanabhan KP, Moore DJ, Subramanyan K, et al. Cleansing without compromise: the impact of cleansers on the skin barrier and the technology of mild cleansing. Dermatol Ther. 2004;17(Suppl1):16-25.
8. Effendy I, Maibach HI. Detergent and skin irritation. Clin Dermatol. 1996;14:15-21.
9. Dominquez JG, Balaguer F, Parra JL, et al. The inhibitory effect of some amphoteric surfactants on the irritation potential of alkyl sulfayes. Int J Cosmet Soc. 1981;3(2): 57-68.
10. Draelos Z, Hornby S, Walters RM, et al. Hydrophobically modified polymers can minimize skin irritation potential caused by surfactant based cleansers. J Cosmet Dermatol. 2013;12(4):314-21.
11. Hornby S, Walters RM, Kamath Y, et al. Reduction in skin barrier perturbation by hydrophobically modified polymers. JAAD. 2011;64;2(Suppl 1):AB25.
12. Eichenfield LF, Tom WL, Berger TG, et al. Guidelines of care for the management of atopic dermatitis: section 2. Management and treatment of atopic dermatitis with topical therapies. J Am Acad Dermatol. 2014;71(1):116-32.
13. Tyebkhan G. A study on the pH of commonly used soaps/cleansers available in the Indian market. Indian J Dermatol Venereol Leprol. 2001;67:290-1.

14. Travassos AR, Claes L, Boey L, et al. Non-fragrance allergens in specific cosmetic products. Contact Dermatitis. 2011;65(5):276-85.
15. Boyapati A, Tam M, Tate B, et al. Allergic contact dermatitis to methylisothiazoline: exposure from baby wipes causing hand dermatitis. Australas J Dermatol. 2013;54(4):264-7.
16. Bikowski J. The use of cleansers as therapeutic concomitants in various dermatologic disorders. Cutis. 2001;68: 12-9.
17. Draelos ZD. Skin care for the sensitive skin and rosacea patient: the biofilm and new cleansing technology. Cosmet Dermat. 2006;19(8):520-2.
18. Lakshmi C, Srinivas CR, Anand CV, et al. Irritancy ranking of 31 cleansers in the Indian market in a 24-h patch test. Int J Cosmet Sci. 2008;30:277-83.
19. Johnson AW, Ananthapadmanabhan KP. Bar cleansers. In: Draelos ZD, editor. Cosmetic dermatology- products and procedures. 1st ed. London:Blackwell publishing ltd;2010:77-86.
20. Ertel K, Focht H. Personal cleansers: body washes. In Draelos ZD (Ed). Cosmetic Dermatology: Products and Procedures, 1st edition. London: Wiley-Blackwell; 2010. pp 88-94.
21. Savant SS. Personal care and cosmetic products. In: Savant SS (Ed). Textbook of Dermatosurgery and Cosmetology, 2nd edition. Mumbai: ASCAD; 2005. pp. 500-15.
22. Landau E. Plastic microbeads to be removed from soap. Edition.cnn.com. CNN. 8 Jan 2013. Web. 25 July.
23. Aust D. Nonfoaming and low foaming cleansers. In: Draelos ZD (Ed). Cosmetic Dermatology: Products and Procedures, 1st edition. London: Wiley-Blackwell; 2010. pp. 102-5.
24. Del Rosso JQ. The use of sodium sulfacetamide 10%-sulphur 5% emollient foam in the treatment of acne vulgaris. J Clin Aesthet Dermatol. 2009;2(8):26-9.
25. Leyden JJ, Del Rosso JQ. The effect of benzoyl peroxide 9.8% emollient foam on reduction of Propionibacterium acnes on the back using a short contact therapy approach. J Drugs Dermatol. 2012;11(7):830-3.
26. Telofski LS, Morello AP, Mack Correa MC, et al. The infant skin barrier: can we preserve, protect, and enhance the barrier? Dermatol Res Pract. 2012;2012:198789.
27. Sarkar R, Basu S, Agarwal RK, et al. Skin care for the new born. Indian Paediatrics. 2010;47:593-98.
28. Tyebkhan G. Skin cleansing in neonates and infants-basics of cleansers. Indian J Pediatr. 2002;69:767-9.
29. Goodman G. Cleansing and moisturizing in acne patients. Am J Clin Dermatol. 2009;10(1):1-6.
30. Solomon BA, Shalita AR. Effect of detergents in acne. Clin Dermatol. 1996;14:95-9.
31. Ananthapadmanabhan K, Yang L, Vincent C, et al. A novel technology in mild and moisturizing cleansing liquids. Cosmet Dermatol. 2009;22(6):307-16.
32. Ananthapadmanabhan P, Mukherjee S, Chandar P. Stratum corneum fatty acids: their critical role in preserving barrier integrity during cleansing. Int J Cosmet Sci. 2013;35(4):337-45.
33. Draelos ZD. The effect of ceramide containing skin care products on eczema resolution duration. Cutis. 2008;81(1):87-91.
34. Draelos ZD, Ertel K, Hartwig P, et al. The effect of two skin cleansing systems on moderate xerotic eczema. J Am Acad Dermatol. 2004;5086:883-8.
35. Draelos ZD. Facial hygiene and comprehensive management of rosacea. Cutis. 2004;73(3):183-7.

2
CHAPTER

Moisturizers

Jaishree Sharad, Neha Sud

INTRODUCTION

Moisturizers can be defined as products that help to reduce or treat dry skin by restoring moisture in the skin.

They work by smoothening and soothing dry irritated skin, correcting imperfections, and improving skin tone and texture.

BASIC SCIENCE[1]

Water content of epidermis: Irwin H Blank in the 1950s demonstrated the importance of the stratum corneum (SC) water content. The epidermis has up to 30% water content which if becomes less than 10% is evident as dry skin. Dysfunction of epidermal enzymes, especially stratum corneum chymotryptic enzyme, essential for sloughing off the upper stratum corneal cells ensues at low moisture levels. This disrupts the process of corneodesmolysis, i.e., the gradual proteolytic dissociation of the corneodesmosomes. As a result, the cells slough off as clumps and with more air-skin interfaces created the skin appears dry and scaly.

Natural moisturizing factors (NMFs) and the stratum corneum barrier: The ability to retain water in the epidermis is served by the barrier of overlapping corneocytes and a functional lipid layer, which is composed of a triple lipid bilayer. These lipids are ceramides, cholesterol, and free fatty acids present in the physiological critical molar ratio of 1:1:1.[2] This molar ratio along with the lamellar organization of the lipids is essential for the integrity of the lipid barrier. These lipids are attached to the corneocytes via the ω-hydroxy ceramide bonds and this forms the corneocyte lipid envelope.[3]

The extracellular processing of polar lipids, present in Odland bodies or the lamellar granules, produces neutral ceramides and free fatty acids by the action of sphingomyelinases and phospholipases, respectively. Cholesterol, from the circulation, enters via receptors in the basal layer cells. Steroid sulphatase enzyme then processes cholesterol substrates as they move from the lower to the upper layers of the SC. Optimal functioning of these enzymes of extracellular processing requires an acidic pH. Hence pH is an indirect contributor to barrier function. A small percentage of lipids is also contributed to by the sebaceous glands.

Where the above has been referred to as the dynamic aspect of cutaneous hydration, the static component is the binding of water to the NMFs.[4]

Natural moisturizing factors are natural humectants of the skin. They are intracellular water-soluble low molecular weight compounds that help maintain hydration of the stratum corneum. They comprise of components like, urocanic acid, amino acids, pyrrolidone carboxylic acid and mineral ions, derived from the breakdown of the protein filaggrin.

Hence effectively the SC barrier, corneocytes, and lipid bilayer help limit transepidermal water loss (TEWL) and loss of NMFs from the cells.

Newer insights into this water barrier have been imparted by the discovery of the aquaporin-3 channels, special moisture regulating channels, in the viable epidermis and the presence of tight junctions between the stratum granulosum and SC.[5]

How Do Moisturizers Help?

In the quest to maintain basic hygiene, by cleaning our bodies with soaps and body washes, we inadvertently damage or harm the SC lipid barrier

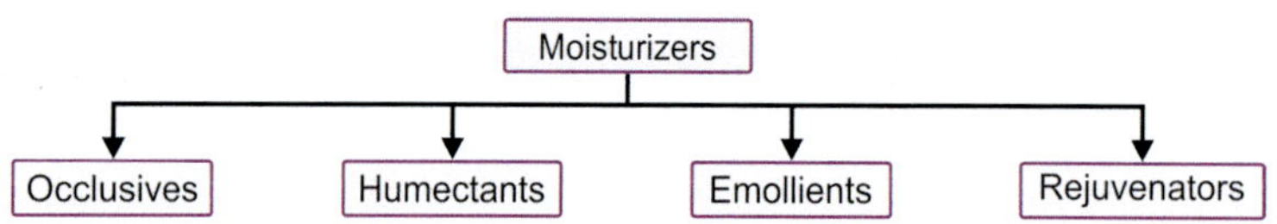

FLOWCHART 1: Key ingredients of moisturizers.

mainly by their surfactant components. This damage is in addition to that incurred by the environment, age, pollutants, drugs, stress, hormones, etc. on the skin. With a damaged barrier, there is increased TEWL and the intracellular NMFs which are water soluble, follow suit. The resultant reduced epidermal water content causes enzyme dysfunction. These changes finally lead to clinically evident dry skin and xerosis.

Moisturizers, stand-alone or incorporated in cleansers, help to cover up the damage caused by cleanser components and also maintain the SC integrity, hence helping to preserve the function of surface enzymes and external appearance of the skin.

The key ingredients and special additives of moisturizers (Flowchart 1), work towards the same and are discussed here.

- Occlusives: The moisture sealers
  - Occlusive agents reduce TEWL by creating a hydrophobic barrier over the skin surface. They are thought to diffuse into the intercellular lipid domains, thus contributing to their efficacy
  - They provide hydration via physical blockage and are more effective when applied to slightly dampened skin
  - Various classes of occusives are shown in table 1[6]
  - Petroleum jelly is undoubtedly the most effective occlusive substance but agents with film-forming properties also exist such as lipophilic (silicones and silicone elastomers) and hydrophilic film-forming agents. The latter consist of very large molecules capable of "capturing" water and forming a film on the surface of the skin stopping water evaporation. They include: Proteins (collagen); complex carbohydrates (glycosaminoglycans: Hyaluronic acid and sulfated sugars); synthetic polymers [carbomer, 2-acrylamido-2-methylpropane sulfonic acid (AMPS®)], and waxes[7]
  - Petroleum jelly, in a minimum concentration of 5%, reduces TEWL by more than 98% and is the most effective occlusive, followed by lanolin, mineral oil, and silicones (e.g., dimethicone), which only reduce TEWL by 20–30%[6]
  - A randomized double-blind controlled trial done by Agero et al. to compare efficacy of virgin coconut oil and mineral oil as a moisturizer, showed effectivity of both oils through significant improvement in skin hydration and increase in skin surface lipid levels. Safety was demonstrated through no significant difference in TEWL and skin pH
  - However, the disadvantage of these occlusive agents is their sticky and/or greasy consistency making them less pleasant to use[8]
  - A balance must exist between the water absorbed and lost from the skin as TEWL. This is important because if the water content of the skin goes above 40%, as can happen with the use of occlusives in body folds or in areas with high humidity, the skin will become macerated. Hence, occlusives are best used with humectants
- Humectants (Box 1): The moisture absorbers
  - Humectants are hygroscopic compounds, which attract water from the environment as well as from dermis into the epidermis
  - They are useful in all skin types in humid climate as they are void of heavier oils
  - In low humidity condition humectants can increase TEWL, making skin drier, so humectants are then used best in conjunction with occlusives

TABLE 1: Different classes of occlusives[6]

Fatty acids	Lanolin acid, stearic acid
Fatty alcohols	Cetyl alcohol, lanolin alcohol, stearyl alcohol
Hydrocarbon oils	Mineral oil, paraffin, petroleum, caprylic/capric triglyceride, silicone derivatives (cyclomethicone, dimethicone), squalene
Polyhydric alcohols	Propylene glycol
Sterols	Cholesterols
Phospholipids	Lecithin
Vegetable waxes	Carnauba, Candelilla

BOX 1 Common substances with humectants properties[6,9]

- Glycerol
- Propylene glycol
- Gelatin
- Honey
- Hyaluronic acid
- Panthenol
- Urea
- Alpha—hydroxy acids (glycolic acid, lactic acid, tartaric acid)
- Sodium pyrrolidone carboxylic acid
- Sodium and ammonium lactate

TABLE 2: Different classes of emollients[6]

Astringent emollients	Dimethicone, cyclomethicone, octyl octanoate
Dry emollients	Isopropyl palmitate, isostearyl alcohol, decyl oleate
Protective emollients	Isopropyl isostearate, diisopropyl dilinoleate
Fatting emollients	Castor oil, jojoba oil, propylene glycol, octyl stearate

  - Many humectants also have emollient properties
  - Glycerine or glycerol was discovered in 1779 by the Swedish chemist Scheele and is among the most effective humectant polyols. Moisturizing properties of glycerol are due to its high degree of hydroxyl groups, which bind and retain water. Beside the moisturizing benefit attributed to its humectant action, it also prevents the SC phase transition and enables the skin lipids to preserve their normal structure even when underhydrated. Furthermore, it shows a keratolytic effect by desmosome degradation, influences the protective function of the skin against irritation and penetration of substances through the SC, reduces tissue scattering, stabilizes skin collagen, and accelerates healing processes. There have been reports of irritation with glycerine though. The purer the source of glycerine, lesser or minimal are the chances of skin irritation[10]
  - Propylene glycol and butylene glycol are other frequently used alcohols with humectant properties. Propylene glycol is often used as a solvent and vehicle for substances unstable or insoluble in water and is regarded as a penetration enhancer[11]
- Emollients (Table 2): The space fillers
  - They are mainly lipids and oils, which lubricate and improve the skin softness, pliability and smoothness by filling the space between corneocytes and restoring the physical barrier function. Emollient lipids are similar to those found naturally in skin. Emollients can be occlusives or humectants. The lubricity of moisturizers is due to emollients.
- Rejuvenators: Dermal boosters
  - These molecules boost and restore the dermal collagen and elastin which gets degraded with age, e.g., copper peptides, growth factors, hyaluronic acid, topical retinoids/retinol
  - They are a part of special additives in the formulation with an antiageing or rejuvenating role.

Additives in Moisturizers

- Emulsifiers: Emulsifiers help suspend two immiscible phases in a preparation. They function like surfactants at the interface of the oil and water phase in an emulsion holding or suspending particles of one phase in the other. The anionic emulsifiers have an irritant potential, of which sodium lauryl sulfate is a classical example, others being the long-chain fatty acids, stearic and palmitic acid. The nonionic and the cationic emulsifiers are overall less irritant but nonetheless all of them are necessary evils in product formulation. Examples are polyethylene glycol (PEG) and PEG compounds, propylene glycol, isopropyl stearate, polysorbate, diethanolamine, triethanolamine, carboxy methyl cellulose, potassium hydroxide, sorbitan stearate, cetearyl alcohol, ceteareth-20, stearyl alcohol and benzalkonium chloride
- Preservatives: Many moisturizers have water as an essential component, hence they carry the inherent risk of bacterial contamination. Preservatives help prevent that and hence increase the shelf-life of the product
- Fragrances: Consumers are easily attracted to products with a better aesthetic appeal over and above their basic functionality. Fragrances help mask the smell of ingredients and also enhance acceptability
- Dyes and pigments: They impart nothing more than visual appeal.

Special Additives

- Lipids: In addition to the above some preparations include lipid molecules like ceramides, pseudo-ceramides, fatty acids and cholesterol, which help in enhancing barrier repair. There are significant barrier benefits if these molecules are used in physiologically relevant proportions in preparations as has been found in various studies.[9,11-13] Of particular significance is their benefit in patients with atopic dermatitis[14,15]

- Antiaging molecules: Mature skin types, evidenced by the presence of fine lines and wrinkles, do well if their daily moisturizer has active antiaging ingredients. There are innumerable molecules in the market and many are being added, with or without supporting evidence and research, into this ever increasing list. Common ones are the alpha hydroxy acids, vitamins, botanicals, etc., which are used individually or in combinations. Many of these repair molecules work best when incorporated in night creams or moisturizers. (These molecules have been discussed in detail in chapter 5 on antiageing cosmeceuticals)
- Sun protection molecules: A sun protectant added to the moisturizing formula helps in serving two purposes with a single application
- Skin lightening molecules: Commonly incorporated skin lightening ingredients are vitamin B3 and vitamin C
- Botanical substances: The rationale to include herbal extracts in moisturizers has not always been based on controlled studies or evidence-based meta-analysis of clinical trials.[16] They are added most of the time for marketing reasons to nurture consumer interest in the perceived benefits of natural ingredients on the skin
  - Aloe (aloe barbadensis miller leaf extract): Evidence to support its role as a moisturizer is lacking although its role in healing of skin ulcers and burn due to its antiinflammatory, antibacterial and vasodilator action has been propounded from time to time[17]
  - Allantoin (comfrey root) is a synthetic derivative known as aluminum dihydroxy allantoinate. It has been marketed for its role as a moisturizer as well as keratolytic. However, supportive studies are lacking[18]
  - Oat meal (Avena sativa) baths for soothing rashes have been part of nursing practice since decades and are considered to be highly relieving to the patient[19]
  - Bioflavinoids, i.e., plant-derived polyphenols are being promoted as topical antioxidants. As a result, they have found a suitable place as an additive to the moisturizers[18]
- Antioxidants:[19] Typical anti oxidants are tocopherols (vit E), butylated hydroxytoluene and alkyl gallates[20]
- Chelating agents:[19] Citric acid, tartaric acid, ethylenediamine-tetraacetic acid, and its salts have limited antioxidant activity themselves, but enhance the efficacy of antioxidants by reacting with heavy metal ions. Such substances are called chelating agents.

Role of Moisturizers

- Moisturizing action:[21-24] This is the most vital action by which they increase the water content of the SC. It also makes the skin surface soft, more extensible and pliable. The moisturizing action of emollients is evident 30 minutes to 1 hour after the use and usually last for 4 hours
- Barrier building action: They help to restore the disrupted brick and mortar model of the epidermis, which serves as a two way barrier to environmental insults and loss of skin moisture
- Antiinflammatory action: Many moisturizers inhibit the production of proinflammatory prostanoids by blocking cyclooxygenase activity, they thus have a soothing effect on inflamed skin[21-24]
- Antimitotic action: Moisturizers containing mineral oils have low-grade antimitotic action on epidermis and thus are useful in inflammatory dermatoses like psoriasis, where there is increased epidermal mitotic activity[21-24]
- Antipruritic action: Emollients downregulate cytokines thus reducing itching. Furthermore, cooling effect following evaporation of water from the skin surface after using water-based moisturizers has an antipruritic effect[21-24]
- Photoprotective action: These days variable sun-protecting agents, like cinnamates, titanium dioxide and zinc oxide are incorporated in the moisturizers providing additional sun protection.
- Miscellaneous action:[21-24]
  - Quality of life improvement: Having a smooth and hydrated skin plays a good role in our social life and psychological satisfaction
  - Antimicrobial action: Act against skin surface microbes
  - Wound healing: Hyaluronic acid is known to play a role.

How to Choose a Moisturizer[25-27]

Pharmacologic and physiologic (e.g., concentration, bioavailability, moisturization effects), as well as patient-based considerations can potentially

TABLE 3: Choice of moisturizer formulations[25-27]

	Ointments	Creams	Gels	Lotion
Composition	Water in oil emulsion in a hydrocarbon or absorption base. Oil:water ration (80:20)	Oil in water (hydrophilic) or water in oil (hydrophobic) w/o contains more than 31% of water	Semisolid emulsion in alcohol base	Powder in water (oil). Liquid formulations with high water content that evaporates to leave a lipid film on the skin
Potency	Strong	Moderate	Strong	Low
Body sites most useful	Nonintertriginous	All sites	Oral, scalp	Scalp, intertriginous
Body sites to avoid	Skin folds, groin, face	Macerated sites	Fissures, erosions, macerated skin	Fissures, erosions
Features	Preservative-free, fragrance-free less chance of contact dermatitis; beneficial in low humidity (<60%); greasy	Less greasy then ointment; high acceptance	Clear, easy to apply, easy absorption nonoily, noncomedogenic	Thinner, nongreasy, cover larger area

TABLE 4: Moisturizer based on skin type

	Normal	Dry	Oily	Sensitive	Mature
Type of moisturizer	Water based, nongreasy, silicone based	Heavier oil based	Water based, noncomedogenic	With soothing ingredients i.e., aloe, chamomile	Petroleum based with antioxidants or alphahydroxy acids

influence the effects of moisturizer ingredients.[28] The specific ingredients in the formula and the properties of the formulation as a whole determine whether the cleanser or moisturizer is truly a mild product and if the product will impact the skin, especially the integrity and function of the SC, in a positive or negative manner.[26]

In general, molecules or ingredients larger than 500 Da can hardly pass through the intact SC.[25] If they are surface molecules like occlusives they serve their purpose well, but for active ingredients which need penetration for physiological effects, this needs to be kept in mind.

Various Dispensing Formulations

Moisturizers can be formulated into a variety of delivery systems (Table 3).

Other factors which determine the choice of a moisturiser:

- Skin type (Table 4)
- Moisturizers for specific body areas (Table 3)
- Age
- Associated skin conditions, hormonal or disease states
- Environmental factors
- Personal preferences.

Individual preferences may be guided by the following factors:

- Tackiness or greasiness of the preparation
- Spreadability
- Fragrance
- Color
- Cost
- Exotic ingredients
- Previous experience.

Ideal Moisturizer

- Reduce and prevent further TEWL
- Restore the lipid barrier
- Absorbed immediately, providing immediate hydration
- Noncomedogenic
- Nonirritant
- Compatible with therapeutic regimens
- Forms stable topical formulations
- Long shelf life.

Instructions and Tips for Moisturizer Use

- To be applied within 3 minutes of bathing.
- For hands, ideally to be used after every wash.

- For feet, best to soak in warm water for 5 minutes and then apply moisturizer before going to bed. Socks can be worn for better absorption
- Moisturize at least twice a day
- Prescribing or picking up the right product: trial and error helps
- Interindividual variations expected
- Face and body products are not interchangeable
- Most exotic ingredients and expensive brands are not always the best
- Customize and make changes according to season.

Coconut oil, used extensively in the tropics, has been shown to be comparable in efficacy and safety to that of mineral oil as a moisturizer for dry skin.[29]

CONCLUSION

The aesthetic goal of moisturization is achieving soft, supple, glowing, healthy looking skin, as subjectively evaluated by the end user.[30] In order to have optimum effect it is conceivable that moisturizers should be tailored with respect to the epidermal abnormality. New biochemical approaches and noninvasive instruments will help in better understanding to meet these ends.

REFERENCES

1. Rawlings AV, Harding CR. Moisturisation and skin barrier function. Dermatol Ther. 2004;17 Suppl 1:43-8.
2. Coderch L, Lopez O, de la Maza A, et al. Ceramides and skin function. Am J Clin Dermatol. 2003;4(2):107-29.
3. Koch PJ, Roop DR, Zhou Z. Cornified envelope and corneocyte-lipid envelope. In: Elias PM, Feingold KR (Eds). Skin Barrier. New York: Taylor & Francis. 2006. pp. 97-110.
4. Marty JP. [NMF and the cosmetology of cutaneous hydration]. Ann Dermatol Venereol. 2002;129(1 Pt 2):131-6.
5. Verdier-Sevrain S, Bonte F. Skin hydration: a review on its molecular mechanisms. J Cosmet Dermatol. 2007;6(2):75-82.
6. Kraft JN, Lynde CW. Moisturizers: what they are and a practical approach to product selection. Skin Therapy Lett. 2005;10(5):1-8.
7. Seite S, Bieber T. Barrier function and microbiotic dysbiosis in atopic dermatitis. Clin Cosmet Investig Dermatol. 2015;8:479-83.
8. Sethi A, Kaur T, Malhotra SK, et al. Moisturizers: the slippery road. Indian J Dermatol. 2016;61(3):279-87.
9. Loden M. The clinical benefit of moisturizers. J Eur Acad Dermatol Venereol. 2005;19:672-88.
10. Fluhr JW, Bornkessel A, Berardesca E. Glycerol—just a moisturizer? Biological and biophysical effects. In: Lodén M, Maibach HI (Eds). Dry Skin and Moisturizers: Chemistry and Function. CRC Press. 2005. pp. 227-43.
11. Flynn TC, Petros J, Clark RE, et al. Dry skin and moisturizers. Clin Dermatol. 2001;19:387-92.
12. Lee YB, Park HJ, Kwon MJ, et al. Beneficial effects of pseudoceramide containing physiologic lipid mixture as a vehicle for topical steroids. Eur J Dermatol. 2011;21:710-6.
13. Takagi Y, Nakagawa H, Higuchi K, et al. Characterization of surfactant induced skin damage through barrier recovery induced by pseudoacylceramides. Dermatology. 2005;211:128-34.
14. Draelos ZD. The effect of ceramide-containing skin care products on eczema resolution duration. Cutis. 2008;81:87-91.
15. Potts RO. Stratum corneum hydration: experimental techniques and interpretations of results. J Soc Cosmet Chem. 1986;37:9-33.
16. Dattner AM. From medical herbalism to phytotherapy in dermatology: back to the future. Dermatol Ther. 2003;16:106-13.
17. Shelton RM. Aloe vera: its chemical and therapeutic properties. Int J Dermatol. 1991;30:679-83.
18. Andreassi M, Stanghellini E, Ettorre A, et al. Antioxidant activity of topically applied lycopene. J Eur Acad Dermatol Venerol. 2004;18:52-5.
19. Wade A, Weller PJ, Kibbe AH. Handbook of Pharmaceuticals Excipients, 3rd edition. London: American Pharmaceutical Association, Washington and Pharmaceutical Press. 2000.
20. Spruit D. The interface of some substances with water vapor loss of human skin. Dermatologica. 1971;142:89-91.
21. Draelos ZD. Moisturizers. In: Draelos ZD (Ed). Cosmetics in Dermatology, 2nd edition. New York: Churchill Livingstone. 1995. pp. 83-96.
22. Marks R. Emollients. London: Martin Dunitz Ltd. 2002.
23. Baumann L. Moisturizing agents. In: Baumann L (Ed). Cosmetic Dermatology: Principles and Practices, 1st edition. New York: Tata McGraw Hill. 2002. pp 93-99.
24. Hawk JLM. Cutaneous photobiology. In: Champion RH, Burton JL, Ebling FJ (Eds). Rook/Wilkinson/Ebling: Textbook of Dermatology, 5th edition. Oxford: Wiley-Blackwell. 1992. pp. 849-66.
25. Tagami H. Location-related differences in structure and function of the stratum corneum with special emphasis on those of the facial skin. Int J Cosmet Sci. 2008;30(6):413-34.
26. Loden M. Role of topical emollients and moisturizers in the treatment of dry skin barrier disorders. Am J Clin Dermatol. 2003;4(11):771-8.
27. Rawlings AV, Canestrari DA, Dobkowski B. Moisturizer technology versus clinical performance. Dermatol Ther. 2004;17:49-56.
28. Lynde C. Moisturizers for the treatment of inflammatory skin conditions. J Drugs Dermatol. 2008;7(11):1038-43.
29. Agero AL, Verallo-Rowell VM. A randomized double blind controlled trial comparing extra virgin coconut oil with mineral oil as a moisturizer for mild to moderate xerosis. Dermatitis. 2004;15(3):109-16.
30. Levin J, Miller R. A guide to the ingredients and potential benefits of over the counter cleansers and moisturizers for rosacea patients. J Clin Aesthet Dermatol. 2011;4(8):31-49.

3 CHAPTER

Sunscreens

Rekha A Sheth, Kshama G Bingewar

INTRODUCTION

Evidence exists that even ancient civilizations sought protection from damaging effects of sun.

Ancient Egyptians considered light skin more attractive than dark skin. They formulated sunscreens by using ingredients such as rice bran, jasmine, and lupine. Recent studies have shown that one of the components of rice bran extract oryzanol has ultraviolet (UV) absorbing properties, jasmine helps repair DNA, and lupine lightens skin. Other cultures have tried their luck at sun protection with varying success. The ancient Greeks used olive oil. Some Native American tribes used *Tsuga canadensis*, a type of pine needle, which was also effective in soothing sunburns. It is surprising that these cultures were able to formulate sunscreens long before the cause of sun damage was understood. In the realm of sun protection, our ancient predecessors proved to be far ahead of their time.[1]

The first commercial chemical sunscreen was introduced in 1928. It contained benzyl salicylate and benzyl cinnamate.

In past few years, significant effort has been put into the development of sunscreens and other photoprotective methods with broad spectrum ultraviolet A (UVA) coverage.

DEFINITION

Sunscreens are pharmaceutical preparations that attenuate UV wavelengths that would otherwise interact with molecules in the skin (chromophores) to generate photochemical reactions leading to photobiologic change.[2]

ULTRAVIOLET LIGHT AND ITS EFFECTS

The UV light and its effects are:

- Solar radiation comprises 5% UV rays, 35% visible light, and 60% infrared rays
- Ultraviolet B ranges from 290 nm to 320 nm
- Ultraviolet A2 ranges from 320 nm to 340 nm
- Ultraviolet A1 ranges from 340 nm to 400 nm
- Visible ranges from 400 nm to 800 nm.

Wavelengths of less than 320 nm are absorbed by stratum corneum and epidermis, while wavelength greater than 320 nm enter the dermis. There is breakdown of cell membrane, lipids, structural proteins, and DNA.

The initial symptom of sun damage is erythema due to vasodilatation in response to cellular damage. Following the appearance of erythema, tanning occurs due to photo-oxidation of melanin, which is immediate pigment darkening effect. Overtime, this cumulative skin damage manifests as photo aging.[3]

SUNSCREEN FILTER CLASSIFICATION

Sunscreen filters can be classified into two types:

1. Organic
2. Inorganic.

Organic (Chemical) Blockers

These are classified as follows in table 1.

Inorganic or Physical Blockers[4]

These are classified as follows in table 2.

TABLE 1: Shows the classification of organic (chemical) blockers

	UVB	UVA2	UVA1
PABA/padimate O	√	–	–
Cinnamate	√	–	–
Salicylates			
Octylsalicylate	√	–	–
Homosalate	√	–	–
Trolamine salicylate	√	–	–
Benzophenones			
Oxybenzone	√	√	–
Sulisobenzone	√	√	√
Dioxybenzone	√	√	–
Others			
Octocrylene	√	–	–
Avobenzone	–	√	√
Menthyl anthranilate (Meradimate)	–	√	–
Ecamsule	√	√	–
Bemotrizinol	√	√	–
Bisoctrizole	√	√	√
Silatriazole	√	√	√
Bisdisulizole	–	√	√
Isoctrizinol	√	√	–
Diethyamino hydroxybenzoyl hexylbenzote	–	√	–

PABA, 4-aminobenzoic acid; UVB, ultraviolet B; UVA2, Ultraviolet A2; UVA1, ultraviolet A1.

TABLE 2: Shows the classification of inorganic or physical blockers

	UVB	UVA2	UVA1
Titanium dioxide	√	√	–
Zinc oxide	√	√	–
Iron oxide	√	√	√ and visible light

UVB, ultraviolet B; UVA2, ultraviolet A2; UVA1, ultraviolet A1.

MECHANISM OF ACTION

Inorganic (Physical Blockers)

Consists of chemical compounds that do not contain carbon atoms in their overall structure. They work by scattering and reflecting UV rays. They are not used up and therefore they stay and act longer on the skin surface.

Organic (Chemical Blockers)

Chemical sunscreens are generally aromatic compounds conjugated with a carbonyl group. These chemicals absorb high-intensity UV rays with excitation to a higher energy state. The energy lost results in conversion of the remaining energy into longer lower energy wavelengths with return to ground state.[5]

ULTRAVIOLET A ORGANIC SUNSCREEN FILTERS

There are three main categories of UVA organic filters. They are:

1. Benzophenones
2. Avobenzone
3. Anthranilates.

Benzophenones

There are three types of benzophenones:

1. Oxybenzone
2. Dioxybenzone
3. Sulisobenzone.

Oxybenzone

- Absorption spectra of oxybenzone are at 288 nm and 325 nm
- Oxybenzone is usually combined with avobenzone to enhance photostability. Oxybenzone is generally used as a secondary sunscreen because it is oily in nature making the sunscreen sticky if used too high in concentration.

Avobenzone

Avobenzone is one of the most common UVA-filters in sunscreens, and is known to be photounstable. The photoprotection capacity is reduced by 50% even on exposure to sunlight for as short as 1 hour, necessitating frequent application.[6] Some of the strategies used to stabilize this filter present some drawbacks like photosensitization reactions. Antioxidants are widely used as cosmetic ingredients that prevent photoaging and complement the photoprotection offered by the UV-filters preventing or reducing photogenerated reactive species. Avobenzone can be stabilized by adding oxybenzone, octocrylene or 2-6 diethylhexyl naphthalate. These ingredients absorb the photon of energy from avobenzone allowing avobenzone to return to a ground state and not undergo photodegradation. This concept of photostabilization is important to ensure the longevity of sunscreens on the skin.

Avobenzone has a strong absorption spectra in UVA1 range at 357 nm.

Sulisobenzone at 286 nm and 324 nm.

Dioxybenzone at 284 nm and 327 nm. These are less commonly used.

Anthranilates

Menthyl anthranilate (meradimate) has its highest absorption at 336 nm. It has a low allergenicity with an excellent safety profile. There are no photodegradation issues. Formulations of anthranilates are stable.

ULTRAVIOLET B ORGANIC SUNSCREEN FILTERS

There are three major UVB organic filters:

1. Para-aminobenzoic acid (PABA) derivatives
2. Salicylates
3. Cinnamates.

Para-aminobenzoic Acid Derivatives

Octyl methyl PABA (Padimate O) with absorption spectrum at 296 nm is rarely used in modern sunscreen formulations.

Salicylates

Salicylates have absorption spectra at 300–310 nm. Salicylates have a safe record in that they are nonsensitizing. They are also excellent solubilizers of other traditionally nonsoluble cosmetic ingredients, including oxybenzone and avobenzone.

Octisalate (Octyl Salicylate)

It has been used in many cosmetic formulations but has been reported to cause photocontact dermatitis.

Homosalate (Homomenthyl Salicylate)

It is used as a standard sunscreen agent in testing of sun protection factors (SPFs) and rarely causes photodermatitis or contact dermatitis.

Trolamine Salicylate

It has been used in hair preparations as a sun-protective agent and is reported to cause photocontact dermatitis.[7]

Cinnamates

Cinnamates are commonly used category in sunscreens with moisturizers and foundations. Octinoxate (octyl methoxy cinnamate) has absorption at 305 nm. It has excellent photostability and is used as an active ingredient.

ECAMSULE

Ecamsule is an organic compound which is added to many sunscreens to filter out UVA rays. It is a benzylidene camphor derivative, many of which are known for their excellent photostability. Absorption range is within the UVA range (320–340 nm). It is only available in select patented sunscreen products.

Although there are a few different UV absorbers with the trade name Mexoryl, only two of them are widely used which were approved. Mexoryl SX (water-soluble) and Mexoryl XL (oil-soluble), together they show a synergistic effect in protection.

It has been shown to prevent photoaging and suppresses carcinogenicity and plays a role in immunosuppression.[8]

Since ecamsule does not cover the entire UV spectrum, it should be combined with other active sunscreen agents to ensure broad spectrum UV protection.[9]

All sunscreens must have an active ingredient disclosure by the guidelines as they are classified as over the counter (OTC) drugs.

Primary sunscreen is used in highest concentration and is listed first under the active ingredient disclosure. Secondary sunscreen is listed second and is next highest in concentration followed by the tertiary and quaternary sunscreens.[3,10]

INORGANIC OR PHYSICAL BLOCKERS

Frequently used inorganic physical sun blockers are zinc oxide (ZnO) and titanium dioxide (TiO_2)

They offer the advantages of high SPF, broad spectrum coverage and reduced potential irritancy to users.[11]

Poor cosmetic acceptance of ZnO and TiO_2 is reduced by using nano sized particles.

Titanium Dioxide

The UV protection spectral range provided by TiO_2 is broad, extending from UVA II to UVB region.

There is a great tendency for TiO_2 particles, particularly nanoparticles, to be nonuniformly distributed and to form clumps, hindering the smooth spreading of the formulation on the skin and thus preventing the formation of an even film over the exposed area and thereby reducing the sunscreen efficiency and the aesthetic attractiveness of the product. Combining chemical UV absorbers with inorganic sunscreens may represent a practical compromise.

Zinc Oxide

Zinc oxide provides better UVA protection.

Zinc oxide also displays photocatalytic activity. There are studies that assess both TiO_2 and ZnO for their ability to act as a bactericidal agent.[11,12]

SUNSCREEN FORMULATION

If a sunscreen ingredient is not properly incorporated into a cosmetic formulation, it will not work no matter how well that ingredient blocks or scatters UV radiation. Also care must be taken to minimize the ingredient interaction between the sunscreen active and the formulation.

Emulsions

- Emulsions are made up of mixture of oils and water and stabilized by an emulsifying ingredient
- Emulsion can be placed into two main categories, oil suspended in water or aqueous phase (o/w) or water suspended in oil (w/o). Water suspended in oil emulsions provide a high sunscreen efficiency as they are very water resistant when compared with O/W emulsion. However, due to lower cost for O/W vehicle it is more widely used. Products that use emulsion include sunscreen creams and lotions
- Emulsions provide an excellent sunscreen film on the skin and still have an elegant film
- One common drawback is their difficulty in stabilization. Overtime, any emulsion product will destabilize and separate into its component oil and water phases. However, with careful formulation efforts and the right emulsifiers, an adequately stable system can be made
- Newer Ultrasheer product further refines the emulsion with use of silica as a mattifier.[13]

Gels

They are thick, clear product with an elegant look that appeals to consumers. Aqueous and hydro alcoholic gels are produced by incorporating acrylic polymers in the system for thickening. Micro emulsions have significantly smaller particles making them transparent and they appear more gel like. Advantage of gels over emulsion is their clarity and unique look. However they are not water resistant. Additionally, these films are not uniform so they may not provide the expected protection. The thickness used in certain gel product can leave a sticky feel on the skin.

Aerosol Sprays

Aerosol sprays are easy to use and have good aesthetic characteristics. They are often oil based so they are expensive and have lower SPF rating. Also they produce a discontinuous film on skin reducing effectiveness.

Mousses

Are essentially emulsion lotions that are put in sealed containers and have a propellant added to them so that the product is released as foam. They are easy to use and have good aesthetic characteristics.

Sticks

- The sticks contain polyvinyl pyrrolidone (PVP)/ hexadecene copolymer, esters, phenyl trimethicone, spherical silica, bismuth oxychloride, mica, and cosmetic waxes
- There are generally three types of cosmetic stick formulations—compressed powder sticks, gel sticks, and wax sticks. Each formulation type has advantages as well as disadvantages over the other forms. For example, compressed powder sticks are often brittle and hard and leave a cosmetically unacceptable dust upon application. Gels, on the other hand, offer excellent aesthetic characteristics but may be unstable due to interaction between the soap gelling agents typically used to solidify the sticks. Wax-based sticks are often cosmetically unacceptable because they are hard, greasy and sticky
- They can be applied in limited areas, such as the lips and around the eyes.

Ointments

These are oily products based on thickened mineral oil formulas. Aesthetically they are not desirable.

Oils

Oils were one of the earliest forms of sunscreens used. Oils are used as formulation vehicles for sunscreen actives. Because most of the sunscreen actives are lipophilic, oils are easy to manufacture.

However, oils have certain drawbacks. Their rapid spread ability results in a thin, transparent film.

This film has a lowered amount of active sunscreen, thus reducing the products overall sun blocking effectiveness.

In general oils have higher costs and aesthetically can feel greasy and leave an unappealing coated feel.

There is also stability issues related to putting an oil-based sunscreen product in certain types of plastic packaging. Products that use this type of formulation are tanning oils. These products are designed to be worn while sunbathing, typically provide minimal UV protection and are used merely to prevent sunburn.[14]

Broad spectrum protection against both UVA and UVB can be achieved by combination of sunscreen filters.

For example avobenzone (long UVA) can be combined with UVB sunscreen (such as octocrylene, homosalate, octisalate) and photostable short UVA sunscreen drugs (such as oxybenzone and ecamsule).

Silatriazole is photostable with two absorption spectra in UVB (303 nm) and UVA range (344 nm). Bisoctrizole is a photostable UVB and UVA blocker active with absorption peaks at 305 nm and 360 nm, respectively.

The performance of a sunscreen depends on the concentration of the filters and the ability to remain on the skin. Increasing the concentration of a sunscreen filter can increase the SPF. For example 3% octyl dimethyl PABA has an SPF of 4 while 4% octyl dimethyl PABA has an SPF of 5. Octyl dimethyl ester of PABA is less water soluble than PABA accounting for its use in water proof sunscreens.

A superior sunscreen can be produced by combining sunscreen agents. A sunscreen containing only 8% octyl dimethyl PABA has an SPF of 8 while combining 8% octyl dimethyl PABA with 3% oxybenzone gives an SPF of 20. Most sunscreens will combine organic and inorganic filters for optimal photoprotection.[3]

SUNSCREEN EFFICACY

Sun Protection Factor

The efficacy of a sunscreen is usually expressed by the SPF, which is defined as the UV energy required to produce a minimal erythema dose (MED) on protected skin, divided by the UV energy required to produce a MED on unprotected skin.

The SPF is calculated as follows:

$$\frac{\text{Minimal erythema dose in sunscreen – protected skin}}{\text{Minimal erythema dose in nonsunscreen – unprotected skin}}$$

TABLE 3: Shows the SPF and proportion of UVB blocked

SPF	Proportion of UVB blocked
10	90%
15	93%
20	95%
30	96.70%
40	97.50%
50	98.30%

SPF, sun protection factors; UVB, ultraviolet B.

TABLE 4: Shows the star rating category and star rating designation

Star rating category	Star rating designation
**	Medium
***	High
****	Higher

A sunscreen with an SPF 10 would allow 10 times as much time in the sun with the same resultant level of erythema as without the product in a given individual (Table 3).

Diffey/Boots

It is the scale of one to four stars corresponding to low, medium, high or very high UVA protection (Table 4).[15]

Ultraviolet A Measurement

Ultraviolet A radiation is measured in terms of persistent pigment darkening (PPD) test and immediate pigment darkening (IPD) test method.

Immediate pigment darkening measures the transient brown color that appears and fades within minutes of UVA exposure in vivo in darker skin types.

Purified Protein Derivative Test

The purified protein derivative (PPD) method has become the most widely used in the past few years. It involves exposure of skin with and without sun protection and observation of pigment response 2–24 hours after the end of UVA exposure; the protection index is determined as the ratio of the dose required to produce a minimally perceptible pigment response on sunscreen-treated skin to the dose for unprotected skin (UVA-PF).[16]

Critical Wavelength Method

In this *in vitro* test, the absorbance of the thin film of the sunscreen is integrated (summed) from 290 nm across the UV wavelengths, until the sum reaches 90% of the total absorbance of the sunscreen in the ultraviolet region (290–400 nm). The wavelength at which the summed absorbance reaches 90% of total absorbance is defined as the critical wavelength (≥ 370) and is considered to be a measure of the breadth of sunscreen protection.[17]

New Rules from Food and Drug Administration

Sunscreen products that pass the broad spectrum test are allowed to be labeled as broad spectrum. These broad spectrum sunscreens protect against both UVA and UVB rays. The SPF value indicates the level of sunburn protection provided by the sunscreen product.[18]

WATER RESISTANCE

Sunscreen water resistance is determined by two 20 minutes water exposure separated by a 20 minutes rest period and concluded by air drying without towel drying. After about total 40 minutes of water contact the SPF of water resistant sunscreen is measured.[19,20]

VERY WATER RESISTANT

- The sunscreen must maintain its SPF over a test cycle including 80 minutes of moderate activity in water
- Not to use labels like waterproof, sunblock or sweat proof as the food and drug administration (FDA) does not believe these are accurate statements[21]
- The patient should be advised to allow drying the sunscreen 20 minutes prior to water contact. Also repeat application ensures good coverage.

METHOD OF APPLICATION

- The current FDA standard recommends 2 mg/cm^2 of skin surface
- The teaspoon rule can be used to guide patients on the appropriate amount of sunscreen required
- Apply more than ½ teaspoon (3 mL) of sunscreen to face, neck and each arm
- Apply more than 1 teaspoon (6 mL) of sunscreen to each leg, 1 teaspoon to front and 1 teaspoon to back of the body[15,22]
- Remember to apply on back of neck, ears, frontal portion of scalp (in case of thinning of hair) and feet.

Reapplication

- Another method recommends that patients apply twice to reduce the skipped areas
- It takes approximately 15 minutes for the skin to absorb sunscreen, hence repeat application 15 minutes later is recommended
- Ideally sunscreen should be reapplied every 2 hours and more frequently during outdoor activities.

ADVERSE EFFECTS

Direct Adverse Effects

- Contact irritant reactions are most common adverse effect. Especially with higher SPF products, several active ingredients may be used in one formulation and at higher concentration increasing the potential for contact reactions.
  Also some products may aggravate pre-existing conditions such as acne rosacea, atopic dermatitis, and seborrheic dermatitis
- Contact allergic dermatitis
- Phototoxic reactions, padimate A was found to be phototoxic and was withdrawn from market
- Photoallergic reaction is a contact allergic reaction due to UVA portion of UV spectrum. Use of potent UVA blocker should minimize this adverse effect.[17]

Indirect Adverse Effects

Vitamin "D" Deficiency

Studies have shown that sunscreen prevented the photoisomerization of 7-dehyrdocholesterol to

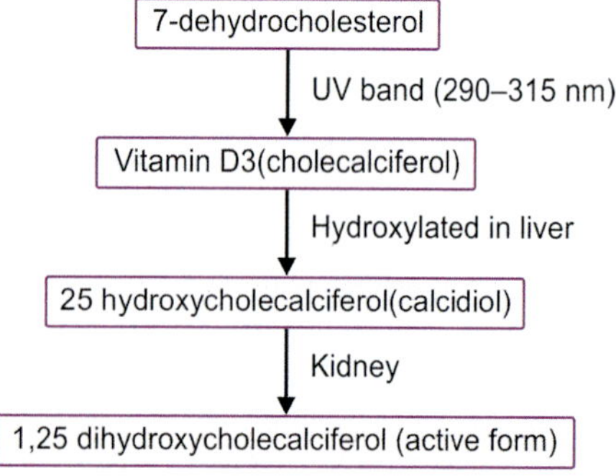

FLOWCHART 1: Synthesis of pre vitamin D in skin.

previtamin D in skin (Flowchart 1). A recent review of all the published evidence concluded that normal usage of sunscreens does not generally result in vitamin D insufficiency. This is primarily due to inadequacies in the application of sunscreen to skin. However, in certain dermatological conditions patients need a stringent photoprotection. For those individuals, a balanced diet and a daily 600 IU vitamin D3 supplement, along with 1 g calcium, is recommended. This recommendation applies especially to elderly individuals who are home bound or dark skinned individuals with modest sun exposure, and those who practice rigorous photoprotection. For persons aged 71 years or older, 800 IU or higher may be recommended.[16,23]

PROTECTION AGAINST VISIBLE LIGHT

Visible light is important phenomenon in solar idiopathic photodermatosis, pale and dark skinned patients with post inflammatory hyperpigmentation and melasma. Organic sunscreen agents like iron oxide, titanium dioxide and zinc oxide can offer some visible range. Large particles are more protective than smaller sized particles.[24]

SYSTEMIC PHOTOPROTECTION

β-carotene, lycopene, ascorbate, tocopherols, and omega 3 polyunsaturated fatty acids are known to provide some systemic photoprotection.[25,26]

PHYSICAL PROTECTION

Sunscreen application does not provide complete protection especially in those individuals who burn easily and tan poorly. Avoiding sun exposure particularly between 10 AM and 4 PM is desirable. One is exposed to UV rays even on cloudy days. Stay in shade whenever possible.

Clothing

The measurement of UV photoprotection of fabric is determined by UV protection factor (UPF). Factors affecting UPF of fabrics:

- Tightly woven fibers (wool and polyester) and thick fibers have higher UPF
- Stretched fibers reduces the UPF
- Closer the fabric to skin less the photoprotection
- Washing shrinks the fabric and reduce gaps between fibers increasing the UPF
- Laundry additive containing UV absorber increases UPF
- Dark colored clothes absorb more visible light than light colored clothes and have greater UPF.[7]

Hats

For additional photoprotection wide brimmed hats are recommended.

Sunglasses

- Sunglasses have been classified into three categories:
  1. Cosmetic sunglasses: Worn as fashion accessories and providing minimal UV protection
  2. General purpose sunglasses: For reducing glare in bright light or in circumstances such as driving in daylight
  3. Special purpose sunglasses: For activities such as skiing, going to the beach.
- Polarizing lenses are helpful in minimizing glare; however, they do not provide added UV-blocking properties
- Darkly tinted lens may cause papillary dilation, allowing the oblique peripheral ray of light to transmit to the eye if the sunglasses are not designed to wrap around the temporal area
- Expensive sunglasses do not necessarily provide better UV protection. Look for sunglasses that meet sunglass standards for a safe level of UV protection.

Make Up

Foundation make up provides SPF 3–4 because of its pigment content for up to four hours after application.

Shade

Staying in shade reduces solar exposure by 50–95%.

Window Glass

It has been well recognized that standard glass filters out UVB, but UVA, visible light, and infrared radiation are still transmitted. With recent developments in the glass industry, additional filters for UVA and infrared radiation can now be incorporated.

Different types of glass available are:

- Clear glass tinted (heat-absorbing) glass
- Reflective glass

- Low-emissivity glass
- Laminated glass
- Ultraviolet-blocking coated glass
- Insulating glass.

Automobile Glass

All windshields of car are made of laminated glass, which blocks the vast portion of UVA radiation. However, side and rear windows are usually made from nonlaminated glass; therefore, a significant level of UVA can pass through. To reduce this, tinted glass or films can be used.[27]

COMMON ISSUES WITH SUNSCREEN COMPLIANCE

- Sunscreens are sticky: The most common factor in noncompliance of sunscreen is stickiness. Sunscreens with higher SPF use combination of actives with mainly w/o formulation and are usually sticky. Once the SPF raises much above 30, the product becomes sticky. A SPF 15 product filters out more than 93% of UV-B radiation, and a SPF 30 product filters out less than 97%. The difference of 4% would not seem significant to most individuals. Hence, it is not mandatory to insist the patient to use highest SPF if compliance is an issue. Lower SPF products provide better aesthetic and compliance
- Sunscreens cause sweating: Chemical sunscreen change UV rays into heat, which is then released from the skin and scattered. This heat causes the feeling of warmth. Physical sunscreen does not produce heat. Selection of proper sunscreen will improve the compliance
- Sunscreen causes acne: The type of acne seen is more of an acneiform eruption (inflammatory papules) which could be suggestive of irritant contact dermatitis. Certain water-resistant sunscreens are occlusive and may block follicular ostia. Avoidance of long wearing sunscreen product may help
- Sunscreens sting when applied: Especially gel sunscreens cause stinging. Creamy sunscreen should be used in such cases. Sunscreen can cause burning sensation when they enter the eye[28]
- The misconception that sunscreen offers total protection is not true. No sunscreen completely blocks the sun.[19]

NANOPARTICLES

Inorganic filters have been widely used in microfine form. Nanoparticles are defined as particles less than 100 nm. *In vitro*, these particles can induce free radical formation in the presence of UV radiation, resulting in cell damage. However, the current evidence shows that these particles remain on the surface of the skin; however, further studies are warranted, especially if these are used on inflamed skin or in infants.[29]

Sunscreen With Infrared Radiation Protection

Infrared radiation comprises infrared radiation type A (IRA) (700–1,400 nm), IRB (1,400–3,000 nm), and IRC (3,000 nm–1 mm). Infrared radiation type B and IRC do not penetrate the skin deeply but IRA does.

Infrared radiation type A irradiation induces the production of intracellular reactive oxygen species, alters the dermal-epidermal junction and modifies the homeostasis of the extracellular matrix of the skin. Based on the experimental conditions used in terms of irradiance and IRA dose, we assume that 1 single hour of sun exposure could be enough to alter skin elasticity, skin firmness and to facilitate wrinkle formation. These results confirm the potential damaging effects of IR and emphasize the need to protect the skin also against IRA radiation. This can be achieved by using light reflectors and/or specific antioxidants.

Antioxidants that are combined are—polypodium leucotomos extract, nicotinamide, afamelanotide, grape seed extract, vitamin E, ubiquinone, and vitamin C.[30-32]

Silicone (Matte Finish) Sunscreens

Silicones provide aesthetic benefits such as unique soft and silky feel, easy and uniform spreading and reduced tackiness. As silicone technology evolves, greater interest has focused on the multifunctional properties of these materials.

In the newest sun care products, silicones also provide substantivity, sebum control, wash-off resistance and enhanced SPF—and they can also help prevent sand from sticking to the skin.

In addition, several classes of silicone materials including silicone acrylate copolymers, elastomers, resins, carbinol fluid, alkylmethylsiloxanes and silicone emulsifiers offer unique formulating advantages.[33-35]

First generation silicone elastomer blends exhibit limitations in formulating with sunscreen actives, such as ethylhexyl methoxycinnamate/ethylhexyl salicylate.

Second-generation silicone organic elastomer such as dimethicone/bis isobutyl PPG-20 cross-polymer exhibits increased compatibility.

Silicones are also noncomedogenic unlike many occlusive lipophilic fatty emollients which promote comedone/acne on skin.[36]

Blemish Balm Creams and Photoprotection

Blemish balm creams have been the rage for the past 3-4 years. The idea was to create a lightweight slightly tinted cream to provide in one product the benefits of a moisturizer, facial foundation, and sunscreen.

The SPF value is mentioned on the packaging (ranging from 10 to 45).

However, there is disparity in SPF mentioned on the product—photostability and photoprotective efficacy.[37]

Effects of Computer Screen and Other Light Sources

Study were conducted on the frequent human exposure to various types of indoor lamps, as well as other light sources like television monitors, tablets and computers, and electronic devices.

It was concluded that the lamps and monitors of commonly used electronic devices do not emit ultraviolet radiation so they pose no health risk for the population.[38]

Melanin as a Sunscreen

The efficacy of melanin as a sunscreen is assumed to be about 1.5-2.0 sun protection factors (SPF); possibly as high as 4 SPF, indicating that melanin absorbs 50-75% of UVR.[39]

Studies on the bacterial-derived melanin has shown significant protection to fibroblast cell and human skin against the UVA radiation. Thus, melanin has the potential to be developed as a sunscreen.[40]

CONCLUSION

Sunscreens have become an important part of a dermatologist's armamentarium of skin care.

REFERENCES

1. Aldahan AS, Shah VV, Mlacker S, et al. The history of sunscreen. JAMA Dermatol. 2015;151(12):1316.
2. Bolognia JL, Jorizzo JL, Schaffer JV. In: Deleo VA (Ed). Sunscreens, 3rd edition, Vol. 2. Elsevier, 2012. pp. 2197-2201.
3. Draelos Z. Cosmetics and Dermatological Problems and Solutions, 3rd edition. New York: Informa Healthcare; 2011. pp. 60-67.
4. Bolognia JL, Jorizzo JL, Schaffer JV. Sunscreens. In: Deleo VA (Ed). 3rd edition, Elsevier; 2012. pp. 2197-2201.
5. Andreassi M, Anselni C. Hot topics on UV filler ingredient. Expert Rev Dermatol. 2011; 6(5):493-499.
6. Bouillon C. Recent advances in sun protection. J Dermatol Sci. 2000;23(Suppl. 1):S57-61.
7. Kullavanijaya P, Lim HW. Photoprotection. J Am Acad Dermatol. 2005;52(6):937-58.
8. Fourtanier A. MexorylSx protects against solar-stimulated UVR-induced photocarcinogenesis in mice. Photochem Photobiol. 1996;64(4):688-93.
9. Levy SB. Sunscreens for photoprotection. Dermatol Ther. 1997;4:59-71.
10. Tuchinda C, Lim HW, Osterwalder U, et al. Novel emerging sunscreen technologies. Dermatol Clin. 2006; 24(1):105-117.
11. Smijs TG, Pavel S. Titanium dioxide and zinc oxide nanoparticles in sunscreens: focus on their safety and effectiveness. Nanotechnol Sci Appl. 2011;4:95-112.
12. Beasley DG, Meyer TA. Characterization of the UVA protection provided by avobenzone, zinc oxide, and titanium dioxide in broad-spectrum sunscreen products. Am J Clin Dermatol. 2010; 11(6):413-21.
13. Tanner PR. Sunscreen product formulation. Dermatol Clin. 2006;24(1):53-62.
14. Schuller and Romanowski. The ABCs of SPFs: An introduction to sun protection products. Sun. 2006;1-9.
15. Cosmeceuticals. In: Draelos Z (Ed). Sunscreens, 2nd edition. Philadelphia, PA: Elsevier Saunders. pp. 145-54.
16. Goldsmith AL, Katz SI, Gilchrest BA, et al. Fitzpatrick's dermatology in general medicine. In: Lim HW. Photoprotection, 8th edition. pp. 2707-13.
17. Moyal D, Galdi A, Oresajo C. Chapter 19: Sunscreen. In: Draelos ZD (Ed). Cosmetic dermatology: product and procedure. Hoboken, NJ: Blackwell publisher; 2010. pp. 144-48.
18. Bolognia, Daniel J. DeNoon. New sunscreen, Health News.
19. Baumann LS. Chapter 29: Sunscreens cosmetic dermatology. Cosmetic Dermatology: Principles and Practice, 2nd edition. New York: McGraw-Hill Education; 2009. pp. 245-55.
20. Draelos ZD. A dermatologist's perspective on the final sunscreen monograph. J Am Acad Dermatol. 2001;44(1):109-10.
21. Bolognia JL, Jorizzo JL, Schaffer JV. Section 19, Chapter 132, sunscreens. Dermatology, Bolognia Series, 3rd edition, Vol. 2. Philadelphia: Elsevier Saunders; 2012. pp. 2197-201.

22. Shneider J. The teaspoon rule of applying sunscreen. Arch Dermatol. 2002;138(6):838-9.
23. Ross AC, Manson JE, Abrams SA, et al. The 2011 report on dietary reference intakes for calcium and vitamin D from the Institute of Medicine: what clinicians need to know. J Clin Endocrinol Metab. 2011;96(1):53-8.
24. Rai R, Srinivas CR. Photoprotection. Indian J Dermatol Venereol Leprol. 2007;73(2):73-9.
25. Bissonette R, Allas S, Moyal D, et al. Comparison of UVA protection afforded by high sun protection factor sunscreens. J Am Acad Dermatol. 2000;43(6):1036.
26. Bissonnette R. Update on sunscreens. Skin Therapy Lett. 2008;13(6):5-7.
27. Tuchinda C, Srivannaboon S, Lim HW. Photoprotection by window glass, automobile glass, and sunglasses. J Am Acad Dermatol. 2006;54(5):845-54.
28. Draelos Z. Chapter 20: Body photoprotection. Cosmetics and Dermatological Problems and Solutions, 3rd edition. CRC Press; 2011. pp. 141-47.
29. Wolff K, Goldsmith L, Katz S, et al. Fitzpatrick's Dermatology in General Medicine, 8th edition, New York, NY: McGraw-Hill; 2001. pp. 2707-2713.
30. Robert C, Bonnet M, Marques S, et al. Low to moderate doses of infrared A irradiation impair extracellular matrix homeostasis of the skin and contribute to skin photodamage. Skin Pharmacol Physiol. 2015;28(4):196-204.
31. Grether-Beck S, Marini A, Jaenicke T, et al. Effective photoprotection of human skin against infrared A radiation by topically applied antioxidants: results from a vehicle controlled, double-blind, randomized study. Photochem Photobiol. 2015;91(1):248-50.
32. Lim HW, Arellano-Mendoza MI, Stengel F, et al. Current challenges in photoprotection. J Am Acad Dermatol. 2017;76(3S1):S91-9.
33. I Van Reeth, J Blakely. Use of current and new test methods to demonstrate the benefits of alkylmethylsiloxanes in suncare products, presented at the European UV Sunfilter Conference, Paris, France, November 3-4, 1999.
34. I Van Reeth, F Dahman, J Hannington. Alkylmethylsiloxanes as SPF enhancers; relationship between effects and physico-chemical properties, presented at the 19th IFSCC Congress, Sydney, Australia, October 22-25, 1996.
35. Van Reeth I, S Postiaux S, Van Dort H. Silicones bring multifunctional performance to sun care. Cosmet Toiletries. 2006;121(10):41-54.
36. Dayan N. Handbook of formulating dermal applications: a definitive practical guide. Hoboken, NJ: John Wiley & Sons; 2016.
37. Couteau C, Paparis E, Coiffard LJ. BB creams and their photoprotective effect. Pharm Dev Technol. 2016;21(1):39-42.
38. Duarte IAG, Hafner M de FS, Malvestiti AA. Ultraviolet radiation emitted by lamps, TVs, tablets and computers: are there risks for the population? Anais Brasileiros de Dermatologia. 2015;90(4):595-97.
39. Brenner M, Hearing VJ. The Protective Role of Melanin Against UV Damage in Human Skin. Photochemistry and photobiology. 2008;84(3):539-49.
40. Geng J, Tang W, Wan X, et al. Photoprotection of bacterial-derived melanin against ultraviolet A-induced cell death and its potential application as an active sunscreen. Journal of the European Academy of Dermatology and Venereology. 2008;22:852-58.

4 CHAPTER

Skin Lightening Agents

Rekha A Sheth, Neetu Gehi

INTRODUCTION

Hyperpigmentation is a common problem among Indian population. Hyperpigmentation not only affects the appearance but can also affect the quality of life, especially in a society where whiter skin is considered to be the hallmark of beauty. The treatment of hyperpigmentation is challenging and often discouraging. There is a huge market for skin lightening products in the Indian market.

The cosmetic and the pharmaceutical market is flooded with lightening products each claiming to be the best but with limited clinical evidence to support their claim. There is a dire need for natural skin lightening agents (SLA) in view of:

- High tolerance
- Efficacy
- Easy accessibility
- Cosmetic appeal
- Safe long-term use.

Among the various skin lightening agents, hydroquinone, kojic acid, retinoids, azelaic acid and the alpha-hydroxy acids have been most widely studied. Many preparations combine multiple ingredients in one formulation with the concept of inhibiting pigment production by interrupting melanogenesis at different stages of melanin synthesis.

This chapter aims at giving a brief overview of the various skin-lightening agents.

MELANIN SYNTHESIS PATHWAY (FLOWCHART 1 AND BOX 1)

Different mechanism of skin lightening agents:

- Tyrosinase inhibition
- Inhibition of melanosome transfer

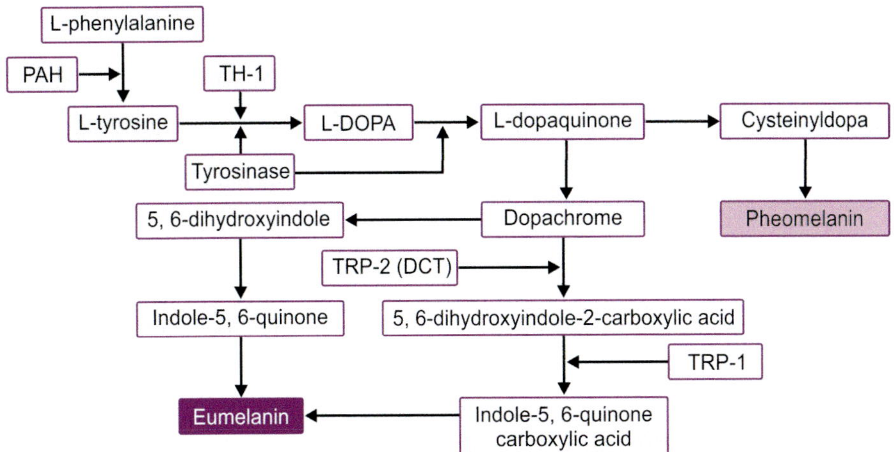

PAH, phenylalanine hydroxylase; TH-1, tyrosinase hydroxylase 1; L-DOPA, levodopa; TRP, tyrosinase related protein; DCT, dopachrome tautomerase.

FLOWCHART 1: Melanin synthesis pathway.

- Epidermal turnover
- Antioxidants
- Flavonoid like agents
- Conjugate to improve the stability and effect of skin lightening agents.

BOX 1 Depigmenting Agents and reported effect on the melanin synthetic pathway[1]

Before melanin synthesis

1. Tyrosinase transcription:
   - Tretinoin

During melanin synthesis

1. Tyrosinase inhibition:
   - Hydroquinone
   - 4-hydroxyanisole
   - 4-S-CAP and derivatives
   - Kojic acid
   - Azelaic acid
   - Arbutin
   - Aloesin
   - Emblica
   - Tyrostat
2. Peroxidase inhibition:
   - Phenols
3. Product reduction and ROS scavengers:
   - Ascorbic acid
   - Ascorbic acid palmitate

After melanin synthesis

1. Tyrosinase degradation:
   - Linoleic acid
   - Alpha-linolenic acid
2. Inhibition of melanosome transfer:
   - Serine protease inhibitors
   - Lecithins
   - Neoglycoproteins
   - Soybean/milk extracts
   - Niacinamide
3. Skin turnover acceleration:
   - Glycolic acid
   - Lactic acid
   - Linoleic acid
   - Retinoic acid
   - Liquiritin
   - Helix aspersa muller

4-S-CAP, 4-S-cystaminylphenol; ROS, reactive oxygen species

SLA WHICH ACT THROUGH TYROSINASE INHIBITION

Hydroquinone

It is one of the oldest and most widely used compounds in the treatment of hyperpigmentation with maximum clinical studies. It is available either as a pharmaceutical or as a cosmeceutical agent.

Mechanism of Action

- It inhibits tyrosinase by binding to the enzyme or by interaction with molecules at the enzymes active site
- It also inhibits DNA and RNA synthesis,[2] as well as degrades melanosomes
- Hydroquinone (HQ) is available commonly in 2% and 4% strength. Various combinations are available in the market. The common ones include:
  - Kligman's formula:[3] 5% HQ + 0.1% tretinoin + 0.1% dexamethasone (tretinoin enhances penetration of HQ, while dexamethasone decreases the irritation and inflammation caused by HQ and also, decreases melanin synthesis by inhibiting metabolic activity)
  - Modified Kligman's formula: HQ 2–4% + tretinoin + low-potency fluorinated steroid, fluocinolone acetonide is effective and safe in the treatment of hyperpigmentation.
- Hydroquinone can also be combined with many other agents like glycolic acid, vitamin C, retinol etc.

Side Effects

- Common side effects reported are skin irritation and contact dermatitis
- Exogenous ochronosis: Hydroquinone has received scrutiny because of its risk of exogenous ochronosis which is severe but a rare side effect. Exogenous ochronosis is the development of sooty hyperpigmentation interspersed with guttate hypopigmentation in the treatment area and is difficult to reverse. It has three clinical stages: Stage I-erythema and mild hyperpigmentation, Stage II-hyperpigmentation, caviar-like lesions and scanty atrophy, and stage III-Papulonodular lesions.[4] It is prevalent among darker individuals, when higher concentration of HQ is used or even when lower concentration of HQ is used for prolonged period. Although the exact cause is not known, some studies suggest that HQ inhibits homogentisic acid oxidase in the dermis thus, causing ochronotic pigment deposition[5]

- Systemic absorption: The other concerns regarding the systemic absorption of hydroquinone is the potential risk from the production of benzene derivatives after hepatic metabolism. These benzene derivatives can cause bone marrow toxicity and exert an anti-apoptotic effect. However, topically applied HQ bypasses the liver.[6] Renal and hepatic adenomas have been reported in animal studies where oral HQ was given. However, no such toxicity has been reported with topical HQ in humans
- There has been no incidence reported till date of any skin or internal organ malignancies as a result of topical HQ application[7]
- The current recommendations for its use are:
    - Use for 6–8 weeks
    - Alternate the use of HQ with one of the alternative agent in 4 months cycle to reduce the side effects and to decrease the risk of ochronosis.

Mequinol

- Mequinol, a derivative of hydroquinone, is chemically known as 4-hydroxyanisole
- It is a substrate of tyrosinase and acts as a competitive inhibitor of melanogenesis[8]
- It is considered safer than HQ as it does not cause melanocytic destruction
- It is US FDA approved and is available in the concentration of 2% in combination with 0.01% tretinoin
- Side effects such as desquamation, burning, and hypopigmentation can be seen post use of this product.

Kojic Acid

It is a fungal metabolite derived from *Aspergillus* and *Penicillium* species.[9] Chemically, it is known as 5-hydroxy-2-hydroxymethyl-pyrone.

Mechanism of Action

It is a potent tyrosinase inhibitor which functions by chelating copper at the enzyme's active site.[10] It also has an antioxidant property. Studies have found it to induce IL-6 production in melanocytes contributing to its anti-melanogenic action.[11] Kojic acid is available in concentrations of 1–4% and can be used one to two times a day for 1–2 months. It is of modest efficacy and is more effective when used in combination with arbutin, glycolic acid, licorice extract, mulberry extract, and vitamin C.

There was a controversy regarding the safety profile of kojic acid due to mutagenicity reported in cell culture studies. Its use was banned in certain countries which was later reintroduced.[7] Few reports of contact sensitivity with kojic acid have also been found.[12]

Azelaic Acid

This naturally occurring dicarboxylic acid is isolated from *Pityrosporum ovale*.

Mechanism of Action

- It is a weak reversible competitive inhibitor of tyrosinase[13,14]
- It interferes with mitochondrial respiration and DNA synthesis in abnormal melanocytes and thus, exerts cytotoxic and antiproliferative effects[15]
- Its lightening effect appears to be selective and is most apparent in highly active melanocytes with minimal effects in normal skin. Hence, it does not induce depigmentation on normally pigmented skin, freckles, senile lentigines, and nevi
- It is available in concentration of 10% and 20%. It is used to treat rosacea, acne, and solar keratoses due to its antioxidant and anti-inflammatory effects.

Side Effects

- It is generally well tolerated
- Side effects include transient erythema and skin irritation which is reversible.

Melatonin

- It is an endogenous hormone secreted by pineal gland in response to sunlight
- It inhibits tyrosinase in melanocytes and inhibits cyclic adenosine monophosphate pathway (AMP) driven processes in the pigment cell. It also has anti-inflammatory effects.

4-n-Butyl Resorcinol

- It is a derivative of resorcinol which has an inhibitory effect against both tyrosinase and tyrosinase-related protein 1 (TRP-1). Studies have shown good efficacy and safety with 4-n-butylresorcinol in patients with melasma[16,17]
- Side effects like skin irritation can be seen if used in higher concentration.

Glutathione

- Glutathione (GSH) is used as a supplement for skin whitening

- It is thiol-tripeptide formed by three amino acids (glutamate, cysteine and glycine).[18] Tomatoes, oranges, asparagus, avocados, walnuts, and whey protein are some of the rich sources of naturally available glutathione.

Mechanism of Action

- Its skin lightening effects result from direct as well as indirect inhibition of tyrosinase enzyme and by switching from eumelanin to pheomelanin. It is also a potent antioxidant
- The major glutathione administration routes available for skin lightening are topical (creams, face washes, soaps, and peels), oral (capsules and sublingual/buccal tablets) and intravenous injections. However, there is paucity of evidence based studies on its efficacy
- Oral glutathione is derived from torula yeast. It is available in a range of 250 to 1,000 mg in combination with ascorbic acid, vitamin E, alpha-lipoic acid, N-acetyl cysteine, grape seed extract etc. Daily recommended dosage is 20-40 mg/kg body weight per day (i.e., 1-2 grams GSH per day) divided into two doses, for skin lightening effects.[19] Bioavailability of oral glutathione is limited as the drug is hydrolyzed by intestinal and hepatic gamma-glutamyl transferase. In a group receiving oral glutathione, reduction in melanin indices was seen[20]
- Because of the poor bioavailability of oral formulations, sublingual formulations have been developed. These are considered safe and are said to be superior in efficacy[21]
- Intravenous injection for skin lightening has been banned by FDA due to incidence of adverse effects like Steven Johnson syndrome and toxic epidermal necrolysis.

Tranexamic Acid (Trans-4-Amino Methylcyclohexanecarboxylic Acid)

- It is a plasmin inhibitor that decreases binding of plasminogen to the keratinocytes, thereby decreasing arachidonic acid and subsequently, prostaglandin causing decreased tyrosinase activity
- Intradermal injection has been found to decrease melasma[22]
- Oral tranexamic acid given in the dosage of 250 mg twice daily for 6 months has shown good results. Minor side effects such as gastrointestinal discomfort and hypomenorrhea were noted[23]
- No long-term studies have been conducted
- It is generally well-tolerated as a topical preparation.

DRUGS WHICH ACT THROUGH SKIN TURNOVER ACCELERATION

Glycolic Acid

Glycolic acid is an alpha-hydroxy acid derived from sugarcane. It is an important cosmeceutical agent used in many skin-lightening products. Glycolic acid peels are commonly used in the treatment of melasma and hyperpigmentation.

Mechanism of Action

At low concentration, it has an epidermal discohesive effect which results in rapid desquamation of pigmented keratinocytes. At higher concentration, it causes epidermolysis.[1] It also enhances the penetration of other topical skin lighteners.

Side Effects

- It can cause irritation and postinflammatory hyperpigmentation especially if a high concentration is used in dark skin individuals. The use of hydroquinone both prior to and after the peel can reduce the risk of pigmentary change
- Glycolic acid is also used in combination with other topical skin-lightening agents as hydroquinone, kojic, and arbutin.

Mandelic Acid

- It is an aromatic alpha-hydroxy acid. Because of its large molecular weight, it causes slow penetration into the skin, and hence less irritation[24]
- It is available in concentration of 2–10% in isolation and also, in combination with other topical vitamins C and E.

Retinoids

- Retinoids are lipophilic vitamin A derivatives, the mechanism of action of which is not completely understood
- They have been found to effectively reduce pigmentation in melasma and postinflammatory pigmentation.

Mechanism of Action

- Retinoids act through multiple mechanisms, by acting both before and during melanin synthesis
- They have been found to inhibit transcription of tyrosinase

- Increase epidermal turnover of keratinocytes → decreases keratinocytes cohesiveness → desquamation → accelerate melanin loss in stratum corneum. This also facilitates better penetration of other lightening agents[25]
- Dispersion of melanin pigment in keratinocytes, causing uniform distribution of melanin in epidermis
- Decreases melanosome transfer to keratinocytes[25]
- Tretinoin (0.025–1%), adapalene (0.1–0.3%), tazarotene are some of the retinoids known to be effective.

Side Effects

- Erythema, dryness, and peeling are few commonly reported side effects especially with tretinoin
- As a monotherapy retinoid takes longer time to act clinically. Better results are obtained in combination with other agents (Kligman formula).[3]

Oligopeptides

Short chained oligopeptides have shown to inhibit tyrosinase activity without any cytotoxic effect. But its use as SLA needs to be studied further.[26,27]

Linoleic Acid

- Unsaturated fatty acids like linoleic acid and alpha-linolenic acid suppress the melanogenesis and tyrosinase activity[28]
- Linoleic acid also stimulates epidermal turnover leading to desquamation of melanin pigment from epidermis
- It is thought that the unsaturated bonds of these molecules can be easily peroxidized, which in combination with increase in epidermal turnover correlate with an inhibitory effect on melanogenesis *in vivo*.

DRUGS WHICH ACT BY PEROXIDASE INHIBITION OR BY ANTIOXIDANT MECHANISM

Vitamin C (Ascorbic Acid)

- It is a very effective antioxidant which rapidly gets oxidized on exposure to air, making it highly unstable.Thus, esters like magnesium-L-ascorbyl-2-phosphate (MAP) are used
- It is found to interfere at different stages of melanogenesis by interacting with copper ions to reduce dopaquinone conversion to DOPA. It also blocks dihydroxyindole-2-carboxylic acid (DHICA) oxidation.[29] It also absorbs UV radiations, preventing free radical formation
- Humans are unable to synthesize vitamin C, hence, they have to acquire it from natural sources. The bioavailability of vitamin C in skin is inadequate when administered orally, hence it should be used topically.[30] Efficacy of topical vitamin C is proportional to its concentration
- Adverse effects such as stinging, burning, yellowish discoloration, urticaria, and erythema multiforme have been reported.[30]

Vitamin E

- It is a fat-soluble antioxidant vitamin present in tissues and plasma. Vitamin C regenerates oxidized vitamin E and thus, the combination has synergistic effect in UV protection[31]
- Topical vitamin E helps in hydration of skin and is an important additive in many cosmeceuticals.

Mechanism of Action

Vitamin E blocks the lipid peroxidation in cells, and hence, helps in photoprotection. It also has antioxidant properties.

Alpha-lipoic Acid (Thioctic Acid)

Alpha-lipoic acid and di-hydro lipoic acid (DHLA) are strong antioxidants which are both water and fat soluble.[32]

It inhibits tyrosinase by chelating copper and decreasing dopa quinone derivative formation.[33] It increases the glutathione (GSH) level which reduces UV radiation sensitivity.[34] Thioctic acid and dihydrolipoic acid block microphthalmia-associated transcription factor (MITF—regulator of melanocyte development) thus inhibiting tyrosinase activity.[35] There have been reports of contact dermatitis.[36]

Hydroxycoumarins

- These are lactones of phenyl propanoic acid with an H-benzopyranone nucleolus
- It inhibits melanogenesis and intracellular glutathione synthesis in melanocytes. It also has an antioxidant action.[37]

Pyruvic Acid

This is an alpha-keto acid found to reduce pigmentation in melasma patients. No side effects have been reported.

Botanicals (Table 1)

In search of newer and more safer skin lightening agents, many plant extracts have been isolated and studied. Botanicals are basically active compounds, that are isolated from plants. Botanical compounds like arbutin, aloesin, flavonoids, hesperidin, licorice, niacinamide and polyphenols, inhibit melanogenesis without any melanocytotoxicity, which makes them safer than other skin lightening agents. There are slew of botanicals, which are extremely promising. But the actives present in different sources of botanicals are extremely variable, depending on the following:

- Plant source: Leaves, roots, fruits, berries, stems, twigs, barks, and flowers
- Growing conditions: Soil composition, amount of available water, climate variations, and plant stress
- Harvesting conditions: Time from harvest to transport, care of plant materials during shipping, and storage conditions prior to manufacture
- Preparation methods: Crushing, grinding, boiling, distilling, pressing, and drying
- Final extract status: Liquid, powder, paste, syrup, and crystal
- Concentration: Sufficient amount of active agent to produce the biologic effect
- The other consideration to be kept in mind is how much of the product is reaching the target tissue
- There are more than 4,000 flavonoids identified in leaves, barks, and flowers
- These are benzopyrene derivatives, which can be classified into flavones, flavanols, isoflavones, flavanones, and anthocyanidins. They can be formulated into nanocapsules so that they reach the active site of melanin synthesis where

TABLE 1: Commonly used botanical skin lightening agents[38]

Name and active constitute	Derived from	Mechanism of action	Comments
Arbutin (β-d-glucopyranoside derivative of hydroquinone) Types: • Alpha arbutin • Beta arbutin Efficiency-(α>>> β)[39]	• Bearberry plant • Cranberry • Blueberry leaves[8]	• Inhibits tyrosinase activity by acting as a molecular mimic to the tyrosine. (It does not suppress tyrosinase synthesis) • Inhibits melanosomes maturation	• Can be used alone or in combination with kojic acid, glycolic acid etc.
Niacinamide (amide form of vitamin B_3)	Root vegetables, yeast	• Reduces melanin transfer[40] • Antioxidant • Anti-inflammatory • Immunomodulation	• Decreases melanin transfer by 35- 68%; significant improvement in 4 weeks. (Bissett et al. 2004)
Aloesin	Aloe vera	• Noncompetitive inhibitor of tyrosinase • Competitive inhibitor of DOPA	• Inhibits UV-induced melanogenesis[1]
Flavonoids-mulberroside F (moracin M-6, 3′-di-O-β-Dglucopyranoside)	Mulberry plant (*Morus alba*)	• Inhibit tyrosinase and L – DOPA oxidation[41] • ROS suppression	–
Licorice extract (flavonoids-Glabiridin Liquiritin[42,43])	Root of Licorice (*Glycyrrhiza glabra*)	• Liquiritin—causes melanin dispersion and increases the epidermal turnover • Glabiridin—inhibits tyrosinase activity without affecting the DNA synthesis	• It also inhibits UVB induce pigmentation and erythema and is widely used in Europe as an anti-inflammatory agent • Trial for melasma using licorice showed good to excellent results in 90% of patients[44]

Contd...

Contd...

Name and active constitute	Derived from	Mechanism of action	Comments
Flavanon glycoside -Hesperidin	Citrus fruits	• Tyrosinase inhibitor • Antioxidant[45]	Protects against UVA-induced fibroblast damage and oxidative collagen damage
Isoflavonon (contains protein Bowman–Birk inhibitor (BBI) and Soybean trypsin inhibitor (STI))	Soy	• Inhibition of protease-activated receptor-2 (PAR-2) pathway by these protease inhibitor, reduces melanosome phagocytosis by keratinocytes and hence, reduces melanin transfer[46]	–
Flavonoids-Procyanidin	French maritime pine (Pycnogenol)	• ROS suppression • Regenerates active forms of vitamins C and E • Tyrosinase inhibition	• Provides potential photoprotection by synthesizing anti-oxidative enzymes and scavenging free radicals • Also, it has antiinflammatory and anti carcinogenic property
Polyphenols	Indian gooseberry or amla (*Phyllanthus emblica*)	• ROS suppression • Tyrosinase inhibition	–
Polyphenols-Ellagic Acid	Strawberry, green tea, eucalyptus	• Tyrosinase inhibition • Inhibit melanocyte proliferation	• Effective lightening agent without any side effects.[47,48] Also, prevent UV-induced pigmentation
Polyphenols-Silymarin	Seeds of the milk thistle plant *Silybum marianum*[49]	Inhibitory effects on melanogenesis. in mouse melanocyte cell lines[50]	–
Green tea polyphenols—epigallocatechin gallate, catechin, epigallocatechin, gallocatechin gallate, and epicatechin gallate[51]	Green tea (*Camellia sinensis*)	• ROS suppression • Anti-inflammatory • Tyrosinase inhibitor	• Guanosine triphosphate given topically or orally acts as antioxidant,[52] anti-inflammatory and anticarcinogenic agents[53]
Polyphenols-ferulic acid and quinic acid	Coffea arabica fruit (coffee berry extract)	ROS suppression	Protective effect against UVB induced pyrimidine dimer formation and inflammation
Chamomile tea extract	Matricaria (*Chamomilla recutita*)	• Antagonizes endothelin receptor binding and thereby inhibiting signaling between keratinocytes and melanocytes • Anti-inflammatory antioxidant property	• These endothelin inhibitors work faster than tyrosinase inhibitor because their mechanism of action is outside the melanocyte cell membrane • Reduces UVB-induced pigmentation[54,55]

Contd...

Contd...

Name and active constitute	Derived from	Mechanism of action	Comments
Polyphenols–resveratrol	• Most plants • Red wine	• Reduces microphthalmia-associated transcription factor (MITF) and tyrosinase activity	
Polyphenols	Daisy flowers (*Bellis perennis*)	• Anti-inflammatory • ROS suppression • Suppresses melanosome transfer	
Polyphenols procyanidin	Grape seed extract (*Vitis vinifera*)	ROS suppression	
Caffeic acid and ferulic acid—*Polypodium leucotomos* extract	Cabbage palm fern (*Phlebodium aureum*)	ROS suppression	
p-Coumaric acid	leaves of Panax ginseng	Inhibit L- tyrosine oxidation	Significantly suppresses melanogenesis
	Western dock (*Rumex occidentalis*)	Tyrosinase inhibition	
	Orchid (*Brassocattleya marcella*)	ROS suppression	

ROS, reactive oxygen species; L-DOPA, levodopa; UVA, ultra violet A.

they exert a strong reducing action, and act as a substrate competitor for the tyrosinase.[23] It also, have antioxidant action.

OTHER EXPERIMENTAL AGENTS

Botanicals like gentisic acid, cinnamic acid, magnolignan (2,2′-dihyroxy 5,5′-dipropyl biphenyl), linoleic acid, etc. are being investigated for their use as skin lightening agent.

There are numerable products available in the commercial market, several of which are of commercial value with no proper governance in regards to the composition and long-term safety studies. Many such whiteners contain toxic mercury such as mercury(II) chloride or ammoniated mercury as the active ingredient. Mercury has been banned in many countries for use in skin whitening because it accumulates on skin and can have serious effects. Studies suggest that long-term use could cause systemic absorption of the substance. Women, especially pregnant and nursing mothers, are at risk of mercury toxicity because of long-term exposure which can cause permanent neurological damage, nephrological disorders, fertility problems, and birth defects. Studies have shown significant accumulation in the ovaries of mice following the application of skin-lightening cream.[16,17,56] As conscientious physicians it is our duty to be aware of such products and warn our patients against their use.

CONCLUSION

The science of melanogenesis and the study of skin lightening agents are at an exciting stage. However, there is too much data that is lacking. It is our duty as dermatologists to scrutinize all the data—especially the clinical studies, that is available for skin lightening agents and decide what is the truth.

Lastly, as dermatologists, evidence-based medicine is the ideal way to go and we should critically scrutinize all the clinical studies that are published—the most reliable being randomized controlled trials.

REFERENCES

1. Rendon MI, Gaviria JI. Skin lightening agents. 2nd edition. In: Drealos ZD, editor. Procedures in Cosmetic Dermatology Series: Cosmeceuticals. Philadelphia:Elsevier Saunders;2009. pp. 145-109.
2. Briganti S, Camera E, Picardo M. Chemical and instrumental approaches to treat hyperpigmentation. Pigment Cell Res. 2003;16:101-10.

3. Kligman AM, Willis I. A new formula for depigmenting human skin. Arch Dermatol.1975;111:40.
4. Bhattar PA, Zawar VP, Godse KV, et al. Exogenous Ochronosis. Indian journal of dermatology. 2015p;60(6):537-543.
5. Talakoub L, Neuhaus IM, Yu SS. Cosmeceuticals. In: Alam M, editor. Requisites in Dermatology Series: Cosmetic Dermatology. New York, NY: Elseiver; 2009. pp. 7-35.
6. Westerhof W, KooyersTJ. Hydroquinone and its analogues in dermatology – a potential health risk. J Cosmet Dermatol. 2005;4:55-9.
7. Nordlund JJ, Grimes PE, Ortonne JP. The safety of hydroquinone. J Eur Acad Dermatol Venereol. 2006;20:781-7.
8. Draelos ZD. Skin lighting preparations and thehydroquinone controversy. Dermatol Ther. 2007;20:308-13.
9. Kim Y-J, Uyama H. Tyrosinase inhibitors and natural synthetic source: structure, inhibition mechanism and perspective for the future. Cell Mol Life Sci. 2005;62:1707-23.
10. Hira Y, Hatae S, Inoue T, et al. Inhibitory effects of kojic acid on melanin formation. In vitro and in vivo studies in black gold fish. JJ pm Cosmet Sci Soc.1982;6:193.
11. Choi H, Kim K , Han J, etal. Kojic acid-induced IL-6 production in human keratinocytes play a role in its anti-melanogenic activity in skin. J Dermatol Sci. 2012;66(3):207-15.
12. Nakayama G, Watanabe N, Nishioka K, et al. Treatment of chloasma with kojic acid cream. J pn J Clin Dermatol.1982;36:715.
13. KimY-J, Uyama H. Tyrosinase inhibitors from natural and synthetic sources:structure,inhibition mechanism and perspective for the future. Cell Mol Life Sci.2005;62:1707-23.
14. Porro NM. Azelaic acid. J Am Acad Dermatol. 1987; 17:1033-41.
15. Fitton A, Goa KL. Azelaic acid. A review of its pharmacological properties and therapeutic efficacy in acne and hyperpigmentary disorders. Drugs.1991;41:780-98.
16. Kolbe L, Mann T, Gerwat W, et al. 4-n-butylresorcinol, a highly effective tyrosinase inhibitor for the topical treatment of hyperpigmentation. J Eur Acad Dermatol Venereol. 2013;27(Suppl 1):19-23.
17. Mohan MNT, Gowda A, Jaiswal AK, et al. Assessment of efficacy safety, and tolerability of 4-n-butylresorcinol 0.3% cream: an Indian multicentric study on melasma. Clin Cosmet Investig Dermatol. 2016;9:21-7.
18. Dickinson DA, Forman HJ. Glutathione in defense and signaling: lessons from a small thiol. Ann N Y Acad Sci. 2002;973:488-504
19. Sidharth S, Daulatabad D, Sarkar R. Glutathione as a skin whitening agent: Facts, myths, evidence and controversies. Indian Journal of Dermatology, Venereology, and Leprology. 2016;82(3): 262
20. Arjinpathana N, Asawanonda P. Glutathione as oral whitening agent: a randomized, double blind, placebo-controlled study. J Dermatolog Treat. 2012;23(2):97-102.
21. Handog C, Handog E, Singzon I, et al. Glutathione as a systemic skin whitening agent via the buccal mucosa: an open-label, single-arm study. JAAD. 2016;74(5):AB17.
22. Lee JH, Park JG, Lim SH, et al. Localized intradermal microinjection of tranexemic acid for treatment of melasma in Asian patients: a preliminary clinical report. Dermatol Surg. 2006;32:626-31.
23. Wu S, Shi H, Wu H, et al. Treatment of melasma with oral administration of Tranexamic acid. Aesthetic Plast Surg. 2012;36(4):964-70.
24. Sarkar R, Chugh S, Garg VK. Newer and upcoming therapies for melasma. Indian J Dermatol Venereol Leprol. 2012;78:417-2.
25. Ortonne JP. Retinoid therapy of pigmented disorders. Dermatol Ther. 2006;19:280-8.
26. Hantash BM, Jimenez F. A split-face, double-blind, randomized and placebo-controlled pilot evaluation of a novel oligopeptide for the treatment of recalcitrant melasma. J Drugs Dermatol. 2009;8(8):732-35.
27. Ubeid AA, Zhao L, Wang Y, et al. Short-sequence oligopeptides with inhibitory activity against Mushroom and human tyrosinase. J Invest Dermatol. 2009;129:2242-49.
28. Ando H, Ryu A, Hashimoto A, et al. Linoleic acid and alpha-linolenic acid lightens ultraviolet-induced hyperpigmentation of skin. Arch Dermatol Res. 1998; 290(7):375-81.
29. Espinal-Perez LE, Moncada B, Castanedo-Cazares JP. A double blind randomized trial of 5% ascorbic acid vs. 4% hydroquinone in melasma. Int J Dermatol. 2004;43: 604 7.
30. Telang PS. Vitamin C in dermatology. Indian Dermatol Online J. 2013;4(2):143-46.
31. Burke KE. Interaction of vitamins C and E as better cosmeceuticals. Dermatol Ther. 2007;20(5):314-21.
32. Kagan VE, Shvedova A, Serbinova E, et al. Dihydrolipolic acid-a universal antioxidant both in membrane & in the aqueous phase. Reduction of peroxyl, ascorbyl & chromanoxyl radicals. Biochem Pharmacol. 1992;44(8):1637-49.
33. Saliou C, Kitazawa M, McLaughlin L, et al. Antioxidant modulate acute solar ultraviolet radiation – induced NF-kappa-B activation in a human keratinocyte cell line. Free Radic Biol Med. 1999;26:174-83.
34. Tyrrell RM, Pidoux M. Correlation between endogenous glutathione content and sensitivity of cultured human skin cells to radiation at defined wave-lengths in the solar ultraviolet range. Photochem Photobial. 1988; 47(3):405-12.
35. Fisher DE. Microphthalmia: a signal responsive transcriptional regulator in development. Pigment Cell Res. 2000;13(suppl 8):145-9.
36. Bergqvist-Karlson A, Thelin I, Bergendorff O. Contact dermatitis to alpha-lipoic acid in an anti-wrinkle cream. Contact Dermatitis. 2006;55:56-7.
37. Yamamura T, Onishi J, Nishiyama T. Anti-melanogenic activity of hydrocoumarins in cultured normal human melanocytes by stimulating intracellular glutathione synthesis. Arch Dermatol Res. 2002;294:349-54.
38. Zhu W, Gao J. The use of botanical extracts as topical skin-lightening agents for the improvement of skin pigmentation disorders. Journal of Investigative Dermatology Symposium Proceedings. 2008;13(1):20-4.

39. Sugimoto K, Nishimura T, Nomura K, et al. Syntheses of alpha-arbutin-glycosides and a comparison of their inhibitory effects with those of alpha-arbutin and arbutin on human tyrosinase. J Cosmet Sci. 2003;51(7): 798-801.
40. Hakozaki T, Minwalla L, Zhuang J, et al. The effect of niacinamide on reducing cutaneous pigmentation and suppression of melanosome transfer. Br J Dermatol. 2002;147:20-31.
41. Hwang JH, Lee BM. Inhibitory effects of plant extracts on tyrosinase, L-DOPA oxidation,and melanin synthesis. J Toxicol Environ Health A. 2007;70:393-407
42. Amer M, Metwalli M. Topical liquiritin improves melasma. Int J Dermatol. 2003;39:299-301.
43. Leyden JJ, Shergill B, Micali G, et al. Natural options for management of hyperpigmentation. J Eur Acad Dermatol Venereol. 2011;25(10):1140-45.
44. Rico MJ. Rising drug costs: the impact on dermatology. Skin Therapy Letter. 2000;5(4):1-2,5.
45. Lee HJ, Lee WJ, Chang SE, et al. Hisperidin, A popular antioxidant inhibits melanogenesis via Erk1/2 mediated MIFT Degradation. Int J Mol Sci. 2015;16(8):18384-95.
46. Paine C, Sharlow E, Liebel F, et al. An alternative approach to depigmentation by soybean extracts via inhibition of thePAR-2 pathway. J Invest Dermatol. 2001:116:587-95.
47. Yoshimura M, Watanabe Y, Kasai K, et al. Inhibitory effect of an ellagic acid-rich pomegranate extract on tyrosinase activity and ultraviolet-induced pigmentation. Bio sci Biotechnol Biochem. 2005;69:2368-73.
48. Shimogaki H, Tanaka Y, Tamai H, et al. In vitro and in vivo evaluation of ellagic acid on melanogenesis inhibition. Int J CosmetSci. 2000;22:291-303.
49. Svobodov'a A, Psotova J, Walterova D. Natural phenolics in the prevention of UV induced skin damage a review. Biomed Pap Med Fac Univ Palacky Olomouc Czech Repub. 2003;147:137-45.
50. Choo SJ, Ryoo IJ, Kim YH, et al. Silymarin inhibits melanin synthesis in melanocyte cells. J Pharm Pharmacol. 2009;61:663-7.
51. Sato K, Toriyama M. Depigmenting effect of catechins. Molecules. 2009;14:4425-32.
52. Hsu S. Green tea and the skin. J Am Acad Dermatol. 2005;52:1049-59.
53. Khan N, Mukhtar H. Tea polyphenols for health promotion. Life Sci. 2007;81:519.
54. Ando H, Matsui MS, Ichihashi M. Qasi-drugs developed in Japan for the prevention or treatment of hyperpigmentation disorders. Int J Mol Sci. 2010;11: 2566-75.
55. Ichihashi M, Kobayashi A, Okuda M, et al. Effect of Chamomilla extract application on UV-induced pigmentation. Nishinihon J Dermatol. 1999;41:475-80.
56. Al-Saleh I, Shinwari N, Al-Amodi M. Accumulation of mercury in ovaries of mice after the application of skin-lightening creams. Biol Trace Elem Res. 2009;131(1):43-54.

5

CHAPTER

Antiaging Cosmeceuticals

Jaishree Sharad, Neha Sud

INTRODUCTION

From times immemorial, people have fantasized about regaining the vitality and vigor of youth by a dip in the fountain of youth. Young age is associated with beauty, charm, and old age with debility, wrinkled, and sagging skin. Baby boomers are aging and they want to look perfect.

Cutaneous ageing is the end result of intrinsic and extrinsic factors working in tandem. At the helm of these is photodamage or sun induced damage. Tell tale signs of environmental and biological insults on our skin appear with passing years (Box 1). Corresponding to what is seen on the skin surface are changes which can be discerned histopathologically (Table 1) and at a functional level too (Box 2).

BOX 1 Features of photoaged skin[1]

- Dryness (roughness)
- Pigmentation
  - Irregular pigmentation
  - Diffuse hyperpigmentation
  - Freckling
  - Lentigines
- Inelasticity
- Telangiectasia
- Wrinkling
  - Fine surface lines
  - Deep furrows
- Comedones
- Sebaceous hyperplasia
- Appendages
  - Depigmentation of hair
  - Loss of hair
  - Terminal to vellus hair
  - Dystrophic/ thickened/ discoloured nail plates
- Guttate hypomelanosis
- Venous lakes
- Purpura (easy bruising)
- Stellate pseudoscars
- Seborrheic and actinic keratoses

TABLE 1: Histopathological changes in aging skin[2,3]

Epidermis	Dermis
• Variable/ decreased thickness • Variable cell size and shape • Occasional nuclear atypia • Fewer melanocytes	• Flattened dermal-epidermal junction • Dermal atrophy • Dermal elastosis, upper reticular dermis • Reduced type I, III collagen • Fragmented elastic fibres • Decreased hyaluronic acid • Increased glycosaminoglycans and matrix metalloproteinases • Fewer fibroblasts/Langerhans cells/mast cells • Fewer blood vessels • Shortened capillary loops • Reduced eccrine glands • Increased size of sebaceous glands

BOX 2 Functions of human skin that decline with age

- Barrier function
- Cell replacement
- Chemical clearance
- DNA repair
- Epidermal hydration
- Immune responsiveness
- Mechanical protection
- Sebum production
- Sensory perception
- Sweat production
- Thermoregulation
- Vitamin D production
- Wound healing

Antiaging cosmeceutics have active molecules that help correct or slow these age related changes. Prevention and protection start with the following strategies that slow down photodamage:[4]

- Preventing sun exposure: Wide-brimmed hat, clothing, umbrella
- Prevention of ultraviolet (UV) penetration into skin: Physical and chemical sunscreens
- Prevention/reduction of inflammation: Anti-inflammatory compounds (e.g., cyclooxygenase inhibitors, inhibitors of cytokine generation)
- Scavenging and quenching of reactive oxygen species (ROS): Antioxidants
- Inhibition of neutrophil elastase activity to prevent extracellular matrix damage
- Inhibition of matrix metalloproteinase (MMP) expression (e.g., by retinoids) and activity (e.g., by natural and synthetic inhibitors).

TOPICAL ANTIAGING COSMECEUTICALS

Antiaging topicals or the age defying molecules work well as the first step to tackle ageing changes, especially for people who prefer a noninvasive approach (Fig. 1). They need to be started at an early age to help prevent or slow down the signs of aging. The list of topical antiaging cosmeceuticals is:

- Prescription molecules
  - Retinoids
  - Alpha-hydroxy acids
- Antioxidants
  - Vitamins
  - Botanicals
  - Miscellaneous
- Cell regulators
  - Growth factors
  - Cytokines
- Peptides
- Sunscreens
- Future molecules.

PRESCRIPTION MOLECULES

Retinoids[4-9]

In the 1960s, Albert Kligman pioneered research in antiaging and the end result were molecules called retinoids, of which retinoic acid is still considered the gold standard in antiaging topical therapy.

Retinoids are vitamin A derivatives, natural, and synthetic. Being lipophilic compounds they can easily penetrate the skin and bring effect by activating RARαβγ and RXRαβγ receptors and modulating genes controlling cell differentiation and proliferation, leading to younger looking skin with a smooth texture. They inhibit MMPs or collagenases from breaking down collagen, interfere with melanogenesis, and improve dermal vasculature, while also stimulating new collagen deposition. They also promote renewal of epidermal cells with expansion of cell layers, increased epidermal and dermal mucin, and the down growth of rete ridges, restoring the undulating dermoepidermal interphase and improve the skin's water barrier properties. Collagen

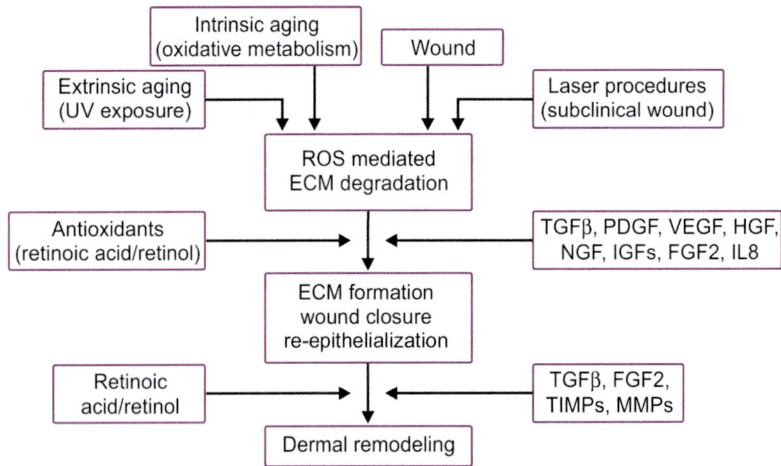

UV, ultraviolet; ROS, reactive oxygen species; ECM, extracellular matrix; TGFβ, transforming growth factor beta; PDGF, platelet-derived growth factor; VEGF, vascular endothelial growth factor; HGF, hepatocyte growth factor; NGF, nerve growth factor; IGFs, insulin-like growth factor; MMPs, matrix metalloproteinases; FGF2, fibroblast growth factor-2; IL8, interleukin 8; TIMPs, tissue inhibitors of metalloproteinases.

FIG. 1: A pictorial representation of site of action of antiaging molecules.

organization continues to improve and elastosis continues to decrease on continued use. In addition, they are free radical scavengers and have antioxidant activity and stimulate fibroblast proliferation. Some key retinoids include retinoic acid (tretinoin), retinaldehyde, retinol and retinyl esters; with progressively decreasing biological activity. Isotretinoin is the 13-cis isomer of retinoic acid. Retinaldehyde is an intermediate in the conversion of retinol (vitamin A) to retinoic acid (the active form). In a review of retinoid-based cosmeceuticals, Babamiri et al. concluded that retinaldehyde-based cosmeceuticals have the most beneficial effect in aging skin as per large randomized-controlled trials (RCTs).[10] They are ideal for the treatment of sun induced aging or photodamage, but have a tendency to increase sun sensitivity so they should always be used at night, with a sunscreen during the day. Side effects may include some irritation with dry scaly red skin.

Randomized-controlled trials have shown tretinoin cream to be safe and effective in patients of moderate to severe photodamage and causes a significant increase in facial procollagen 1C terminal a marker of procollagen synthesis.[11]

Preparations containing nanosomes of pro-retinol A have also been introduced with claims of instant retautening of the skin and wrinkle reduction.[12]

Alpha-hydroxy Acids[5,13]

They are organic carboxylic acids and are also commonly called the fruit acids. They improve skin texture, hydration, and reduce signs of skin aging. One hypothesis on their mechanism of action is by their Ca chelating property.[14] Keratinocyte discohesion (low concentrations) and epidermolysis (higher concentrations) follows. Basal keratinocyte stimulation, thicker epidermis, and dermal fibroblast stimulation, increased collagen and glycosaminoglycans (GAGs), with a probable antioxidant action are mechanisms by which they help play a role as antiaging molecules. Common alpha-hydroxy acids (AHAs) include:

- Citric acid (from citrus fruits)
- Glycolic acid (from sugarcane)
- Lactic acid (from fermented milk)
- Malic acid (from unripened apples)
- Mandelic acid (from bitter almonds)
- Tartaric acid (from fermented grapes), and
- Pyruvic acid.

Of the above hydroxy acids, glycolic acid is the one most commonly found in cosmeceuticals in the range of 6–12% (generally below 15%).

Beta-hydroxy Acids

Salicylic acid (SA) is a β-hydroxy acid. Lipohydroxy acid (LHA) is a SA derivative with an additional fatty chain which enhances its anti-inflammatory, antibacterial, anticomedogenic, and exfoliative properties even at low concentrations.[15]

Polyhydroxy Acids and Bionic Acids[16-18]

These are a new generation of AHAs that provide similar effects but do not cause the sensory irritation responses that can limit the use of classical AHAs. Polyhydroxy acids (PHAs) are AHAs that contain multiple hydroxyl groups, as the name signals ("poly" "hydroxyl"), on the molecule, and bionics are PHAs with an additional sugar molecule attached to the PHA structure.

They are compatible in patients with sensitive skin, rosacea,[19] atopic dermatitis, and postprocedure, providing moisturization and humectant properties enhancing barrier function. Antioxidant and chelating properties make them safe for use even in the daytime. Bionic acids (BAs) in addition inhibit MMP enzymes in skin, providing a preventative antiaging benefit.[20] They improve tolerability and enhance efficacy when used in conjunction with retinoids, azelaic acid, benzoyl peroxide and hydroquinone. Gluconolactone, a PHA, can be formulated with oxidative drugs, such as benzoyl peroxide, to help reduce irritation potential and erythema caused by the oxidative drug.[21,22] In addition, it enhances epidermal cell turnover.

Bionic acids are commonly obtained from their disaccharide through chemical or enzymatic oxidation; for example, lactobionic acid is obtained from lactose, maltobionic acid from maltose, and cellobionic acid from cellobiose. Maltobionic is a plant derived newer BA and, like lactobionic acid, is gentle and nonirritating, a strong humectant and an antioxidant chelator.[23]

Antioxidants

Antioxidants in skin care products:

- Vitamins: A, B3, C, E
- Lipoic acids
- Coenzyme Q10 (ubiquinone)
- Glucopyranosides
- Polyphenols
- Cysteine
- Glutathione
- Allantoin
- Furfuryladenine
- Dimethylaminoethanol

- Uric acid
- Carnosine
- Spin traps
- Melatonin
- Catalase
- Superoxide dismutase
- Peroxidase
- Panthenol.

The application of antioxidants in the form of cosmeceuticals should aim to support a physiologically balanced oxidation status in the skin.[24]

These molecules are most effective as a combination of topical and oral products.

Vitamin C (l-Ascorbic Acid) and Vitamin E[5,25-27]

Ascorbic acid is a naturally occurring antioxidant found in citrus fruits and leafy green vegetables. It is hydrophilic, so skin penetration is low. When applied to the skin vitamin C counteracts the acute redness, sunburn and tanning, as well as chronic effects of UV exposure. This has been corroborated in studies too.[28] Formulation challenges in topical cosmeceuticals include providing a high concentration, i.e., at least 10%, of the nonesterified optical isomer of vitamin C which is adequately stabilized, as on exposure to air L-ascorbic acid converts to inactive brown dihydroascorbic acid. Vitamin C regenerates oxidized vitamin E and also stimulates neocollagenesis. Vitamin C or ascorbic acid and its derivatives, magnesium ascorbyl phosphate (MAP) and ascorbyl tetra isopalmitate, are used extensively in topical antiaging cocktails. Vitamin E also has properties akin to vitamin C, and in a combination their effect manifests multifold.[29] Vitamin E has poor skin penetration and primarily prevents oxidation of cell wall lipids.

Ferulic Acid[30]

Ferulic acid (FA) is a potent antioxidant present in the cell walls of grains, fruits, and vegetables. It stabilizes formulations that contain vitamin C and E and also doubles its photoprotection properties. Ferulic acid is a precursor to ethyl ferulate, a molecule that has been shown to be more effective in scavenging ROS generated from activated leucocytes than FA, with lower spreadability.

Niacinamide (Vitamin B3)[31,3]

This molecule is a potent, well tolerated antioxidant with action on both pigmentation and wrinkles. Niacinamide decreases protein glycation and acts as an nonirritant exfoliant. It improves the lipid barrier function by increasing biosynthesis of ceramides. Niacinamide also enhances repair of UV radiation-induced deoxyribonucleic acid (DNA) damage.

Alphalipoic Acids[5,33]

Both alphalipoic acid and its reduced form dihydrolipoate are potent scavengers with anti-inflammatory properties. It also has a role in stabilizing vitamin C and E in preparations and an exfoliant action.

Ubiquinone and Idebenone[9]

Coenzyme Q10 is an essential component of the mitochondrial respiratory chain and forms an important defense against superoxide radicals. Ubiquinone (from ubiquitous, i.e., universally found) is naturally derived whereas idebenone is a low molecular weight synthetic derivative. As idebenone is a smaller molecule its penetration into the skin on application is much better. Also, nanostructured lipid carriers enhance skin permeation along with increasing the stability of idebenone.[34]

Used twice a day over 6 weeks 0.5–1% idebenone lotion was effective in reducing fine lines and wrinkles with improvement in skin hydration.

Botanicals[7,35]

These are an exhaustive list of molecules and are encountered as one of the most frequent ingredients in antiaging cosmeceuticals.

Some of the common natural antioxidants are shown in box 3.

Essential fatty acids (EFAs) are building blocks of cellular membranes which allow efficient transportation of nutrients from the extracellular space into the intracellular environment where metabolism takes place. Rosehip seed oil (*Rosa mosqueta*) which is high in EFAs smoothens wrinkles by hydrating the skin and slows new signs of aging.[39]

Other topical antioxidants include leaf wax of Eucalyptus and *Prunus*, the seeds of black rice, leaves of barley, sesame seeds, rosemary green tea, turmeric, beta-carotene, coral extracts, aloe, and so forth.

Tea[40,41]

Green, black, white, oolong tea are derived from the tea plant, leaves and buds, but by different processing, oxidation, and fermentation steps. Black tea is fermented and green tea is not. They are known

BOX 3 Botanical antioxidants and their sources[36-38]

- Flavones
  - Rutin (apples, blueberries)
  - Quercetin (apples, blueberries)
  - Hesperidin (lemons, oranges)
  - Diosmin (lemons, oranges)
  - Isoflavones (soybean)
  - silydin (silymarin)
- Xanthones
  - Mangiferin (mango plant)
  - Mangostin (bilberry plant)
- Carotenoids
  - Astaxanthin (marine algae)
  - Lutein (tomatoes)
  - Lycopene (tomatoes)
- Polyphenols
  - Rosmarinic acid (rosemary)
  - Hypericin (St John's wort)
  - Ellagic acid (pomegranate fruit)
  - Chlorogenic acid (blueberry leaf)
  - Oleuropein (olive leaf)
  - Curcumin (tumeric root)
  - Pycnogenol (marine pine bark)
  - Terpenoids (ginkobiloba)
  - Procyanidins (grape seed)
  - Epigallocatechin (green tea)

to be high in antioxidant activity; this property is imparted by ingredients called polyphenolic catechins. White tea has higher levels of the same compared to green tea. Green tea offers antioxidant, anti-inflammatory and anticarcinogenic properties with both topical and systemic administration. Research has found that of the many catechins in tea, epicatechin, epigallocatechin, epicatechin-3-gallate, epigallocatechin-3-gallate (EGCG), the main active ingredient in green tea is EGCG and it works well as an anti-inflammatory, antioxidant, and sunscreen.

Topical green tea applied to human skin has been shown to provide a photoprotective effect, reduce the number of sunburn cells, protect epidermal Langerhans cells from UV damage, and reduce the DNA damage that formed after UV radiation.

Black tea has a much lower content of catechins than green tea, but a higher content of other flavonoids, such as quercetin, theaflavin, and kaempferol.

It is generally accepted that 5% green tea extract or polyphenols in the 90% range is an effective concentration in topical preparations.

Curcumin

Procured from the tuberous rhizome turmeric it has tetrahydrocurcumin a polyphenol antioxidant. It has been used as a preservative and antiseptic. Slight burning sensation is possible on application.

Grape Seed Extract[42]

Procured from *Vitis vinifera*, a polyphenol-rich antioxidant, and claimed to have higher antioxidant capacity than vitamin C and E.

Oligomeric proanthocyanidins, polyphenols, in grape seeds helps in wound contraction and closure. It also enhances sun protection.

Soy[35]

The major components of soy are phospholipids (45–60%) and essential fatty oils (30–35%) while the minor components include the most active compounds, such as isoflavones and the proteases soybean trypsin inhibitor and Bowman-Birk inhibitor.

Soy isoflavones, genistein and daidzein are potent phytoestrogens hence useful in postmenopausal women with thin skin and reduced collagen.

Soy stimulates the production GAGs and HA in aging skin. Collagen stimulation is not only in part because of the soy isoflavones, genistein and daidzein, but other ingredients in soy, such as saponins, may play a larger role.

Topical application of soy has been used to reduce hyperpigmentation, enhance skin elasticity, control oil production, moisturize the skin, and delay hair regrowth. It also has antioxidant properties and the ability to reduce photoaging.

Coffeeberry[7,43]

Polyphenols constitute the active ingredients in coffeeberry, the fruit of the coffee plant (*Coffea arabica*). Its use leads to overall improvement in fine lines, wrinkles, and skin pigmentation. *In vitro* testing showed coffee berry to have the highest antioxidative activity when compared to green tea extract, pomegranate extract, vitamin C, and vitamin E.

Silymarin

A flavonoid antioxidant with silybin, silydianin and silychristine. Has role topically in photosensitive individuals.

Oatmeal[7,44]

Colloidal oatmeal is a natural product derived from oat grains (Avena sativa). This FDA-approved compounds antioxidant constituents are avenanthramides, polyphenols, which reduce proinflammatory cytokines and transcription factors, reduce histamine induced pruritus, and UVB-induced erythema. It cleanses, moisturizes, provides barrier protection and has anti-inflammatory properties.

Lycopenes[7]

Lycopenes are carotenoids and are predominantly found in tomatoes. When applied before UVA exposure, it prevents apoptosis, reduces inflammation, and diminishes expression of enzymes implicated in carcinogenesis. They have an ability to regenerate vitamin E. In an *in vitro* study on human fibroblasts it was shown to have photoprotective properties only in combination with vitamin E.[45]

Chamomile

Chamomile or *Matricaria recutita* is a traditional herb which has been used for centuries with active ingredients including terpenoids, flavonoids, hydroxycoumarins, mono- and oligosaccharides, and mucilages. It has been shown to diminish the signs of photodamage, reduce pruritus, and ameliorate skin texture and elasticity with purported antioxidant activity in chemical assays.[46]

Aloe[47]

Its anti-inflammatory properties and ability to soften the skin, brought about by active ingredients like SA, magnesium lactate, and gel polysaccharides make place for it in loads of skin creams.

Pycnogenol[48]

This is an extract from the French maritime pine bark (*Pinus pinaster*). It has photoprotective, anti-inflammatory, antioxidant, antimicrobial, and anticarcinogenic effects attributed to active ingredients that include proanthocyanidins. It also converts vitamin C radical to its active form and raises levels of glutathione and other free radical scavengers.

Allantoin

It is extracted from the comfrey root. It helps induce cell proliferation.

Tea Tree Oil[49]

Tea tree oil (TTO) is obtained by steam distillation from the Australian native plant *Melaleuca alternifolia*. Terpinen-4-ol is a major TTO component which exhibits strong antimicrobial and anti-inflammatory properties. Tea tree oil also exerts antioxidant activity.

Feverfew[50]

Parthenolide, a sensitizer, free extract of feverfew in a study showed to significantly reduce erythema versus placebo 24 hours post UV exposure. It was shown to possess ability to scavenge free radicals, preserve endogenous antioxidant levels, reduce DNA damage and induce DNA repair enzymes, which can help repair damaged DNA.

Mushroom Extract[51]

It is capable of accelerating the skin turnover rate and repairing dermal molecular components that provide structure and elasticity to the skin.

Marine Algae[52,53]

Based on their pigment formation the marine algae can be divided into: Green algae (Chlorophyta), brown algae (Phaeophyta), and red algae (Rhodophyta). The latter two are primarily used in cosmeceutical products. Marine algae or seaweeds are rich in fiber, ω-3 fatty acids, essential amino acids, and vitamins A, B, C, and E. Bioactive cosmeceutical ingredients in marine algae include: Phlorotannins, sulphated polysaccharides, carotenoid pigments (fucoxanthin, astaxanthin), and fucosterol and tyrosinase inhibitors. The majority of the investigations on the metabolites derived from brown algae have revealed their multipotential benefits including the following in relevance to the skin—antioxidant, anti-inflammatory, antitumor, anti-allergic properties, as well as their role in hyaluronidase enzyme inhibition, and MMPs inhibition activity. They also modulate sebaceous gland activity. Oral fucoxanthin, isolated from *Laminaria japonica*, has been reported to negatively regulate melanogenesis factor at transcriptional level.[54] Fucosterol, a phytosterol in brown algae, elevates the activities of free radical scavenging enzymes such as superoxide dismutase, catalase, and glutathione peroxidase in addition to its antidiabetic and cholesterol reducing properties.[52,55] Phloroglucinol derivatives, a common secondary metabolite constituent of brown algae, possess tyrosinase inhibitory activity due to their ability to chelate copper in this enzyme.[56,57] Apart from cell wall polysaccharides, the different matrix polysaccharides including fucoidan, carrageenan, alginate, and agar have been isolated and identified as texture-improving agents in cosmeceutical products. Marine algae extracts have been employed in the topical delivery systems as marinosomes and photosomes. Marinosomes are liposomes based on a natural marine lipid extract containing high ratio of polyunsaturated fatty acids like, eicosapentaenoic acid and docosahexaenoic acid. Their use in cosmeceuticals is associated with a variety of benefits with respect to prevention and treatment of inflammatory skin disorders.[58] Photosomes are incorporated in sun-care product to protect the sun-exposed skin by releasing a photoreactivating enzyme extracted from a marine plant *Anacystis nidulans*. Photosomes on light activation reverse the cell DNA damage, reducing immune suppression, and cancer induction.[59] Microalgae are unicellular colorful algae, a rich source of bioactive proteins, vitamins, minerals, and carotenoid pigments, zeaxanthin, and their extracts have been used widely in cosmetic preparations.

Melatonin

Melatonin was initially isolated (N1-acetyl-5-methoxytryptamine) from Bovine Pineal and significantly high concentrations are also found in the skin. In skin a melatoninergic antioxdatative system (MAS) has been discovered that regulates skin homeostasis preventing the harmful consequences of UV solar skin damage i.e., skin aging and skin cancer.[60]

Because of its broad antioxidant and radical scavenger properties, melatonin may act as a protective agent against UV-mediated damage in the skin. Clinical studies have indicated that melatonin is able to prevent sun damage only when it is administrated before UV irradiation in relevant concentrations directly at the irradiation site upon UV exposure.[61-64]

Cell Regulators[65,66]

Cell regulators, growth factors and cytokines, which are commonly found in cosmeceutical products are enumerated in table 2 with their actions.

Growth factors are important and guide tissue remodeling in wound healing. On the other hand, their values are reduced in intrinsic and extrinsic aging along with fibroblasts number and activity. So supplementing them would mean reversal of the damage. They can be obtained from cultured human fetal fibroblasts biotechnologically. Growth factors and cytokines found within processed skin-cell proteins from cultured fetal dermal fibroblasts include the nerve growth factor, epidermal growth factor, fibroblast growth factor, macrophage colony stimulating factor, IL-1, 6, 8,10, 12, 13, TGFβ1, PDGF, TIMP-1,2, TNf-α and the like. A study assessing the effect of topical growth factors, on photodamaged skin found that 11 of the 14 study patients showed clinical improvement in at least one facial area. The periorbital region showed a statistically significant improvement in the depth and number of textural irregularities or fine lines. Biopsies revealed new collagen formation in the grenz zone (37% increases in thickness) and thickening of the epidermis by 27%.[68] Other studies have corroborated this effect on aging.[69,70]

Kinetin (N-furfuryladenine growth factor) is a plant growth factor that has shown antiaging effects on skin on topical application. It acts by inhibiting the formation and by scavenging ROS.[9]

It has a synergistic antiaging effect with niacinamide.[71]

Peptides[72,73,74]

Peptides, namely small amino acid sequences, and proteins have an effect on stimulation of collagen production or downregulation of collagenase activity and modulation of cell proliferation, cell migration, inflammation, angiogenesis, and melanogenesis. They are of three types:

1. Signal peptides: Fragments of elastin and collagen activate fibroblasts and stimulate healing, increase collagen formation and improve skin appearance
2. Neurotransmitter affecting peptides: Interfere with neurotransmitter release with resultant decrease in muscle movement
3. Carrier peptides: Deliver trace elements like copper into skin which activates enzymatic pathway of wound healing and enhanced collagen production.

The most stable and widely used signal peptide is lysine-threonine-threonine-lysine-serine (KTTKS) found on type I procollagen.

These molecules penetrate the skin poorly. Linking of KTTKS to palmitic acid (pal-KTTKS) or their application following microneedling to bypass the stratum corneum barrier can enhance penetration.

Investigators in a 12-week, double-blind, placebo-controlled, split-face, randomized clinical study of 93 Caucasian women found that a moisturizer containing pal-KTTKS was well tolerated and significantly reduced fine lines by both qualitative technical and expert grader image analysis.[75]

The tri-peptide GHK (glycyl-L-histidyl-L-lysine) helps deliver copper to the cells by readily complexing with it.[76] Enzymes like superoxide dismutase and lysyl oxidase require copper as a cofactor. It

TABLE 2: Cell regulators in cosmeceutical products[67]

Cell regulator	Subtype	Action
Growth factors	Fibroblast growth factor	Activates fibroblasts, angiogenic, induces collagen synthesis
	Heparin binding-epidermal growth factor	Keratinocyte and fibroblast mitogen
	Hepatocyte growth factor	Tissue regeneration and wound healing
	Insulin-like growth factor	Activates fibroblasts and endothelial cells
	Placenta growth factor	Activates fibroblasts, promotes endothelial growth
	Platelet-derived growth factor	Induces fibroblast migration, fibroblast mitogen, matrix production
	Transforming growth factor-β1	Induces keratinocyte, fibroblast and macrophage migration, and angiogenesis Initiates collagen and fibronectin synthesis; modulates degradation of matrix proteins
	Transforming growth factor-β	Induces keratinocyte, fibroblast, and macrophage migration; initiates collagen and fibronectin synthesis
	Transforming growth factor-β3	Antiscarring
	Vascular endothelial growth factor	Inhibits collagen and hyaluronic acid degradation
Cytokines	Interleukin (IL)-1α and 1-β	Activates growth factor expression in macrophages, keratinocytes, and fibroblasts
	IL-1ra	Anti-inflammatory
	IL-10	Anti-inflammatory
	IL-13	Anti-inflammatory
	Tumor necrosis factor-α	Activates growth factor expression in macrophages, keratinocytes, and fibroblasts

was found that copper-complexed GHK-Cu suppresses inflammation by decreasing the level of transforming growth factor β and TNF-α. Tri-peptide GHK also reduces oxidative damage by modulating iron levels and by quenching toxic products of fatty acid peroxidation. It serves as the chemoattractant for inflammatory and endothelial cells and increases fibroblast proliferation.[77]

Palmitoyl tetrapeptide-7 is able to downregulate IL-6 *in vitro* in both resting and inflamed cells. Many cosmetics include this as an ingredient, with claims of increased skin firmness, smoothness, and elasticity.

Acetyl hexapeptide-3, a neurotransmitter inhibiting peptide, is patterned from the N-terminal end of the protein SNAP-25.

In a randomized placebo-controlled study on 60 Chinese patients by Wang et al. Argireline (a synthetic hexapeptide) showed an anti-wrinkle efficacy of 48.9%, compared with 0% in the placebo group in the subjective analysis. In the objective evaluation, the parameters of roughness were all decreased in the argireline group ($p < 0.01$), while no decrease was obvious in the placebo group ($p > 0.05$).[78] Different peptides used as cosmeceutical ingredients are shown in table 3.

Future Molecules

Ribonucleic Acid[79]

There has been ongoing research into genes controlling aging and how ribonucleic acid interference (RNAi) can benefit the development of antiaging cosmeceuticals. Ribonucleic acid here is used to block or inactivate a target gene. The study of genomics has helped identify potential targets for this approach. Delivery remains a major hurdle for these molecules, oligonucleotides can be injected directly or vectors, like viruses, used. Ribonucleic acids have been employed as small interference RNA and micro RNA as antiaging cosmeceutical ingredients.

Stem Cells[80,81]

Stem cell therapy has spelled a new boom in antiaging therapy. A stem cell is a sort of unprogrammed cell that has the potential to become any type of cell in an

TABLE 3: Peptides used as cosmeceutical ingredients[67]

Antiaging effect	Peptide type	Peptide	Mechanism
Wrinkle and fine line reduction	Signal	Arg-gly-asp-ser	• Increases cell-cell cohesion
		Oligopeptide-20	• Increases collagen I and III, fibronectin, and elastin
		Pal-KTTKS	• Inhibits glycoasaminoglycan formation
		Pal-KT	• Induces differentiation of epidermis, BM zone, and fibroblasts • Increases collagen I, collagen IV, and fibronectin
		Amino acids val-gly-val-ala-pro-gly	• Stimulates fibroblast proliferation
	Carrier and signal	Glycyl-L-histidyl-L-lysine	• Enhances collagen production • Cu complex inhibits TIMP-1 and 2, increases levels of MMP-1 and 2, and increases synthesis of dermatan sulfate and heparin sulfate
	Enzyme inhibiting	Tyr-tyr-arg-ala-asp-asp-ala	• Inhibits procollagen C proteinase
Wrinkle improvement, firming	Signal	AcTP1	• Increases collagen I and lumican synthesis
		AcTP2	• Stimulates keratinocyte growth and syndecan-1 synthesis
		T10-C	• Mimics decorin • Increases collagen fiber uniformity and enhances cohesion
Skin firming	Signal	Peptamide-6	• Increases collagen synthesis • Upregulates growth factors
Skin whitening	Signal	PKEK	• Reduces IL-6, IL-8, tumor necrosis factor-α, melanocyte-stimulating hormone, tyrosinase

ACTP1, acetyl tetrapepide-9; AcTP2, acetyl tetrapepide-11; Pal-KT, palmitoyl-lysine-threonine; Pal-KTTKS, palmitoyl pentapeptide-4; T10-C, tripeptide-10 citrulline.

organ or in the body. The embryonic stem cells are pluripotent, i.e., they can differentiate into any cell type in the body. Whereas, the skin stem cells, which reside in the basal layer of the epidermis only form epidermal cells. With age their numbers dwindle and they are not able to replenish the superficial layers as optimally with daughter cells. This reduced regeneration and proliferation capacity runs in parallel with aging changes in the skin. To replace these cells from outside remains a viable option using embryonic stem cells.

Cell therapy is a novel treatment where genetically engineered cells can be introduced to replace aged cells in the body. They overcome limitations of gene therapy and RNAi.

Stem cells exert a direct cellular and a paracrine effect. They synthesize and secrete a variety of extracellular matrix proteins, cytokines, growth factors, and other bioactive proteins that govern their own functioning and also contribute to the healing process.[82,83,84]

The use of human embryonic stem cells in cosmeceuticals has been shrouded in the controversy of ethical issues.

Adipose derived stem cells surpass the issue by their easy accessibility and ready abundance. Their soluble factors have shown stimulation of both collagen synthesis and migration of dermal fibroblasts with increase in angiogenesis, improving wrinkling and accelerating wound healing in animal models. In addition, there is inhibition of melanogenesis and protection of dermal fibroblasts from oxidative stress induced by chemicals and UVB irradiation.[85] Further research and reviews will ascertain if this beneficial effect is carried on to human skin.

Plant extracts, plant stem cells and plant stem cell extracts, seemingly same, are all different. The first and the last are what have been used in cosmeceutical preparations. The former have been used in cheaper preparations with the downside of lacking standardization, contamination with pesticides and heavy metals, and being ineffective or having non-reproducible results. Plant stem cell extracts on the other hand are obtained from plant stem cells which have been cultured in the lab under standardized conditions after sterilizing the plant part of origin. It does not contain plant stem cells per se but their filtered, homogenized, centrifuged, and lyophilized extracts, which are then incorporated in different formulations. They provide pure, standardized ingredients with dose consistency. Extracts have been prepared and used from grape fruit seeds, lilac leaf, swiss green apple, berries; strawberry, raspberry, blueberries. It has been seen that wild plant extracts have a higher antioxidant action. These stem cells have been shown to protect the skins internal antioxidant system, protecting the human stem cells in the basal layer from free radical induced DNA damage and reversing the effects of photoageing.[86,87] Though there are not many peer reviewed studies on the clinical efficacy of these individual extracts the industry sponsored ones have shown improvement in wrinkle depth and stimulation of skin cell proliferation.[88]

The Klotho Gene[89]

Klotho gene, named after the Greek goddess *Klotho,* was first discovered in mice. It was shown that dysfunction of this gene causes premature aging symptoms and short-life span of the mice.

This gene codes for many things including a transmembrane protein inhibiting phosphorylation of insulin-like growth factor 1.

The transmembrane form of *Klotho* protein functions as a co-receptor for FGF23 and regulates phosphate, calcium, and vitamin D metabolism. The extracellular domain of *Klotho* protein is shed and secreted into the systemic circulation where it functions as an endocrine factor. The secreted *Klotho* protein controls multiple ion channels and growth factor signaling pathways including insulin, IGF-1, and WNT, potentially participating in biology of cancer and stem cells. Identification of the common molecular basis for these multiple functions of *Klotho* will be of particular importance to understand the antiaging properties of *Klotho*.

There have been claims by the cosmetic industry that red snow algae from the Swiss Alps increase the expression of *Klotho gene* in human cells, thus promoting antiaging processes in the cells. However, there are no scientific studies to confirm this.

CONCLUSION

Recent research on the impact of chronic psychological stress on the HPA axis, the autonomic system, and the renin angiotensin system has shown that prolonged activation of these pathways can result in immune dysfunction, oxidative stress, and DNA damage. This opens up a whole new Pandora's box for future research for novel antiaging molecules.

There are new innovative antiaging molecules being added each day but we need to keep in mind, Kligmans question: Are there published, peer-reviewed, double-blind, placebo-controlled, statistically significant, clinical trials to substantiate the efficacy claim of the product?

Well not many, so our choice should be guided by evidence and peer experience before considering them the new elixirs of youth.

For cosmeceuticals clinical efficacy can be guided by the following factors:[72]

- Ability to maintain integrity of the active ingredient
- Ability to deliver it in a biologically active form
- Ability to reach the target site in sufficient quantity to exert an effect
- Ability to release properly from the carrier vehicle
- Ability to exert a biological effect through a known mechanism.

REFERENCES

1. Yaar M, Gilchrest BA. Aging of skin. In: Goldsmith AL, Stephen KI, Barbara GA, et al., editors. Fitzpatrick's dermatology in general medicine. 8th ed. United States: McGraw-Hill; 2012. pp. 1213-20.
2. Wlaschek M, Tantcheva-Poor I, Naderi L, et al. Solar UV irradiation and dermal photoageing. J Photochem Photobiol B. 2001;63(1-3):41-51.
3. Premlatha S, Sarveswari KN. The skin at different ages. In: Valia RG, Valia AR, editors. IADVL textbook of dermatology. 3rd ed. Vol 1. Mumbai: Bhalani Publishing House; 2008. pp. 122-28.
4. Pillai S, Oresaio C, Hayward J. Ultraviolet radiation and skin aging: Roles of reactive oxygen species, inflammation and protease activation, and strategies for prevention of inflammation induced matrix degradation - a review. Int J Cosmet Sci. 2005;27(1):17-34.
5. Sorg O, Antille C, Kaya G, et al. Retinoids in cosmeceuticals. Dermatol Ther. 2006;19(5):289-96.
6. Bhawan J. Short and long term histological effects of topical tretinoin on photodamaged skin. Int J Dermatol. 1998;37(4):286-92.
7. Reszko AE, Berson D, Lupo MP. Cosmeceuticals: Practical applications. Dermatol Clin. 2009;27(3):401-16.
8. Stratigos AJ, Katsambas AD. The role of topical retinoids in the treatment of photoageing. Drugs. 2005;65(8):1061-72.

9. Vedamurthy M. Anti-aging therapies. Indian J Dermat Venerol Leprol. 2006;72:183-6.
10. Babamiri K, Nassab R. Cosmeceuticals: The evidence behind the retinoids. Aesthet Surg J. 2010;30(1):74-7.
11. Kang S, Bergfeld W, Gottlieb AB, et al. Long term efficacy and safety of tretinoin emollient cream 0.05% in the treatment of photodamaged facial skin: A two year, randomized, placebo controlled trial. Am J Clin Dermatol. 2015;6(4):245-53.
12. Lohani A, Verma A, Joshi H, et al. Nanotechnology based cosmeceuticals. ISRN Dermatol. 2014;2014:843687.
13. Shah RA. Cosmeceuticals. In: Savant SS, editor. Textbook of dermatosurgery and cosmetology. 2nd ed. Mumbai: ASCAD; 2005. pp. 519-24.
14. Wang X. A theory for the mechanism of action of the alpha hydroxy acids applied to the skin. Med Hypotheses. 1999;53(5):380-2.
15. Corcuff P, Fiat F, Minondo AM, et al. A comparative ultrastructural study of hydroxy acids induced desquamation. Eur J Dermatol. 2002;12(4):39-43.
16. Grimes PE, Green BA, Wildnauer RH, et al. The use of polyhydroxy acids (PHAs) in photoaged skin. Cutis. 2004;73(2):3-13.
17. Green BA, Yu RJ, Van Scott EJ. Clinical and cosmeceutical uses of hydroxyacids. Clin Dermatol. 2009;27(5):495-501.
18. Sharad J. Polyhydroxy acids. In: Khunger N, Sachdev M, Baumann L, editors. Cosmeceuticals - focus on skin of color 2014. New Delhi: Kontentworx Publishers; 2014.
19. Draelos ZD, Green BA, Edison BL. An evaluation of a polyhydroxy acid skin care regimen in combination with azelaic acid 15% gel in rosacea patients. J Cosmet Dermatol. 2006;5:23-9.
20. Thibodeau A. Metalloproteinase inhibitors. Cosmet Toil. 2000;115:75-6.
21. Kakita LS, Green BA. A review of the physical and chemical properties of alpha-hydroxyacids (AHAs) and polyhydroxy acids (PHAs) and their therapeutic use in pharmacologics. J Am Acad Dermatol. 2006;54: AB107.
22. Hunt MJ, Barnetson RS. A comparative study of gluconolactone versus benzoyl peroxide in the treatment of acne. Australian J Dermatol. 1992;33:131-4.
23. Yu RJ, Van Scott EJ. α-hydroxyacids, polyhydroxy acids, aldobionic acids and their topical actions. In: Baran R, Maibach HI, editors. Textbook of cosmetic dermatology. 3rd ed. New York: Taylor & Francis; 2005. pp. 77-93.
24. Wolfle U, Seelinger G, Bauer G, et al. Reactive molecule species and antioxidative mechanisms in normal skin and skin aging. Skin Pharmacol Physiol. 2014;27(6):316-32.
25. Burke KE. Interaction of vitamins C and E as better cosmeceuticals. Dermatol Ther. 2007;20(5):314-21.
26. Stamford NP. Stability, transdermal penetration, and cutaneous effects of ascorbic acid and its derivatives. J Cosmet Dermatol. 2012;11(4):310-7.
27. Farris PK. Topical vitamin C: A useful agent for treating photoageing and other dermatological conditions. Dermatol Surg. 2005;31(7 pt2):814-7.
28. Humbert PG, Haftek M, Creidi P, et al. Topical ascorbic acid on photoaged skin. Clinical, topographical and ultrastructural evaluation: Double blind study verses placebo. Exp Dermatol. 2003;12(3):237-44.
29. Lin JY, Selim MA, Shea CR, et al. UV photoprotection by combination topical antioxidants vitamin C and E. J Am Acad Dermatol. 2003;48(6):866-74.
30. Murray JC, Burch JA, Streilein RD, et al. A topical antioxidant solution containing vitamins C and E stabilized by ferulic acid provides protection for human skin against damage caused by ultraviolet irradiation. J Am Acad Dermatol. 2008;59(3):418-25.
31. Bissett DL, Oblong JE, Berge CA. Niacinamide: A B vitamin that improves aging facial skin appearance. Dermatol Surg. 2005;31(7 pt. 2):860-5.
32. Tanno O, Ota Y, Kitamura N, et al. Nicotinamide increases biosynthesis of ceramides as well as other stratum corneum lipids to improve the epidermal permeability barrier. Br J Dermatol. 2000;143(3):524-31.
33. Beitner H. Randomized, placebo controlled, double blind study on the clinical efficacy of a cream containing 5% alpha lipoid acid related to photoageing of facial skin. Br J Dermatol. 2003;149(4):841-9.
34. Mc Daniel DH, Neudecker BA, DiNardo JC, et al. Idebenone: A new antioxidant-part I. Relative assessment of oxidative stress protection capacity compared to commonly known antioxidants. J Cosmet Dermatol. 2005;4(1):10-7.
35. Stallings AF, Lupo MP. Practical uses of botanicals in skin care. J Clin Aesthet Dermatol. 2009;2(1):36-40.
36. Alam M, et al. Cosmetic dermatology. Elsevier Saunders; 2009. pp. 13-6.
37. Draelos ZD. Cosmeceuticals. Elsevier Saunders; 2009. pp. 129-35.
38. Baumann L. Cosmetic dermatology. 2nd ed. McGraw Hill; 2009. pp. 292-305.
39. Datta HS, Mitra SK, Paramesh R, et al. Theories and management of aging: Modern and ayurveda perspectives. Evid Based Complement Alt Med. 2011;2011:528527.
40. Elmets CA, Singh D, Tubesing K, et al. Cutaneous photoprotection from ultraviolet injury by green tea polyphenols. J Am Acad Dermatol. 2001;44(3):425-32.
41. Chiu AE, Chan JL, Kern DG, et al. Double blinded, placebo controlled trial of green tea extracts in the clinical and histologic appearance of photoageing skin. Dermatol Surg. 2005;31(7 pt2):855-60.
42. Cornacchione S, Sadick NS, Neveu M, et al. In vivo skin antioxidant effect of a new combination based on a specific vitis vinifera shoot extract and a biotechnological extract. J Drugs Dermatol. 2007;6(6 suppl.):s8-13.
43. Farris P. Idebenone, green tea, and coffee berry extract: new and innovative antioxidants. Dermatol Ther. 2007;20(5):322-9.
44. Kurtz ES, Wallo W. Colloidal oatmeal: History chemistry and chemical properties. J Drugs Dermatol. 2007;6(2):167-70.
45. Andreassi M, Stanghellini E, Ettorre A, et al. Antioxidant activity of topically applied lycopene. J Eur Acad Dermatol Venereol. 2004;18(1):52-5.

46. Lee KG, Shibamoto T. Determination of antioxidantpotential of volatile extracts from various herbs and spices. J Agric Food Chem. 2002;50(17):4947-52.
47. Choi S, Lee SK, Kim JE, et al. Aloesin inhibits hyperpigmentation induced by UV radiation. Clin Exp Dermatol. 2002;27(6):513-5.
48. Rohdewald P. A review of the French maritime pinebark extract (Pycnogenol), a herbal medication with diverse clinical pharmacology. Int J Clin Pharmacol Ther. 2002;40(4):158-68.
49. Pazyar N, Yaghoobi R, Bagherani N, et al. A review of applications of tea tree oil in dermatology. Int J Dermatol. 2013;52(7):784-90.
50. Bowe WP. Cosmetic benefits of natural ingredients: mushrooms, feverfew, tea, and wheat complex. J Drugs Dermatol. 2013;12(9 Suppl.):s133-6.
51. Thomas NV, Kim SK. Beneficial effects of marine algal compounds in cosmeceuticals. Mr Drugs. 2013;11:146-64.
52. Kim SK. Marine cosmeceuticals. J Cos Dermatol. 2014;13:56-67.
53. Fitton JH, Irhimeh M, Falk N. Macroalgalfucoidan extracts: A new opportunity for marine cosmetics. Cosmet Toiletries. 2007;122:55-64.
54. Shimoda H, Tanaka J, Shan SJ, et al. Anti-pigmentary activity of fucoxanthin and its influence on skin mRNA expression of melanogenic molecules. J Pharm Pharmacol Res. 2010;62:1137-45.
55. Cabello-Pasini A, Victoria-Cota N, Macias-Carranza V, et al. Clarification of wines using polysaccharides extracted from seaweeds. Am J Enol Vitic. 2005;56:52-9.
56. Kang HS, Kim HR, Byun DS, et al. Tyrosinase inhibitors isolated from the edible brown alga Ecklonia stolonifera. Arch Pharm Res. 2004;27:1226-32.
57. Cha SH, Ko SC, Kim D, et al. Screening of marine algae for potential tyrosinase inhibitor: Those inhibitors reduced tyrosinase activity and melanin synthesis in zebrafish. J Dermatol. 2011;38:354-63.
58. Moussaoui N, Cansell M, Denizot A. Marinosomes marine lipid-based liposomes: Physical characterization and potential applications in cosmetics. Int J Pharm. 2002;242:361-5.
59. Patravale VB, Mandawgade SD. Novel cosmetic delivery systems: An application update. Int J Cosmetic Sci. 2008;30:19-33.
60. Kleszczynski K, Fischer TW. Melatonin and human skin aging. Dermatoendocrinol. 2012;4(3):245-52.
61. Bangha E, Elsner P, Kistler GS. Suppression of UV-induced erythema by topical treatment with melatonin (N-aceryl-5-merhoxytrypramine). A dose response study. Arch Dermatol Res. 1996;288:522-6.
62. Dreher F, Gabard B, Schwindt DA, et al. Topical melatonin in combination with vitamins E and C protects skin from ultraviolet-induced eryrhema: A human study in vivo. Br J Derrnatol. 1998;139:332-9.
63. Lee KS, Lee WS, Suh SI, et al, Melatonin reduces ultraviolet-B induced cell damages and polyamine levels in human skin fibroblasts in culture. Exp Mol Med. 2003;35:263-8.
64. Ryoo YW, Suh SI, Mun KC, et al. The effects of the melatonin on ultraviolet-B irradiated cultured dermal fibroblasts. J Dermarcl Sci. 2001;27:162-9.
65. Fitzpatrick RE. Endogenous growth factors as cosmeceuticals. Dermatol Surg. 2005;31(7 pt. 2):827-31.
66. Sundaram H, Mehta RC, Norine JA, et al. Topically applied physiologically balanced growth factors: A new paradigm of skin rejuvenation. J Drugs Dermatol. 2009;8(5 Suppl Skin Rejuvenation):4-13.
67. Malerich S, Berson D. Next generation cosmeceuticals: The latest in peptides, growth factors, cytokines and stem cells. Dermatol Clin. 2014;32(1):13-21.
68. Fitzpatrick RE, Rostan EF. Reversal of photodamage with topical growth factors: A pilot study. J Cosmet Laser Ther. 2003;5(1):25-34.
69. Lupo ML, Cohen JL, Rendon MI. Novel eye cream containing a mixture of human growth factors and cytokines for periorbital skin rejuvenation. J Drugs Dermatol. 2007;6(7):725-9.
70. Hussain M, Phelps R, Goldberg DJ. Clinical, histologic, and ultrastructural changes after use of human growth factor and cytokine skin cream for the treatment of skin rejuvenation. J Cosmet Laser Ther. 2008;10(2):104-9.
71. Chiu PC, Chan CC, Lin HM, et al. The clinical anti-aging effects of topical kinetin and niacinamide in Asians: A randomized double bind, placebo-controlled, split face comparative trial. J Cosmet Dermatol. 2007;6(4):243-9.
72. Lupo MP. Cosmeceutical peptides. Dermatol Surg. 2005;31(7):832-6.
73. Fields K, Falla TJ, Rodan K, et al. Bioactive peptides: signaling the future. J Cosmet Dermatol. 2009;8(1):8-13.
74. Zhang L, Falla TJ. Cosmeceuticals and peptides. Clin Dermatol. 2009;27(5):485-94.
75. Robinson LR, Fitzgerald NC, Doughty DG, et al. Topical palmitoyl pentapeptide provides improvement in photoaged human facial skin. Int J Cosmet Sci. 2005:27;155-60.
76. Pickart L, Freedman JH, Loker WJ, et al. Growth modulating plasma tripeptide may function by facilitating copper uptake into the cells. Nature. 1980;288(5792):715-7.
77. Gruchlik A, Jurzak M, Chodurek E, et al. Effect of Gly-Gly-His, Gly-His-Lys and their copper complexes on TNF-alpha-dependent IL-6 secretion in normal human dermal fibroblasts. Acta Pol Pharm. 2012;69(6):1303-6.
78. Wang Y, Wang M, Xiao S, et al. The anti-wrinkle efficacy of argireline, a synthetic hexapeptide, in Chinese subjects: a randomized, placebo controlled study. Am J Clin Dermatol. 2013;14(2):147-53.
79. Zhang P, Chen J, Li T, et al. Use of small RNA as anti-aging cosmeceuticals. J Cosmet Sci. 2013;64(6):455-68.
80. Draelos ZD. Plant stem cells and skin care. Cosmet Dermatol. 2012;25(9):395-96.
81. Zacharias DG, Nelson TJ, Mueller PS, et al. The science and ethics of induced pluripotency: What will become of embryonic stem cells? Mayo Clinic Proc. 2011;86(7):634-40.
82. Cha J, Falanga V. Stem cells in cutaneous wound healing. Clin Dermatol. 2007;25:73-8.

83. Lee MJ, Kim J, Lee KI, et al. Enhancement of wound healing by secretory factors of endothelial precursor cells derived from human embryonic stem cells. Cytotherapy. 2011;13(2):165-78.
84. Wu Y, Wang J, Scott PG, et al. Bone marrow-derived stem cells in wound healing: A review. Wound Repair Regen. 2007;15(Suppl 1):S18-S26.
85. Kim JH, Jung M, Kim HS, et al. Adipose derived stem cells as a new therapeutic modality for aging skin. Exp Dermatol. 2011;20(5):383-7.
86. Mantena SK, Katiyar SK. Grape seed proanthocyanidins inhibit UV-radiation-induced oxidative stress and activation of MAPK and NF-κB signaling in human epidermal keratinocytes. Free Radic Biol Med. 2006;40(9):1603-14.
87. Zhao J, Wang J, Chen Y, et al. Anti-tumor- promoting activity of a polyphenolic fraction isolated from grape seeds in the mouse skin two-stage initiation-promotion protocol and identification of procyanidin B5-3′- gallate as the most effective antioxidant constituent. Carcinogenesis. 1999;20(9):1737-45.
88. Schmid D, Schürch P, Blum P, et al. Plant stem cell extract for longevity of skin and hair. SOFW J. 2008;134(5):30-35.
89. Kuro-o M. Klotho and aging. Biochimica et biophysica Acta. 2009;1790(10):1049-58.

6
CHAPTER

Lip Care and Cosmetics

Zoe D Draelos

INTRODUCTION

From historical inceptions, lips remain a prominent part of the face distinguishing youth from maturity and male from female. They are necessary for speaking, eating, and kissing representing a major portal for the entry of disease into the body. Anatomically, the lips consist of transitional epithelium between skin and oral mucosa. Lips remain the primary site of dermatologic disease from cheilitis to leukokeratosis oris to actinic cheilitis to leukoplakia to squamous cell carcinoma. Lips are common female adornment site as well. This chapter examines lip care and lip cosmetics for the dermatologist.

HISTORY

The image of female beauty includes well-structured, symmetrical lips. While the lip area is naturally rich in pheomelanin with a rich vascular supply, both imparting a redness hue, cosmetic adornment to highlight the lips can be traced to antiquity with persistence into modern culture. Lip cosmetics have been identified as early as 7,000 BC with the Sumerians praising the lips of both the sexes in the royal lineage. This adornment has been passed on from centuries, from Egyptians to Babylonians to Romans to present day people. In those times, hybrid saffron or brazilwood was used to stain the lips a red color.

Modern lipstick was not introduced until 1920 when beeswax, tallow, and pigment were combined to make a red tube that could be stroked over the lips. What truly revolutionized lipstick was the invention of the push up holder still used today for easy storage and application of the lipstick either in private or public. Females of all ages find lip cosmetics an indispensable part of facial adornment.

BASIC ANATOMY

The anatomy of the lips is presented in figure 1. The upper lip is typically smaller than the lower lip and well-proportioned lips begin at one end and end at the other end of the pupil. The dip in the central upper lip is known as the philtrum and the reddish part of the lip between the keratinized skin and oral mucosa is termed as the vermilion.

As lips age, they thin out and loose their classical shape because of subcutaneous fat loss, which simultaneously occurs over the entire face.[1] It is the fat that gives the lips their plump angelica look in children, a child reveals lips that protrude from the face as compared. A 70-year-old woman shows flat and depressed lips. This flattened lip profile further goes downhill cosmetically with loss of teeth and bony gum structures, giving it to the classical Cupid's bow shape. The lip muscles remain same throughout life but the loss of subcutaneous fat from the lips cannot be recovered.

Some of the beauty of the lips can be restored through the use of lip moisturizers, known as lip balm and lip gloss. The size of the lips can be cosmetically

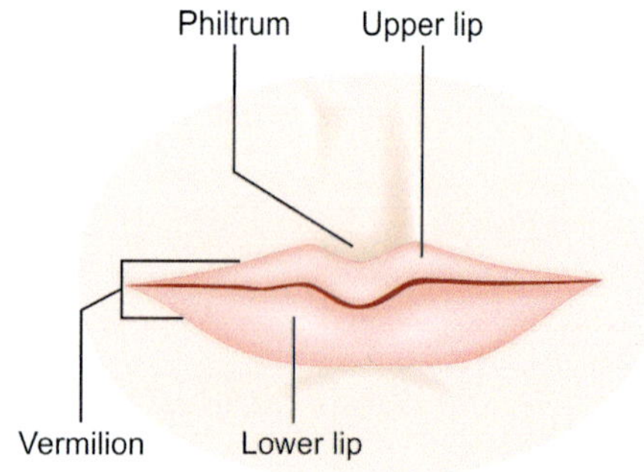

FIG. 1: Lip anatomy.

improved through the use of lip cosmetics and the structure of the lip can be restored through the use of injectable fillers. The remainder of this chapter will focus on lip beautification through topical and injectable product use.

LIP CARE

The transitional skin that forms the lips possesses a precarious barrier that is easily compromised. The lips possess modified sebaceous glands, but caustic food and repeated wetting followed by drying can damage the lips creating the need for moisturizers. Lip moisturizers are commonly known as balms due to the high wax content required for the product to stay on the lips, a quality labeled substantivity. If the moisturizing qualities of a lip balm are combined with the aesthetic properties of a colored cosmetic, the product is known as a lipstick. The discussion now turns to the formulation and use of lip balms, squeeze tube lip moisturizers, and lip glosses.[2]

Lip Balms

Lip moisturizers, sometimes known as lip balms, are commonly used for the treatment of chapped lips. These transparent products form a film over the lips which act as an occlusive moisturizer and prevent loss of water from the transitional mucosa. Transepidermal water loss from the lips is higher than keratinized skin requiring an intact barrier to lower water loss and maintain the lips disease free. Lip balms usually are a mixture of oil, dimethicone, and wax, in varying proportions. Higher wax containing formulations are stiffer and can be formed into a round cylinder that is rubbed over the lips to apply the product. The wax cylinder is encased in a plastic roll-up tube that pushes the wax column up as the product is used. The waxes commonly employed are the natural carnauba and candela waxes sometimes combined with synthetic waxes. Stiffer products with higher wax content leave a thicker film on the lips while the lower wax content products leave a thinner film. The type of film desired depends on the aesthetic requirements of the patient and the amount of lip dryness present.

Some of the newer lip balms incorporate dimethicone, which is silicone based. Dimethicone is listed on the skin protectant monograph in the United States (US) allowing lip balms containing this ingredient to be listed as over-the-counter (OTC) drugs. These products contain a product labeling that lists an active ingredient, which is silicone, in combination with the other waxes and oils in traditional lip balm formulations. Dimethicone is popular in lip balms because it allows more robust marketing claims and better aesthetics by cutting down on the waxy stiff feel of some older lip balm formulations.

Lip balms can provide other benefits to the lips besides decreasing water loss. Organic sunscreens, listed in the sunscreen monograph in the US, may also be incorporated allowing the lip balm to provide photoprotection. Most lip balms constitute a sun protection factor (SPF) between 15–30, because a higher concentration of organic filters gives the product an unpalatable bitter taste consumers will not tolerate. Nevertheless, lip balms containing sunscreen filters provide photoprotection in actinic cheilitis, leukoplakia, or lip cancer; but contact allergy can occur.[3,4] There is some concern regarding the safety of ingesting organic sunscreen filters, so consumers should minimize the use of these products when the lip is not applied during the day. For example, an excellent time to allow the vermilion to repair is at night when the lips are at rest from speaking and eating. Nighttime lip balm applications should not contain sunscreen to minimize exposure.

One of the consumer concerns aired regarding frequent consistent lip balm use is their theorized addictive potential. Some claim addiction to lip balm and feel the urge to reapply it at all times. While this area remains controversial, some investigations done in this area revealed that patients were addicted to the waxy feel of the lip balm on the lips and not the lip balm per se, pointing to a more sensory than a functional addiction. The lip balm created a warm moist feel initially after application, which disappeared as the product got removed during speaking and eating. This necessitated the frequent reapplication to maintain the same aesthetic feel of the product.

Squeeze Tube Lip Moisturizers

A new variation on lip balms packaged in a roll-up tube is a lip moisturizer packaged in a squeeze tube with a slatted tip and a small dispensing orifice (Fig. 2). These squeeze tube lip moisturizers do not contain the higher concentration of waxes found in lip balms, instead they are based on petrolatum. A thin petrolatum film is rubbed over the lips after a small amount is dispensed from the orifice onto the slanted applicator. This formulation may also contain dimethicone, in which case it also is classified as an OTC drug. The dimethicone minimizes the sticky feel of the petrolatum and many consumers find this beneficial.

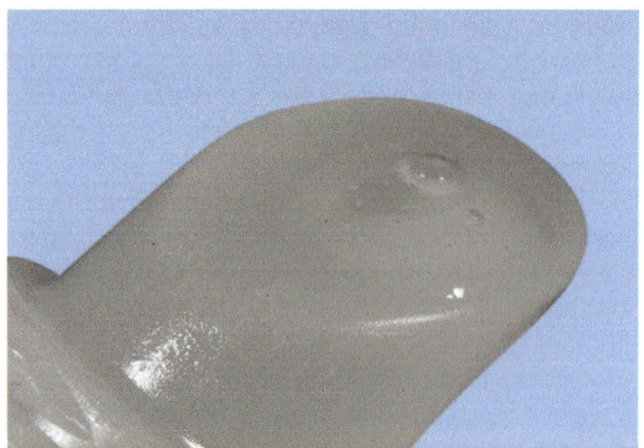

FIG. 2: This angled tip plastic applicator has a small orifice for the application of lip moisturizer products.

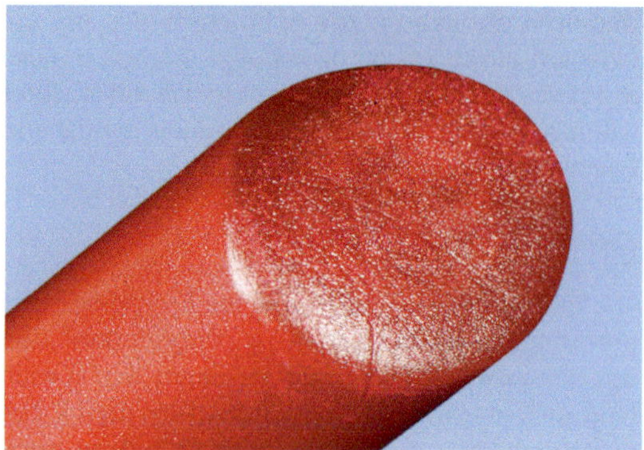

FIG. 3: Pigmented lipsticks can be used for both adornment and camouflage.

Lip Glosses

Another entity in the lineage is the lip gloss, which differs from lip balm as it does not contain waxes, but only oils and dimethicone. Lip gloss is chosen by adolescent age group as a first cosmetic as it adds shine, smell, and taste to the lips, but lacks moisturization. It migrates off rapidly, making it less preferable for adults plus some oils used in the gloss may be comedogenic. Lip gloss has bounced back as film forming polymer of lipsticks, leading us to the next topic of lip cosmetics.

LIP COSMETICS

The previously discussed lip products have focused on lip moisturization, but the adornment of the lips with color and texture is also a popular fashion statement. Lip cosmetics include lipsticks, lip stains, and polymer lipsticks.

Lipstick Structurization

It is an elongated tube shape rod of color, mixed in a blend of oils, waxes and fats, packaged, and presented in a roll-up tube (Fig. 3). Ratio of oils and waxes varies in the final product. Numerous varieties are there, like, lipstick designed to hide lip imperfections must be long wearing. Waxes used are to make the lip color stay on the lip. Waxes used in lipstick formulations are white beeswax, candelilla wax, carnauba wax, ozokerite wax, lanolin wax, ceresin wax, and other synthetic waxes. Lipsticks have a combination of abovementioned waxes, which are blend to get the desired melting point followed by addition of oils to soften the wax and enhance shining of lips. Oils which are used include castor oil, white mineral oil, lanolin oil, hydrogenated vegetable oils, or oleyl alcohol. These also help in pigment dispersion.

A variety of coloring agents are used with oils and waxes. In the recent times, the safety of these coloring agents is being questioned after a group of consumer safety and people announced the possibility of high lead levels in lipsticks. Hence, US Food and Drug Administration (FDA) approved colors that should be used in lipsticks. The US FDA has done division of coloring agents into three groups: (1) Food, drug, and cosmetic (fd and c), colors, (2) drug and cosmetic (d and c) colors, and (3) external drug and cosmetic colors. With only the earlier two permitted for usage in lipsticks and the latter is restricted for use in locations where they are not likely to enter the mouth.

Lip Stains

A special type of lipstick is a lip stain, which is the basis for the long wearing lipsticks. These products contain ineffaceable or indelible color agents including bromo acids, such as fluoresceins, halogenated fluoresceins, and related water-insoluble dyes. The most commonly used one is acid eosin, which happens to be a tetrabromo derivative of fluorescein. Acid eosin, also known as bromo acid or d and c red number 21, is naturally colored orange, but changes to a red salt at a pH of 4, which changes the orange lipstick to a vivid long-lasting indelible red stain, accounting for red color of all long-lasting lipsticks.

The major issue with these long wearing lipsticks is desiccation of lips and precipitation of cheilitis. For the same reason, these lipsticks should be used in combination with lip moisturizing products previously discussed.

Polymer Film Lipsticks

Another way to keep the color stay for long on the lips is creating polymer films; they are the newest addition to lipstick market. They are packaged in a bi-way fashion where one end holds he lip color and the other end contains a lip gloss or balm. The application is done in the same order as well, pigmented polymer first followed by lip gloss or balm and these products stay on until peeled off or rubbed off.

These are excellent for use for people desiring lip product for camouflage reasons as they form an opaque film, covering pigmentation or vascular abnormalities of the lip. Another layer of camouflage can be added by putting a creamy opaque lipstick on top for moisturization and shine.

Lip Liners

Lip liners are thin pigmented rods encased in wood or placed in an automatic pencil-type holder. The articulation remains same as lipsticks, except the fact that stiffer waxes with higher melting points are used with minimal oil creating an extremely hard rod that applies a thick layer of pigment to the lips. Lip liners define the outer edge of lips and valuable in reconstruction of a normal lip contour. The thick wax layer prevents creamier lip products from bleeding.[5] The lip liner shade is one or two shades darker than the lipstick.

Lip liners are irreplaceable in people who need lip definition or lip enhancement. They are also used to carve out temporary lines for lip filler injections. However, they also act as allergic contact dermatitis agents.[6]

Opaque Lipsticks

Opaque lip cosmetics are used on polymer lip products so as to prevent inevitable lip dryness.[7] They are also agents of camouflage for patients requiring the same. The opaqueness is credited to the incorporation of high levels of titanium dioxide in the lipstick, which provides excellent coverage. It is formulated as a fine powder so as to enable smoother application. It also adds color brightness to lip cosmetics so that it can be used to create pastel shades. Opaque lipsticks offer a superlative degree of lip protection for people with actinic cheilitis. They wholesomely protect the lip's transitional mucosa postcryosurgery or lip advancement for reconstruction following lip cancer surgery.

LIP COSMETICS AND ALLERGIC CONTACT DERMATITIS

Application of lipstick can sometimes cause allergic contact dermatitis.[8] The lipstick ingredients reported to cause allergic contact dermatitis include: Ricinoleic acid,[9] benzoic acid,[10] Lithol Rubin BCA (pigment red 57-1),[11] microcrystalline wax,[12] oxybenzone,[13] propyl gallate,[14] and C18 aliphatic compounds.[15]

Castor oil is the most common cause of allergic contact dermatitis which is almost found in all lipsticks. It is used to dissolve bromo acid dyes,[16-18] however the bromo acid dye eosin (d and c red number 21), is also a cause of allergic contact dermatitis.[19] Castor oil allergy is the cause of allergic contact dermatitis in patients having allergy to many different types and brands of lipstick.[20] The best alternative is one of the polymer lipsticks as these products do not contain castor oil.

LIP PLUMPERS

Full and well-defined lips impart a sense of youth, health, and attractiveness hence women fascinate to have plumper more luscious looking fuller lips. Lip plumpers first appeared in the market in 2000 and they have become increasingly popular in the last few years.

Lip plumpers are cosmetic agents aimed to create the appearance of increased lip volume. It is usually available in the form of a cream or regular lip gloss. Lip plumpers are also available in different colors so it can be used as lipstick.

Lip plumper generally contains hyaluronic acid, collagen microparticles of the marine sponge, emollients, tripeptide palmitoyl-glycyl-L-histidyl-L-lysine (Pal-GHK) complex, niacin, essential fatty acids, essential oils of cinnamon, cayenne pepper (*Capsicum frutescens*), ginger, menthol, etc.

The mechanisms by which lip plumpers act are varied, and include skin hydration by which there is appearance of increased lip volume. Hyaluronic acid is a glycosaminoglycan, and has ability to retain water molecules thereby providing moisturizing and plumping effect. Collagen, a high-molecular weight humectant, holds water in the stratum corneum and increases the degree of skin humidity.[21] Collagen microparticles of the marine sponge are commonly found in lip plumpers. Moreover, the GHK tripeptide is found to enhance the expression of extracellular matrix macromolecules, such as collagen and glycosaminoglycans.[22] This tripeptide has been introduced recently into skin care products, including lip plumpers. The other mechanism is vasodilation secondary to either irritant contact dermatitis or nonimmunologic contact urticaria by ingredients such as essential oils of cinnamon, cayenne pepper, ginger, menthol, etc. that are classified as both irritants and urticariants.[23,24] In irritant dermatitis, vasodilation occurs after nociceptors trigger the release of substance P.[25] In nonimmunologic contact urticaria, vasodilation most likely occurs secondary to prostaglandin metabolism.[26,27] Lip plumpers may also achieve vasodilation through compounds that have direct vasodilatory effects, such as niacin or vitamin B3, and L-arginine, an amino acid that is converted to nitric oxide, a potent vasodilator.[28]

Lip plumpers generally pose no threat to the lips and have been used by women to plump up their lips. Lip plumpers usually have a stingy sensation. It might cause severe burning sensations and redness if there is allergy to certain ingredients present in the plumpers.

CONCLUSION

Lipsticks are useful for cosmetic adornment, but can also be used by the dermatologist to facilitate the healing of a variety of lip conditions. For example, actinic cheilitis can be minimized by using a sunscreen-containing lip balm or an opaque lipstick. Remember that an opaque lipstick has an unlimited SPF, since the transitional lip mucosa is completely protected. Lip abnormalities can be minimized by selecting a polymer lip product combined with a lip liner. Finally, patients who experience problems with lip swelling following the use of lipsticks may be allergic to castor oil. Lipsticks and lip balms are to the lips what hand cream is to the hands. Both are important therapeutic adjuvants in the treatment of dermatologic disease.

REFERENCES

1. Lévêque JL, Goubanova E. Influence of age on the lips and perioral skin. Dermatology. 2004;208(4):307-13.
2. Engasser PG. Lip cosmetics. Dermatol Clin. 2000;18(4): 641-9.
3. Schram SE, Glesne LA, Warshaw EM. Allergic contact cheilitis from benzophenone-3 in lip balm and fragrance/flavorings. Dermatitis. 2007;18(4):221-4.
4. Wilson AG, White IR, Kirby JD. Allergic contact dermatitis from propyl gallate in a lip balm. Contact Dermatitis. 1989;20(2):145-6.
5. Ryu JS, Park SG, Kwak TJ, et al. Improving lip wrinkles: lipstick-related image analysis. Skin Res Technol. 2005; 11(3):157-64.
6. Angelini E, Marinaro C, Carrozzo AM, et al. Allergic contact dermatitis of the lip margins from para-tertiary-butylphenol in a lip liner. Contact Dermatitis. 1993;28(3):146-8.
7. Schena D, Fantuzzi F, Girolomoni G. Contact allergy in chronic eczematous lip dermatitis. Eur J Dermatol. 2008;18(6):688-92.
8. Zug KA, Kornik R, Belsito DV, et al. Patch-testing North American lip dermatitis patients: data from the North American Contact Dermatitis Group, 2001 to 2004. Dermatitis. 2008;19(4):202-8.
9. Sai S. Lipstick dermatitis caused by ricinoleic acid. Contact Dermatitis. 1983;9(6):524.
10. Calnan CD. Amyldimethylamino benzoic acid causing lipstick dermatitis. Contact Dermatitis. 1980;6(3):233.
11. Hayakawa R, Fujimoto Y, Kaniwa M. Allergic pigmented lip dermatitis from lithol rubine BCA. Am J Contact Dermatitis. 1994;5:34-7.
12. de Darko E, Osmundsen PE. Allergic contact dermatitis to Lipcare lipstick. Contact Dermatitis. 1984;11(1):46.
13. Aguirre A, Izu R, Gardeazabal J, et al. Allergic contact cheilitis from a lipstick containing oxybenzone. Contact Dermatitis. 1992;27(4):267-8.
14. Cronin E. Lipstick dermatitis due to propyl gallate. Contact Dermatitis. 1980;6(3):213-4.
15. Hayakawa R, Matsunaga K, Suzuki M, et al. Lipstick dermatitis due to C18 aliphatic compounds. Contact Dermatitis. 1987;16(4):215-9.
16. Sai S. Lipstick dermatitis caused by castor oil. Contact Dermatitis. 1983;9(1):75.
17. Brandle I, Boujnah-Khouadja A, Foussereau J. Allergy to castor oil. Contact Dermatitis. 1983;9:424-5.
18. Andersen KE, Nielsen R. Lipstick dermatitis related to castor oil. Contact Dermatitis. 1984;11(4):253-4.
19. Calnan CD. Allergic sensitivity to eosin. Acta Allergol. 1959;13:493-9.
20. le Coz CJ, Ball C. Recurrent allergic contact dermatitis and cheilitis due to castor oil. Contact Dermatitis. 2000;42(2):114-5.
21. Swatschek D, Schatton W, Kellermann J, et al. Marine sponge collagen: isolation, characterization and effects on the skin parameters surface-pH, moisture and sebum. Eur J Pharm Biopharm. 2002;53(1):107-13.
22. Maquart FX, Bellon G, Chaqour B, et al. In vivo stimulation of connective tissue accumulation by the tripeptide-copper complex glycyl-L-histidyl-L-lysine-Cu2+ in rat experimental wounds. J Clin Invest. 1993;92(5):2368-76.
23. Brancaccio RR, Alvarez MS. Contact allergy to food. Dermatol Ther. 2004;17(4):302-13.
24. Cleenewerck MB, Martin P. Food. In: Chew AL, Maibach HI (Eds). Irritant Dermatitis. New York: Springer; 2006. pp. 285-316.
25. Kydonieus AF, Willie JJ. Biochemical Modulation of Skin Reactions: Transdermals, Topicals, Cosmetics. New York: CRC press; 2000.
26. Morrow JD, Minton TA, Awad JA, et al. Release of markedly increased quantities of prostaglandin D2 from the skin in vivo in humans following the application of sorbic acid. Arch Dermatol. 1994;130(11):1408-12.
27. Bashir SJ, Maibach HI. Contact urticaria syndrome. In: Chew AL, Maibach HI (Eds). Irritant Dermatitis. New York: Springer; 2006. pp. 63-70.
28. Lundberg JO, Weitzberg E, Gladwin MT. The nitrate-nitrite-nitric oxide pathway in physiology and therapeutics. Nat Rev Drug Discov. 2008;7(2):156-67.

7
CHAPTER

Salon Nail Procedures and Associated Dermatoses

Jaishree Sharad, Neha Sud

INTRODUCTION

Well-groomed nails have come of age. The use of nail color in Chinese and Indian civilizations, thousands of years back, may have inspired the nail lacquer market in the 1930s when starlets and stars started flaunting bright nail lacquer. But it has evolved over the years with product innovations like quick dry lacquers, soak off gels, and others. The present day nail care too has extended much beyond the original French manicure to artificial nail extensions, shellacs, embellishments, nail tattoos, three dimensional texture finishes and much more lies in the pipeline.[1]

NAIL STRUCTURE (FIG. 1)

The nail plate is dead hardened keratin. Any changes on the plate as a result of disease or manipulation will remain till the plate is shed or cut. Also the tissue surrounding the nail is vulnerable to any products applied to the nail for adornment because of their close proximity to the plate. The cuticle and hyponychium are the sentries of the nail. Damage to them may result in the entry of infection from the dorsal nail plate to the proximal nail fold or nail matrix and the nail bed, respectively. These will be discussed under the relevant parts.

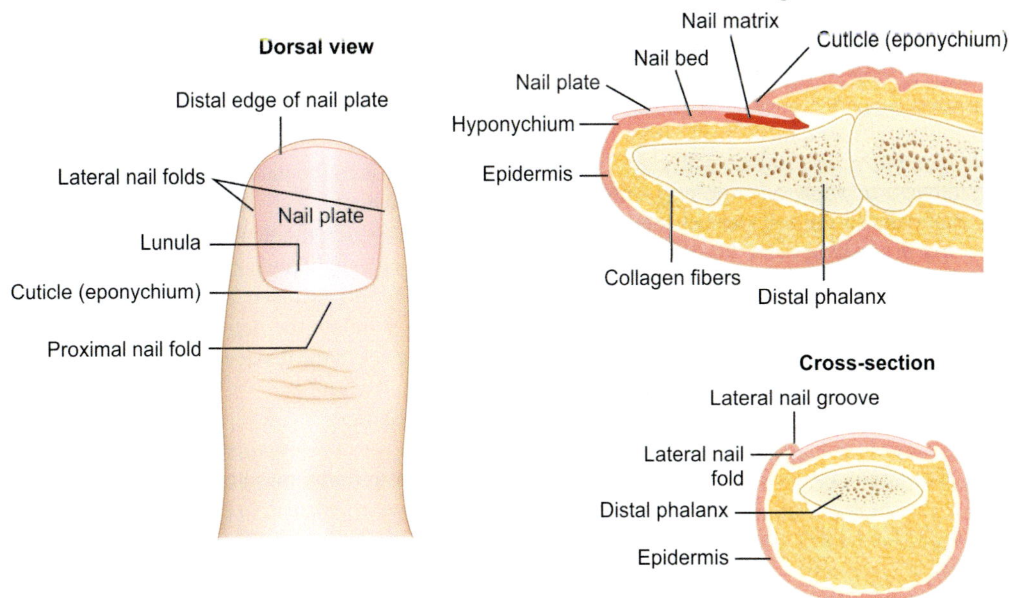

FIG. 1: Nail structure.

SALON PROCEDURES

Manicure or Pedicure

Manicure, the basic essential in nail salons, is the professional grooming of the nails of the hand. Analogous to manicure, pedicure is the term used for toenails. The various steps for both the sites remain the same, though on the feet it also encompasses the trimming and pairing of calluses and corns if any.

Basic Steps Followed

1. *Soaking and cleaning:* This process helps to remove the nail and skin surface of any dirt and grime, and, debris from under the nail plate. The skin absorbs in moisture and becomes soft, so do the nail plates. This makes cutting the nail plate or filing it easy, reducing the chances of nail plate splitting and onychoschizia.
2. *Trimming and shaping the nails:* If possible it is better to only file the nails and not cut them. In either case the direction should be maintained perpendicular to the nail plate. In addition filing should be done in one direction only. These tips help circumvent any damage to the nail plate. Nail shape trends change with each passing season. They are best cut with a minimal curve at the free margin. Manipulating the medial and lateral edge at the free margin should be avoided to reduce the chances of ingrown nails, toenails especially. They should be kept flat. Pointy nails, or nails with an acute arc extending beyond the finger tips are more prone to trauma with resultant chipping and onycholysis.
3. *Cuticle curing:* This is one step that should be skipped in nail grooming if possible. Cutting or pushing the cuticle back from its distal attachment on the dorsal nail plate helps the manicurist to apply an even and smooth layer of nail paint in the last step. But this process of cutting or pushing back the cuticle, by a cutter or an orange stick or metallic cuticle pusher, can open up the proximal nail fold and the nail matrix underneath to bacterial, fungal and viral pathogens. This can lead to acute paronychia and repeated infections eventually to chronic paronychia, beau's lines, injury to the proximal nail fold and onychodystrophy. Even the keratolytic chemical cuticle removers can irritate the nail fold and initiate paronychia.[2] Common chemicals used are 2-5% sodium or potassium hydroxide, tri/tetra sodium phosphate and quaternary ammonium compounds with urea. They work by breaking the disulphide bonds of cystine and therefore soften keratin.[3] They have a tendency of softening the nail plates in addition.
4. *Filing the nail plate surface:* This step helps in the better adhesion of the enamel to the nail plate. Excessive filing can lead to thinning of the nail plate and should be avoided. It has been shown that filing as much as just 5% of the surface maybe enough for this purpose. The surface of the nail plate can be also buffed with creams containing abrasives and waxes to give smoothness and shine to the nail plate, respectively. But either ways it thins the plate and weakens the bed. Hence, electric files or abraders with less than 180 grit and removing more than 5% of the cell layers should be avoided.[4] Alternately a coat of primer can provide the needed adhesion between the plate and the overlay material.
5. *Massage:* As a part of the manicure/pedicure, the forearms and hands and the lower legs and feet are also massaged.
6. *Application of nail polish:* This is the last step. Modern day nail polish was formulated in 1920 by the Charles Revson Company, which today is known as Revlon.[5] In the present day constituents of an enamel vary from brand to brand. The basic ingredients with what purpose they serve are shown in table 1. Three types of coats are generally applied in a manicure.
   i. The base coat: Fills in the irregularities on the surface of the nail plate and makes a smooth base on which to apply the colored enamel. It is colorless/transparent.
   ii. The color enamel coat: Preferred color enamel is applied as 2-3 layers.
   iii. The top coat: This topmost glossy coat gives sheen to the nail paint and also makes it chip resistant.

For a French manicure nail enamel in a neutral color, beige or light pink, is applied over the nail plate proximally and the distal 1-2 mm rim in painted with white to simulate the natural nail.[6] Alternately, the undersurface of the distal end is marked with a white pencil (nail white).

Nail hardeners can be applied as a base coat for the purpose of strengthening the nail plate. They may contain titanium-silicone-zirconium polymers, polytef, nylon, calcium, and biotin.[2]

A manicure or a pedicure can help conceal nail plate surface irregularities like ridging, beau's lines, pitting, and onychorrhexis with nail fillers or lacquer-based nail enamels. Nail bed abnormalities, splinter

TABLE 1: Constituents of nail polish[3-10]

	Component	%	Example	Function
1.	Film forming agent	15%	• Nitrocellulose—most common	• Shiny, tough, waterproof, nontoxic film that adheres well to the nail plate
2.	Thermoplastic resin	7%	• Toluene sulphonamide formaldehyde resin • Polyvinyl butyral • Methacrylate polymers • Vinyl polymers	• Allows adhesion between nail and polish. Provides hardness, gloss, and improves flow
3.	Plasticizer	7%	• Dibutyl phthalate[a] • Camphor • Triphenyl phosphate • Trimethyl pentanyl diisobutyrate • Acetyl tributyl citrate • Ethyl tosylamide • Sucrose benzoate	• Improves flexibility, prevents shrinkage, and makes polish chip resistant
4.	Solvent extender	70%	• Toluene • Butyl acetate • Ethyl acetate • Toluene and isopropyl alcohol	• Allows other components to remain liquid
5.	Pigment	0–1%	• Organic or inorganic colors	• Increases attractiveness and appeal of the nail polish
6.	Thixotropic agents/ Suspending agents	1%	• Stearalkonium hectronite • Stearalkonium bentonite	• Control flow and help in color dispersion
7.	Special additives	–	• Chopped metals (Al, Au, and Ag) Fish scales, guanine, and titanium dioxide coated mica • Bismuth oxychloride • Magnetic enamels containing iron powder • Nylon/rayon fibers	• Give metallic shine/shimmer or frosted effect • Iridescence • Magnetic designs manipulated by magnet in wet state • Help in nail plate strengthening
8.	Color stabilizers (Akin to sunscreens)	–	• Benzophenone-1 • Etocrylene	• Prevent color fading on ultraviolet exposure

[a]Banned in 2004 in the European Union, no longer widely used.[5]

hemorrhages, onycholysis, and salmon patches can be camouflaged in a similar fashion.[11]

Nail lacquers can help dry brittle nails, resulting because of reduced nail plate water content (<16%), by sealing in the moisture.[4]

Problems Related to Manicure or Pedicure

These issues or concerns can be grouped as follows:

1. *Material related:* Starting from the first step; soaking and cleaning the skin in antiseptic soapy solution may lead to dry skin, and allergic or irritant contact dermatitis. The surfactant in soap may lead to dryness of the skin. Dettol, an antiseptic brand commonly used in India, containing chloroxylenol, if added to water can lead to allergic contact dermatitis (ACD) in sensitized individuals. In general salons should refrain from using antiseptics in the cleaning water and use only mild cleansers. Chemical cuticle removers can lead to an irritant or an allergic contact dermatitis. If the latter is

suspected then an open patch test using a 2% aqueous concentration can be used to discern the same.[4] The constituents of a nail polish with their function and the problems faced are discussed in tables 1 and 2, respectively.

Up to 3% of the population has nail polish allergy.[3] Allergic contact dermatitis to nail lacquer has most commonly been established to be due to the free formaldehyde in toluene sulfonamide formaldehyde resin (TFSR) which is to the tune of 0.2–0.5%.[6] The reaction can be both to the dry and wet polish.[18,19] Individual testing can be accomplished by testing with 10% resin in petrolatum. Hypoallergenic nonsensitizing products contain alkyl polyester resins, but with a lesser longevity of polish wear.[20]

Brittleness due to drying and dehydration of the nail plate, wrongly attributed to nail polish use, actually results from the use of the nail polish removers that are alcohol- or acetone-based solvents and inherently drying.[21] They can also lead to an irritant effect because of their dehydrating and defatting effect on the skin. In severe cases an irritant paronychia may also result.[2] ACD is primarily as a result of botanical extracts and fragrances in the removers.[12] An open patch test 10% in olive oil can help discern the same.

2. Procedure/technique related: Discussed in table 3
3. Equipment related: Nail salons should maintain a basic standard of hygiene. All implements used on clients should be regularly sterilized after each use. Cleaning them in a ultrasonic cleaner followed by soaking for 10 minutes in a solution of 2% glutaraldehyde or benzyl alconium chloride should be the norm.[6]

TABLE 2: Reactions to components and side effects of nail polish use

	Side effect	Cause	Comments	Treatment
1.	Staining of the nail plate-yellow/red[6]	Keratin staining with pigments in nail polish	More with pigments D and C reds nos. 6, 7, 34, and 5 lake[7]	• Self-limiting, 2 weeks. For cases with prolonged use and staining, wait till nail grows out and then cut • Apply base coat to protect nail
		Some nail hardeners[12]	Formalin, dimethyl urea, glyoxal	Cycle between hardening and non-hardening base coat weekly
2.	ACD (1–3%)[13-15]	TFSR resin, formaldehyde, and other sensitizers in hardeners	Limited to periungual area or distant spread to area of contact, eyelids, face, and neck[16]	• Steroid cream or ointment, with or without antibiotic, application twice a day • Oral steroids, short course, in severe cases • Use of TFSR-free (epoxy or phthalic-polyester based products)[2]
		Nickel (Ni)	Metallic beads in the nail polish	• As above
3.	ICD	Nail polish remover, solvents in the nail polish, chemical cuticle removers	Periungual tissue involved	Steroid ointment with/without antibiotic
4.	Keratin granulations	Localized friable white patches on the plate due to prolonged enamel wear	D/d SWO, do potassium hydroxide preparation (KOH)	
5.	Increased bacterial carriage[1]	Under chipped nail polish	Advisable not to wear chipped polish for long	Remove chipped polish and maintain nail hygiene
6.	Onycholysis[15,17]	Nail hardeners	High concentrations of formaldehyde resin	Use lacquers with lower concentration (1–2%) of formaldehyde resin

ACD, allergic contact dermatitis; ICD, irritant contact dermatitis; TFSR, toluene sulfonamide formaldehyde resin; D/d, differential diagnosis; SWO, superficial white onychomycosis.

TABLE 3: Manicure: Procedure- or technique-related problems[3]

	Procedure	Function	Problem	Cause
1.	Clipping nails	Reduce length, give shape to nails	• Onychoschizia, • Ingrown nails, paronychia	• Direction not perpendicular to nail • Cutting the medial and lateral ends too low
2.	Filing	Trim and shape nails	Onychoschizia	• Not maintaining perpendicular direction • Using to and fro movement
		Smoothening the dorsal surface of nail plate, helps in better adhesion of nail product	Thinning and weakening of the nail plate	More than 5% of the surface abraded/filed
3.	Pushing the cuticle proximally	Helps in even application of lacquer later	Hang nails, irregular cuticle, detachment of cuticle from nail plate, resultant paronychia, beau's lines/onychodystrophy, onychomycosis	• Damage to cuticle • Entry of microorganisms following loss of protective cuticle
4.	Direct manipulation of the periungual tissues	Removing debris, smoothening edges	Cuts and bleeds, subungual hemorrhages, entry of microorganisms, and infection	• Direct trauma to the tissue • Careless technique • Destruction of protective seal of the hyponychium
5.	Massage of hands/legs	Gentle massage to relax the muscles and hydrate the skin with emollients	Folliculitis	Too vigorous a massage
6.	Pairing corns and calluses	Smoothen and even out skin	Cuts in the skin and bleeding	Poorly performed procedure
7.	Nail enamel application	Gives a smooth glossy and attractive look to the nails	Nail granulations[6] (D/d superficial white onychomycosis, potassium hydroxide mount of scrapings helpful)	• Applying new polish on old to cover up chipping or smoothening old layer of enamel • More common where primer base coat used

D/d, differential diagnosis

Another option is to use disposable files. Some clients do carry their own filers and this should be encouraged.

Filters of pedicure tubs and baths if not thoroughly cleaned after use become laden with debris and are home for infective organisms like *Mycobacterium sp.* There have been reports of spread of mycobacterial infections, *Mycobacterium fortuitum*, after pedicures in salons.[22] Chances of acquiring infection increase if there is an injury or an abridged epidermal cover that provides a portal of entry for the infective organisms. The incubation period is generally around 2 weeks or more. These infections may present as furunculosis over the treated area or may spread proximally in a sporotrichoid fashion.[23] The lesions may look like tiny spider bites to begin with and then become fluctuant abscesses that heal with pigmentation and scarring. Treatment involves antibiotics, usually a combination depending on the cultured organism, given over several months. The average duration for treatment in Winthrop's patient review [24] was 4 months, though treatment may invariably last longer.

It has been suggested that the tub filters should be cleansed thoroughly and frequently and a bleach solution circulated for 15 minutes to prevent transmission of infections.

There is also probability of spread of other bacterial, fungal (*Candida*, dermatophyte) and viral infections (herpes, verrucae, hepatitis) with unsterilized implements.[25]

Nail Adornments

Tiny jewels in various shapes and sizes are applied to the nondried nail polish, which helps them to adhere and stay in place.

Nail Enhancements

Plastic Nail Tips

Plastic nails are applied on the nail plate to give an impression of long-shaped plates extending well beyond the natural plate or as preference be. They come in either ready to use forms with the adhesive in place or as plastic tips where adhesive needs to be applied on the plate and then the tip pressed for a few seconds to hold it in place. The basic steps of tip application are enumerated in table 4.

These tips may work as part of adjunctive management in patients with nail plate surface and structural abnormalities, e.g. in brachyonychia they can give an illusion of length. Though, as a word of caution, they should not to be used as a camouflage if nail infection is suspected.

Fibers of linen, cotton, wool, paper, silk, or fiberglass as nail wraps may be applied on a layer of cyanoacrylate glue on the natural plate or artificial tip. Another protective layer of glue is applied on top or saturated with clear nail polish, which once dry is followed by shaping of the nail. These nail wraps provide additional strength to the nail plate. They are also available as home use kits.

Allergic contact dermatitis to the adhesives, methyl 2-cynoacrylate and ethyl 2-cynoacrylate, is a known entity.[26] Sensitization can be prevented by careful application technique, avoiding contact with the nail folds or surrounding skin. Other problems encountered include the increased onycholytic tendency of the artificial tips given their nonresilience compared to the natural nail plate. These separated tips can home bacteria, which can be an evident scare for health care professionals who can act as carriers for *Candida, Pseudomonas, Klebsiella*, and the like.

Nail Sculptures

This three-dimensional art of covering, shaping, and creating nails involves the curing of methacrylates (liquid monomers and powdered polymers) in the presence of an organic peroxide (benzoyl peroxide) and accelerator. The composition of these acrylic systems is shown in table 5. This formable acrylic is coated on the entire length of the dehydrated natural plate or the artificial tip after the initial coat of a primer. Primers provide adhesion between the nail plate and the overlay material and are mostly propriety mixtures and may contain corrosive acids.[11] Excess can spill onto the nail folds and result in burns if not applied carefully.

If extension of the overlay beyond the limits of the natural nail plate is desired, then a template is placed, later removed, on which the coating in applied. Nonstick Teflon@ or Mylar@ coated paper serves the purpose of the template.[4]

The polymerization of the applied product takes a total of 24–48 hours, though majority (up to 95%)

TABLE 4: Steps for basic nail extension application[4,7]

	Procedure	Purpose
1.	Filing the nail plate	Roughening the plate surface for better adhesion
2.	Application of decolorized iodine or antiseptic dehydrator (isopropyl alcohol)	Prevent fungal infection between the artificial tip and the natural plate
3.	Application of adhesive, cyanoacrylate glue	Holds the nail extension securely on the nail plate
4.	Application of artificial plastic plate	Give length to nail, cover up nail plate surface defects
5.	Cutting and filing the plate	To get desired length and shape
6.	Applying formable acrylic	To cover the remaining nail plate, give smooth surface, if need be
7.	Drilling the nail or filing the undersurface	To make the undersurface smooth
8.	Apply polish and adornments	To make nails attractive

TABLE 5: Composition of acrylic systems[4,12]

1.	Acrylic monomers – liquid system	Ethyl methacrylate	60–95%	–
		Di/tri methacrylate monomers	3–5%	Help cross linking and improve durability
		Dimethyl tolyamine Tertiary aromatic amines	0.75–1.25%	Catalyst
		Ultraviolet (UV) stabilizers	–	–
		Plasticizers	–	Impart flexibility
		Hydroquinone Methyl ether hydroquinone Pyrogallol	+/–	Reaction inhibitors
2.	Acrylic polymers – powder system	Methyl/ethyl methacrylate polymer	50–80 μm beads	–
		Benzoyl peroxide	1–2%	Polymerization initiator
		Titanium dioxide	+/–	Opacifiers
		Colorants	+/–	–

is completed in the first 5-10 minutes itself.[11] Once the polymer hardens shaping and buffing for the final effect follow. This sculpture can then be covered with lacquer and other adornments or left as is after buffing it to a shine.

Differentiation from natural nails can be a daunting task for well executed jobs in the hands of an expert manicurist, nevertheless, these are high maintenance prostheses, any chipping and loosening requires timely clipping and application of fresh acrylic lest infections supervene. As the natural nail plate grows over a period of time the proximal end of the sculpture also requires "filling" covering up the new nail plate proximally with the polymer. A two-three weekly inspection, repair, and filling in is imperative.

Sensitization remains an issue, though the trick lies in the careful application, no-touch technique, of the cured polymer before hardening. Methyl methacrylate was banned by the Food and Drug Administration in 1974 from acrylic nail preparations given the chances of increased allergic reactions with its use.[27] Other acrylate monomers do have a similar propensity albeit to a lesser severity. Clients can be tested for reactions by wearing the sculpture/enhancement on only one nail before embarking on the process for all the nails. This also familiarizes them with the care demanded for such procedures. If there is a history of allergy or it is suspected to the various adhesives or resins, then patch testing is the best tool in the hand of a dermatologist, results of which help guide and counsel the patient with regard to avoidance of products and procedures. Methyl methacrylate monomer can be tested in the liquid form in 10% olive oil, or as acid esters as 1% and 5% in olive oil or petrolatum.[28] Many products do not contain methyl methacrylate monomer any longer but the other methacrylates are also strong sensitizers. Several articles suggest screening for acrylate allergy by patch testing to ethyl methacrylate.[29] The dermatitis vis-a-vis to nail polish resins can be limited to the nail folds and areas surrounding the nail plates or can be more extensive involving other areas of the hand, eyelids, face, and neck. For patients using sculptured nails and suffering from allergic paronychia, patch testing with a recently recommended panel of 10 acrylates may provide them with alternative products to use.[30,31]

Photobonded Nails[32]

Instead of letting the acrylates in the nail sculptures polymerize on their own the process can be hastened by exposure to a magnesium light. This process takes 1-2 minutes for curing compared to 24-48 hours with acrylics.

Ultraviolet Cured Gel Nails

In contrast to acrylics, gel nails cure faster on exposure to ultraviolet (UV) light or UV emitting lamps. Gel nails (Table 6) are chip resistant and easy to use, even at home. Unlike the acrylic overlays, here gel primers are used and the gel is then applied as three coats. Preceding prep is the same. Each step/layer involves photocuring before going ahead. The hands for this are placed in UVA emitting hand

TABLE 6: Constituents of gel nails[12]

1.	Urethane acrylate oligomers	75–95%
2.	Cross linking monomers	–
3.	Photoinitiaters	1–4%
4.	Catalyst- dimethyl tolyamine	0.75–1.25%

lamps. As per recommendations the skin of the hands should be protected with sunscreens and a white cloth during exposure and the client and manicurist should be wear protective eyewear. After arching, cleansing, and shaping the last layer of gel gloss is applied. Maintenance is like for acrylic nails, with filling in required every 2 weeks.

Ultraviolet Cured Shellacs

They are the answer to easy and quick to use gel nails. They are a mix of gel and nail polish. Shellacs unlike lacquers have a base of polymerization photoinitiators and UV curable methacrylates or acrylate oligomers/monomers.[8] Photocuring is done for 1–3 minutes, after two coats of each, base polymer, pigment polymer and clear coats, with low intensity UVA emitting or LED lamps. They have a high durability of up to 4–6 weeks. They are also chip resistant and do not smudge.

Problems and side effects related to nail enhancements and adornment use are summarized in table 7.

TABLE 7: Problems encountered with nail enhancements/sculptures/adornments[8,23,33-40]

	Adverse effect	Cause	Treatment
1.	Allergic contact dermatitis	This reaction can occur to the adhesives, ultraviolet (UV) cured gel or the adornments or jewels	• Prevent periungual skin exposure to chemicals
		Nickel (Ni)- in artificial nail plates, nail jewels and other adornments. Also in metallic pigment nail polish	• Remove source • Steroid containing creams and ointments, with or without antibiotic, twice a day application • Use nickel-free adornments
		Acrylic monomers in gel nails	• As above
		Cyanoacrylate glues: Methyl/ethyl cyanoacrylate	• As above
2.	Paronychia/ erythema/pruritic vesicles	• Methacrylates • Improper procedure damaging cuticles • Excessive water exposure	• Removal of artificial nails • Steroid + antibiotic cream for application • Antifungal to be added if yeast present, mostly in chronic cases • Reduce wet work, limit use of removers, use acetone free products
3.	Thinning of nail plate	Occlusion preventing oxygen diffusion to the nail plate	• Give lacquer free periods for the nails • Oral biotin and vitamin supplementation
4.	Onycholysis	Inflexible artificial tips extending beyond digit tips, more prone	Keep length well within digit tip margin
		Shearing force while removing the artificial nail tip	Don't use nails as tools
		Probing beneath distal nail plate	Gentle removal after soaking in solvent solution
		Strong irritants like methacrylic acid primers	Topical antifungals and antibacterials, for secondary fungal or pseudomonal infection
		Also seen on use of cyanoacrylate based adhesives	Avoid strong irritants

Contd...

Contd...

	Adverse effect	Cause	Treatment
5.	Photo-onycholysis	• Photobonding • Patients taking photosensitizing drugs like doxycycline	• Topical antifungals and antibacterials, for secondary fungal or pseudomonal infection
6.	Nail pitting/dry and rough nail plate surface/ lustureless nails	• Trauma while removing the nail enhancements/adornments	• Emolliation with petroleum jelly • Glycolic peels (70%) for dry/rough/ lustureless plates
7.	Onychodystrophy	• Chronic paronychia with damage to the nail matrix and changes on the nail plate • Strong irritant/allergic reactions damaging the nail matrix	• Prevention and treatment as mentioned above
8.	Paresthesias: burning/tingling/ numbness	• Acrylic exposure • Photobonding	
9.	Increased bacterial carriage	• Risk to *Candida* and *Pseudomonas* carriage under onycholytic artificial tips	• Maintain length up to finger tips only • Remove onycholytic tips • Topical antifungals and antibacterial drops
10.	Brittle, fragile nails	• Primers	• Avoid repeated and frequent contact with water • Urea and alpha hydroxyl acid containing emollients, repeated application • Oral supplementation, iron, biotin, cysteine may help
11.	Temporary or permanent loss of nails	• Secondary to drug or chemical induced onycholysis or photo-onycholysis • Traumatic due to shearing force of artificial tips	
12.	Macular degeneration5	• Eye exposure to UV light from lamps for curing, leading to damage to lutein pigment	• Wear protective eyewear
13.	Nonmelanoma skin cancer	• Photoexposure of normal skin of hands to UV light from lamps. Rare	• Protect skin with sunscreen and white cloth

Medical Indications for Nail Enhancements[2,5,12]

Tendency to sensitization and other side effects cannot ostracize the use of nail care procedures. It is important to understand areas where a dermatologist can advise his patients to go ahead with the above techniques. It is important to be empathetic to patient concerns. These procedures can serve as a camouflage, helping conceal unsightly, diseased or ageing nails. This can help boost patient confidence, esteem and social interactions. Some areas where they can be considered are:

- Ridging of nails: Lacquer-based enamels help fill in the grooves and give smooth surface finish.
- Brachyonychia or nail shape abnormalities: Overlays/artificial tips can give illusion of length and pleasing shape
- Other nail plate abnormalities (pitting, onycho-rrhexis)
- Subungual hemorrhages/splinter hemorrhages
- Salmon patches/onycholysis

- Onychophagia: Artificial nails can help break the habit
- Brittle and soft nails: Shellacs help reinforce the nail and seal in the moisture
- Fragile and weak nails: Protective shell of lacquers, shellacs and other enhancements helps
- To tide over the interim period before medical treatment for nail dystrophy shows effect.

Workplace Safety

Technicians handling or working with nail cosmetics are inadvertently exposed to the chemicals therein. Be it direct contact while application or use, or as a result of inhalation of fumes and filing dust. They need to be well aware of the harmful and sensitizing potential of products and ingredients in their occupational environment.[41,42] Precautions like good ventilation, wearing gloves and masks, careful use using no touch technique, washing hands thoroughly after each procedure and avoiding contact with dusts and fillings, which may contain uncured monomer, can circumvent many of the adverse effects that can result from exposure to these chemicals.[43] The main issues faced are outlined in table 8.

Another factor to be kept in mind is that once sensitized to an occupational sensitizer, e.g. acrylates, there may be cross reactions triggering allergic reactions with other acrylic compounds in different settings away from work on re-exposure.[43]

Ultraviolet exposure to the eyes while curing of shellacs/nail gels may damage the lutein pigment in the eye and result in macular degeneration necessitating the use of protective eyewear even for the manicurists.

Tips on nail salon choice/visit are:

- Salons with technicians having practical training
- Check on proper sterilization of manicure equipment—autoclaving/chemical sterilization. If in doubt always ask
- Good personal hygiene levels for technicians; neat and clean appearance and washing hands before procedures
- Overall salon cleanliness
- Carry your own implements especially filers
- Avoid shaving or waxing legs and arms 24 hours before a manicure or pedicure
- Avoid visiting salons when active skin infection on hands and feet
- Ask the manicurist not to manipulate the cuticle or cut dead skin around the nail.

TABLE 8: Workplace issues for nail salon technicians[44-49]

1.	Contact sensitization
2.	Irritant reactions
3.	As a result of inhalation: • Throat irritation • Asthma • Rhinitis
4.	Trembling of hands
5.	Drowsiness/dizziness
6.	Macular degeneration in the eye
7.	Mild cognitive and neurosensory changes

CONCLUSION

Beauty pundits have used the lipstick index as a yardstick to measure the growth of economy. The nail polish index is sure to usurp this status the lipstick had. Easy availability and affordability have helped it form a niche of its own with nail salons sprouting all over and many new easy to use home kits. But care has to be taken in lieu of the numerous new nail art technologies and myriad products stocking shelves of drug and departmental stores. The salon technicians need to be trained to maintain the basic standards of hygiene, use careful technique along with use of products with established safety profiles. Dermatologists too need to keep abreast of the latest techniques and products introduced for the nails and their potential risks. Allergic contact dermatitis is by far the most common side effect of nail cosmetics. Though research is directed to hypoallergenic, nonsensitizing products, cheaper alternates and fakes are always rampant in the market. Their use can definitely be harmful and people should be familiarized with these potential side effects.

REFERENCES

1. Rich P. Nail cosmetics. Dermatol Clin. 2006;24(3):393-9.
2. Dahdah MJ, Scher RK. Nail diseases related to nail cosmetics. Dermatol Clin. 2006;24(2):233-9.
3. Moosavi M, Scher RK. Nail care products. Clin Dermatol. 2001;19(4):445-8.
4. Jefferson J, Rich P. Update on nail cosmetics. Dermatol Ther. 2012;25(6):481-90.
5. Madnani NA, Khan KJ. Nail cosmetics. Indian J Dermatol Venereol Leprol. 2012;78(3):309-17.
6. Iorizzo M, Piraccini BM, Tosti A. Nail cosmetics in nail disorders. J Cosmet Dermatol. 2007;6(1):53-8.
7. Draelos ZD. Nail cosmetic issues. Dermatol Clinics. 2000;18(4):675-83.
8. Bryson PH, Sirdesai SJ. Colored nail cosmetics and hardeners. In: Draelos ZD. (Ed). Cosmetic dermatology

products and procedures, 1st edition. Hoboken, NJ: Wiley-Blackwell; 2010. pp. 206-13.

9. Liden C, Berg M, Farm G, et al. Nail varnish allergy with far reaching consequences. Br J Dermatol. 1993;128(1):57-62.
10. Scher RK. Cosmetics and ancillary preparations for the care of nails. J Am Acad Dermatol. 1982; 6(4 Pt 1):523-8.
11. Rich P. Nail cosmetics and camouflaging techniques. Dermatol Ther. 2001;14(3):228-36.
12. Schoon D. Cosmetic prostheses as artificial nail enhancements. In: Draelos ZD. (Ed). Cosmetic dermatology products and procedures, 1st edition. Hoboken, NJ: Wiley-Blackwell; 2010. pp. 215-21.
13. Fuchs T, Gutgesell C. Is contact allergy to toluene sulphonamide-formaldehyde resin common? Br J Dermatol. 1996;135(6):1003-17.
14. Sainio EL, Engstrom K, Henriks-Eckerman ML, et al. Allergenic ingredients in nail polishes. Contact Dermatitis. 1997;37(4):155-62.
15. Norton L. Common and uncommon reactions to formaldehyde containing nail hardeners. Semin Dermatol. 1991;10(1):29.
16. Baran R. Nail cosmetics: allergies and irritations. Am J Clin Dermatol. 2002;3(8):547-55.
17. Helsing P, Austad J, Talberg HJ. Onycholysis induced by nail hardener. Contact Dermatitis. 2007;57(4):280-1.
18. Hausen BM, Milbrodt M, Koenig WA. The allergens of nail polish: allergenic constituents of common nail polish and toluene sulfonamide-formaldehyde resin (TSFR). Contact Dermatitis. 1995;33(3):157-64.
19. Tosti A, Guerra L, Vincenzi C, et al. Contact sensitization caused by toluene sulfonamide-formaldehyde resins in women who use nail cosmetics. Am J Contact Dermatitis. 1993;4:150-3.
20. Giorgini S, Brusi C, Francalanci S, et al. Prevention of allergic contact dermatitis from nail varnishes and hardeners. Contact Dermatitis 1994;31(5):325-6.
21. Draelos ZD. Nail cosmetics. E-medicine/Specialities/Dermatology. 2001:1-10.
22. Chang RM, Hare HQ, Rich P. Treating cosmetically induced nail problems. Dermatol Ther. 2007;20(1):54-9.
23. Sniezek PJ, Graham BS, Busch HB, et al. Rapidly growing mycobacterial infections after pedicures. Arch Dermatol. 2003;139(5):629-34.
24. Winthrop KL, Abrams M, Yakrus M, et al. An outbreak of furunculosis associated with foot- baths at a nail salon. N Engl J Med. 2002;346(18):1366-71.
25. Sekula SA. Nail salons can be risky business. Arch Dermatol. 2002;138(3):414-15.
26. Methyl 2-cyanoacrylate and ethyl 2-cyanoacrylate [MAK Value Documentation, 1999]. The MAK Collection for Occupational Health and Safety. Germany: Wiley-VCH; 2012. pp. 234-47.
27. Maio P, Carvalho R, Amaro C, et al. Letter: allergic contact dermatitis from sculptured acrylic nails: special presentation with a possible airborne pattern. Dermatol Online J. 2012;18(2):13.
28. Baran R, Dawber RPR. The nail and cosmetics. In: Samman PD, Fenton DA (Eds). The nails in disease. 4th edition. Chicago: Year book publishers; 1986. p. 129.
29. Koppula SV, Fellman JH, Storrs FJ, et al. Screening allergens for acrylate dermatitis associated with artificial nails. Am J Contact Derm. 1995;6:78-85.
30. Constandt L, Hecke EV, Naeyaert JM, et al. Screening for contact allergy to artificial nails. Contact Dermatitis. 2005;52(2):73-7.
31. Movad CM, Ferringer T. Allergic contact dermatitis from acrylates in artificial nails. Dermatitis.2004;15(1):51-3.
32. Lazarov A. Sensitization to acrylates is a common adverse reaction to artificial fingernails. J Eur Acad Dermatol Venereol. 2007;21(2):169-74.
33. Kanerva L, Lauerma A, Estlander T, et al. Occupational allergic contact dermatitis caused by photobonded sculptured nails and a review of methacrylates in nail cosmetics. Am J Contact Dermat. 1996;7(2):109-15.
34. Hemmer W, Focke M, Wantke F, et al. Allergic contact dermatitis to artificial fingernails prepared from UV light cured acrylates. J Am Acad Dermatol. 1996;35 (3 pt1):377-80.
35. Fisher A. Adverse nail reactions and paraesthesia from photobonded acrylate sculptured acrylic nails." Cutis. 1990:45:293-4.
36. Drucker AM, Pratt MD. Acrylate contact allergy: patient characteristics and evaluation of screening allergens. Dermatitis. 2011;22(2):98-101.
37. Lawry M, Rich P. The nail apparatus: a guide for basic and clinical science. Curr Probl Dermatol. 1999;11(5):202-4.
38. Militello G. Contact and primary irritant dermatitis of the nail unit diagnosis and treatment. Dermatol Ther. 2007;20(1):47-53.
39. Scheinfeld N, Dahdah MJ, Scher R. Vitamins and minerals: their role in nail health and disease. J Drugs Dermatol. 2007;6(8):782-7.
40. Cashman MW, Sloan SB. Nutrition and nail disease. Clin Dermatol. 2010;28(4):420-5.
41. Baran R. Pathology induced by the application of cosmetics to the nails. In: Frost P, Horwitz SN (Eds). Cosmetics for the dermatologist. Philadelphia: CV Mosby; 1982. p. 182.
42. Daniel CR. Simple onycholysis. In: Scher RK, Daniel CR (Eds). Nails: diagnosis, therapy, surgery, 3rd edition. Philadelphia: Elsevier Saunders; 2005. pp. 97-8.
43. Lazar P. Reactions to nail hardeners. Arch Dermatol. 1966;94(4):446-8.
44. Cruz MJ, Baudrier T, Cunha AP, et al. Severe onychodystrophy caused by allergic contact dermatitis to acrylates in artificial nails. Cutan Ocul Toxicol. 2011;30(4):323-4.
45. Slodownik D, Williams JD, Tate BJ. Prolonged paresthesia due to sculpted acrylic nails. Contact Dermatitis. 2007; 56(5):298-9.
46. Jeanes A, Green J. Nail art: a review of current infection control issues. J Hosp Infect. 2001;49(2):139 -42.
47. Hochman LG, Scher RK, Meyerson MS. Brittle nails: response to daily biotin supplementation. Cutis. 1993; 51(4):303-5.
48. MacFarlane DF, Alonso CA. Occurrence of nonmelanoma skin cancers on the hands after UV nail light exposure. Arch Dermatol. 2009;145(4):447-9.
49. National Institute of Occupational Safety and Health (NIOSH). Controlling chemical hazards during the application of artificial fingernails. Appl Occup Environ Hyg. 2001;16(5):509-11.

8

CHAPTER

Hair Cosmeceuticals

Jaishree Sharad, Vrushali Rane

INTRODUCTION

Hair reflects the state of mind, financial, professional, and social status and finally the health status, both positively and negatively irrespective of ethnic, cultural, and economic differences. This chapter attempts to understand the formulation and functioning of commonly used hair products.

PROPERTIES OF HAIR AND ITS ROLE IN HAIR APPEARANCE

The appearance and perception of hair is determined by its interaction with light and the physical and chemical properties of cuticle, cortex, and medulla.[1]

Optical Properties

The cortex carries the bulk of melanin and is responsible for the reflection and refraction of incident light that in turn determines the color of hair. Medulla also contributes to the color of hair. A newly formed unpigmented hair with no medulla appears yellowish rather than white, due to the intrinsic color of dense and well organized arrangement of keratin fibers.[1]

Chemical Properties

The production of melanin pigment is genetically determined and it is of two types: (i) Eumelanin—Brown to black; and (ii) Pheomelanin—Yellow-red to red. The ratio of eumelanin and pheomelanin, and their distribution determine the color of hair.[2]

Electrical Properties

Static electricity causes repulsion between individual hairs.[2] Static electricity is determined by several factors such as combing, surface of hair, ambient climate, etc. Combing increases the static electricity. Like charges in adjoining hair can even cause matting of hair and a haircut would be the only solution.[2]

Mechanical Properties

The configuration of hair fibers within the hair shaft determines its tensile strength and ease of breakage. Black hair are generally most elliptical in shape and Asian hair are circular. Extremely curled black hair is more fragile than Asiatic hair.[2,3] Curled hair is also more sensitive to hairdressing procedures like ironing, coloring, and chemical straightening.[2,3]

HAIR COSMETICS

Hair cosmetics have been classified into those used for cleansing and health of the hair and those for styling. While shampoos and conditioners constitute the former, hair cosmetics/styling agents constitute the latter.

Hair Shampoo

Shampoo is a specially designed formulation to remove sebum, desquamated corneocytes, sweat, fungal residue, styling products if any, and pollution residue from the scalp and hair.[4]

Chemical Composition

A shampoo comprises of constituents like detergents, foam inducing agents, thickeners, opacifiers, fragrances, preservatives, additives, sequestering agents, and in some cases inbuilt conditioners.

Detergents

The cleansing action of a shampoo is attributed to synthetic amphiphilic detergents. They comprise of both lipophilic and hydrophilic moieties.[3] While the lipophilic terminal binds to the oil and dust, the hydrophilic site binds to water and helps removal of the shampoo that has bonded with the oil and dust during rinsing.[5,6] There are four types of detergents based on their chemical properties: (i) Anionics, (ii) Cationics, (iii) Amphoterics, and (iv) Nonionic/natural surfactants.[7,8] Depending on the desired output of varying amounts of each of cleansing, foaming, and conditioning, these detergents are combined.

Anionic detergents: They are so named because of their negative charge and are best at removing dirt and sebum from scalp, but leave the hair dry and unmanageable due to static intershaft friction.[3]

For example, lauryl sulfates, laureth sulfates, sarcosines, and sulfosuccinates.[9] Lauryl sulfates are popular as they produce rich foam and work in hard water but leave hair dry. Laureth sulfates are less harsh on the hair. Both lauryl and laureth sulfates are primary detergents in shampoos. Sarcosines are used as secondary detergents, they are not that good at cleansing but very good at conditioning. Sulfosuccinates are strong detergents and accompany the lauryl sulfates and sulfonates as adjuvants.

Cationic detergents: Just as anionic detergents are negatively charged, cationic detergents are positively charged molecules making them relatively hydrophobic and less foam producing. They generally form a constituent of daily shampoos and chemically treated hair where mild cleansing is expected.[10]

Nonionic detergents:[9] For example, polyoxyethylene fatty alcohols and sorbitol esters, alkanolamides.

They have no charge on them and are generally additive with other detergents.

Amphoteric detergents[9]: For example, betaines, sultaines, and imidazolinium.

They have both positive and negatively charged groups and switch from cationic to anionic state depending on the pH. They are soft on the hair and are a constituent of shampoos for chemically treated and fine hair. They have an added advantage of being "no cry" shampoos and are a popular constituent of baby shampoos.

Additives[9]

In addition to the detergents, some additives are present in a shampoo which include foam inducing agents (for better spreadability), thickeners (to increase viscosity), opacifiers, fragrances, and sequestering agents (chelating agents to prevent forming scum as seen with soap). These agents are added to a shampoo to enhance aesthetic appeal and not for cleansing purpose.

Commercial Preparations

Despite having similar ingredients, shampoos vary because of the varied combination of the ingredients to suit different cleansing needs and hair types. They are named for common understanding. For example, normal shampoo, dry hair shampoo, daily use shampoo, volumizing shampoo, deep cleansing shampoo, baby (no tears) shampoo, shampoo for long hair or limp hair, shampoo for curly coarse hair, shampoo for chemically treated hair, sulfate free shampoo, 2 in 1 conditioning shampoo, etc. (Table 1).[11-15]

Shampoos and Hair Damage

Hair damage because of shampoo is very rare as it has a very short contact time with the skin.

Hair loss complained after a particular shampoo is generally attributed to repeated blow drying, vigorous towel drying, and wet combing of chemically treated and fine hair rather than the shampoo itself. However, long term use of strong detergents on fine hair can gradually dissolve a surface membrane of the cuticular layer or even the structural lipids.[16]

Allergic contact dermatitis is another rare complication with the use of shampoos; culprits being formalin, parabens, hexachlorophene, and miranols.[9] These can be affirmed by patch testing.

With a huge consumer market, it is essential that the dermatologist guide his/her patient to not fall prey to the wide gimmicks and help select a suitable shampoo.

Hair Conditioners

With the advent of a myriad of hair styling agents and chemical treatments for hair and repeated use of shampoo to wash off these stylants, often one is left with dry, frizzy, unmanageable hair. Hair conditioners make the hair feel softer, manageable, and increase the hair shine[1,17] and are a constant accompaniment with shampoos. The primary role of a conditioner is to deposit positive ions and reduce the negative charge on the hair.[9] Conditioners depending on their size and properties also fill gaps between cuticular cells giving rise to a smoother cuticular surface, adding shine to the hair.[9,11,15] Split ends or trichoptilosis is also temporarily mended by conditioners by the same principle.[9] However, all of these effects are short lasting and last only till the next shampooing.

TABLE 1: Types of shampoo with its other characteristic features

Type of shampoo	Type of hair	Detergent	Cleansing	Conditioning
Normal	Normal untreated hair, Men	Lauryl sulfate	Good	Mild
Dry	Dry	Mild detergents with conditioning agents like hydrolyzed animal protein	Mild	Good
Baby[11]	Babies/fine hair	Amphoterics	Mild	Mild
2 in 1[12,13]	Dry hair	Amphoterics/anionics (sulfosuccinate) with added conditioning agents	Good	Excellent
Oily	Oily	Lauryl sulfates, sulfosuccinates	Excellent	Minimal/none
Damaged hair	Chemically treated hair	Mild detergents with conditioning agents like hydrolyzed animal protein	Mild	Good
Colored hair	Colored hair	Cationic surfactants with conditioning agents like hydrolyzed animal protein	Mild	Good
Deep cleansing	Frequent users of gels, sprays	Similar to oily hair shampoos	Excellent	Mild/none
Everyday			Mild	Mild
Ethnic shampoos[14]	Black patients, coarse curly hair	Similar to 2 in 1 shampoo	Good	Excellent
Antidandruff[15]		Added coal tar, selenium sulfide, ketoconazole, zinc pyrithione, sulfur, and salicylic acid	Mild	Mild

Hair Surface Properties and Damage

Hair fiber consists of a central medulla followed by cortex. The cortex is responsible for the tensile strength of the hair.[18,19] The cortex is surrounded by multiple layers of cells called the cuticle which determines the cosmetic appearance of hair, i.e. shine, softness, and manageability. Hair styling agents, frequent shampooing, wet combing, reverse combing, and aggressive toweling of wet hair damages the cuticle giving a flyaway rough appearance of hair.[16]

Hair surface damage is not limited to chemical treatments or styling agents but also because of chemical properties of hair. The surface of hair is negatively charged which contributes to repulsive charges between neighboring strands of hair which is increased by combing. This is attributed to the oxidation of cysteine to cysteine-S-sulfonate and cysteic acid by ultraviolet light.[20,21] These negative charges increase from the root of the hair to its tip.[16] Also terminal hair/tips of hair are more subjective to combing, increasing the friction further. Chemical treatments (perming/coloring) cause both cortex and cuticular damage. They introduce more negative charges, increasing the friction, and unmanageability of the hair.[19,22-26]

Chemical Classification

Conditioning agents are classified based on their chemical characteristics as follows—cationic surfactants or quaternary ammonium compounds, cationic polymers, proteins, and silicones.

Cationic surfactants or quaternary ammonium compounds: For example, stearalkonium chloride, cetrimonium chloride, and trimethylammonium chloride.

These deposit positive charges on the hair surface, reduce the buildup of static charge, and reduce intershaft repulsion.[16] Also the more negative charge on the hair, the more deposition of conditioner will occur. This was evidenced when bleached hair showed more proportion of the conditioner as compared to virgin hair.[16] Cetrimonium chloride is a light to medium conditioning agent while trimethylammonium chloride is a much deeper conditioning agent.[27-31] Detangling and substantivity improve from monoacetyl to diacetyl to triacetyl quats.[16] They are also present in conditioning shampoos, however, the efficacy of a cationic surfactant is identified by its hydrophobicity and shampoos with ionic detergents are not chemically compatible with them. So these conditioning shampoos use detergent soluble quats albeit with milder conditioning properties. An exception is octyl dimonium chloride with good substantivity and conditioning but is also water soluble.[32]

Cationic polymers: For example, polyquaternium 6, 7, 10, 11, and 16.

Also known as film forming conditioners, they reduce the static electricity not by adding positive charges but by coating away the negative charges with a thin polymer coating around the hair.[33] It also increases the light reflection that adds to the luster of the hair.[9] However, being cationic, they are also positively charged and if the charge density is high, once deposited they might be difficult to remove with shampooing.[34,35] This often contributes to the greasiness of hair due to overconditioning, more so seen in chemically treated hair.[34-36]

Protein containing conditioners:[9] These act by virtue of penetration in the fractured areas of hair shafts that are damaged by chemicals and procedures.

Silicones: For example, dimethicone (dimethyl siloxanes), amodimethicone, cyclomethicone, and dimethicone copolyol.

They have revolutionized the market of hair conditioners since their entry from the last 2 decades.[16] They act by forming a thin film giving a sheen[37,38] and reduce static electricity without any greasiness.[16] Yahagi demonstrated that conditioning efficacy of silicones was greater than cationic surfactants.[39] Also, coexistence of silicones with the cationic surfactants and cationic polymers increased the conditioning efficacy.[16] Silicone and dimethicone provide the maximum conditioning while cyclomethicone and dimethicone copolyol are the weaker agents.

Additives/Auxiliary Ingredients[16]

These are the agents added to a conditioner to improve the aesthetic appeal and for long-term preservation of its efficacy. These include preservatives, thickeners (hydroxyethyl cellulose), polyamides, plasticizers, emulsifying agents (ethoxylated fatty alcohols and esters), fragrances, humectants (propylene glycol, honey, and glycerin chitosan), and vitamins.

Commercial Preparations[9]

Conditioners are available as postshampoo conditioners, leave-on conditioners, deep conditioners, and hair rinses.

Postshampoo conditioners: They are the most commonly used conditioners for home used on wet hair, typically left for 5–10 minutes after a shampoo and then rinsed off.

Leave-on conditioners: They are suited for both home and salon use after hair is dry. They are best suited for curly or coarse hair but make fine hair look limp and greasy. Also, increased substantivity may make it difficult to rinse off in subsequent shampooing.

Hair rinses: They are similar to postshampoo conditioners, however, they do not condition and only help in detangling.

Deep conditioners: These are generally meant for salon use for extremely dry and damaged hair. They are applied to hair for 30 minutes to an hour followed by steam to enhance its penetration before being rinsed off.

Understanding the needs of different hair and advising the right conditioner is the role of a dermatologist. Short straight hair needs only static control while curly coarse hair requires both static control and easy combing. Fine hair needs a light conditioner while bleached or chemically treated hair requires a stronger agent.

HAIR GROOMING COSMETICS

With extensive marketing of hairstyling, the use of styling products is logarithmically rising. The onus of educating a patient about the potential damage due to overzealous use of hair cosmetics lies on dermatologists.

All styling products are used with an intention to set the hair in a particular style. There are different types of styling products depending on the type of hair that determine how long the hair will remain in that style. Some styling agents have an additional role to impart shine to the hair or to detangle the hair. Generally, they contain synthetic film forming polymers and other additives depending on the role of the product. Some additives are mentioned as here in Table 2.[2]

Hair Gel

Hair gel is an alcohol based styling aid that is used to keep hair in place. On application to wet hair, it dries completely keeping the hair in a stiff shape. It is useful for creating volume in curly hair, building height in hairstyles, and stabilizing frizzy hair. Because of its water content, it can be easily

TABLE 2: Major additives of hair grooming

Octylacrylamide/acrylates/ butylaminoethyl methacrylate copolymer/poly(vinyl methyl ether) maleic anhydrous-5.0 film formaldehyde ethyl ester/polyquaternium-4/ polyquaternium-11	Film forming agent
Glycols	Plasticizers
Dimethyl phthalate (phthalates)	Plasticizers
Cetearyl octanoate	Plasticizers
Lanolin	Conditioner
Silicon	Conditioner
Fragrance	Fragrance
Ethanol/deionized water/ isobutane/propane	Solvent
Dimethicone copolyol	Styling ease
Isosteareth-10, lauramide DEA	Foam stabilizers
Paraben, hydantoin	Preservative
Isobutane/propane blend	Propellant

removed by rinsing. Recently alcohol-free gels are commercially available which is ideal for dry hair as alcohol on evaporation takes away the moisture from the hair. Depending on their stiffening potential, they are further classified into styling gel, to emphasize on a style, and sculpturing gel for stiffening effect or styling for thick unruly hair.[9]

Hair Creams

Hair creams are used on dry or damp hair to stabilize frizzy hair without the greasiness or stiffness of hair gels. They are best used for thick and curly hair as fine hair would appear limp because of its moisturizing properties.

Hair Mousse

They are variants of hair gel but in a foam base and are meant for thin, limp hair. They can be applied to both dry and damp hair. It is not as strong as gel but less sticky and adds less weight to the hair.

Hair Wax[40]

Hair waxes are thick textured hairstyling products used to assist holding of dry hair while remaining pliable. Wax based products do not dry and hence, hair does not stay stiff. This allows the user to restyle the hair several times a day without disturbing its stability. However, styles created by hair wax can be easily spoilt as opposed to a stiff styling hair gel. Because, they are wax based, they are difficult to rinse off.

Pomade

While some consider them synonymous with hair wax, they are oil based, more greasy products that may cause pomade acne.[9] Water based pomades are softer, nongreasy, and claimed to be non-comedogenic.

Brilliantines

They are the liquid counterpart of pomades minus the oil buildup, although, the traditional ones contain mineral oils and may cause the same side effects as of pomades.[9]

Oil Sheen Spray

They are variants of pomades but in a spray form (aerosolized oil) with a major concentration of conditioners.[9]

Hairspray

Hairsprays are sprayed onto dry hair after styling to maintain the state of styled hair.[9] The spray deposits millions of droplets on the surface of hair, which settle at points where the hair fibers are intersecting each other forming temporary bonds/ joints. As the solvent evaporate and the hair dries, these bonds become stronger and rigid and resist the movement of hair over each other. These bonds break on exposure to water or ambient humidity. Hair sprays are also available as pump sprays and aerosol sprays. While the older pump sprays used butyl and ethyl esters of poly (vinyl/methylether/ maleic anhydride) copolymers, the newer ones use octylacrylamide/acrylates/methacrylate copolymers. Aerosol hairsprays use vinyl acetate/crotonates/ neodecanoate.[2] Fine or limp hair benefit from hair spray as it does not weigh down the hair.

Hair Serum

A popular styling product for thick locks that helps reduce frizz and is also a thermal protective agent. It also imparts sheen because of silicone and various oils.

Hair volumizers are constituents that are used to temporarily add volume to thin, limp, and fine hair. They are not used independently but generally an additive to shampoos and hair sprays. Hair volumizers attract moisture from the ambient climate, causing swelling of the hair making it look apparently thicker.

Hair styling aids should be chosen as per the thickness of hair, length, density, and surface properties of hair. Short, fine hair are best styled by waxes or strong gels. Heavier products like, hair creams and nonwater-based pomades should be avoided for thinning hair.

Hair Oils

Hair oils have been an integral part of almost every Indian household as the secret of thick, dark, lustrous, and voluminous hair. Hair oils are supposed to seal the gap between the cuticular cells causing lubrication and imparting shine. The seal also prevents the penetration of the aggressive detergents, hairstyling agents, and other cosmetics into the follicle and causing damage.[41] However, that depends on the penetration potential of the hair. Rele and Mohile in 2003,[42] compared the properties of mineral oil, coconut oil, and sunflower oil on hair with regards to their penetration power. Among the three oils, coconut oil was the only oil found to penetrate the hair. Coconut oil is a triglyceride of lauric acid (principal fatty acid) with low molecular weight and straight linear chain and coupled with its high affinity for hair proteins, it was found to be the only oil which could reduce the hair protein loss. Mineral oil, by virtue of its chemical structure, does not penetrate. Sunflower oil has a bulky molecular structure with limited penetration of hair. Moroccan argan oil has become a very popular hair cosmetic with superior moisturizing properties.[41] Argan fruits are left to dry and it kernels are extracted to source the oil.[43] Although, literature speaks of its use in chronic conditions such as atherosclerosis and psoriasis, there is not enough evidence of its role in hair fall prevention.[44,45] In another study, peppermint oil caused faster hair growth as compared to minoxidil in androgenetic alopecia.[46] Peppermint oil acted by restoring the vascularity of dermal papilla and menthol, an important constituent acted as a penetration enhancer. More research needs to be done in hair oils as primary evidence looks promising as effective and economical in maintaining hair health and possibly in reducing hair breakage.

HAIR COSMETICS AND HAIR DAMAGE

Hair cosmetics come with their share of side effects, either due to skin contact or directly on the hair.

- Damage due to contact with skin:
  - Irritant reaction: This is because of inadvertent contact with skin during hair dying and bleaching procedures ranging from erythema to actual burns.[2] Irritant effect is attributed to disturbance in the lipophilic component of the stratum corneum by the hair cosmetic. The effect can extend deeper and denature protein as well[2]
  - Allergic contact dermatitis: More common than irritant reactions are chronic allergic contact dermatitis. It may be limited to the margins of the hair or even spread to the face, chest, and back. Pigmentation noticed on sides of forehead is commonly noted in some patients with known dye allergy. The common culprits in hair cosmetics that act as skin sensitizers are:[19] Shampoos (surfactants, zinc pyrithione, and hydroxyquinolines), hair dyes (p-phenylenediamine, resorcinol), hair gels (lanolin, parabens), hair lotions (quinone, resorcinol), and deodorants (hydroxyquinolines, Irgasan DP 300). Transient but reversible hair loss may be associated with contact dermatitis[1,23]
  - Chemical burn: Although rare, chemical burns/scald injury of scalp skin can happen on contact with hair coloring agents and permanent waving solutions or their neutralizers[2]
  - Physical burn: These are generally iatrogenic injuries. Heated rollers or ironing apparatus, use of flammable liquids in close proximity to a fire source are avoidable injuries.[2]
- Damage due to effect on hair:
  - Cuticle damage: Any procedure such as perming, straightening, coloring, or bleaching that can potentially alter the chemical properties of hair invariably causes cuticle damage. This not only affects the physical appearance of hair but also makes it fragile and prone to breakage[2]
  - Hair breakage: It could be due to actual physical trauma such as tight rollers or increased tensile force on hair during ironing or continued assault of the cuticle finally breaking down the tough cortex[2]
  - Chignon alopecia: Permanent hair loss/thinning may result from chronic assaults to

the hair also known as chignon alopecia and frontoliminal alopecia[2]

- Faulty color of hair: This generally happens with repeated dying. The hair shaft can be damaged by previous permanent waving or bleaching making it more permeable to some dyes, leading to faulty colors, e.g. green color from azo dyes, green hair from copper metallic salts, and red hair from chino form[2]
- Bird nest hair: Although this can happen to physically damaged hair due to any cause, anyone subjecting their hair to a lot of chemical procedures should be aware of this condition. It results in a mass of hair that cannot be untangled and essentially needs to be cut.[1]

CONCLUSION

It is imperative for every dermatologist to stay abreast of the technological advances in the field of hair cosmetics to address all the hair related issues of their patients.

REFERENCES

1. Dawber RP, Van Neste D. Hair and Scalp Disorders, 2nd edition. London: Martin Dunitz Ltd; 1995.
2. Naste W, Kahre S. Hair care products. In: Maibach BP (Ed). Handbook of Cosmetic Science and Technology, 2nd edition. New York: Marcel Dekker; 2001. pp. 575-605.
3. Draelos ZD. Nonmedicated grooming products and beauty treatments. In: Draelos ZD (Ed). Hair and Scalp Diseases; 2008. pp. 59-72.
4. Robbins CR. Interaction of shampoo and creme rinse ingredients with human hair. In: Robbins CR (Ed). Chemical and Physical Behavior of Human Hair, 2nd edition. New York: Springer-Verlag; 1988. pp. 122-67.
5. Zviak C, Vanlerberghe G. Scalp and hair hygiene. In: Zviak C (Ed). The Science of Hair Care. New York: Marcel Dekker; 1986. pp. 49-86.
6. Fox C. An introduction to the formulation of shampoos. Cosmet Toilet. 1988;103:25-58.
7. Powers DH. Shampoos. In: Balsam MS, Gershon SD, Reiger MM, Sagarin E, Strianse SJ (Eds). Cosmetics Science and Technology, 2nd edition. New York: Wiley-Interscience; 1972. pp. 73-116.
8. Tokiwa F, Hayashi S, Okumura T. Hair and surfactants. In: Kobori T, Montagna W (Eds). Biology and Disease of the Hair. Baltimore: University Park Press; 1975. pp. 631-40.
9. Draelos ZD. Hair Care: An Illustrated Dermatology Handbook. North Carolina: Taylor and Francis; 2005.
10. Bouillon C. Shampoos and hair conditioners. Clin Dermatol. 1988;6:83-92.
11. Wilkinson JB, Moore RJ. Harry's Cosmeticology. New York: Chemical Publishing; 1982. pp. 457-8.
12. Hunting AL. Can there be cleaning and conditioning in the same product? Cosmet Toilet. 1988;103:73-8.
13. Gruber J, Lamoureux B, Joshi N, et al. The use of X-ray fluorescent spectroscopy to study the influence of cationic polymers on silicone oil deposition from shampoo. J Cosmet Sci. 2001;52:131-6.
14. Brooks G, Burmeister F. Black hair care ingredients. Cosmet Toilet. 1988;103:93-6.
15. Spoor HJ. Shampoos. Cutis. 1973;12:671-2.
16. Reich C, Su D. Hair conditioners. In: Maibach BP. Handbook of Cosmetic Science and Technology, 2nd edition. New York: Marcel Dekker; 2001. pp. 331-46.
17. Lunn AC, Evans RE. The electrostatic properties of human hair. J Soc Cosmet Chem. 1977;28:549-69.
18. Robbins CR, Crawford RJ. Cuticle damage and the tensile properties of human hair. J Soc Cosmet Chem. 1991;42:59.
19. Robbins CR. Chemical and Physical Behavior of Human Hair, 3rd edition. New York: Springer-Verlag; 1994. p. 301.
20. Robbins CR, Bahl MK. Analysis of hair by electron spectroscopy for chemical analysis. J Soc Cosmet Chem. 1984;35:379-90.
21. Stranick MA. Determination of negative binding sites on hair surfaces using XPS and Ba^{2+} labeling. Surface Interface Anal. 1996;24:522-8.
22. Jachowicz J. Hair damage and attempts to its repair. J Soc Cosmet Chem. 1987;38:263-86.
23. Tate ML, Kamath YK, Ruetsch SB, et al. Quantification and prevention of hair damage. J Soc Cosmet Chem. 1993;44:347-71.
24. Horiuchi T. Nature of damaged hair. Cosmet Toilet. 1978;93:65-77.
25. Kaplin IJ, Schwann A, Zahn H. Effects of cosmetic treatments on the ultrastructure of hair. Cosmet Toilet. 1982;97:22-6.
26. Sandhu SS, Ramachandran R, Robbins CR. A simple and sensitive method using protein loss measurements to evaluate damage to human hair during combing. J Soc Cosmet Chem. 1995;46:39-52.
27. Jurczyk MF, Berger DR, Damaso GR. Quaternary ammonium salt: applications in hair conditioners. Cosmet Toilet. 1991;106:63-8.
28. Finkelstein P, Laden K. The mechanism of conditioning of hair with alkyl quaternary ammonium compounds. Appl Poly Symp. 1971;18:673-80.
29. Jachowicz J. Fingerprinting of cosmetic formulations by dynamic electrokinetic and permeability analysis. II. Hair conditioners. J Soc Cosmet Chem. 1995;46:100-16.
30. Spiess E. The influence of chemical structure on performance in hair care preparations. Parfumerie Kosmetik. 1991;72(6):370-4.
31. Yahagi K, Hoshino N, Hirota H. Solution behavior of new cationic surfactants derived from Guerbet alcohols and their use in hair conditioners. Int J Cosmet Sci. 1991;13:221-34.
32. Jurczyk MF. A new quaternary conditioner for damaged hair. Cosmet Toilet. 1991;106:91-5.

33. Rook A. The clinical importance of 'weathering' in human hair. Br J Dermatol. 1976;95:111-12.
34. Reich C. Hair cleansers. In: Rieger MM, Rhein LD (Eds). Surfactants in Cosmetics, 2nd edition. New York: Marcel Dekker; 1997. p. 373.
35. Sykes AR, Hammes PA. The use of Merquat polymers in cosmetics. Drug Cosmet Ind. 1980;1:62-6.
36. Faucher JA, Goddard ED. Influence of surfactants on the sorption of a cationic polymer by keratinous substrates. J Colloid Int Sci. 1976;55(2):313-9.
37. Tango Y, Shimmoto K. Development of a device to measure human hair luster. J Cosmet Sci. 2001;52:237-50.
38. Robinson VN. A study of damaged hair. J Soc Cosmet Chem. 1976;27:155-61.
39. Yahagi K. Silicones as conditioning agents in shampoos. J Soc Cosmet Chem. 1992;43:275-84.
40. Madnani N, Khan K. Hair cosmetics. Indian J Dermatol Venereol Leprol. 2013;79:654-67.
41. Gavazzoni Dias MF. Hair cosmetics: an overview. Int J Trichology. 2015;7(1):2-15.
42. Rele AS, Mohile RB. Effect of mineral oil, sunflower oil, and coconut oil on prevention of hair damage. J Cosmet Sci. 2003;54:175-92.
43. Harhar H, Gharby S, Kartah BE, et al. Long argan fruit drying time is detrimental for argan oil quality. Nat Prod Commun. 2010;5:1799-802.
44. Aidoud A, Ammouche A, Garrido M, et al. Effect of lycopene-enriched olive and argan oils upon lipid serum parameters in Wistar rats. J Sci Food Agric. 2014;94:2943-50.
45. El Abbassi A, Khalid N, Zbakh H, et al. Physicochemical characteristics, nutritional properties, and health benefits of argan oil: a review. Crit Rev Food Sci Nutr. 2014;54:1401-14.
46. Oh JY, Park MA, Kim YC. Peppermint oil promotes hair growth without toxic signs. Toxicol Res. 2014;30(4):297-304.

9

CHAPTER

Salon Hair Procedures

Jaishree Sharad, Jasmine M Gandhi

INTRODUCTION

Salon hair procedures are getting more and more popular by the day. The quest for lustrous, nonfrizzy, and voluminous hair has created a huge market for these procedures. Hair coloring, straightening, and perming are the other procedures which make the hair dry, frizzy, thin, brittle, and unruly as a result of which people get lured into doing keratin, cysteine, and other salon therapies.

In the market, a range of products are available today, which include shampoos, conditioners, serums, hair styling products, and hair nourishing products to choose from, for the daily needs. Apart from these, hair can be modified with the use of blow dryers, straighteners, curlers, and artificial extensions or through different salon procedures like hair coloring, chemical straightening, keratin, cysteine treatment, and perming. However, the hair shaft damage caused by all these products disrupts the overlapping cuticles, making hair vulnerable to breakage.

ANATOMY

Hair consists of two structures: (i) The hair follicle inside the skin and (ii) the shaft. Hair shaft is made up of cuticles, cortex, and medulla from outside to the center.

The thickest portion of hair shaft is cortex. It is made up of approximately 50–60% of microfibrils embedded into a matrix. Alpha-keratin intermediate filaments (α-KIF) is a major structural component of the cortex and is an obligate heteropolymer, containing type 1 and 2 polypeptide chain. Sixteen KIF forms one microfibril.[1] Cortex plays an important role in maintaining the physical and mechanical properties of hair.

The cuticle is the outermost protective layer having 5–10 overlapping cells, made up of compact cuticular keratin and high sulfur proteins. The visible length of each cuticle is about 50 lm with 0.3–0.5 lm in thickness. Cuticle has various sublamellar structures (the epicuticle, A-layer, exocuticle, endocuticle, and inner layer) and the cell membrane complex. The outermost hydrophobic cell layer is the epicuticle that defenses hair against water. Beneath this, is the A-layer, which is rich in cysteine. The oxidation of thiol groups of these adjacent cysteine residues form disulfide bonds, which give structural strength and rigidity to the cuticle. The B-layer also called the exocuticle lies immediately below, trailed by the endocuticle which has the least cysteine content. This layer swells up by absorbing water, allowing change in the physical properties of hair. The cellular membrane complex (CMC) separates each cell from the one below. Eighteen methyleicosanoic acid (18-MEA) is an important lipid component of this hydrophobic layer.[2] The integrity and properties of the cuticle layers are crucial in protecting the inner cortex from physical and chemical insults and in maintaining integrity of the hair shaft.[3] Damage to the cuticle by various physical and chemical processes lifts the free margins of the cuticular cells, eventually leading to exposure of the cortex and fracture of the hair shaft.

Alpha-keratin, assumes a helical structure, constituting of amino acids in long sequences (>300).

Two such helical pairs then coil around each other, to form a coiled-coil in a left-handed fashion. A pair of such coiled-coil structures attracts each other and sticks together. These four with another similar structure of four constitute to form a hair filament. The sulfur group belonging to cysteine, an amino acid, can form sulfide bonds. Based on the number of interactions between filaments, the coils become tighter as noted in a curly hair. This shows that straight hair has lesser interactions than curly hair.

HAIR COLORING

The natural color of hair is determined by its melanin content. Both the amount of melanin and the proportions of eumelanin and pheomelanin (individually or mixed) control the final hair color. A second major contributor to hair color is age. With aging, hair becomes gray due to absence of melanin pigments. Inhibition of tyrosinase activity and accumulation of metabolites in melanocytes may contribute to graying.

Many hair coloring formulations are available in the market for consumer usage. Hair coloring molecules can act as temporary, semipermanent, or permanent, based on their molecular size.[4,5]

TYPES OF HAIR DYE

- Gradual hair dye
- Temporary
- Semipermanent
- Demipermanent
- Permanent.

Gradual Hair Dye

Also called metallic/progressive hair dye, these dyes contains salts of metals (lead, silver, and bismuth) in a liquid form that get deposited on the hair shaft as sulfides and oxides. Large molecules of temporary hair dyes cannot penetrate hair cortex; hence repeated application is needed to get the desired shade. It is useful in individuals allergic to paraphenylenediamine (PPD). The messy application and not so perfect shades of color are some of the disadvantages of gradual hair dye. For example, vegetal (non-PPD), and Indigo leaf powder.

Temporary Hair Dye

There are a significant number of people who desire a color change for a single event, and wish to remove that color at the following shampoo; for them temporary hair color can be beneficial. These are textile acid dyes (FDC and DC) blue, red, green, and violet. Mechanism of action involves deposition of acid dyes on the surface of the hair. As these dyes have little affinity for hair, precipitation is required to deposit the dye and cationic surfactants or cationic polymers do that. For example, silver shampoo.

Semi-permanent Hair Dye

It is available as a preformed water-soluble mixture.[6] Dye components comprise yellow to orange ortho and paranitroanilines, violet to blue amino and hydroxyl anthraquinones, and yellow to violet nitrophenylenediamines. Major use of semi-permanent colorants is for the limited gray hair coverage (<30% gray) because of its low intensity. The dye gets diffused into the hair cortex because of low molecules, without any chemical reactions; therefore causes little or no damage. The product is applied on wet hair and rinsed off after 20 minutes. A conditioner is used post shampooing. As the name suggests, color gets reduced with each wash and is completely washed off in six to eight washes.

Demi-permanent Hair Dye[4,7,8]

Demi-permanent dye contains lower concentration of hydrogen peroxide (H_2O_2) (2%) compared to permanent hair dye[4] and does not contain ammonia, causing less irritation to the scalp, and damage to the hair shaft. It can create more color change and last longer than semi-permanent. This type of dye can last for 12–24 washes before completely washing out. It adds darker color to hair, and so is beneficial for covering gray hair covering gray hair but it may not lighten hair significantly due to the small amount of peroxide. L'Oréal Paris Crème Gloss color, Wella Color Charm Demipermanent color, and Garnier HerbaShine Color Crème are the few demi-permanent dye available in Indian market.

Permanent Hair Dye

Permanent dyes are the most commonly used hair dyes because of their longevity. A wide range of dyes are available which can produce lighter or darker shades than the natural hair color. These contain dye precursors [PPD or paratoluenediamine (PTD)], H_2O_2, and couplers with or without ammonia.[4,9] Entry of hair dyes into the cortex is facilitated by ammonia. This is done by alkaline agents like sodium carbonate and ethanolamine present in ammonia free dyes. The final pH achieved is 8–9 (Flowchart 1).

VEGETABLE DYE

Henna (*Lawsonia alba*) is a natural organic substance. The active ingredient in henna is 2-hydroxy-1,4-naphthoquinone, which is obtained by treating henna leaves with sodium bicarbonate. For example, vegetal (contains henna and other herbs).

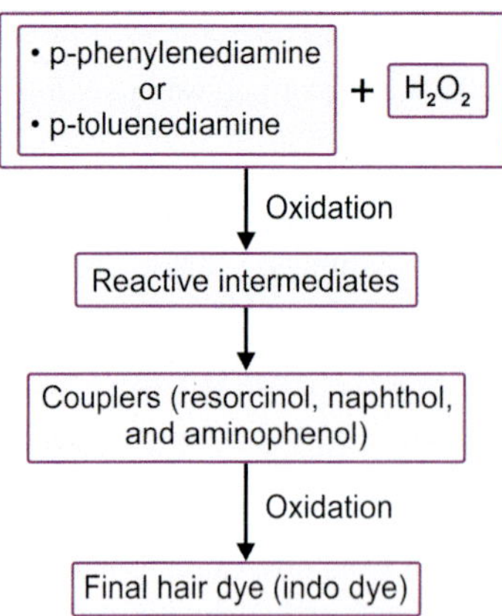

FLOWCHART 1: Mechanism of action of permanent hair dyes.

Indigofera tinctoria is another natural dye available as a green powder for commercial use.

ADVERSE EFFECTS

- Structural damage: Hair dyes damage 18-MEA, an important hydrophobic layer, making the hair more coarse and dull.[10] Paraphenylenediamine induces apoptosis of cells and thus contributes to hair fall.[11]
- Contact dermatitis:[12] The PPD in hair dye is mainly responsible for the irritant or allergic contact dermatitis. Ammonia-free dyes, although gentler to the hair shaft, do not prevent PPD reaction. Photoallergic dermatitis and dye-induced depigmentation which tend to run along the hairline have also been observed. This is more apparent with subsequent applications of the dye. Hence, it is important to do patch tests before using a hair dye.
  Options for individuals allergic to PPD:
  - Semipermanent
  - Dyes containing PTD
  - Metallic dyes
  - Pure henna
- Erythema multiforme, lymphomatoid reaction, and anaphylaxis are other uncommon adverse reactions following hair dye application.[13]
- Past studies show that certain chemicals in permanent hair dyes are structurally similar to aromatic amines and are known to cause bladder cancer. However, recent studies do not support any co-relation between the use of hair dye and malignancies of the bladder.[14-16]

SAFETY REGULATIONS FOR HAIR DYE

The permissible concentration of hair dye substances in oxidative hair dyes should not exceed 2% according to the European Commission directive regulation of 2009.

HAIR STRAIGHTENING

Different hair straightening procedures are available to ensure straight, shiny, and silky hair. The basic principle in straightening involves breaking down the disulfide bonds between the keratin filament and re-arranging and reforming these bonds.

Temporary Hair Straightening

Also called hair pressing method, temporary hair straightening is achieved using a flat iron. Small strips of hair are passed through heated tongs to achieve straight hair and the same process is repeated in all the hair sections.[3,17] The heat temporarily breaks and then reforms the hydrogen bonds in the cortex. Excess heat may damage the hair.[18,19] Hair serum is advisable to be used before this procedure to minimize hair damage from excess heat acquired. Trichorrhexis nodosa is the most common hair shaft anomaly caused due to heat damage to the hair.[20]

Semipermanent Straightening[21]

It is also called lanthionization, as cysteine bonds convert to lanthionine using chemical relaxers in this procedure.

Strong alkaline agents are used as chemical relaxers. These are:

- Sodium/potassium hydroxide (1.5–3.5%) (lye based)
- Guanidine/lithium hydroxide (no lye relaxers).

The pH of these straighteners is high (between 12.5 and 14) causing irritation to eyes, hands, and scalp and hence, should only be handled by trained professionals.

Higher pH of the solution lifts the outer cuticles favoring the entry of alkaline agents into the endocuticle.[22]

A chemical reaction that occurs between alkalis and cysteine, forms lanthionine which is a stable thioester crosslink.

Alkalis + Keratin cysteine → Lanthionine.[23]

Japanese Hair Straightening

Also called thermal reconditioning, this process involves supercontraction and transformation of alpha keratin proteins into amorphous proteins using a reducing agent named thioglycolic acid.

Advantages of thioglycolate over lye-based reducer:

- Ammonium thioglycolate, instead of disrupting the entire cysteine protein, only weakens the cysteine bond causing no lanthionization with 90% retention of the initial cysteine content[24]
- Less protein loss than hydroxides
- Less caustic (pH—9-9.5)

Therefore, in this procedure, cysteine bonds are weakened using thioglycolate followed by flat iron use to achieve permanent straightening. Later, H_2O_2 is used to neutralize thioglycolate.

Basic hair straightening procedure involves three main steps:

1. First step (reducing phase): It involves application of softening agent to the wet partitioned hair sections, followed by combing the hair sections to restructure the position of disulfide bonds. The solution is left on for half an hour. The hair is checked in between for the degree of softening. Once the desired softening is achieved, the hair is rinsed and conditioned
2. Second step: The hair is then "ironed" and a neutralizer is applied. Neutralizer is kept on for 20 minutes
3. Third step: The hair is again rinsed and dried and ironed.

The next hair wash and conditioning is advised after 24 hours.

The two terms that are very popular nowadays are: (i) Hair rebonding and (ii) hair smoothening. Both procedures are quite similar. Smoothening is 70-80% straightening that gives a natural look while rebonding is 100% straightening that gives poker straight hair. Results last for 10-12 months and 6-8 months for rebonding and smoothening, respectively. Use of hot iron is more in rebonding as compared to that in smoothening. As the name suggests, hair rebonding breaks down original hair bonds with the use of chemical relaxers and they are then rearranged by the use of neutralizer and hot iron.

Use of specialized shampoos and deep conditioning is advised postprocedure to ensure minimal damage to the hair.

Even when performed correctly, straightening causes irreplaceable damage to hydrophobic 18-MEA layer, which reduces the tensile strength. This makes hair more porous leading to loss of proteins and moisture, resulting in dry, brittle hair, and severe hair fall.[25-27]

A study done by Shetty et al., on post straightening hair damage showed following adverse effects: Frizzy hair in 67%, dandruff in 61%, hair loss and thinning in 47% and 40%, respectively, graying of hair in 22%, and split ends in 17%.[23]

A research done by Dias TC et al. showed beneficial effect with the addition of conditioning agent to the straightening solution, in terms of less protein loss and improvement of the resistance to breakage. Conditioning agents like Jojoba oil and lauryl methicone showed the best results.[28]

It is best to avoid repeated and frequent sessions, as damage by successive straightening is additive.

KERATIN TREATMENT

"Chemical relaxers" is the name given to the traditional hair straighteners, which are often responsible for dry and frizzy hair due to which keratin and cysteine treatments have emerged. Keratin treatments became popular in Brazil as early as 2003 and hence they are popularly also known as Brazilian keratin treatments.[29] Brazilian keratin treatment gives more natural looking, smooth, and shiny hair than chemical relaxers.

Major component of keratin therapy is formaldehyde as the hair is remodeled straight by disruption of hydrogen bonds in keratin by water and precisely aligned crosslinking of the newly formed keratin filaments by formaldehyde, resulting in straight hair.

The solution is applied to the hair and after a gap of 20-30 minutes, the hair is subjected twice to hot iron to incorporate the solution into the hair shaft. Strong smell, burning, and watering of eyes are common complaints experienced by customers because of formaldehyde.

The International Agency for Research on Cancer classifies formaldehyde as a human carcinogen and the recommendation is that salon hair products should not have more than 2% formaldehyde.[30]

CYSTEINE THERAPY

Due to serious health concerns associated with formaldehyde and hair damage caused with chemical relaxers, safer options are becoming popular. Carbocysteine is one such treatment which is a combination of glyoxylic acid + cysteine + acetic acid. It has become popular as formaldehyde free treatment. The glyoxylic acid actually belongs to the aldehyde group, albeit in small concentrations.

HAIR PERMING[9,30]

The process of chemically treating for rather permanent curls is called perming; another synonym for the same is permanent waving, which is achieved by relaxing, rearranging, and refixing the bonds.[3]

The polypeptide chains are interlinked using disulfide bonds. Thiol compounds are used in perm, as reducing agents, which are achieved by breaking the sulfide bond, each with a hydrogen atom. Polypeptide chains then assume a new shape. With the help of H_2O_2, the earlier broken bonds among the peptide chain are reformed by "oxidation" process, whence the disulfide bonds are reformed after removing the hydrogen atoms, which then result in water molecules. It is important to carefully rinse and thoroughly blot the hair before neutralizing the thiol compound, since the extent of oxidation may lighten the hair color.

The solution containing ammonium thioglycolate, also known as perm salt, is applied to the hair and kept for 20 minutes. This is then neutralized using an oxidizing agent (H_2O_2) and left on for 15 minutes on the hair strands that are rolled around the rollers and upto 5 minutes after removing all the rollers. The disulfide bonds are reformed and the hair comes off the rod with a curl. The hair is then rinsed. Shampooing is done after 2 days. The curls usually open a bit in a few weeks.

HAIR SPA

Hair spa has become the most preferred treatment for malnourished, dry, brittle, and rough hair with split ends. This procedure involves deep conditioning to nourish each strand of hair and includes five steps: (i) Massaging, (ii) steaming, (iii) washing, (iv) conditioning, and (v) applying hair mask. After shampooing, a spa cream is applied to all hair strands by making small partitions, after which hair strands are covered with a hot towel or steam is given to increase the absorption which is followed by massaging and washing after 20 minutes. Hot drying is avoided after spa treatment. Though hair spa is becoming more popular with each passing day, the science behind it is not fully known. More scientific studies are required to comment on its long-term effects on hair.

CONCLUSION

There is no significant clinical research published on all the therapies. However, as dermatologists, we should be aware of the pros and cons of these salon procedures to be able to guide our patients. The need for good evidenced based data remains.

REFERENCES

1. Wolfram LJ. Human hair: a unique physicochemical composite. J Am Acad Dermatol. 2003;48(6 Suppl): S106-14.
2. Swift JA. Human hair cuticle: Biologically conspired to the owner's advantage. J Soc Cosmet Chem. 1999;50(1): 23-47.
3. Bolduc C, Shapiro J. Hair care products: waving, straightening, conditioning, and coloring. Clin Dermatol. 2001;19(4):431-6.
4. Neuser F, Schlatter H. Hair dyes. In: Draelos ZD (Ed). Cosmetic Dermatology: Products and Procedures. USA: Duke University School of Medicine; 2010. pp. 256-310.
5. Harrison S, Sinclair R. Hair colouring, permanent styling and hair structure. J Cosmet Dermatol. 2003;2(3-4):180-5.
6. Corbett JF. Hair dyes – their chemistry and toxicology. Cosmet Toilet. 1976;91:21-8.
7. Guerra-Tapia A, Gonzalez-Guerra E. Hair cosmetics: dyes. Actas Dermosifiliogr. 2014;105(9):833-9.
8. Gray J. The World of Hair Colour: A Scientific Companion, 1st edition. Croatia: Thompson Learning; 2004.
9. Draelos ZK. Hair cosmetics. Dermatol Clin. 1991;9(1):19-27.
10. Chye SM, Tiong YL, Yip WK, et al. Apoptosis induced by para-phenylenediamine involves formation of ROS and activation of p38 and JNK in chang liver cells. Environ Toxicol. 2014;29(9):981-90.
11. Ishida W, Makino T, Shimizu T. Severe hair loss of the scalp due to a hair dye containing Para phenylenediamine. ISRN Dermatol. 2011;2011:947284.
12. Koley S, Sarkar J, Choudhary S, et al. Erythema multiforme following application of hair dye. Indian J Dermatol. 2012;57(3):230-2.
13. Mavroleon G, Begishvili B, Frew AJ. Anaphylaxis to hair dye: A case report. Clin Exp Allergy. 1998;28(1): 121-2.
14. Shafer N, Shafer RW. Potential of carcinogenic effects of hair dyes. N Y State J Med. 1976;76(3):394-6.
15. Saitta P, Cook CE, Messina JL, et al. Is there a true concern regarding the use of hair dye and malignancy development?: A review of the epidemiological evidence relating personal hair dye use to the risk of malignancy. J Clin Aesthet Dermatol. 2013;6(1):39-46.
16. Bolt HM, Golka K. The debate on carcinogenicity of permanent hair dyes: New insights. Crit Rev Toxicol. 2007;37(6):521-36.
17. Quinn CR, Quinn TM, Kelly AP. Hair care practices in African American women. Cutis. 2003;72(4):280-2, 285-9.
18. Gummer CL. Evaluation techniques. In: McMichael AJ, Hordinsky MK (Eds). Hair and Scalp Diseases: Medical, Surgical, and Cosmetic Treatments. New York: Informa Healthcare; 2008.
19. Whiting DA, Dy LC. Office diagnosis of hair shaft defects. Semin Cutan Med Surg. 2006;25(1):24-34.
20. Price VH. Structural Anomalies of the Hair Shaft. Berlin Heidelberg: Springer; 1990. pp. 363-422.
21. Gavazzoni Dias MF. Hair cosmetics: An overview. Int J Trichology. 2015;7(1):2-15.

22. Schueller R, Romanowski P. The science of reactive hair-care products: A review of changing natural hair appearences. Cosmet Toiletries. 1998;113(5):39-46.
23. Shetty VH, Shetty NJ, Nair DG. Chemical hair relaxers have adverse effects a myth or reality. Int J Trichology. 2013;5(1):26-8.
24. Wong M, Wis-Surel G, Epps J. Mechanism of hair straightening. J Soc Cosmet Chemists. 1994;45(6):347-52.
25. Smith RS, Shear G. Corneal alkali burns arising from accidental instillation of a hair straightener. Am J Ophthalmol. 1975;79(4):602-5.
26. Swee W, Klontz KC, Lambert LA. A nationwide outbreak of alopecia associated with the use of a hair-relaxing formulation. Arch Dermatol. 2000;136(9):1104-8.
27. Nicholson AG, Harland CC, Bull RH, et al. Chemically induced cosmetic alopecia. Br J Dermatol. 1993;128(5): 537-41.
28. Dias TC, Baby AR, Kaneko TM, et al. Protective effect of conditioning agents on Afro-ethnic hair chemically treated with thioglycolate-based straightening emulsion. J Cosmet Dermatol. 2008;7(2):120-6.
29. Weathersby C, McMichael A. Brazilian keratin hair treatment: a review. J Cosmet Dermatol. 2013;12(2):144-8.
30. Maneli MH, Smith P, Khumalo NP. Elevated formaldehyde concentration in "Brazilian keratin type" hair-straightening products: A cross-sectional study. J Am Acad Dermatol. 2014;70(2):276-80.

2

SECTION

BOTULINUM TOXIN

10
CHAPTER

Science of Botulinum Toxin

Rasya Dixit

INTRODUCTION

Botulinum toxin (BoNT or BTX) is an exotoxin derived from *Clostridium botulinum*.[1] The dreadful neurotoxin which causes botulism, but offers a treatment option for multiple medical and cosmetic indications, has made this bacterium as one of the serendipitous discoveries in medical history. This discovery and development of this dangerous toxin into a medical remedy is a journey through medical history.

HISTORY

The story of "botulinum" begins in the late 1700s where the Napoleonic wars (1795–1813) led to poor sanitary measures in rural Europe's food production. This led to an outbreak of severe food poisoning-related deaths in the community of Stuttgart.[2] The primary source was linked to the food, namely the half cooked sausages which were being consumed during the wars. In 1802, the government of Stuttgart undertook various measures to prevent the consumption of these sausages. The health authorities attributed these deaths to a substance called prussic acid[3] and the name "botulism" was coined for this disease derived from Latin for sausage.[4]

Finally, the medical community was asked for their opinion. The first report of suspicion of a zoonic or organic poison came from Wilhelm Gottfried von Ploucquet.[2] Then Autenrieth described the clinical symptoms of foodborne botulism. He collected the works of the case officers and described the symptoms of diarrhea, double vision, and dilation of the iris as the symptoms of this condition, the so called sausage poisoning.[2]

Assisting Autenrieth with their reports were JG Steinbuch and Justinus Kerner, two medical officers working independently reported similar observations. These observations were published by Autenrieth.[5]

The first series of cases about BoNT poisoning was published in 1817 by Kerner.[6] He then intensified his toxin research and started animal experiments as well as experimentation on himself. He wanted to isolate the toxin from the sausages which he called the "fatty toxin." The results of his work was published as a monograph, which contained the clinical examination, summary, and even postmortem results of 155 patient with probable botulism. As a result of his experiments, Kerner made several important observations about this toxin. He postulated that the toxin developed under anaerobic conditions. He even deduced that the toxin acted by interruption of signal transmission in the peripheral nervous systems, the sympathetic and parasympathetic nervous systems, leaving the sensory nervous system intact.

Kerner also accurately described all the clinical neurological symptoms of botulism including vomiting, dysphagia, intestinal cramps, mydriasis, ptosis, and respiratory distress.[5] He was also the first to suggest therapeutic opportunities using the toxin in lowering sympathetic activity in movement disorders as well as hypersecretion of body fluids such as sweat.[6] Though his attempts to isolate the toxin failed, Kerner also suspected that the toxin was a protein of infectious origin. For the prevention of sausage poisoning, he advocated that the sausages should be boiled long enough, and stored under dry and aerobic conditions.

DISCOVERY OF THE BACTERIUM

Robert Koch (1843–1910) was the first scientist to associate certain diseases to microorganisms. He is credited with the discoveries of anthrax, cholera, and tuberculosis. In 1895, there was an outbreak of botulism in the Belgium. Émile van Ermengem (1851–1922), a microbiologist who trained under Koch, was the first to correlate botulism with a bacterium found in the postmortem tissue of the victims with a bacterium seen in raw pork.[7,8] The isolated bacterium was named *Bacillus botulinus*.[8]

DISCOVERY OF THE TOXIN

It was not till the 1920s that the pure isolate of botulinum toxin A (BoNT A or BTX A) was isolated by Dr. Hermann Sommer from California.[9] Seeding the need for biological warfare, research on this toxin took a macabre turn, when during World War II, the American strategic office ordered the manufacture of the toxin in a manner suitable for biological warfare. The plan was to assassinate high level Japanese officials by slipping these capsules into their food with the help of Chinese prostitutes. However, the project failed as the animal testing of this batch of toxin that was done on donkeys failed.[9,10]

However, research into the toxin and its properties continued, and in 1946, Dr. Edward Schantz and his colleagues at the US Army campus were able to isolate large quantities of purified BoNT. It was not until 1972 when the Biological Toxins and Weapons Convention Treaty was signed by more than 100 countries that the United States declared that all their biological weapons stocks would be destroyed.[11] All research oriented toward biological warfare stopped at Fort Detrick.

Dr. Schantz moved to the University of Wisconsin, where he continued his research into botulism and other foodborne toxins for medical use. His batch containing 200 mg of twice crystallized toxin was approved for human use by Food and Drug Administration (FDA) in 1978, and the same preparation retained its toxicity and was in use till 1997.[12] This was because biological drugs need a batch-wise approval from FDA. So it was till 1997, the same batch or 150 mg of toxin was used in over 250,000 treatments in humans. In 1997, the FDA approved a new bulk toxin source for the manufacture of BTX A.[13]

A THERAPEUTIC BREAKTHROUGH

Dr. Vernon Brooks triggered the renewed interest in BTX as a therapeutic agent, when he injected BoNT A into a hyperactive muscle and induced a temporary paralysis of the same by blocking the release of acetylcholine (Ach) from motor nerve endings.[14] Then came the work of Dr. Alan Scott, an ophthalmologist who found that small amounts of BTX was able to correct strabismus in animal models.[15] Over a period of next two decades, Dr. Scott and Dr. Schantz collaborated to develop BoNT A for human use.[14] In 1978, when the FDA approved the batch for human use. Between 1980 and 1990, a master batch record was written for the manufacture of medical grade BoNT, and in 1991 a pharmaceutical company called Allergan bought the research findings and renamed the agent as Botoxä.

Meanwhile, when the ophthalmologists were injecting toxin into the periocular muscles, neurologists recognized the potential benefits of the toxin in blockage of involuntary muscle contractions in larger muscle groups. In 1989, the FDA approved BoNT A for the treatment of involuntary muscle contractions, strabismus, blepharospasm, and hemifacial spasm. To see the complete list of treatment indications, refer box 1.[16-19]

Canadian ophthalmologist Jean Carruthers, in 1987, made an observation in her patients treated for blepharospasm with BoNT A. The frown lines had markedly disappeared. Together with her

BOX 1 The different commercially available preparations of botulinum toxin

Botulinum toxin A

- OnabotulinumtoxinA (BOTOX®; Allergan; Irvine, CA, USA) BoNT A
- AbobotulinumtoxinA (Dysport®; Ipsen; Paris, France)
- IncobotulinumtoxinA (Xeomin®; Merz Pharmaceuticals, Frankfurt, Germany)
- CS-BOT (Chiba Serum Institute; Chiba, Japan)
- Chinese BTX-A (Prosigne®; Lanzhou Biological Products Institute, China)

Botulinum toxin B

- Myobloc/Neurobloc (US World Meds, Louisville, KY, USA)
- The different toxins differ in potency and doses cannot be interchanged for one other.[20] For example, clinically u of BoNT A is equal to 3 units of Dysport®[21]
- Studies of Xeomin® and Prosigne® use unit dosing comparable (1:1) with BOTOX®[22,23]
- Botulinum toxin B is marketed in the United States as rimabotulinumB (MyoBloc®). This preparation is a ready-to-use solution that does not require reconstitution; it is available in three vial sizes (i.e., 2,500 U, 5,000 U, and 10,000 U) and is stable for up to 21 months in refrigerator storage
- 1 U of BoNT A is equal to 50–100 U of MyoBloc®

dermatologist husband Alistair Carruthers, she had discovered a treatment that would revolutionize the world of medical aesthetics and antiaging treatments. In 1996, and later 1998, the first publications listing the use of this toxin in medical aesthetic practice came out.[24,25] To this day, multiple cosmetic and noncosmetic indications of the toxin have been described, and the search to find further clinical applications goes on.

PHYSIOLOGY

Clostridium botulinum elaborates seven antigenically different exotoxins (A, B, C1, D, E, F, and G) from seven different serotypes. Type A is the most potent toxin, followed by types B and F toxin. Types A, B, and E are commonly associated with systemic botulism in humans.[26] Type C is toxic to the cell but not the neuron. Only Type A and Type B are available commercially.

Biological activity of the toxin is measured in mouse units, mouse LD50 (lethal dose, 50%) or simply a unit. This is the dose of toxin needed to kill half the test mouse population after injection.[27,28] While LD50 calculations for humans are projections from primate data, 2,700–3,000 mouse units is the dose usually cited as the lethal dose for a 70 kg human.[29]

All the exotoxins are produced as a relatively inactive molecule of molecular weight around 150 kDA. The unique part of this molecule is that the neurotoxin itself is a zinc binding metalloprotease. This single chain polypeptide undergoes endogenous cleavage inside the bacterium to yield an active molecule with a heavy chain of about 100 kDA heavy chain and a light chain of 50 kD (also known as the endopeptidase, associated with an atom of zinc). A disulfide bond, in complex with hemagglutinin and nontoxin-nonhemagglutinin proteins, holds the heavy and light chains together.[30] The size of the neurotoxin depends on the serotype and the associated nontoxic accessory proteins or neurotoxin associated proteins (NAPs). Both the proteins are cosynthesized by the bacteria and spontaneously associate with each other. The size and molecular weight may determine the distance of diffusion of toxin from the point of injection.

ROLE OF NEUROTOXIN-ASSOCIATED PROTEINS

Neurotoxin-associated proteins are produced by the bacteria along with the neurotoxin. They may serve critical roles in protecting the core neurotoxin from conditions such as proteolytic enzymes, environmental stress, or pH changes especially the digestive enzymes.[31] Their role in intramuscular injections is less clear; however, they may serve to protect the core toxin from muscle proteases following intramuscular injection. Antibodies have also been described to NAPs; however, these are non-neutralizing antibodies, and do not have an effect on efficacy. Though the role of NAPs in clinical efficacy has not been evaluated, one of the important differences between the commercially available botulinum type A products is the amount of NAPs they contain.

Neurotoxic activation happens in two steps, the first is the cleavage of the parent chain between aminoacid 449 and 449 which gives rise to the light and heavy chains connected by the disulfide bond. In this form, the protein is internalized by the target cell, where the disulfide bond is reduced and the molecule is activated.[32] The integrity of the disulfide bond is essential for the toxins biological activity.

MECHANISM OF ACTION

Following intramuscular injection, BTX causes the stoppage of release of the Ach from the presynaptic nerve terminal. This blocks the neuromuscular signaling causing a denervation of the muscle. Muscle function returns after 12 weeks as nerve terminals sprout and reconnect with the endplate. Through a process of binding, internalization, translocation, and cleavage, the toxin exerts its inhibition on neuromuscular junction of smooth and striated muscle and the autonomic nerve terminals that innervates glands (Figs 1 and 2).

Dissociation

Dissociation of the 150 kDa neurotoxin from the NAPs is the first step in the mechanism of BoNT action. This dissociation is a function of pH and ionic strength. Eisele et al. have proposed that this dissociation happens inside the vial no sooner than the saline is added for reconstitution, and the naked neuroprotein was released from its associated complex in less than 1 minute with a change to physiological pH.[33]

Binding

The heavy (H) chain of the toxin binds to the receptors at the presynaptic surface of the neurones by a two receptor interaction between the botulinum

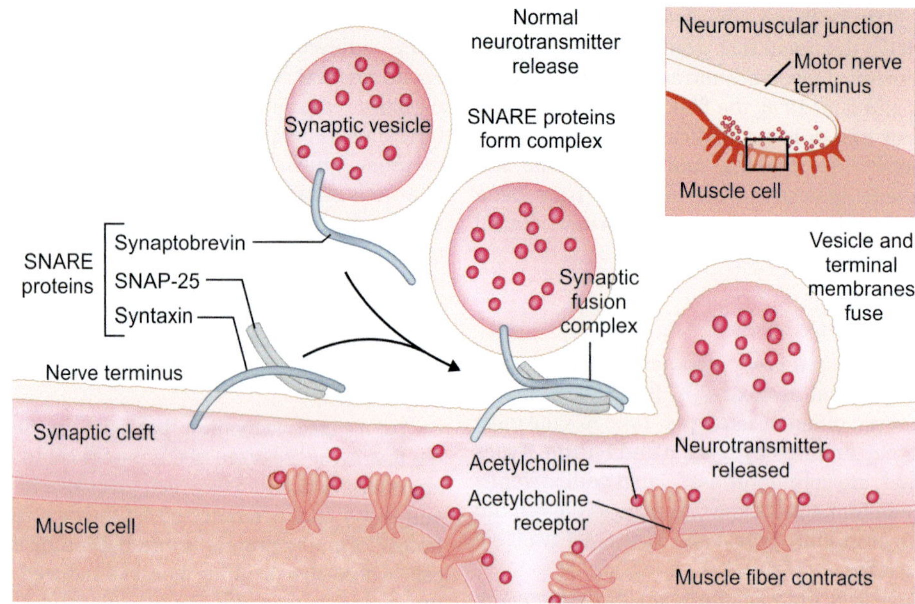

SNAP, synaptosomal-associated protein; SNARE, Soluble N-ethylmaleimide-sensitive factor attachment protein receptor.

FIG. 1: Mechanism of action of botulinum neurotoxins.

molecule and its target cell. Then the synaptic vesicle 2 (SV2) interacts with the heavy chain and the toxin-receptor complex is endocytosed and enters the neuronal cytoplasm.[34,35]

Internalization

Once bound to SV2, the receptor-toxin complex is endocytosed. Inside these vesicles, the peptide toxin folds on itself due to the pH change as the proton pumps in the endocytosomal wall lower the pH.[36] The endopeptidase on the heavy chain cleaves the disulfide bond between the heavy and the light and the toxin escapes into the cytoplasm of the neuron through the lipid bilayer of the endosome.

Cleavage

In the neuronal cytoplasm, the light (L) chain interacts with its target proteins in the SNARE complex. This complex normally enables calcium mediated exocytosis of the neurotransmitters. The light chain contains proteases, which cleave one or more proteins in the SNARE complex, making them inactive. Different BoNT serotypes have distinct SNARE protein targets. For example, BoNT A cleaves synaptosomal-associated protein (SNAP 25), botulinum toxin B (BoNT B) cleaves synaptobrevin or vesicle-associated membrane protein (VAMP).[37]

Recovery from the Action of Botulinum Toxin

The neuromuscular signaling is not permanently blocked by BTX. The inactive muscle sends growth factors to signal the silenced nerve. Axonal sprouts arise from the nerve endings and make immature synapses with the muscle. Over time, complete activity returns to the neuromuscular junction. This return in function signals the end of clinical result.

Lowe et al. and Dmochowski et al. observed that the duration of clinical efficacy was 3–4 months in skeletal muscle, and in contrast was longer than 6 months in tissues innervated by autonomic nervous system. The reason for this clinical difference is unknown.[38,39]

Botulinum toxin has also been used for the treatment of migraine and headache. Here, the mechanism of action is postulated to be the inhibition of secretion of several neurochemicals that stimulate nociceptive receptors including glutamate, substance P, and calcitonin gene related peptide (CGRP).[40] Morenilla-Palao and colleagues showed that BoNT A treatment causes a downregulation of transient receptor potential vanilloid type 1, which is known to be activated by capsaicin, protons, and noxious heat.[41]

Botulinum toxin does not work as an anesthetic as it does not affect the A beta or A delta fibers which

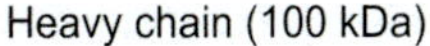

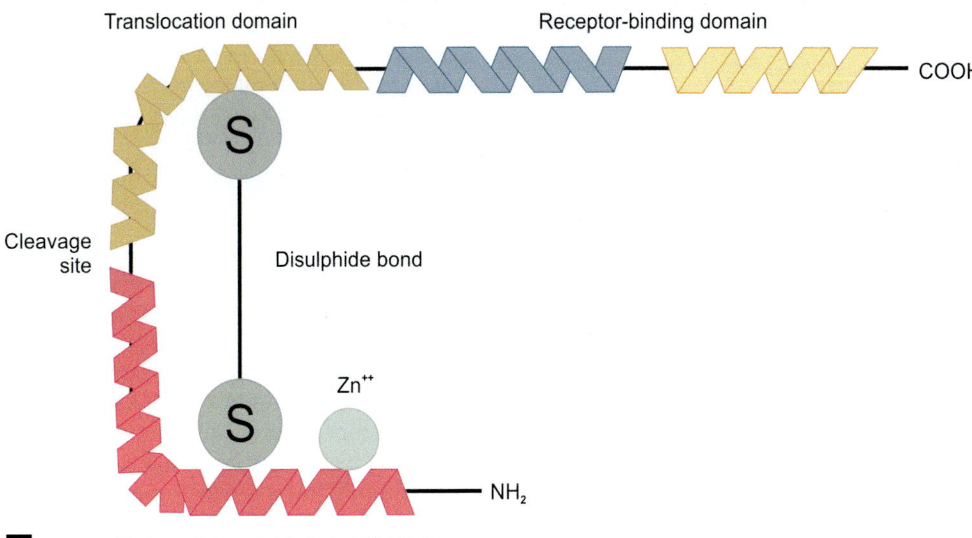

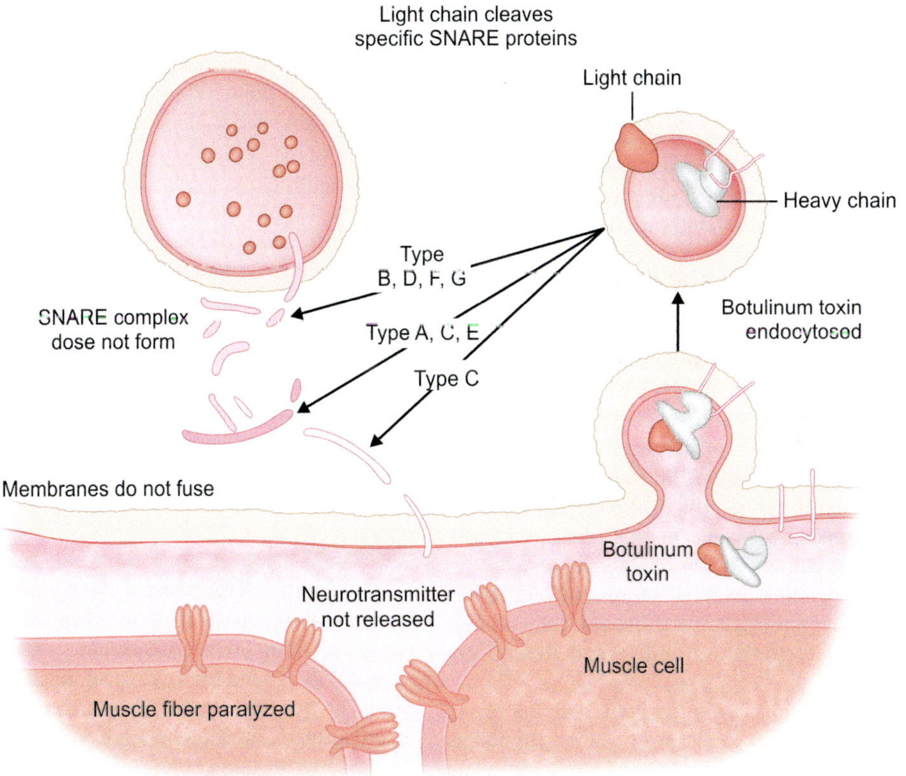

SNARE, Soluble N-ethylmaleimide-sensitive factor attachment protein receptor.

FIG. 2: Molecular structure of botulinum toxin type A. Once the botulinum neurotoxin is injected, the toxin is endocytosed. The heavy chain then is cleaved from the light chain through the zinc-dependent endopeptidase. Then the light chains are released into the cytoplasm, where the specific SNARE proteins are cleaved. This stops the formation of the SNARE complex, which in turn means that the acetyl choline is not released from the vesicles.

carry information of touch, pressure, and pain, as these fibers do not release neurochemicals at their ends.

MANUFACTURING

The production of BoNT begins with the fermentation of *Clostridium* bacterium in an anaerobic environment, which releases the toxin into the bacterial broth. Then, the neurotoxin is purified from the bacterial broth. Each manufacturer has their own proprietary method of purification of the bacterial contents, resulting in their unique product. In order to stablize the toxin, excipients are added. They help to prevent protein aggregation and cryoprotectant. It also prevents loss from surface adsorption. Finally, the product is dried with freezing (Dysport®, Ipsen, Inc.) or vacuum dried (Botox®, Allergan). Botulinum neurotoxin B is stable in solution and is not dried.

BOTULINUM TOXIN FORMULATIONS

Botulinum toxin formulations differ by their molecular weight, protein size, serotype strain, and preparation/purification process. These factors affect the onset of action, longevity of effect, and the chances of diffusion. Box 1 lists the various commercially available preparations of BoNT, it sums up the comparison of different commercially available preparations of botulinum toxin.

RECONSTITUTION AND STORAGE

Botox® is available in a sterile vial in lyophilized form. It is recommended to be stored in at or below –5°C. The BTX is reconstituted with sterile 0.9% NaCl.

As Botox® is thought to be sensitive to agitation or frothing during reconstitution with NaCl care has to be taken during dilution. Saline is introduced by just plunging the needle of the syringe into the cap and the saline enters the vial due to vaccum. This process allows for us to determine whether the vial is vaccum sealed (if saline does not enter the vial by negative pressure, discard the vial) and also prevent frothing and inadvertent denaturing of protein.

Dilution of Botox® is often done with 2.5 mL of diluent being added to 100 units. Most physicians prefer this as it gives 4 U to every 0.1 mL. However, other dilutions can be used as per the treating physicians discretion. More dilute the solution; more is the diffusion of the toxin.

Once reconstituted, Botox® has to be used within 4 hours or stored at 4–8°. Do not freeze the reconstituted toxin. On keeping the toxin at room temperature, the toxin loses potency gradually with loss of up to 50% of potency within 14 hours. Refreezing the toxin can cause a loss of up to 70% and these are not recommended to be used as the efficacy may be unpredicatable.[42]

PHARMACOLOGY

Upon injection, BoNT requires 24–72 hours to take effect, possibly this is the time needed for the action at the neuromuscular junction. It may rarely take up to 5 days for results of toxin to be observed, and often the results last up to 24 weeks.

The time to reinjection can vary depending on the indication and the dose used. A study evaluating onabotulinum toxin and abobotulinumtoxin on glabellar lines showed the effect lasted for 3–4 months.[43] This is similar to most other cosmetic indications of the toxin. However, in the case of masseter hypertrophy, the improvement is seen after 6–8 weeks and results last for 6–12 months.

The neurotoxin needs to be injected into the target muscle precisely for the patient to benefit from the results and the physician to get predictable results each time. So a knowledge of anatomy is invaluable. Also it is important to understand the potential diffusion of various formulations of BoTX A. Abobotulinum had a greater diffusion when compared to onabotulinum.[44] Botulinum toxin B has the maximum local and systemic diffusion, and hence has a higher number of associated side effects. The other factors which affect diffusion are muscle selection, dose, and dilution. The more dilute the toxin, the more propensity it has to diffuse. So in an area or indication where there is high risk of side effects from toxin diffusion, BoNT can be diluted in a smaller volume of NaCl giving lesser risk of diffusion related side effects.

IMMUNOLOGY

Botulinum toxin group of toxins have been effective in the management of many chronic conditions, requiring long term treatment, with repeated neurotoxin treatment over prolonged periods of time. The development of resistance can be a major disadvantage as this toxin needs to be administered repeatedly. The toxin behaves as an antigen, as it is a foreign protein, and upon repeated exposure, there is an development of antibody response. Critchfield and Janovich have described the various factors for the development of antibody response to any antigen.

Two different types of antibodies develop after exposure to botulinum neurotoxin—neutralizing antibodies and nonneutralizing antibodies. Neutralizing antibodies have been described against the heavy chain of the molecule; however, neutralizing antibodies that bind to all the epitopes of the core have been described as well.[45]

In sufficient titres, these can inhibit the toxin by blocking its interaction with the neuronal receptors. The nonneutralizing antibodies are produced against the accessory proteins (NAPs) and they do not affect the efficacy of the toxin. In toxins containing NAPs, the NAPs may actually shield the core sites of the toxin and prevent neutralizing antibodies from developing.[46]

Factors That Predispose to the Development of Antibodies

The original toxin source which was initially used as a source for manufacturing neurotoxin contained 25 ng of neurotoxin per 100 U.[47] In 1997, when the updated bulk source for neurotoxin was made available the content fell to 5 ng/100 U. This has resulted in a significant decrease in immunogenicity.

The 150 kDa core of BoNT which is produced by the bacteria with is actually inactive also forms a target for development of antibodies. This inactive antigen needs to be kept as a minimum during the manufacturing process to keep the antigenicity low. To become activated, BoNT toxins are cleaved by the use of a protease.[47] The BoNT A is approximately 95% nicked endogenously before it is released from the cell; however, it is not the same with BoNT B. So during the manufacturing process, the BoNT B goes through more exposure to proteases. Despite this, 25-20% of product may stay inactive. This may explain the higher immunogenicity with BoNT B.[48]

Greene et al. postulated that large doses of BoNT A, (>250 U) and repeated "booster" injections could lead to development of antibodies.[49] This is understandable because resistance is more common in patients receiving larger doses of toxin for the treatment, as resistance is more common for patients receiving larger doses of toxin for therapeutic use (for example cervical dystonias) versus those that target smaller muscle groups (blepharospasm). Lange et al. reported that in secondary nonresponders, with a frequency between injections less than 2 months were more likely to have higher levels of neutralizing antibodies than those who had received injection at intervals longer than 4 months.[50]

RESISTANCE IN COSMETIC APPLICATIONS

In cosmetic use, BoNT is often used at lower doses than that for therapeutic use. Studies across the various toxins serotypes showed neutralizing antibodies in 0.13–1.4% of patients. However, there was no reduction in efficacy noted.[51-53]

IMMUNOGENICITY VERSUS CLINICAL NONRESPONSE

The immunogenicity of a protein is its ability to produce or stimulate an antibody response. However, it has to be differentiated from a clinical nonresponse. The clinical nonresponse may be primary, where the toxin fails to produce result in the patient from the first treatment itself, or secondary; where the patient responds at first, and then loses responsiveness with subsequent treatments. The secondary nonresponse may be due to the formation of the antibodies. However, the clinical nonresponse may not always be present even if neutralizing antibodies are present.[51]

It is important to look at technical details such as inadequate dosing, incorrect injection techniques, or improper identification of the muscle groups before looking for neutralizing antibodies. Changes in the indications and patient nonsatisfaction with results may in fact be a cause of secondary nonresponse.[54]

CONCLUSION

Botulinum toxin tops the charts as one of the most common cosmetic treatments world over, and has made the journey from deadly poison to a therapeutic treatment. Newer indications and formulations continue to emerge and the dermatologist should familiarize and equip themselves with current guidelines for treatment.

REFERENCES

1. Simpson LL. The origin, structure, and pharmacological activity of botulinum toxin. Pharmacol Rev. 1981;33(3):155-88.
2. Erbguth FJ, Naumann M. Historical aspects of botulinum toxin: Justinus Kerner (1786-1862) and the "sausage poison". Neurology. 1999;53(8):1850-3.
3. Erbguth FJ. Historical notes on botulism, Clostridium botulinum, botulinum toxin, and the idea of the therapeutic use of the toxin. Mov Disord. 2004;19(Supp. 8):S2-6.
4. Torrens JK. Clostridium botulinum was named because of association with 'sausage poisoning. BMJ. 1998; 316(7125):151.

5. Erbguth FJ, Naumann M. On the first systematic descriptions of botulism and botulinum toxin by Justinus Kerner (1786-1862). J Hist Neurosci. 2000;9(2):218-20.
6. Erbguth FJ. Historical note on the therapeutic use of botulinum toxin in neurological disorders. J Neurol Neurosurg Psychiat. 1996;60(2):151.
7. Gunn RA. Botulism: from van Ermengem to the present. A comment. Rev Infect Dis. 1979;1(4):720-1.
8. van Ermengem E. Classics in infectious diseases. A new anaerobic bacillus and its relation to botulism. Rev Infect Dis. 1979;1(4):701-19. (Originally published as 'Ueber einen neuen anaeroben Bacillus und seine Beziehungen zum Botulismus' in Zeitschrift fur Hygiene und Infektionskrankheiten 1897;26:1-56.)
9. Sotos JG. Botulinum toxin in biowarfare. JAMA. 2001; 285(21):2716.
10. Lamb A. Biological weapons: the facts not the fiction. Clin Med. 2001;1(6):502-4.
11. Meyler Z, Cooper G. History and mechanism of action. In: Cooper G (Ed). Therapeutic Uses of Botulinum Toxin. Berlin: Springer; 2017.
12. Klein AW. Cosmetic therapy with botulinum toxin, Anecdotal memoirs. Dermatol Surg. 1996;22(9):757-9
13. Kopera D. Botulinum toxin historical aspects: from food poisoning to pharmaceutical. Int J Dermatol. 2011; 50(8):976-80
14. Ting PT, Freiman A. The story of Clostridium botulinum: from food poisoning to Botox. Clin Med. 2004; 4(3):258-61.
15. Scott AB, Rosenbaum A, Collins CC. Pharmacologic weakening of extraocular muscles. Invest Ophthalmol. 1973;12(12):924-7.
16. Mahant N, Clouston PD, Lorentz IT. The current use of botulinum toxin. J Clin Neurosci. 2000;7(5):389-94.
17. Jankovic J, Brin MF. Botulinum toxin: historical perspective and potential new indications. Muscle Nerve Suppl. 1997;6:S129-45.
18. Binder WJ, Brin MF, Blitzer A, et al.. Botulinum toxin type A (BOTOX) for treatment of migraine. Semin Cutan Med Surg. 2001;20(2):93-100.
19. Verheyden J, Blitzer A, Brin MF. Other noncosmetic uses of BOTOX. Semin Cutan Med Surg. 2001;20(2):121-6.
20. Carruthers A, Kiene K, Carruthers J. Botulinum A exotoxin use in clinical dermatology. J Am Acad Dermatol. 1996;34(5 Pt. 1):788-97.
21. Carruthers A, Carruthers J. History of the cosmetic use of Botulinum A exotoxin. Dermatol Surg. 1998;24(11):1168-70.
22. Ellenhorn MJ, Barceloux DG. (Eds). Diagnosis and treatment of human poisoning. In Medical Toxicology. New York, NY: Elsevier; 1988. pp. 1185-7.
23. Dressler D. Botulinum Toxin Therapy. Stuttgart: Georg Thieme Verlag; 2000.
24. Brin MF, Aoki KR. Botulinum toxin type A: Pharmacology. In: Simpson DM, Mayer NH (Eds). Spasticity: Etiology, Evaluation, Management and the Role of Botulinum Toxin. New York: We Move Publications; 2002. pp. 100-9.
25. Muthane UB, Panikar JN. Botulinum toxins: Pharmacology and its current therapeutic evidence for use. Neurol India. 2003;51(4):455-60.
26. Brin MF. Botulinum toxin: chemistry, pharmacology, toxicity, and immunology. Muscle Nerve Suppl. 1997;6:S146-68.
27. Kukreja RV, Singh BR. Comparative role of neurotoxin-associated proteins in the structural stability and endopeptidase activity of botulinum neurotoxin complex types A and E. Biochemistry. 2007;46(49):14316-24.
28. Huang W, Foster JA, Rogachefsky AS. Pharmacology of botulinum toxin. J Am Acad Dermatol. 2000;43(2 Part 1):249-59.
29. Eisele KH, Fink K, Martin V, et al. Studies on dissociation of botulinum neurotoxin Type A complexes. Toxicon. 2011;57(4):555-65.
30. Rummel A. Double receptor anchorage of botulinum neurotoxins accounts for their exquisite neurospecificity. Curr Top Microbiol Immunol. 2013;364:61-90.
31. Peng L, Tepp WH, Johnson EA, et al. Botulinum neurotoxin D uses synaptic vesicle protein SV2 and gangliosides as receptors. PLoS Pathog. 2011;7(3):e1002008.
32. Yamashiro DJ, Fluss SR, Maxfield FR. Acidification of endocytic vesicles by an ATP-dependent proton pump. J Cell Biol. 1983;97(3):929-34.
33. Sikorra S, Henke T, Galli T, et al. Substrate recognition mechanism of VAMP/Synaptobrevin-cleaving clostridial neurotoxins. J Biol Chem. 2008;283(30):21145-52.
34. Lowe NJ, Lowe P. Botulinum toxins for facial lines: a concise review. Dermatol Ther. 2012;2(1);14.
35. Dmochowski R, Chapple C, Nitti VW, et al. Efficacy and safety of onabotulinum toxin A for idiopathic overactive bladder: a double-blind, placebo controlled, randomized, dose ranging trial. J Urol. 2010;184(6):2416-22.
36. Luvisetto S, Gazerani P, Cianchetti C, Pavone F. Botulinum toxin type A as a therapeutic agent against headache and related disorders. Toxins 2015;7(9):3818-44.
37. Morenilla-Palao C, Planells-Cases R, Garcia-Sanz N, et al. Regulated exocytosis contributes to protein kinase C potentiation of vanilloid receptor activity. J Biol Chem. 2004;279(24):25665-72.
38. Brin MF. Botulinum toxin: chemistry, pharmacology, toxicity, and immunology. Muscle Nerve Suppl. 1997;6:S146-68.
39. Wohlfarth K, Schwandt I, Wegner F, et al. Biological activity of two botulinum toxin type A complexes (Dysport and Botox) in volunteers: a double-blind, randomized, dose-ranging study. J Neurol. 2008;255(12):1932-9.
40. Rieder CR, Schestatsky P, Socal MP, et al. A double-blind, randomized, crossover study of prosigne versus botox in patients with blepharospasm and hemifacial spasm. Clin Neuropharmacol. 2007;30(1):39-42.
41. Wohlfarth K, Müller C, Sassin I, et al. Neurophysiological double-blind trial of a botulinum neurotoxin type a free of complexing proteins. Clin Neuropharmacol. 2007; 30(2):86-94.
42. Ranoux D, Gury C, Fondarai J, et al. Therapy with Botulinum Toxin. J Neurol Neurosurg Psychiatry. 2002;72:459-62.
43. Carruthers A, Carruthers J, Said S. Dose-ranging study of botulinum toxin type A in the treatment of glabellar rhytids in females. Dermatol Surg. 2005;31(4):414-22.
44. Trinidade de Almeida AR, Marques E, et al. Pilot study comparing the diffusion of two formulations

of botulinum toxin type A in patients with forehead hyperhidrosis. Dermatol Surg. 2007;33(Suppl. 1):S37-43.

45. Dolimbek BZ, Aoki KR, Steward LE, et al. Mapping of the regions on the heavy chain of botulinum neurotoxin A (BoNT/A) recognized by antibodies of cervical dystonia patients with immunoresistance to BoNT/A. Mol Immunol. 2007;44(5):1029-41.
46. Göschel H, Wohlfarth K, Frevert J, et al. Botulinum A toxin therapy: neutralizing and nonneutralizing antibodies--therapeutic consequences. Exp Neurol. 1997;147(1):96-102.
47. Jankovic J, Vuong KD, Ahsan J. Comparison of efficacy and immunogenicity of original versus current botulinum toxin in cervical dystonia. Neurology. 2003;60(7):1186-8.
48. Jankovic J, Hunter C, Dolimbek BZ, et al. Clinico-immunologic aspects of botulinum toxin type B treatment of cervical dystonia. Neurology. 2006;67(12):2233-5.
49. Greene P, Fahn S, Diamond B. Development of resistance to botulinum toxin type A in patients with torticollis. Mov Disord. 1994;9:213-17.
50. Lange O, Bigalke H, Dengler R, et al. Neutralizing antibodies and secondary therapy failure after treatment with botulinum toxin type A: much ado about nothing? Clin Neuropharmacol. 2009;32(4):213-8.
51. Carruthers A, Carruthers J, Lowe N, et al. One-year, randomised, multicenter, two-period study of the safety and efficacy of repeated treatments with botulinum toxin type A in patients with glabellar lines. J Clin Res. 2004;7:1-20.
52. Monheit GD, Cohen JL, Reloxin Investigational Group. Long-term safety of repeated administrations of a new formulation of botulinum toxin type A in the treatment of glabellar lines: interim analysis from an open-label extension study. J Am Acad Dermatol. 2009;61(3):421-5.
53. Imhof M, Kühne UJ.A phase III study of incobotulinumtoxinA in the treatment of glabellar frown lines. J Clin Aesthet Dermatol. 2011;4(10):28-34.
54. Brin MF, Dressler D, Aoki KR. Pharmacology of botulinum toxin therapy. In: Brin MF, Cornella C, Jankovic J (Eds). Dystonia: Etiology, Clinical Features, and Treatment. Philadelphia, PA: Lippincott Williams & Wilkins; 2004. pp. 93-112.

11

CHAPTER

Patient Selection, Dilution, and Storage

Jaishree Sharad

INTRODUCTION

Botulinum toxin injections are among the top treatments done in aesthetic practice.

Successful outcomes of botulinum toxin injections depend on the injector's expertise, thorough knowledge of the muscle anatomy, interaction between the muscles, and careful patient selection. When trying to reduce or paralyze the activity of a certain muscle or group of muscles, there could be a secondary compensatory mechanism by other adjacent muscles. The most important goal should be to be able to soften the dynamic lines and wrinkles caused due to hyperactivity of muscles, keeping the face as natural as possible.

RECONSTITUTION (VIDEO 1)[1,2]

Each vial of onabotulinum toxin and incobotulinum toxin contains 100 U of toxin, 0.5 mg of human albumin, and 0.9 mg of sodium chloride in a sterilized, vacuum-dried form without a preservative.

Volumes varying between 1 and 10 cc can be used to dilute the toxin for a 100 U vial.

It has been seen that with higher dilution, the diffusion is more and duration of action is less.

The consensus recommendation for dilution by Carruthers matches a survey by Dr Klein. Both recommend to reconstitute the powder in each vial of 100 units of botulinum toxin with 2.5 mL of 0.9% nonpreserved saline to attain a final concentration of 4.0 U/0.1 mL.

Required amount of diluent (usually 2.5 cc of nonpreserved 0.9% normal saline), is taken in a sterile syringe and the needle is gently inserted into the vial containing 100 units of botulinum toxin. The needle is plunged through the rubber stopper by removing the top seal flap. Avoid opening the seal of the vial. The vacuum in the vial allows the saline to penetrate into the vial without having to push the plunger of the syringe. Once all the diluent is sucked, the syringe is separated from the needle, the needle still plunged into the vial. The vial is rotated between the palms of the hands, gently to mix in the diluent and the toxin. The needle is then removed and discarded (Fig. 1).

A few studies have reported that dilution with preserved saline was as safe and effective as dilution with nonpreserved saline for the treatment of upper face wrinkles which are dynamic as well as for essential blepharospasm. Moreover, the treatment was less painful. This was probably due to the anesthetic properties of benzyl alcohol contained in the preserved saline.[3,4] Another study done for axillary hyperhidrosis showed that dilution with 2% lidocaine chlorhydrate was less painful and as effective as dilution with saline.[5]

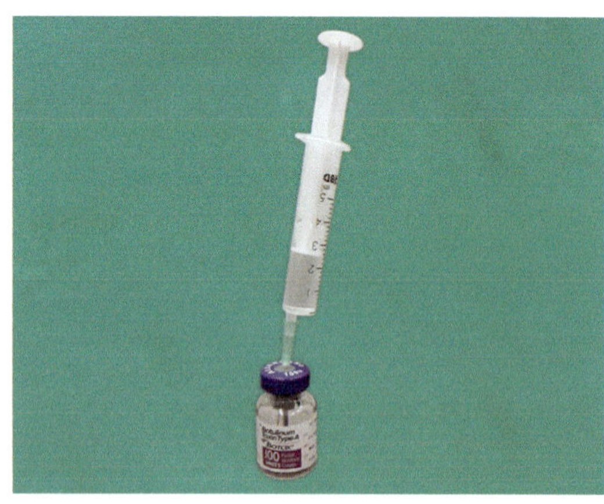

FIG. 1: Reconstitution of botulinum toxin.

Some important points to remember when reconstituting:

- Check the box for untampered seal and date of manufacture/expiry date
- Note down date and time when vial opened
- Remove any air bubbles from the syringe to get a correct measure of the diluent
- Keep in mind the fact that if needle with hub is used, there is an extra volume of diluent in the hub in addition to that measured
- If the diluent is not pulled in by the vacuum in the vial, you must not use the vial, just discard it
- Reconstituted botulinum toxin should be clear, colorless and free of particulate matter.

STORAGE[1,6,7]

Botulinum toxin is available in various preparations by various pharmaceutical companies.

It is important to know about the various products before one chooses to do a treatment. Onabotulinum toxin A (Botox®; Allergan) is available in vials of 50 and 100 units. Each vial has vacuum dried neurotoxin complex which needs to be diluted with normal saline for use. The vacuum dried vial is stored in a refrigerator at 2-8°C temperature. An unopened vial can be stored for up to 3 years.

Unopened vials of incobotulinum toxin A (Xeomin) can be stored at room temperature 20–25°C, in a refrigerator at 2–8°C, or in a freezer at -20° to -10°C for up to 3 years.

Abobotulinum toxin or Dysport® comes in a plastic hinged box containing two glass vials. It is a freeze-dried powder that clumps at the bottom of the vial. Dysport® does not have to be stored in a deep freeze but, once reconstituted, it must be kept at 2–8° centigrade. Reconstituted Dysport® should not be frozen.

Reconstituted onabotulinum toxin A and reconstituted incobotulinum toxin A should be stored in a refrigerator at 2–8°C. Reconstituted toxin retains its original potency for up to 6 weeks when refrigerated and in a frozen state for up to 6 months.

There is an increased risk of bacterial contamination and colonization of the solution if remained unused for a long time when normal saline is used without a preservative.

There is greater efficacy with freshly reconstituted botulinum toxin.

DIFFUSION

Spread of the toxin depends on the size of needle, technique of injection, and volume of injection. While spread occurs immediately after the injection, diffusion occurs as the toxin passively moves away from the injection site over many days. The mimic muscles of the face share an intimate relationship among themselves. In order to prevent untoward spread and diffusion to another muscle other than the targeted muscle, one must use lower volumes and higher concentrations of the toxin.[8] A higher dilution can cause greater diffusion with the effect staying for a shorter span of time.

ONSET AND DURATION OF ACTION[9]

The onset of action is about 12–72 hours after injection but the peak effect is seen at 1–2 weeks. The effects of the toxin plateau for about 3 months and then start waning. Patients usually require reinjection every 4 to 6 months.

A study conducted by Carruthers which evaluated the efficacy of onabotulinum toxin A (Botox) for the treatment of glabellar lines showed that the rate of response at maximal frown lasted for 3 months in 75% of patients and in 25% up to 4 months. Similarly, a study using abobotulinum toxin A (Dysport) with a 50-U dose showed that the effect lasted anywhere from 3 to 4 months.[10]

In case of masseter hypertrophy, the maximal cosmetic benefit is seen around 6–8 weeks after injecting the botulinum toxin and the effect lasts for 8–12 months.

PATIENT SELECTION

A careful history and examination is mandatory.

All contraindications (Box 1) should be kept in mind during patient selection.

Neuromuscular blockage is monitored by facial nerve stimulation of the orbicularis oculi by

BOX 1 Contraindications of botulinum toxin[7]

- Absolute:
  - Infection at the injection site
  - Pregnancy and lactation
  - Hypersensitivity to any of the components of botulinum toxin (toxin itself, human albumin, sodium chloride, sodium succinate, and lactose)
- Relative:
  - Neuromuscular disorders like myasthenia gravis, Lambert–Eaton syndrome
  - Concomitant use of aminoglycosides, cholinesterase inhibitors, penicillamine, calcium channel blockers, quinidine, and cholinesterase inhibitors

anesthesiologists frequently. Hence they must be informed should the patient need general anesthesia after having botulinum toxin injections. Peripheral ulnar nerve stimulation of the adductor pollicis muscle can be used as an alternative way to monitor neuromuscular blockage.[11]

Patients should be made aware that deep, static rhytides which occur as a result of chronologic aging or actinic damage do not improve. They would see an improvement in all dynamic wrinkles.[12]

Proper examination is a must in order to understand the muscle anatomy of the patient's face. The positioning of muscles and their relation to adjacent muscles need to be carefully understood. Asymmetries should be looked for and the patient made aware of such asymmetries before the treatment. Injections should not be given if the patient has any important event within a week of the treatment in case of bruising or any untoward effect.

Older patients tend to use certain muscles more frequently in order to compensate for weaker muscles or lax skin, e.g., to overcome ptosis of the eyebrows, they may use the frontalis more. So, one should be cautious while injecting this patient's frontalis muscle. Patients with excessive lower eyelid skin or prominent fat pads under the eye should not be treated with botulinum toxin. Adjunctive cosmetic procedures such as blepharoplasty are better options for these patients.[13-15]

ABSOLUTE CONTRAINDICATIONS

- Presence of any infection at the proposed site of injections
- Hypersensitivity to botulinum toxin, human albumin, or saline.
- Pregnant or lactating women (botulinum toxin is classified as a pregnancy category C drug). There have been no reports of any side effects on fetuses of patients who were injected with botulinum toxin in the first few months of pregnancy. Only one patient was reported to have had a miscarriage but she had history of previous spontaneous abortions.[16] There are no studies showing the effect of toxin in human milk or on the infant's nervous system. But it is better to avoid botulinum toxin during lactation to be safe[17]

RELATIVE CONTRAINDICATIONS

- Patients suffering from a neuromuscular disorder (e.g., myasthenia gravis, Lambert-Eaton syndrome)
- Patients on medications that can interfere with neuromuscular transmission and amplify the effects of botulinum toxin (e.g., aminoglycosides, penicillamine, quinine, and calcium channel blockers)
- People with unrealistic expectations or body dysmorphic disorders: They need to be counseled before injecting them with botulinum toxin.

INDICATIONS

The indications for botulinum toxin are given in box 2.

PRETREATMENT COUNSELING[7]

It is important to counsel a patient before injecting botulinum toxin. Understanding the patient's needs and planning the treatment leads to a happy patient. The patient must be explained the following points:

- The onset of action is as early as 24 to 48 hours but may take up to 1 to 10 days
- Treatments may last from 3 to 5 months depending on the facial area, dose, and formulation
- Injections need to be repeated once the effects of botulinum toxin wane away
- The aim of treatment should be to make the lines softer rather than trying to make the lines disappear
- Static lines do not respond to botulinum toxin, only dynamic lines can be erased temporarily
- Deep folds and wrinkles present at rest, sagging skin, and skin laxity cannot be treated with botulinum toxin
- The dosage should be calculated during the assessment and the patient should be made aware of the cost during the counseling session itself
- The doses differ in every individual as well as on both the sides of the face. This will depend entirely on the muscle anatomy, the muscle bulk, and the asymmetries

BOX 2 Indications for botulinum toxin[7]

- Forehead lines
- Glabellar or frown lines
- Crow's feet
- Eyebrow lift
- Bunny's lines or nasal scrunch lines
- Nasal tip elevation
- Gummy smile
- Perioral rhytides
- Marionette lines
- Popply chin
- Platysmal bands
- Nefertiti lift
- Masseter hypertrophy
- Calf muscles hypertrophy
- Temporal hypertrophy
- Trapezius muscle hypertrophy

- Time the injections in such a way that the patient has enough days to recover in case of a bruise or untoward effect. Never inject a patient who has an important event within a week of treatment
- Low doses should be injected in case of actors, singers, and performers who are dependent on facial expressions for their livelihood. A frozen expression would not be appreciated in their profession and may even cost them their job.

CONSENT AND PHOTOGRAPHY

A written informed consent is mandatory. The consent form should include the nature of botulinum toxin to be used, the longevity, and the risk of possible complications. The consent form should also mention that the patient has no history of any contraindications for botulinum toxin.

Pretreatment photographs both in front and profile views help in assessment of the treatment sites and determine asymmetries if any. They also help in comparison with posttreatment photographs. A standard camera should be used and there should be adequate lighting. The lights should be just in front and above the area to be photographed. Avoid reflections and shadows on the treatment site. Always ensure the same lighting is used every time. All makeup should be removed, the hair should be pinned back, and a clean background (white or black) should be used. Photographs should be taken at rest and in motion, i.e., asking the patient to make the necessary expressions. For example, take a picture after asking the patient to give a big smile in order to see the crow's feet. Also take a picture at rest to see if he/she has any static lines. This will help us to assess the anatomy of muscles at rest and at maximum contraction. Precise delineation of the natural muscle movement and corresponding facial rhytides may be achieved by marking the area to be injected while the patient is seated upright.

PREPARING THE PATIENT TO GET OPTIMAL RESULTS

Nonsteroidal anti-inflammatory drugs (NSAIDs), vitamin E, *Ginkgo biloba*, green tea, and various herbs and supplements which act as blood thinners should be avoided for a week before the injection in order to prevent bruising. Turmeric, cinnamon, and cayenne peppers are also known to cause thinning of blood and hence excessive use of these spices should be avoided too. Patients on aspirin and other blood thinners due to medical ailments need to be cautioned that they may bruise and that the bruise may take a week or two to subside.

Topical anesthesia in the form of prilocaine and lidocaine is used in patients who have a low threshold to pain. Ice packs can also be used to numb the skin prior to injection. Sometimes, just talking to the patient while injecting allays their anxiety.

CARE DURING THE PROCEDURE

After the photographs are taken, the area to be treated is cleaned with chlorhexidine sulfate and alcohol. The patient is asked to demonstrate various expressions and the muscles to be injected are delineated. The points to be injected are marked with an eyeliner or a lip liner pencil.

Botulinum toxin should be filled in 1 mL tuberculin or insulin syringes with 30–32 gauge needles. Not more than 10 units should be filled per syringe. More than four to six pricks with the same needle will cause blunting of the needle and cause pain. The syringes should be for single use only. Do not reintroduce the same needle again into the vial.

The injection should be given while the patient is in a comfortable sitting position. Good lighting is another important factor.

Care should be taken not to overdose the patient. The aim should be to soften the lines and wrinkles rather than making them disappear completely. A touch up can always be done a week to 10 days later if needed.

POSTTREATMENT CARE

- Ask the patient not to lie down or bend for 5–6 hours postinjection
- Do not massage the area
- Avoid heavy exercise for about 24 hours
- Avoid facials and massages for 2 weeks post-treatment
- Avoid radiofrequency treatments for 4 weeks posttreatment.

CONCLUSION

Careful reconstitution and storage will result in accurate efficacy and better results with lesser chances of untoward complications or diffusion. Pre - treatment planning will help to decide on the accurate dosage, to check for asymmetries and also give the patient an estimate of the cost involved. Post treatment care is important in order to prevent bruising, asymmetries, diffusion.

REFERENCES

1. Klein AW. Dilution and storage of botulinum toxin. Dermatol Surg. 1998;24(11):1179-80.
2. Carruthers J, Fagien S, Matarasso SL, et al. Consensus recommendations on the use of botulinum toxin type a in facial aesthetics. Plast Reconstr Surg. 2004;114(6 Suppl):1S-22.
3. Alam M, Dover JS, Arndt KA. Pain associated with injection of botulinum A exotoxin reconstituted using isotonic sodium chloride with and without preservative: a double-blind, randomized controlled trial. Arch Dermatol. 2002;138(4):510-4.
4. Kwiat DM, Bersani TA, Bersani A. Increased patient comfort utilizing botulinum toxin type a reconstituted with preserved versus nonpreserved saline. Ophthal Plast Reconstr Surg. 2004;20(3):186-9.
5. Vadoud-Seyedi J, Simonart T. Treatment of axillary hyperhidrosis with botulinum toxin type A reconstituted in lidocaine or in normal saline: a randomized, side-by-side, double-blind study. Br J Dermatol. 2007;156(5):986-9.
6. Hexsel DM, De Almeida AT, Rutowitsch M, et al. Multicenter, double-blind study of the efficacy of injections with botulinum toxin type A reconstituted up to six consecutive weeks before application. Dermatol Surg. 2003;29(5):523-9.
7. Sharad J. Botulinum toxin. In: Viswanath V, Gopalani V (Eds). Cosmetic Dermatology: A Practical and Evidence-Based Approach. New Delhi: CBS Publishers and Distributors; 2016.
8. Klein AW. Complications, adverse reactions, and insights with the use of botulinum toxin. Dermatol Surg. 2003;29(5):549-56.
9. Flynn TC. Botulinum toxin: examining duration of effect in facial aesthetic applications. Am J Clin Dermatol. 2010;11(3):183-99.
10. Carruthers JD, Lowe NJ, Menter MA, et al. Double-blind, placebo-controlled study of the safety and efficacy of botulinum toxin type A for patients with glabellar lines. Plast Reconstr Surg. 2003;112(4):1089-98.
11. Ward SJ, Harrop-Griffiths W. Botox injections and monitoring neuromuscular blockade. Anaesthesia. 2006;61(7):726.
12. de Sa Earp AP, Marmur ES. The five D's of botulinum toxin: doses, dilution, diffusion, duration and dogma. J Cosmet Laser Ther. 2008;10(2):93-102.
13. Carruthers A, Carruthers J. Clinical indications and injection technique for the cosmetic use of botulinum A exotoxin. Dermatol Surg. 1998;24(11):1189-94.
14. Shetty MK. Cosmetic uses of botulinum toxin. In: Mysore V (Ed). ACSI Textbook on Cutaneous and Aesthetic Surgery. New Delhi: Jaypee Brothers Medical Publishers (P) Ltd; 2012. pp. 607-12.
15. Carruthers A, Carruthers J. Upper face treatment. In: Carruthers A, Carruthers J (Eds). Botulinum Toxin: Procedures in Cosmetic Dermatology, 2nd edition. Philadelphia: Elsevier; 2008. p. 32.
16. Morgan JC, Iyer SS, Moser ET, et al. Botulinum toxin A during pregnancy: a survey of treating physicians. J Neurol Neurosurg Psychiatry. 2006;77(1):117-9.
17. de Oliveira Monteiro E. Botulinum toxin and pregnancy. Skinmed. 2006;5(6):308.

12

CHAPTER

Facial Anatomy Relevant for the Application of Botulinum Toxin

Renita Lourdhurajan

INTRODUCTION

Botulinum toxin (BoNT) works at the neuromuscular junction, by blocking the secretion of acetylcholine, thus causing a chemical denervation of the target muscle. Since the outcome of the treatment depends very specifically on the correct amount of toxin reaching the exact location in the muscle, a thorough understanding of the anatomy of the target muscles becomes imperative. This chapter reviews the anatomy and applied significance of the muscles that are amenable to treatment with botulinum toxin A (BoNT A), listed below in table 1. Muscles of the face are shown in figure 1.

Some muscles, namely the levator labii superioris alaeque nasi (LLSAN), depressor anguli oris (DAO), and mentalis are figuratively called 3D muscles,[1] as their location may vary from superficial to deep at different points along the length of the muscle—deep, at the bony origin to superficial at the cutaneous insertion. This is a very important characteristic, as correct placement of injections at the preferred depth as dictated by anatomy, is crucial to avoid complications, but also to deliver the best results. On one hand, inadvertently injecting a neighboring muscle may cause complications, but on the other, inadequately treating the target muscle may give suboptimal results leading to dissatisfied patients and frustrated injectors. It is therefore important to assess each muscle from the following standpoints—its action, extent, orientation, and composition; functional interplay with neighboring muscles; area of concentration of the motor end plates; depth from the surface and variability of this depth; surface anatomy of nearby vessels and nerves, and racial variations.

TABLE 1: Muscles that are amenable to treatment with BoNTA

	Muscle	Principal action	Indication for botulinum toxin
Upper face	Frontalis	Brow elevation	Transverse forehead lines
	Corrugator supercilii	Brow depression	Vertical frown lines/Glabellar lines
	Procerus	Brow depression	Transverse glabellar lines
	Orbicularis oculi	Eyelid closure	Crow's feet, bunny lines, brow lift
Lower face	Nasalis	Flaring of nostrils	Nostril flare, bunny lines
	Depressor septi nasi	Depression of nasal tip	Nasal tip droop
	Levator labii superioris alaeque nasi	Upper lip elevation	Gummy smile, bunny lines
	Orbicularis oris	Mouth closure, protrusion of lips	Vertical lip lines
	Depressor anguli oris	Depression of oral commissures	Marionette lines
	Mentalis	Elevation and protrusion of the lower lip	Chin dimpling
	Masseter	Masticator	Masseter hypertrophy
	Platysma	Retraction and depression of the lower lip	Vertical platysmal bands, necklace lines
Other	Gastrocnemius	Plantarflexion, leg flexion at knee	Calf contouring

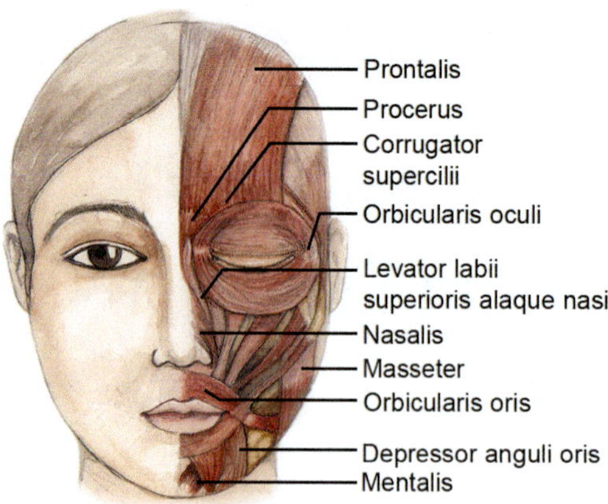

FIG. 1: Muscles of the face.

TABLE OF MUSCLES

Facial muscles that are amenable to treatment with BoNT can be grouped as those of the upper and the lower face, respectively (Table 1).

FRONTALIS

The frontalis is a bilaterally symmetrical muscle that elevates the eyebrows. The muscle is mostly composed of vertical fibers, which when they contract, produce the horizontal forehead lines. The frontalis occurs in one of two patterns—a broad contiguous sheet across the entire breadth of the forehead, on contraction leading to long, unbroken transverse lines, and the second pattern showing two discrete muscle bellies[2,3] (Fig. 2).

TABLE 2: Muscles of the face

Muscle	Origin	Insertion
Frontalis	Galea aponeurotica	Skin of the forehead, interdigitating with fibers of the procerus, the corrugator supercilii, and the orbicularis oculi
Corrugator supercilii	Medial supraorbital ridge	Skin of the forehead, merging with fibers of the frontalis
Procerus	Periosteum of inferior nasal bone and adjacent cartilage	Glabellar skin, merging with fibers of the frontalis
Orbicularis oculi	Nasal part of the frontal bone, the medial palpebral ligament and the frontal process of the maxilla	At the origin itself
Nasalis	Alar fibers from the maxilla and the transverse nasal fibers originate from the nasal bone	Alar fibers insert into the alar facial crease and external skin, adjacent to the alar crease. The transverse nasal fibers insert into the skin, bilaterally, just above the nasal ala
Depressor septi nasi	Maxillary periosteum adjacent to incisor fossa	Nasal septum
Levator labii superioris alaeque nasi	Frontal process of the maxilla	Skin of the upper lip and the lateral nostril
Orbicularis oris	Modiolus, mandible, and maxilla near the incisor fossae	Skin of the lips and skin of the opposite side
Depressor anguli oris	Oblique line of the mandible	Modiolus
Mentalis	Incisor fossa of the mandible	Skin of the chin
Masseter	Zygomatic arch	Masseter tuberosity
Platysma	Outer aspect of the superficial thoracic fascia	The pars labialis inserts into the lateral half of the lower lip the pars mandibularis inserts into the lower border of the mandibular body, and the pars modiolus inserts into the modiolar musculature, and the overlying cutaneous tissue
Gastrocnemius	The medial and the lateral heads of the muscle originate from the medial and lateral femoral condyles, respectively	Into the calcaneum at the heel as the Achilles tendon, together with the fibers of the soleus

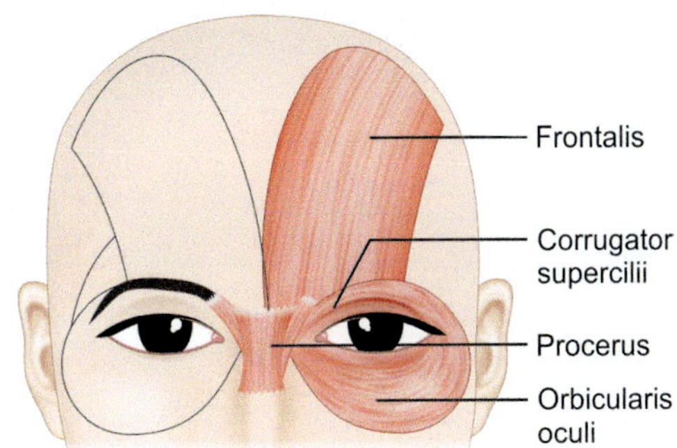

FIG. 2: Muscles of the forehead, and periocular region.

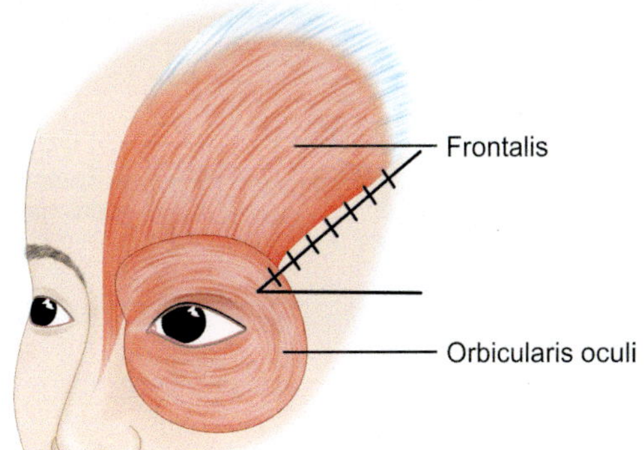

FIG. 3: Overlap of the lateral frontalis with orbicularis oculi fibres.

The frontalis muscle originates from the galea aponeurotica along the coronal suture, forming the anterior half of the occipitofrontalis muscle.[3-5] The muscle has no bony attachments, and its fibers run forward to insert inferiorly. The medial frontalis fibers become contiguous with the procerus fibers, the intermediate fibers interdigitate with those of the orbicularis oculi and the corrugator supercilii, and the lateral fibers merge with those of the orbicularis oculi over the zygomatic process of the frontal bone.[6]

As one of the most easily accessible muscles available for BoNT treatment, the frontalis does not need much surface anatomical assistance. Except, an important anatomical point is the lateral border of the frontalis, which must be addressed when treating the forehead lines.[7] The lateral border overlaps the orbicularis oculi along the caudal 2 cm, and tends to be located within 1 cm on either side of a line drawn from the most protuberant part of the frontotemporal region along the orbit (Fig. 3).

This anatomical landmark is useful in avoiding a Mephisto/Samurai/Spock appearance, due to unopposed elevation of the untreated lateral frontalis, when only the medial fibers are targeted.

The muscle is located at an average depth of 3-5 mm beneath the skin, with a range of 2-7 mm.[4] Gender difference exist,[8] with the depth being 1 mm more in men as compared to women.[4] Also, the medial borders of the frontalis tend to be more vertically oriented in women as compared to men. Racial differences may also exist with larger frontal facial movements and higher wrinkle scores in Caucasian over Asian subjects.[9]

PROCERUS

The procerus is one of the depressors that counters the brow elevation of the frontalis. It pulls the medial eyebrow downward, thereby contributing to squinting and frowning with the formation of horizontal wrinkles in the glabellar region.[3] Its fibers originate in the tendinous periosteum over the inferior nasal bone and the adjacent cartilage. A pyramid-shaped muscle, its fibers insert into the glabellar cutaneous tissue, merging with the fibers of the frontalis muscle. Less than a mm thick, the procerus lies at a depth of 2–3 mm beneath the skin.[4] The length of the muscle varies between sexes, at 16 mm in males to 19 mm in females.[4]

CORRUGATOR SUPERCILII

These muscles depress the brow, pulling it inward and downward, producing a frowning and/or squinting appearance. Recent data show that the muscle has two bellies, an oblique belly, and lying deeper to it, a transverse belly.[10] The oblique belly again can have one of two forms: a narrow vertical and a broad triangular type (Fig 4). The corrugator supercilii muscle is said to have its apex at the point of its origin at the medial supraorbital ridge, and its broader base where it inserts into the skin of the forehead, its fibers closely interdigitating with those of the frontalis.

The vertical height of the muscle varied between races ranging from 21 mm to 30 mm in Caucasians versus 13 mm to 33 mm in Koreans. Also, the distance of the thickest portion of the muscle from the midline was variable; these differences must be kept in mind while choosing the optimal site for injection.[10]

The base or the tail of the muscle is often variable at its insertion with a much smaller muscle mass than at the apex or at the body, and so is not always a reliable area for injection of toxin. An area at or near

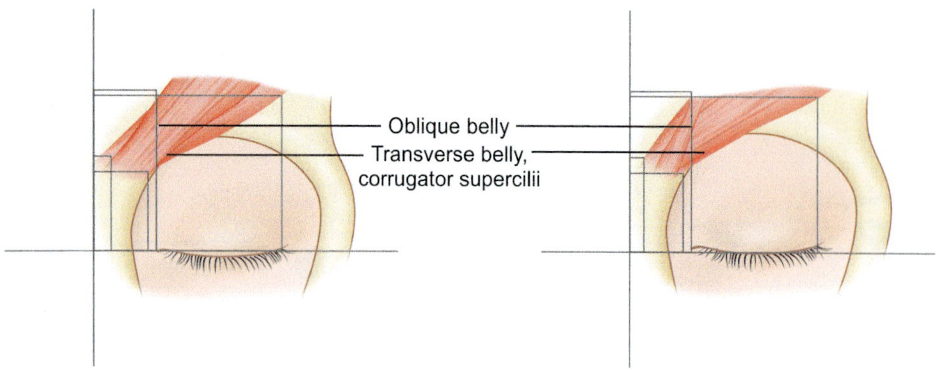

FIG. 4: Anatomical variations of the corrugator supercilia (supercilii) muscle.

the apex would be a more preferred site in order to target both the bellies of the muscle.[10] The muscle is located at an average depth of 4–6 mm under the skin, going from deep to superficial from origin to insertion.[4]

ORBICULARIS OCULI

A complex muscle with a high concentration of fast fibers,[6] the orbicularis oculi muscle has four components: (1) the orbital, (2) the preseptal, (3) the pretarsal, and (4) the lacrimal parts. Considered as an eyelid sphincter, the orbital part contributes to powerful closure of the eyelids. Other actions include depression of the lateral brow, and a small contribution to cheek elevation, particularly on the lateral aspects.[3]

The arrangement of its fibers in the form of a circle contributes to horizontal wrinkles at the 3 o'clock and 9 o'clock positions, and vertical wrinkling at the 6 o'clock and 12 o'clock positions.[4] These fibers arise from the nasal part of the frontal bone, the medial palpebral ligament, and the frontal process of the maxilla, to loop around concentrically in the orbit and terminate eventually at the origin itself, thus contributing to the sphincteric action mentioned above (Fig. 2). The orbital part also extends for some distance into the skin around the orbit, interdigitating with the neighboring muscles.[2,3]

DEPRESSOR SUPERCILII

A small muscle that lies parallel to the procerus muscle, the depressor supercilii depresses the medial eyebrows, and thus helps in eyelid closure and in frowning. Its fibers originate from the bony processes adjacent to the medial canthus, and travel up about 1-1.5 cm, to insert into the skin of the brow.[4]

NASALIS

Wrinkles around the upper part of the nose called the nasociliary wrinkles are contributed by a number of muscles: the orbicularis oculi, the nasalis, the LLSAN, the depressor septi, and the zygomaticus major and minor muscles.[11] These wrinkles or rhytides can be classified based on the muscle contribution as follows: Nasal rhytides where the nasalis muscle is the only contributor, nasoalar rhytides with an input from the LLSAN in addition to the nasalis, nasoorbicular, where the participating muscles are the nasalis and the orbicularis oculi, and the nasociliary rhytides, when all the rhytide subgroups are involved. The nasalis can easily be targeted with BoNT, improving these wrinkles, which may often be exacerbated when the crow's feet and the glabellar complex have been treated, but not the nasal wrinkles. Studies have shown that it is important to target all contributing muscles, as over 60% of subjects had inadequate response of the nasociliary wrinkles when the nasalis alone was targeted.[11]

There are two parts to the nasalis, a transverse part and an alar part (Fig. 5). The former is also called the compressor naris and the latter, the dilator naris—the function of these muscles can easily be surmised from these self-explanatory names. The former contributes to the nasociliary wrinkles, and the latter, to the nasal flare.

The alar fibers originate from the maxilla and insert into the alar facial crease and external skin, adjacent to the alar crease. The transverse nasal fibers originate from the nasal bone, and proceed downward and laterally to insert into the skin, bilaterally, just above the nasal ala.[11]

Traditionally, the dilator naris, or the alar nasalis is said to have an anterior and a posterior part. More recent Asian cadaver studies describe the dilator

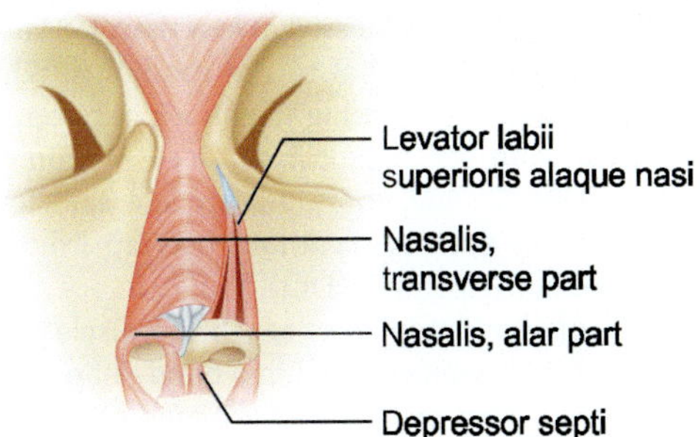

FIG. 5: Nasalis, Levator Labii Superioris Alaque Nasi, Depressor Septi Nasi.

naris anterior as being somewhat distinct from the nasalis itself. These studies have characterized the origin of the dilator naris anterior as being from the frontolateral aspect of the lateral crus of the greater alar cartilage and the adjacent aspect of the accessory alar cartilage with the insertion into the skin above the alar groove.[12] Also, a new component, the dilator naris vestibularis muscle, situated between the external and the vestibular skin of the alar lobule, has been characterized. At this location, this muscle covers almost the entire surface of the ala, and has been speculated to contribute significantly to the shape and the flare of the ala.[12]

These differences simply underscore the racial differences in facial shape—with Asian noses described to have an acute nasolabial angle, a shorter columella, a lower dorsum, and a more bulbous tip than Caucasian counterparts.[13] In noses which were more flared, the muscle masses of the dilators was found to be larger, than in the straight types.[13]

Asian cadavers showed variation related to the vector of nostril orientation. Horizontal nostrils revealed insertion into the medial crura footplates, with variable insertion into the columella and vestibular skin or membranous septum. Vertical nostrils did not exhibit an abundant musculature, and thus the question is posed as to whether nostril shape influences or is influenced by the depressor septi nasi muscle.

DEPRESSOR SEPTI NASI

The position of the tip of the nose is dictated by the depressor septi muscle, activity of which can make a drooping nasal tip more prominent.[11,14] Relaxing this muscle with BoNT allows lifting of the tip of the nose, also called a medical rhinoplasty.[15] Given the racial differences mentioned above, lifting of the nasal tip is a much favored treatment among Asians.

The origin of this muscle seems to have a few variations, with the consensus that the muscle fibers arise from the maxillary periosteum, with or without contributions from the orbicularis oculi muscle.[16] The input from the orbicularis muscle was found to be different across races.

LEVATOR LABII SUPERIORIS ALAQUE NASI

The levator labii superioris alaeque nasi is the main muscle responsible for causing the *gummy smile.* An additional role for the LLSAN is related to its two parts—the nasal portion causes the nostril to dilate, and the labial portion is an upper lip elevator. The LLSAN also contributes to the depth of nasolabial fold in the upper third and plays a role in the formation of bunny lines along with the nasalis.[1-3] The LLSAN originates in the frontal process of the maxilla and runs vertically down to its insertion in the skin of the upper lip and the lateral nostril, the labial and the nasal portions, respectively. Superiorly, the LLSAN relates to the orbicularis oculi, and inferiorly, to the orbicularis oris, and laterally to the levator labii superioris muscles.

As a 3D muscle, the LLSAN can be accessed at two different depths. At its bony origin, the LLSAN can be reached at a depth of about 3 mm, just medial to the levator labii superioris muscle at the level of the emergence of the infraorbital nerve through the infraorbital foramen. Inferiorly and more superficially, the muscle can be reached at a subdermal plane at a point lateral to the nostril above the nasolabial fold.[1]

ORBICULARIS ORIS

Another sphincter-like muscle similar to the orbicularis oculi, the orbicularis oris is made up of concentrically arranged fibers, to form a complete ring around the oral cavity. The actions include mouth closure and forward protrusion of the lips, as in a pout.[1-3]

There are two parts that join at the modiolus, an upper and a lower, each composed of two portions, a pars marginalis and a pars peripheralis. The pars marginalis which contributes to the sphincter action of the orbicularis oris muscles arcs under the free border of the lips and communicates with its counterpart at the corners of the mouth, reaching to insert into the red lip dermis of the other side. The curved shape of the lips is attributed to the anterior position and function of the pars marginalis, which helps in compressing the lips and pulling them inward. Located a little posterior in the cutaneous lip is the pars peripheralis, again the fibers reach above and below to insert into the dermis of the opposite side at the mouth corners. The accentuation of the fine perioral wrinkles is attributed to the contraction of the pars peripheralis.[1]

The maximum concentration of the motor end plates on the lower lip was found to be along the vermilion border, at the midline of each half of the lower lip[17] (Fig. 6).

DEPRESSOR ANGULI ORIS

Another 3D muscle,[1] the DAO acts to depress the oral commissures, or the corners of the mouth, as well as to dilate the mouth. Arising deep from the oblique line of the mandible, the fibers of the DAO end superficially at the modiolus,[18] which is nothing but a mobile muscular mass formed by the convergence of fibers of the following muscles: The zygomaticus major, orbicularis oris, risorius, buccinators, and the levator anguli oris muscles, in addition to the DAO as just mentioned.[19] The course of the muscle fibers varies between individuals, from straight to almost curved, as shown in mapping studies.[17]

Overactivity of the DAO pulls the modiolus down giving the face, a sad, tired or angry appearance. Chemoimmobilization of the DAO allows the counteracting muscles, namely the levator anguli oris and the zygomaticus major, to elevate the corner of the mouth, however, this involves some risk. This is due to the intimate relationship of the DAO, medially to the orbicularis oris and the depressor labii inferioris, and laterally to the zygomaticus major, risorius, and the platysma muscles, and the close interaction of all these muscles at the modiolus. Also the medial border of the DAO which runs deep to the depressor labii inferioris muscle seems to be connected with the fibers of the latter in a good proportion of studied specimens.[20]

Cadaver studies suggest the following surface anatomical landmarks to identify the safe area of the DAO. From a sagittal line drawn along the modiolus, the DAO is located at less than 45° lateral and less than 30° medial to the modiolus, which can be located by palpating the cheek between the cutaneous and the mucosal surfaces. Within this triangle (Fig. 7), the fibers present are said to be only those of the DAO, without overlap from the depressor labii inferioris (DLI).[19]

The motor endplates of this muscle were identified to be concentrated in a band-shaped area which runs across the muscle from medial to lateral, located just caudal to the midpoint between the modiolus and lower mandibular border[17] (Fig. 6).

Another important landmark to consider is the mental foramen, which has been shown to be located in the middle third between the cheilion and the inferior mandibular border, lying under the DAO.[21] When targeting this end plate rich area, it is important to avoid injecting directly into the mental foramen to avoid damage to the mental nerve, so a location just inferior to the mental foramen is suggested.

MENTALIS

The mentalis acts as an elevator of the lower lip, aids in lip protrusion, and also causes chin dimpling. As a 3D muscle, the mentalis has a deep location at its origin superiorly at the mandible, and a superficial location at its insertion into the medial chin. Laterally the muscle lies in relation to the DLI, and medially, together with its twin, forms a V-shaped triangle. The motor end plates are concentrated in an area that lies around the second quarter of the distance between the inferior vermilion border of the lower lip to the inferior border of the mandible[17] (Fig. 6)

MASSETER

The masseter is one of the muscles of mastication, the others being the temporalis and the pterygoids. This

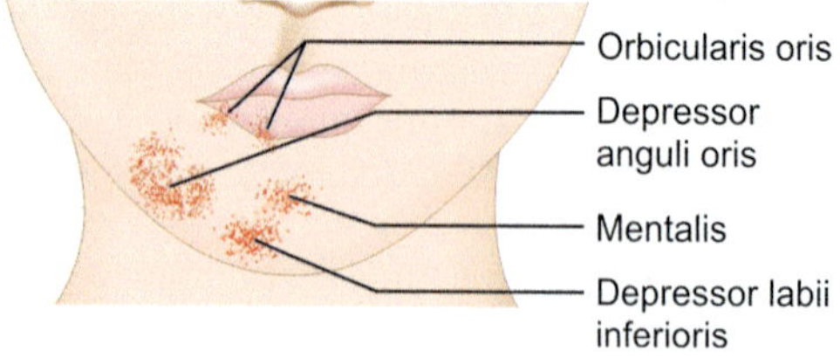

FIG. 6: Motor end plate concentrations of muscles around the mouth.

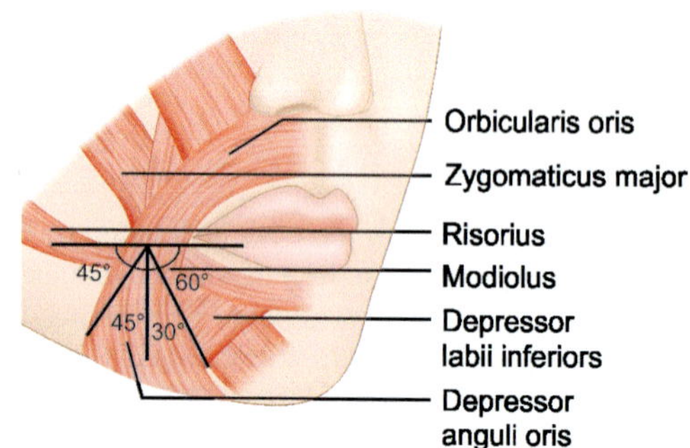

FIG. 7: Muscles in the modiolar complex.

muscle aids in elevating the mandible, with some contribution to the side-to-side movement of the jaw. It is covered by a thick aponeurosis, and extends from the zygomatic bone and its arch to the ramus, angle, and the coronoid process of the mandible. Earlier thought to have two parts namely, the pars superficialis and the pars profunda,[1] the masseter is more recently thought to have three distinct muscle layers, based on cadaver dissection analyses.[22] Accordingly, the muscle was found to have a superficial, middle, and a deep layer, the myofibers being arranged in different directions within each of these layers. The superficial layer originated from the anterior part of the zygomatic arch, while the middle and posterior layers originated from the posterior part of the zygomatic arch, with all three layers inserting into the masseter tuberosity. While the layers were discrete in the upper two-thirds of the mandibular ramus, more caudally, they were fused intimately. The motor end plates are said to be concentration in the central area of the lower half of the muscle, thereby making this region the target of the BoNT injection.[17] This also holds good from a point of safety.[23] More precisely, cadaver studies suggest an area, located 5 cm inferior to the orbitomeatal line, and 1 cm anterior and posterior to a vertical line which connects the tip of the angle of the mandible to the midpoint of the orbitomeatal line, as being an effective target for injection (Fig. 8).[24] This location is also considered safe as it avoids injection into important surrounding structures, such as the parotid gland, marginal mandibular nerve, and branches of the facial nerve such as the buccal.

To aid more accurate placement of the toxin, five patterns of masseter hypertrophy have recently been characterized, based on the specific layer of the masseter that has undergone hypertrophy, and the combinations thereof.[22] Type I is an evenly contracted masseter, and is termed 'minimal.' Type II called 'mono' is characterized by a local, single longitudinal bulge, and was noted to be the most common type. 'Double' or type III presents as two separate longitudinal bulges of equal or differing height and type IV or 'triple' with three longitudinal bulges. Finally, type V or 'excessive' denotes, as the name suggests, a massive, single bulge. Understanding the components of the hypertrophy, helps in placing the injections well within the muscle, thereby reducing the involvement of the nearby risorius[25] or the buccinators which can lead to unpleasant outcomes.

PLATYSMA

The platysma muscle runs beneath the thin subcutaneous tissue of the neck, and depresses the oral commissures, working together with the DAO. The muscle originates from the upper aspect of the superficial thoracic fascia, and can be differentiated into three parts based on the site of insertion of its fibers[18] (Fig. 9). The pars labialis inserts into the lateral half of the lower lip, passing beneath the DAO muscle fibers, the pars mandibularis inserts into the lower border of the mandibular body, and the pars modiolus inserts into the modiolar musculature, and the overlying cutaneous tissue.[1-3,18]

Hyperactivity of the anterior platysma fibers produces the vertical cervical platysma bands.[18] When holding the bands between the fingers, the muscle belly is accessed at a depth of 3–4 mm.[1] Women have a thinner plastyma than men.

The thyroid cartilage is a useful anatomical landmark when treating the platysma, as an injection of BoNT into the thin platysma muscle below this level, can spread into the nearby muscles leading to dysphagia and/or dysphonia.[1]

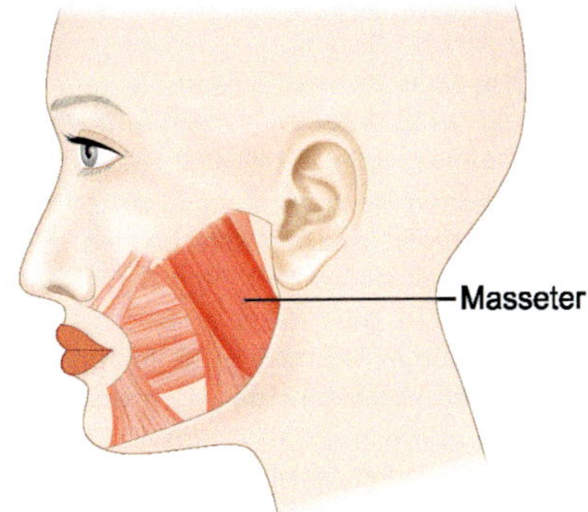

FIG. 8: Masseter muscle.

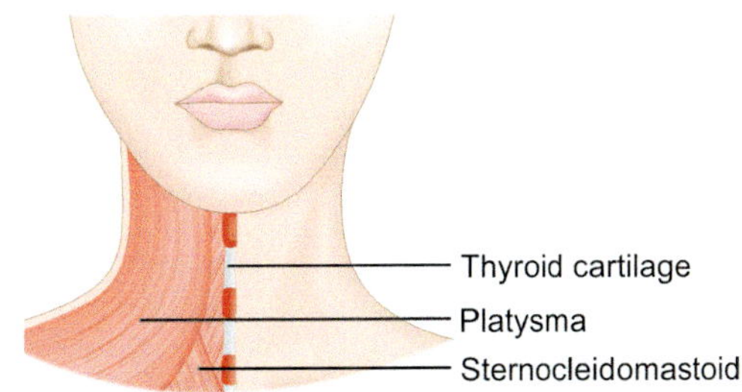

FIG. 9: Platysma.

GASTROCNEMIUS

This is a relatively newer aesthetic indication, included in the Asian Consensus Guidelines, which underlines its popularity in this part of the world. The shape of the calf is attributable to the soleus and the gastrocnemius muscles. Being more superficially located, the gastrocnemius contributes to the superficial posterior contour of the leg. A hypertrophy of this muscle is said to produce the undesirable appearance of thick, stocky looking legs, further quantified by the inelegant eponym of 'radish legs.'[26] This has been sought to be addressed with surgical denervation or even with a resection of the medial head of the muscle, said to be functionally redundant.[27,28] More recently, BoNT has been used to reduce the bulk of the medial, and more recently, the lateral heads of the gastrocnemius muscle, thereby providing a less invasive option than surgery, in the quest for slender looking legs.[26]

The medial and the lateral heads of the muscle originate from the medial and lateral femoral condyles, respectively (Fig. 10). The insertion is into the calcaneum at the heel as the Achilles tendon, together with the fibers of the soleus. The muscle may be made more prominent by asking the patient to stand on his/her toes, and the injections are then directed at the area of maximum bulk.

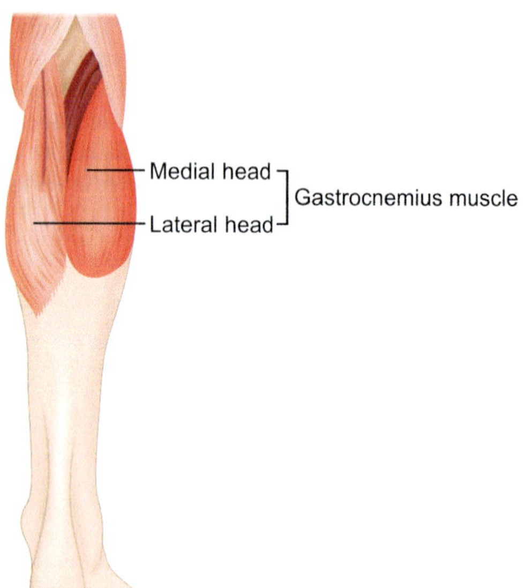

FIG. 10: Gastrocnemius.

CONCLUSION

A good knowledge of the anatomy remains a non-negotiable criterion for the successful performance of neurotoxin injections. Anatomy, much like every other medical discipline, continues to evolve, making it mandatory for practitioners to update their knowledge regularly. Racial and gender differences, nuances in injection technique, and the need-driven focus on newer areas of treatment, all are reasons to revisit the anatomical ground rules. A trend toward more cadaver studies and newer tools for better visualization, characterization, and localization of anatomical structures makes this continuous learning process an enjoyable one.

REFERENCES

1. Trevidic P, Sykes J, Criollo-Lamilla G. Anatomy of the lower face and botulinum toxin injections. Plast Reconstr Surg. 2015;136(5 Suppl.): 84S-91S.
2. Petrus G, Lewis D, Maas C. Anatomic considerations for treatment with botulinum toxin. Facial Plast Surg Clin North Am. 2007;15(1):1-9.
3. Jaishree Sharad (2016) Botulinum Toxin in Vishalakshi Vishwanath ed. Cosmetic Dermatology, A Practical and Evidence-Based Approach. New Delhi, CBS Publisher and Distributor.
4. Lorenc Z, Smith S, Nestor M, et al. Understanding the functional anatomy of the frontalis and glabellar complex for optimal aesthetic botulinum toxin type A therapy. Aesthetic Plast Surg. 2013;37(5):975-83.
5. Dorizas A, Krueger N, Sadick N. Aesthetic uses of the botulinum toxin. Dermatol Clin. 2014;32(1):23-36.
6. Kwang H. Surgical anatomy of the upper eyelid relating to upper blepharoplasty or blepharoptosis surgery. Anat Cell Biol. 2013;46(2): 93-100.
7. Choi Y, Won S, Lee J, et al. Characterizing the lateral border of the frontalis for safe and effective injection of botulinum toxin. Aesthet Surg J. 2016;36(3): 344-8.
8. KeaneyT, Alster T. Botulinum toxin in men: review of relevant anatomy and clinical trial data. Dermatol Surg. 2013;39(10):1434-43.
9. Ahn B, Kim Y, Kim H, et al. Consensus recommendations on the aesthetic usage of botulinum toxin type A in Asians. Dermatol Surg. 2013;39(12):1843-60.
10. Yang H, Kim H. Anatomical study of the corrugator supercilii muscle and its clinical implication with botulinum toxin A injection. Surg Radiol Anat. 2013; 35(9):817-21.
11. Tamura B, Odo M, Chang B, et al. Treatment of nasal wrinkles with botulinum toxin. Dermatol Surg. 2005; 31(3):271-5.
12. Hur M, Hu K, Youn K, et al. New anatomical profile of the nasal musculature: dilator naris vestibularis, dilator naris anterior, and alar part of the nasalis. Clin Anat. 2011;24(2):162-7.

13. Chun K, Kang H, Han S, et al. Anatomy of the alar lobule in the Asian nose. J Plast Reconstr Aesthet Surg. 2008;61(4):400-7.
14. Cigna E, Sorvillo V, Stefanizzi G, et al. The use of botulinum toxin in the treatment of plunging nose: cosmetic results and a functional serendipity. Clin Ter. 2014;164(2):e107-13.
15. Redaelli A. Medical rhinoplasty with hyaluronic acid and botulinum toxin A: a very simple and quite effective technique. J Cosmet Dermatol. 2008;73:10-20.
16. Sinno S, Chang J, Saadeh P, et al. Anatomy and surgical treatment of the depressor septi nasi muscle: a systematic review. Plast Reconstr Surg. 2015;135(5): 838e-48e.
17. Lapatki B, Oostenveld R, Van Djik J, et al. Topographical characteristics of motor units of the lower facial musculature revealed by means of high-density surface EMG. J Neurophysiol. 2006;95(1):342-54.
18. Goldman A, Wollina U. Elevation of the corner of the mouth using botulinum toxin type A. J Cutan Aesthet Surg. 2010;3(3):145-50.
19. Choi Y, Kim J, Gil Y, et al. Anatomical considerations regarding the location and boundary of the depressor Anguli oris muscle with reference to botulinum toxin injection. Plast Reconstr Surg. 2014;134(5):917-21.
20. Hur M, Kim H, Lee K. An anatomic study of the medial fibers of depressor anguli oris muscle passing deep to the depressor labii inferioris muscle. J Craniofac Surg. 2014;25(2):614-6.
21. Hur M, Hu K, Cho J, et al. Topography and location of the depressor anguli oris muscle with a reference to the mental foramen. Surg Radiol Anat. 2008;30(5):403-7.
22. Xie Y, Zhou J, Li H, et al. Classification of masseter hypertrophy for tailored botulinum toxin type A treatment. Plast Reconstr Surg. 2014;134(2):209e-18e.
23. Klein F, Brenner F, Sato M, et al. Lower facial remodeling with botulinum toxin type A for the treatment of masseter hypertrophy. An Bras Dermatol. 2014:89(6):878-84.
24. Kaya B, Apaydin N, Loykas M, et al. The topographic anatomy of the masseteric nerve: a cadaveric study with an emphasis on the effective zone of botulinum toxin A injections in masseter. J Plast Reconstr Aesthet Surg. 2014;67(12):1663-8.
25. Hwang K. Discussion on the risorius muscle: anatomic considerations with reference to botulinum neurotoxin injection for masseteric hypertroph. Dermatol Surg. 2014;40(12):1340-1.
26. Han K, Joo Y, Moon S, et al. Botulinum toxin A treatment for contouring of the lower leg. J Dermatolog Treat. 2006;17(4):250-54.
27. Lee H, Lee D, Park Y, et al. Botulinum toxin A for aesthetic contouring of enlarged medial gastrocnemius muscle. Dermatol Surg. 2004;30(6):867-71.
28. Wang H, Lin S, Xu D, et al. Anatomic study of selective neurectomy of gastrocnemius muscle for calf reduction in Chinese. J Plast Reconstr Aesthet Surg. 2013;66(6):e162-5.

13

CHAPTER

Upper Face Indications

Jaishree Sharad

INTRODUCTION

The face is divided into "horizontal thirds" from trichion to glabella (upper face), glabella to subnasale (midface), and subnasale to menton (lower face).

Forehead lines, crow's feet, and frown lines can be best treated with botulinum toxin making it the most sought after aesthetic procedure when it comes to the upper face.

A clear understanding of the anatomy, especially that of the muscles and their relationship with each other, makes it easy to inject botulinum toxin and give pleasant cosmetic results.

GLABELLAR COMPLEX AND VERTICAL FROWN LINES

The glabella is the area between the two eyebrows and its contraction causes the appearance of two lines between the brows called the frown lines. Frown lines are associated with negative feelings such as worry, irritation, anger, frustration, or tiredness.[1]

The corrugators, depressor supercilii, procerus, medial fibers of orbicularis oculi, and lower fibers of frontalis muscle are all responsible for hyperkinetic lines between the eyebrows forming unaesthetic horizontal, vertical, and oblique frown lines or wrinkles.[2]

When these frown lines become more prominent and form a constant expression on the face, one looks worried even if he or she is happy. Although fractional and nonablative devices, radiofrequency tightening, and chemical peels have been described to treat these lines, chemodenervation with botulinum toxin is the best treatment option for treating dynamic frown lines.

Glabellar lines may differ in appearance with gender (larger muscle mass and thicker skin in men), age, ethnicity, solar exposure, or physical activity.[3-7]

Interpersonal differences in facial animation and expressions that are typical of each person result in variations in the contraction patterns for the same area during facial animation in different patients.

Muscles Involved

Corrugator supercilii, procerus, and depressor supercilii are the primary muscles that are responsible for frown lines.

In addition to these muscles, the lower medial fibers of frontalis and medial fibers of the orbicularis oculi may interdigitate with those of the corrugator and contribute to frown lines.

Hence, while making a treatment plan, one needs to take into account the interdigitation of muscle fibers and the degree to which their activities are in opposition to anticipate the effect of botulinum toxin type A injection.[3]

Corrugator Supercilii Muscle

This muscle adducts and slightly depresses the eyebrow thus, moving it medially and inferiorly. It originates at the medial supraorbital ridge of the frontal bone, runs obliquely in a superior lateral direction and inserts in the skin, interdigitating with fibers of frontalis. It is deep centrally and gets more superficial at the point of insertion. Contraction of the corrugators cause vertical glabellar crease or frown lines. Contraction of the muscle by way of frowning results in a skin dimple at the point of insertion (Fig. 1).

Procerus

This is a thin depressor muscle that pulls the medial part of the brow down causing horizontal wrinkles on the bridge of the nose. It originates over the

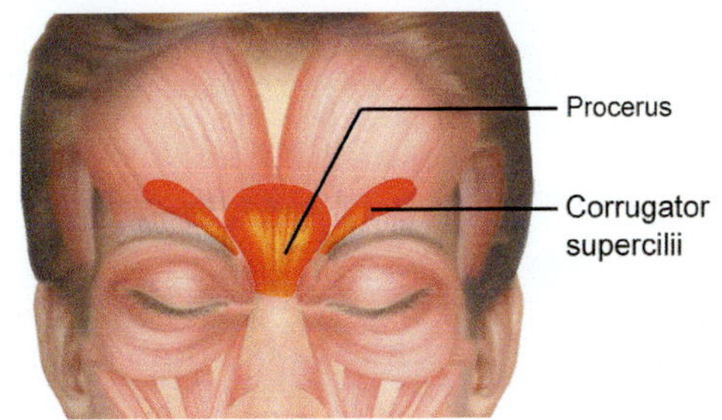

FIG. 1: Corrugator supercilii muscle and procerus muscle.

periosteum of the nasal bone and inserts into the dermis of the glabella (Fig. 1).

Conventional Injection Technique, Sites and Doses (Video 2)

The first point of injection is marked by drawing a line between the origin of the medial brow and the contralateral inner canthus on either side. The center of the procerus muscle lies at intersection of these lines.[8] If the muscle belly is too large, you may choose to have two injection sites in the midline: (i) One at the point mentioned earlier and (ii) The other a centimeter away from it on the procerus muscle. Four to five units of botulinum toxin are injected perpendicularly into the body of the procerus.

Two bilateral injection points are marked on the corrugators above the supraorbital ridge in line with the medial canthus. Inject 3–4 units of neurotoxin, keeping the needle a little more superficial as compared to the first injection into the procerus. Two more points are marked bilaterally 1 cm lateral to the first point for corrugators. Note the dimpling of the corrugators, which is the point of insertion of the muscle and keep medial to it. Also, stay medial to the midpupillary line. Two to three units are injected into each point with only one-third of the needle inserting in as the corrugators insert superficially into the skin. The supratrochlear vessels and nerves lie approximately 3 mm away from the medial canthus . Thus, care should be taken not to inject in this area in order to prevent bruising and pain.

Always place the thumb of the non-dominant hand on the supraorbital ridge in order to prevent injecting into the orbital rim.

It is better to be very conservative while injecting botulinum toxin in elderly patients who may have a reduced or absent orbital septum. Low volume and accurate technique can decrease the risk for ptosis. Large volumes if injected will increase the spread of the neurotoxin from the injection site, increasing the possibility of affecting unwanted muscles. To avoid ptosis, injections should be 1 cm above the eyebrow (Fig. 2).[9]

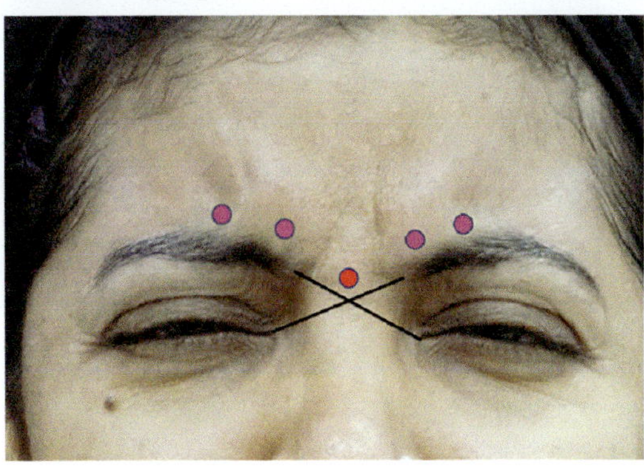

FIG. 2: Injection point for procerus and corrugators.

Patterns of Glabellar Frown Lines

Two studies: (i) One by Kim et al. and (ii) the other by Almeida et al., have shown five wrinkle patterns in the glabella region. These are described as:

1. "U" pattern (Fig. 3)
2. "V" pattern (Fig. 4)
3. "Omega" pattern (Fig. 5)
4. "Inverted omega" pattern (Fig. 6)
5. "Converging arrows" pattern (Fig. 7).

The figures show the injection points in case of these five wrinkle patterns.

This classification system enables a more accurate, individualized treatment with botulinum toxin (Fig. 8). Muscles that are more recruited, hyperkinetic, and/or hypertonic need higher doses or more injection sites. Other less solicited muscles are injected with lower doses or not treated at all.[10,11]

Ethnic Differences

Asians

In treating Asian women, a more conservative approach may be warranted because of their epicanthal folds and the effects on their ability to apply makeup. In these circumstances, three injection points may be sufficient to start with and a total dose of 10 units may be injected. The patient may be re-evaluated in 2 weeks and more units may be injected if required.[3]

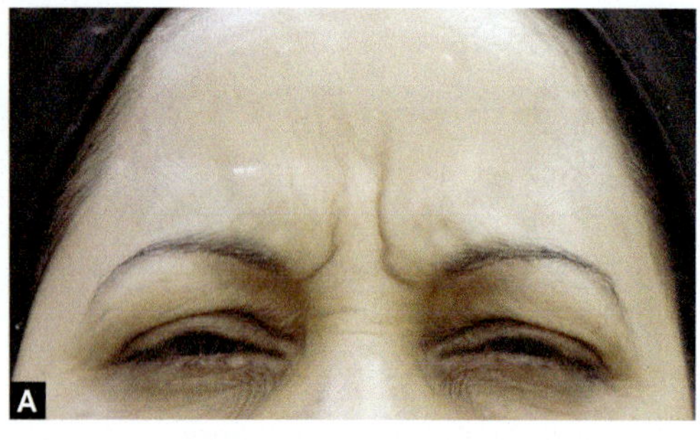

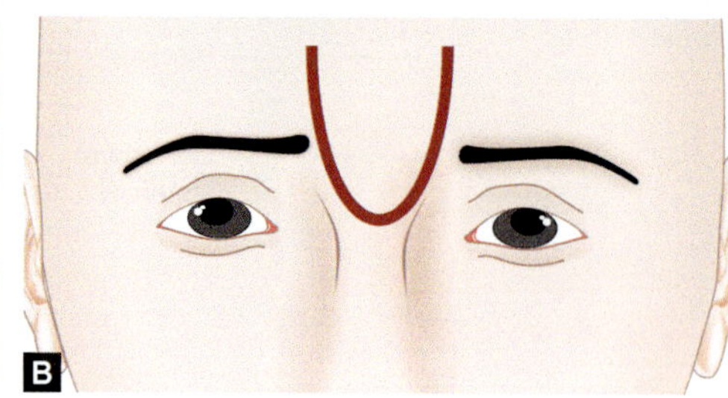

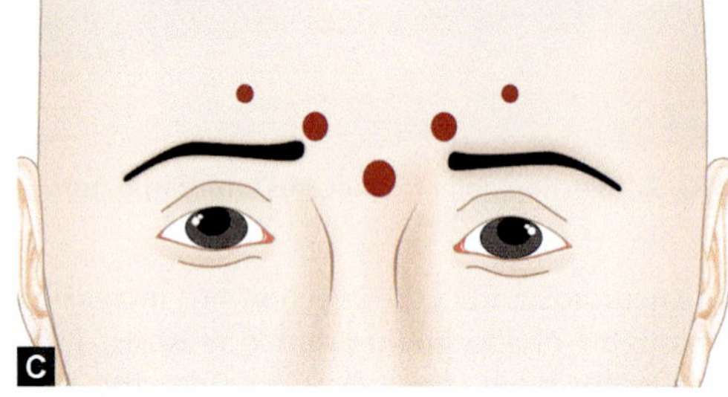

FIG. 3: A, U pattern of frown lines; **B,** schematic diagram of U pattern of frown lines; and **C,** injection points for U pattern of frown lines.

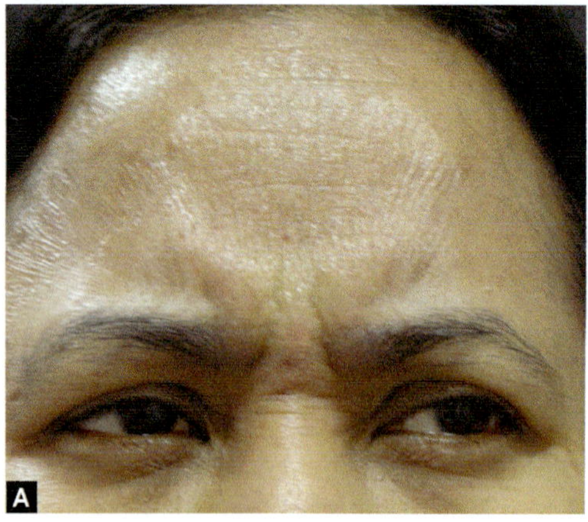

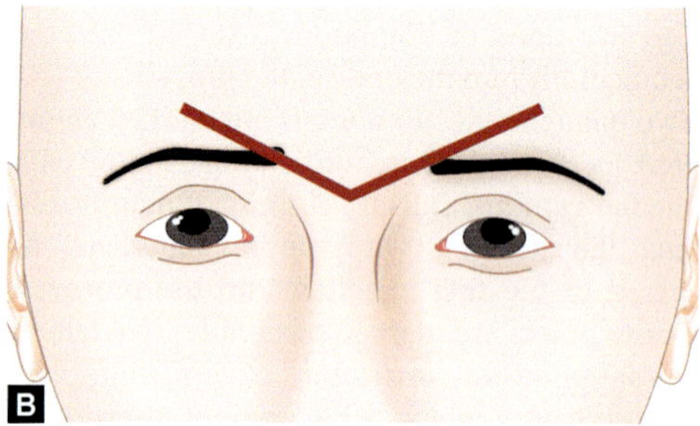

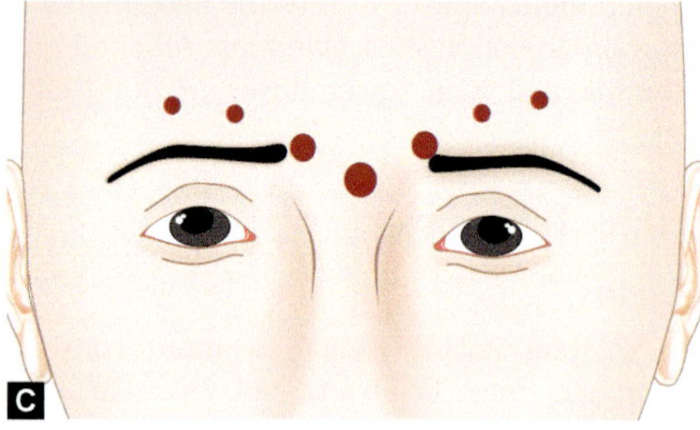

FIG. 4: A, V pattern of frown lines; **B,** schematic diagram of V pattern of frown lines; and **C,** injection points for V pattern of frown lines.

Gender

Men have larger muscle masses on an average. The shape of the male brow tends to be horizontal, whereas the female brow is characterized by a gentle arch. Males tend to have thick sebaceous skin. All these factors call for higher doses of botulinum toxin.

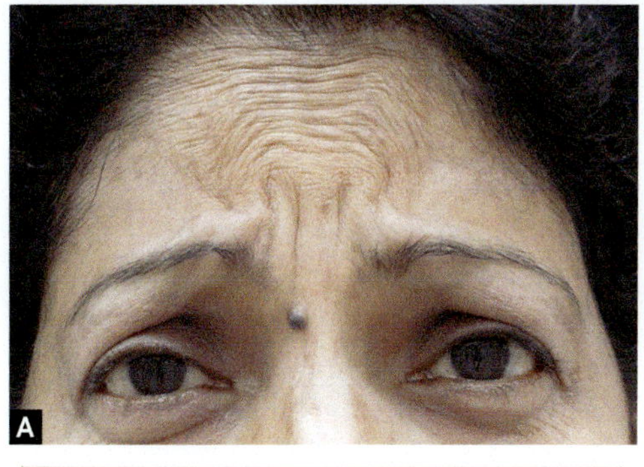
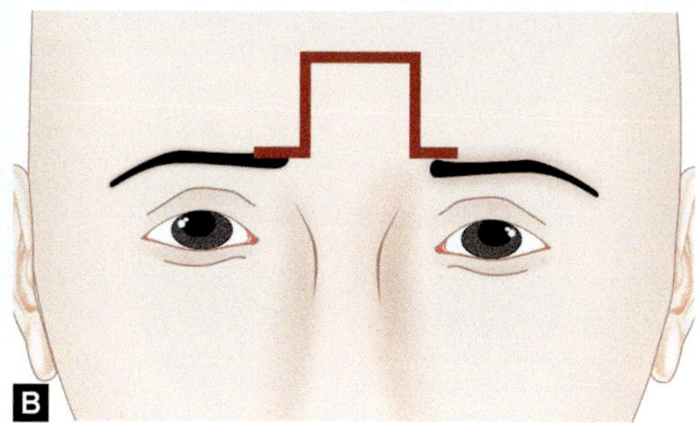
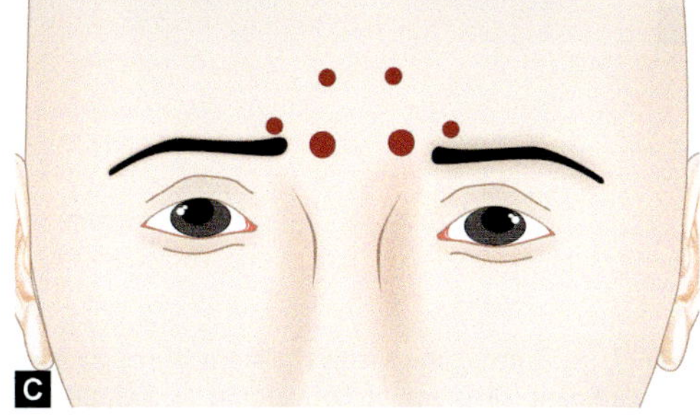

FIG. 5: A, Omega pattern of frown lines; **B,** schematic diagram of omega pattern of frown lines; and **C,** injection points for omega pattern of frown lines.

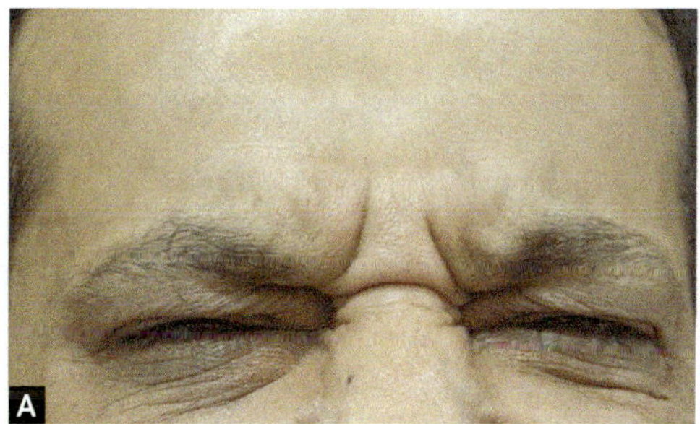
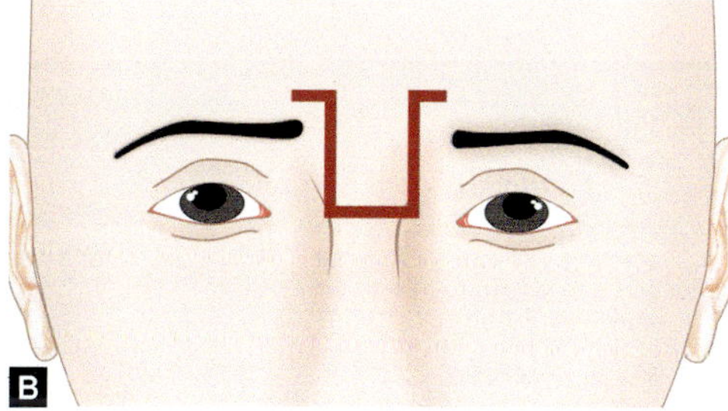
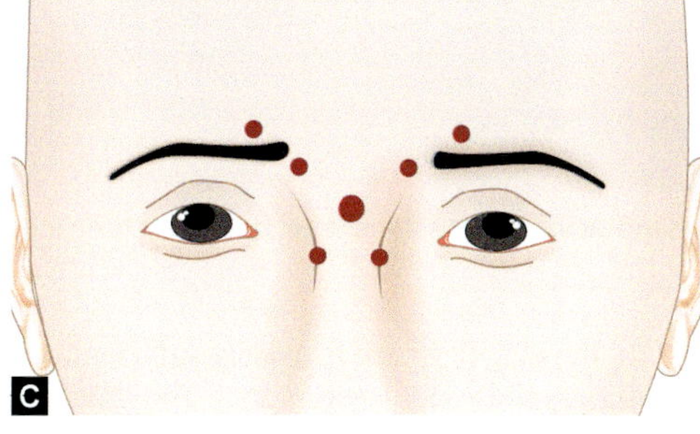

FIG. 6: A, Inverted omega pattern of frown lines; **B,** schematic diagram of inverted omega pattern of frown lines; and **C,** injection points for inverted omega pattern of frown lines.

Complications

- Eyelid ptosis occurs when the botulinum toxin diffuses through the orbital septum into the levator palpebrae superioris muscle which is the upper eyelid elevator muscle. This usually occurs if injections are placed at or under the eyebrows in the vicinity of the midpupillary line or even when one injects the lateral fibers of corrugators too close to the orbital rim with the needle pointed towards the orbital rim. This can occur as early as 48 hours or as late as 7–10 days following injection,

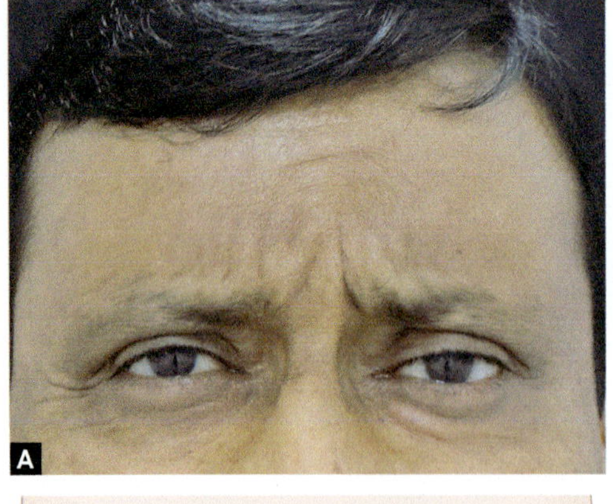
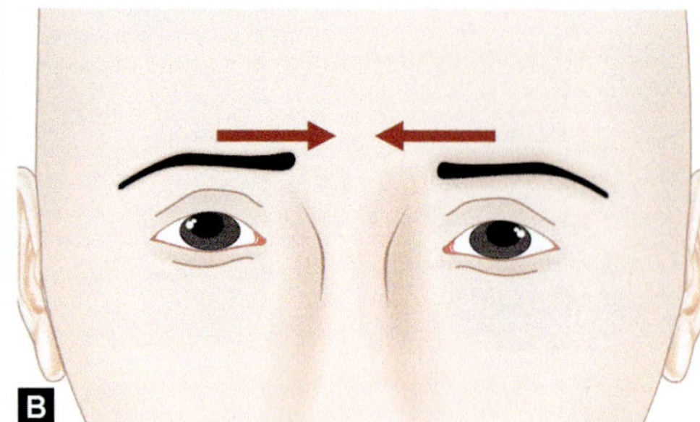
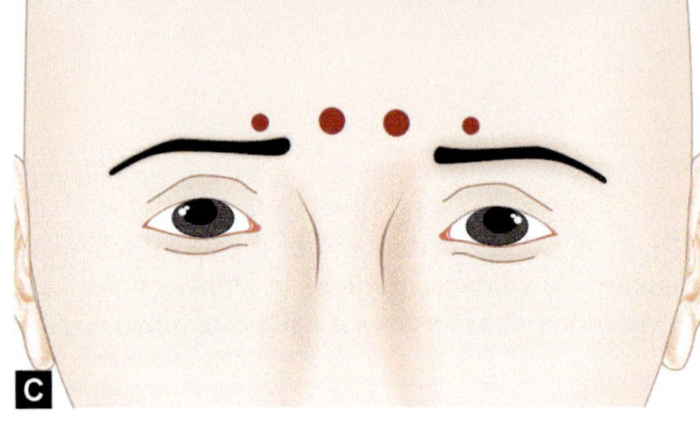

FIG. 7: A, Converging arrows pattern of frown lines; **B,** schematic diagram of converging arrows pattern of frown lines; and **C,** injection points for converging arrows pattern of frown lines.

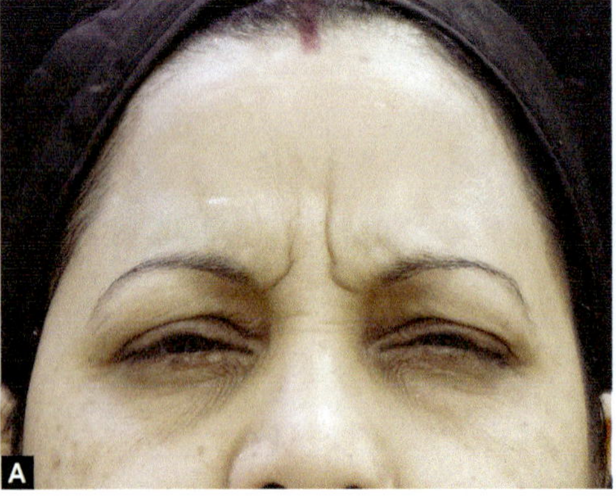
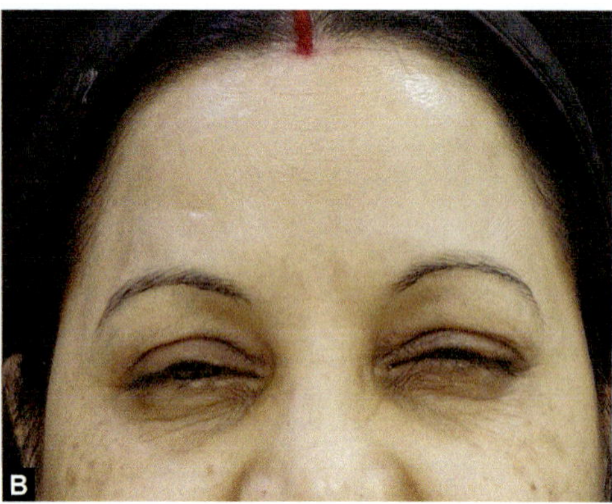

FIG. 8: A, Frown lines before botulinum toxin injection and **B,** Disappearance of frown lines after botulinum toxin injection.

and can persist for up to 2–4 weeks. Lid ptosis can be treated with eye drops in the affected side, however, only temporarily. Alpha-adrenergic agonists ophthalmic eye drops, apraclonidine 0.5% and phenylephrine hydrochloride 2.5% are mydriatic agents. These cause contraction of Muller's muscle, an adrenergic muscle, which is situated beneath the levator muscle of the upper eyelid. This treatment causes 1–2 mm of elevation of the eyelid, which is usually sufficient to make the eyelids look symmetric. The treatment is symptomatic and one to two drops three times a day must be continued until the ptosis resolves (Fig. 9).[9]

- Splayed eyebrows: A higher dose in the glabella causes the medial eyebrows to appear splayed. It is better to inject lower doses and soften the lines rather than trying to make them disappear.

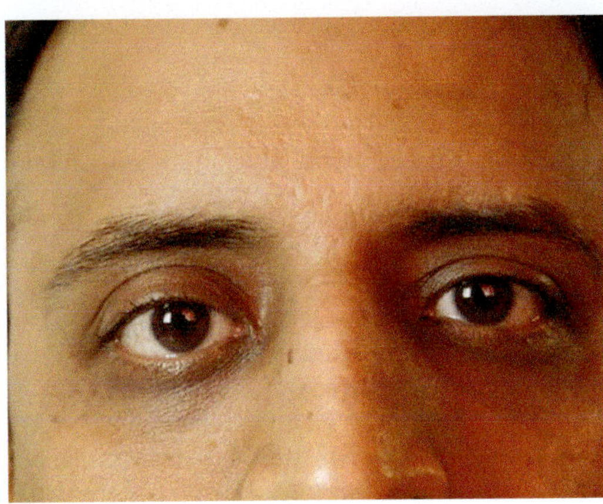

FIG. 9: Complication—lid ptosis.

Tips to Get Optimum Results

- Study the type of brow arch.
- Look for brow asymmetry.
- Look for any pre-existing ptosis.
- Study the muscle mass (usually more in males).
- Study the type of frown lines.
- Assess brow position. In women, make sure to find out whether the brows have been plucked or tattooed.
- Exercise caution in patients who have undergone surgery that can alter the underlying anatomy.
- Recognize the variables that affect required dosage in individuals.
- Always start with lowest required doses. A touch up can be done 2 weeks later.
- Do not aim at paralyzing the muscles completely as it will result in an expressionless face.
- Brow position especially in men may lie below the orbital margin. It is important to avoid injecting into the orbit.
- Never inject with the needle pointing toward the orbital rim. This will prevent accidental injection into the superior oblique muscle which could result in lid ptosis.
- Never inject way too high above the supraorbital ridge as you may end up injecting into the lower fibers of the frontalis.
- Avoid injecting into the corrugators lateral to the midpupillary line.
- Males may need a higher dosage as compared to females due to a higher muscle mass and thicker skin.
- Soft tissue augmentation may be needed to treat static glabellar lines.
- Ask the patient to frown and note the dimpling as the muscle bulk ends. This is the point of insertion of the corrugators. Your last injection point should be medial to this dimpling.
- Make sure you inject at least 0.5 cm above the supraorbital rim. Palpate the supraorbital rim and place the thumb finger of the non-injecting hand over the rim. Digital pressure at the border of the supraorbital ridge while injecting the corrugator also reduces the potential for extravasation of the toxin, avoiding inadvertent weakening of the levator muscle and resulting eyelid ptosis.[9]

HORIZONTAL FOREHEAD LINES

These are horizontal lines which appear on the forehead when one raises the eyebrows as if in question or surprise.

Muscle Involved

Frontalis

The frontalis muscle elevates the eyebrows and the skin of the forehead. It originates on the galea aponeurotica along the coronal suture and inserts on the dermis at the level of the supraorbital ridge of the frontal bone where it interdigitates with fibers of procerus, corrugator supercilii, and orbicularis oculi muscles. The fibers of the frontalis are oriented vertically, hence, the wrinkles of the forehead appear horizontally (Fig. 10).

The key in treating the forehead is to keep a little activity of the frontalis rather than freezing it completely as it is the only brow elevator.

In a study by Carruthers et al., they noted that the frontalis muscle presents significant challenges for the more inexperienced user for several reasons:[12] (i) inter-individual variability in frontalis structural anatomy, (ii) inter-individual variability in frontalis functional (habit/expression) anatomy, (iii) difficulty in treating in isolation because of the potential for eyebrow ptosis on the one hand and failure to efface

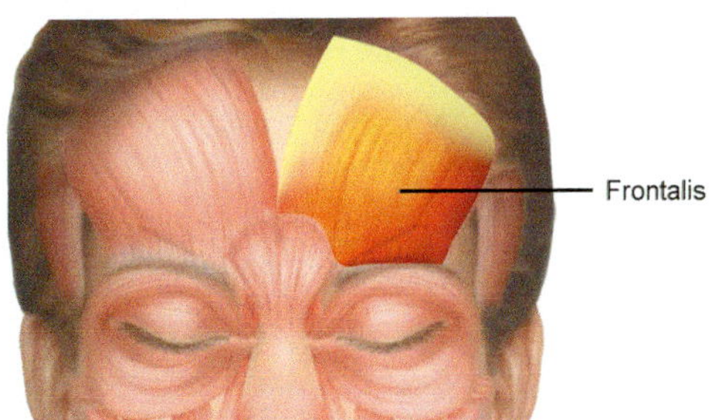

FIG. 10: Frontalis muscle.

lines on the other, and (iv) the potential for overtreating and producing an inanimate appearance.[13]

Conventional Injection Technique, Sites and Doses (Video 3)

In order to contract the forehead muscles, the patient is asked to elevate the eyebrows. The injection points are marked in a "Jacob's ladder" configuration or staggered distribution, 1–2 cm apart. About 1 unit of botulinum toxin is injected into each point and a total of 10–12 units may be injected in males and about 6–8 units in females depending on the muscle thickness (Fig. 11).

Avoid injecting into the lowest fibers of frontalis, i.e., in the lower third of the forehead. Stay 2 cm above the superior orbital rim in order to prevent brow ptosis.

If the patient has a low eyebrow, treatment of the forehead lines should be either avoided, or limited to that portion of the forehead 4 cm or more above the brow.

Some injectors believe in injecting both the frontalis and the depressors simultaneously for a more harmonious result. However, this is an individual decision and will vary from patient to patient depending on the anatomy and age of the patient.

Others are of the opinion that forehead lines should not be treated until 2 weeks after treatment of vertical frown lines, to achieve aesthetic harmony in the upper face.

Older patients with redundant skin under the brow (pseudoptosis) should be approached with caution. In such patients, brow depressors should be treated once the brow ptosis manifests.[11]

A lot of times, older people use their frontalis to raise their eyebrows in order to see. These are the people you should refrain from injecting the frontalis muscle.

Some patients have very fine forehead lines. These people should be treated with fractional lasers, chemical peels etc. before attempting to treat with botulinum toxin.

Patterns

Although, usually depicted as two somewhat fan-shaped bands, the midline fibers overlap substantially in some individuals.[14]

So, two patterns are seen most commonly. One is a broad band of muscle which causes single contiguous transverse forehead lines. The second pattern shows two separate muscle bellies with a central separation. In addition, the medial fibers of the frontalis may be more fibrous than the lateral fibers.[15] Forehead shape also differs between individuals in both vertical and horizontal directions. In addition, some individuals have numerous fine forehead lines, whereas others have a single deep horizontal furrow. Moreover, individuals will also demonstrate a spectrum of variations in habitual facial expression, causing furrows and influencing eyebrow shape. The totality of these anatomic features and their variations play an important role in determining the treatment plan for horizontal forehead rhytides (Figs 12 and 13). Horizontal forehead lines before and after injection is represented in figure 14.

Ethnic Differences

Asians need fewer injections for the forehead as they often have fewer wrinkles in the upper face compared with age-matched Caucasians.[16] There is less use of muscles in facial expression and

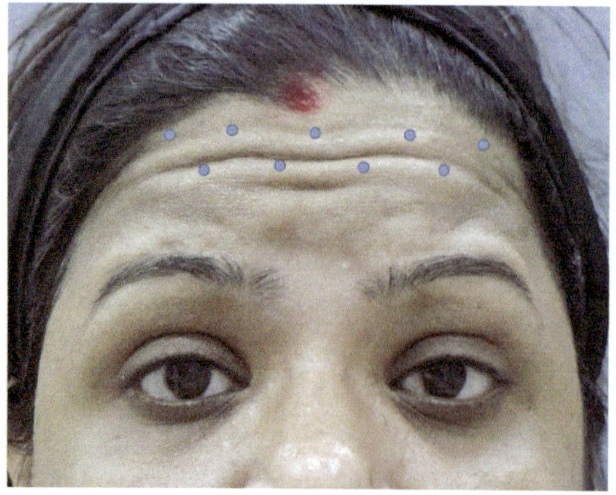

FIG. 11: Injection points for horizontal forehead lines.

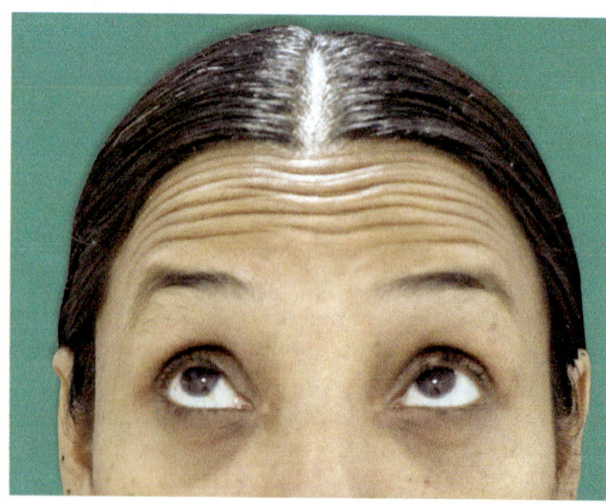

FIG. 12: Horizontal forehead lines: single belly.

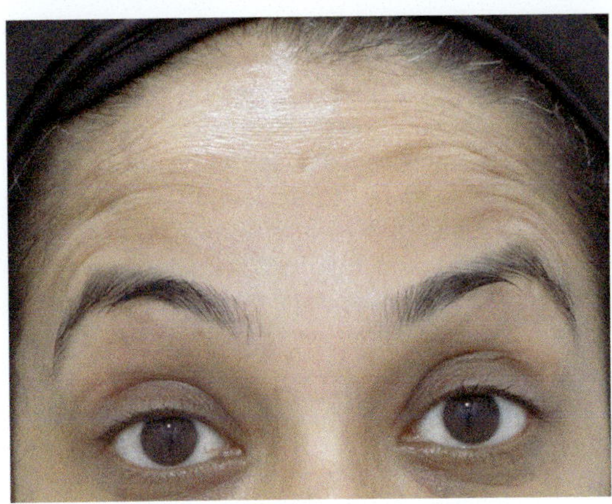

FIG. 13: Horizontal forehead lines: two bellies.

communication in the forehead area in Asians, compared with Caucasians.[17] Finally, Asians tend to have the appearance of "puffy" eyelids, and any inadvertent eyebrow ptosis and heaviness of the brow will exacerbate eyelid heaviness.[18]

Gender Differences

Men have larger muscle masses on an average and will require higher doses. The shape of the male brow tends to be horizontal, whereas the female brow is characterized by a gentle arch. This should be kept in mind as injecting the frontalis can change the shape of the brow.

Complications

- Brow ptosis: By using incorrect injection sites, too high dosages, and by an inappropriate selection of patients.

  Botulinum toxin when injected within 1 cm of the bony superior orbital rim (lower portion of the frontalis) can cause brow ptosis due to unopposed action of the depressors. This can be reduced by injecting the glabellar complex. Lateral brow ptosis can be reduced by injecting 2–3 units of botulinum toxin at the lateral canthus, in order to prevent the pull of the orbicularis oculi downward (Fig. 15).
- Quizzical brow: A quizzical or Spock's brow is seen when the lateral eyebrows arch upward to an excessive extent because of the unopposed pull of the frontalis.[19] This occurs when the lateral fibers of the frontalis muscle have either not been injected or have been underdosed as compared to the medial fibers of frontalis. This may be corrected by injecting 1–2 U of botulinum toxin into the higher fibers of frontalis laterally in line with the Spock's appearance (Fig. 16).
- Ptosis of the upper eyelid: Lid ptosis occurs secondary to downward diffusion of the botulinum toxin into the levator palpebrae superioris. This is usually a result of poor injection technique, when you inject too close to the orbital rim or point your needle toward the orbital rim at or lateral to the midpupillary line. It can also occur due to overdosage of the glabellar complex or the lower fibers of frontalis muscle.
- Lack of expressivity or a mask-like frozen face: It results due to overcorrection of the frontalis muscle. Always inject low doses of botulinum toxin into the frontalis as this is the only brow elevator.
- Appearance of new wrinkles or noticeable glabellar protrusion following botulinum toxin injection on the forehead: This was reported by

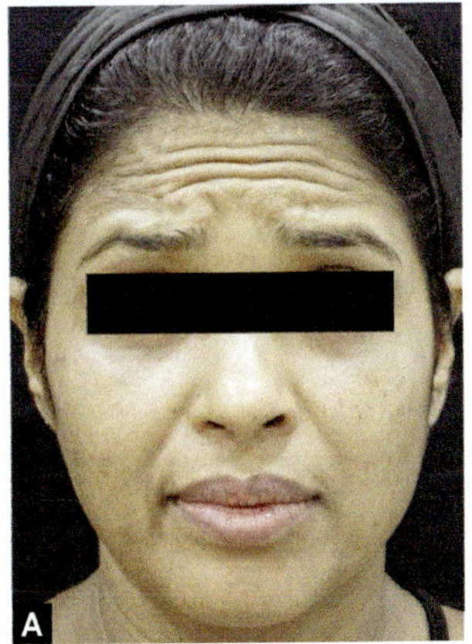

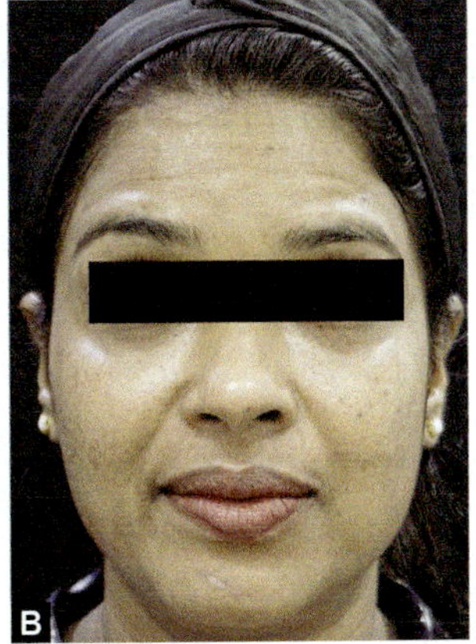

FIG. 14: **A,** Horizontal forehead lines before injection and **B,** horizontal forehead lines after injection.

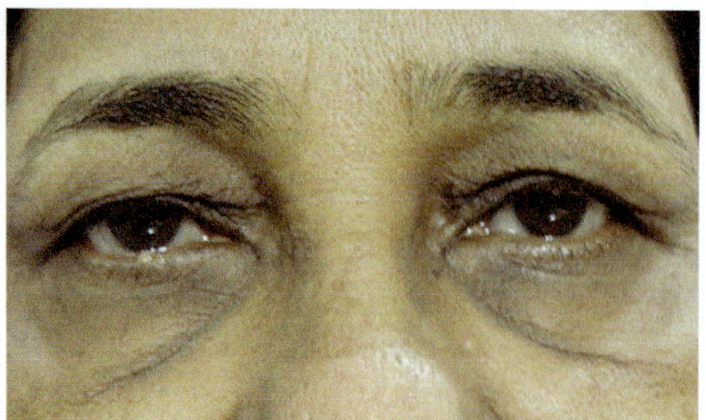

FIG. 15: Brow ptosis.

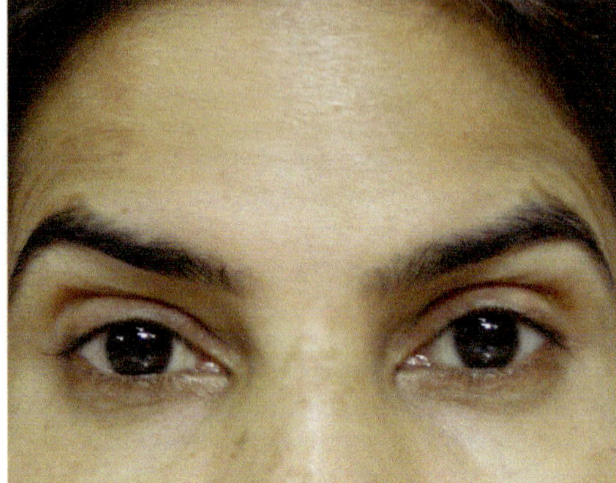

FIG. 16: Spock's brow.

Kang et al. in 2011.[20] Hyperactivity and overcompensation of untreated muscles can cause appearance of new lines or exaggerations of wrinkles. In people frequently using the frontalis muscle to raise their eyebrows or eyelids, exaggeration of previously unidentifiable wrinkles can take place at the border between the paralyzed frontalis muscle and nonparalyzed frontalis muscle. Sometimes, you may see a protrusion in the glabellar area due to hyperactivation of glabellar muscles with weakness of the frontalis muscle. The only way to treat this protrusion or bulge is to inject botulinum toxin into the glabellar complex.

Tips to Get Optimum Results

- Do not inject botulinum toxin into the lower third of the forehead. It is better to stay at least 2 cm above the eyebrow margin to prevent brow ptosis.
- In people with a small forehead, inject higher up on the forehead and keep the doses low to prevent brow ptosis.
- If the patient has a low eyebrow, treatment of the forehead lines should be avoided, or limited to that portion of the forehead 4 cm or more above the brow. The lower 2.5–4 cm of the frontalis muscle moves cephalad to elevate the eyebrows.
- The brow depressors should be treated in individuals with low-set brows or mild brow ptosis, and probably all individuals over 60 years of age. There is upward diffusion of toxin that addresses the lower forehead lines.
- Do not leave the lateral fibers of the frontalis unopposed. This will result in Spock's or quizzical brow.
- Look for brow asymmetries and inject higher up into the frontalis to correct the asymmetry.
- Start with a low dose in the frontalis and avoid using a dose of botulinum toxin A (BTXA) as it will give a frozen appearance.
- Distribute the injection points according to the observed animation and muscle function of the individual patient.

CROW'S FEET

Muscle Involved

Lateral fibers of orbicularis oculi.

Muscle Anatomy (Fig. 17)

This muscle comprises of three parts: (i) the orbital, (ii) palpebral, and (iii) lacrimal parts. The orbital part is the largest and extends onto the face some distance beyond the orbital rim. The orbicularis oculi muscle may be regarded as a sphincter of the eyelids. The orbital part is involved in forced closure, i.e., "screwing up" the eye. The lateral fibers of this muscle act as lateral brow depressors. As the inferior lateral orbicularis fibers curve more medially, the muscle acts as an accessory elevator of the cheek.

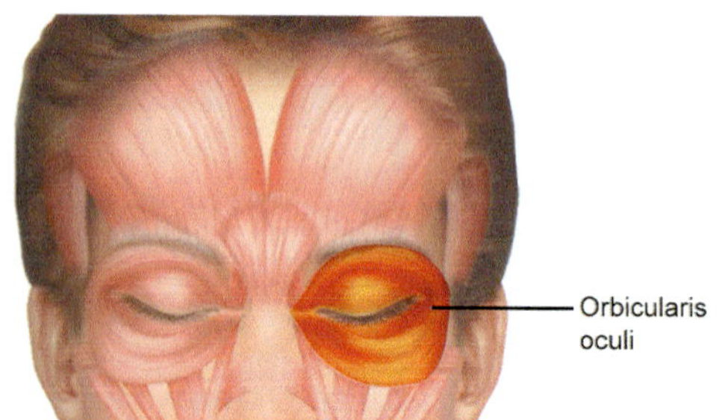

FIG. 17: Orbicularis oculi muscle.

Conventional Injection Technique, Sites and Doses (Fig. 18) (Video 4)

Ask the patient to squint or give a big smile and mark the injection points. Mark 1–4 injection points depending on the pattern of the wrinkles staying 1 cm lateral to the orbital rim. Keep a distance of 1 cm between two injection points. Palpate the zygomatic arch and make sure you stay above the arch. Diffusion into the zygomaticus major or minor muscles can lead to lip ptosis. Stay away from all visible blood vessels in order to prevent obvious bruising. While injecting, the needle should point away from the orbit and should be almost parallel to the skin as the muscle fibers are very superficial in the region. A tiny bleb may be raised as you inject. The recommended dose is 8–10 units per side in females and 10–12 units per side in males.[21]

Patterns of crow's feet lines vary among individuals.[22]

- Type I—Full fan pattern: Wrinkles lateral to the external canthus of the eye, extending from the brow to the zygomatic arch (Fig. 19)
- Type II—Lower fan: Wrinkles lateral to the external canthus of the eye, extending from the line of the external canthus of the eye to the zygomatic arch (absence of wrinkles in the superior lateral region) (Fig. 20)
- Type III—Central fan: Presence of wrinkles in the line of the external canthus only (Fig. 21)
- Type IV—Upper fan: Wrinkles lateral to the external canthus of the eye, extending from external canthus to upper eyebrow (Fig. 22).
  Crow's feet before and after injecting botulinum toxin is represented in figure 23.

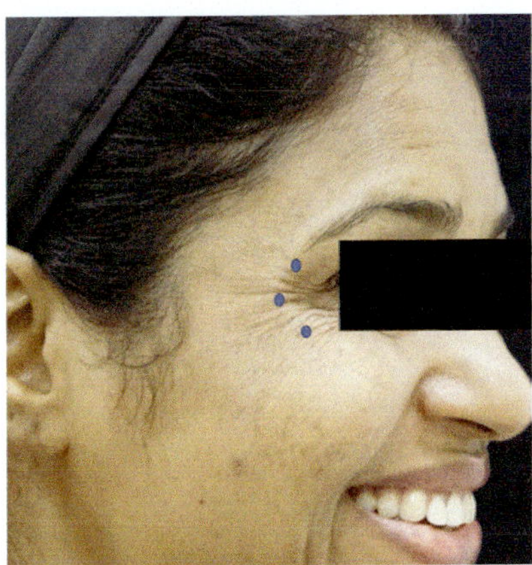

FIG. 18: Injection points for crow's feet.

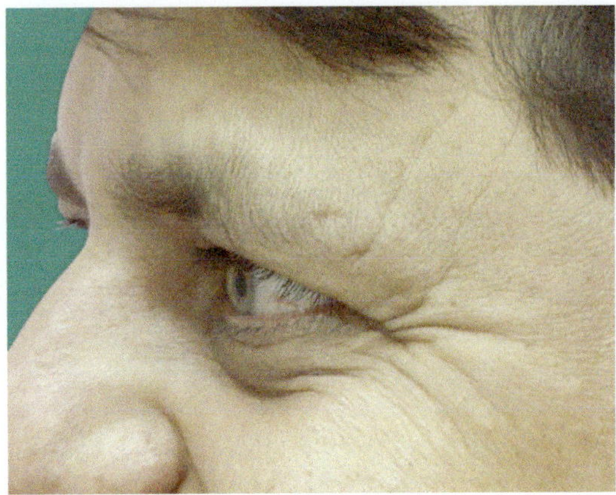

FIG. 19: Full fan crow's feet.

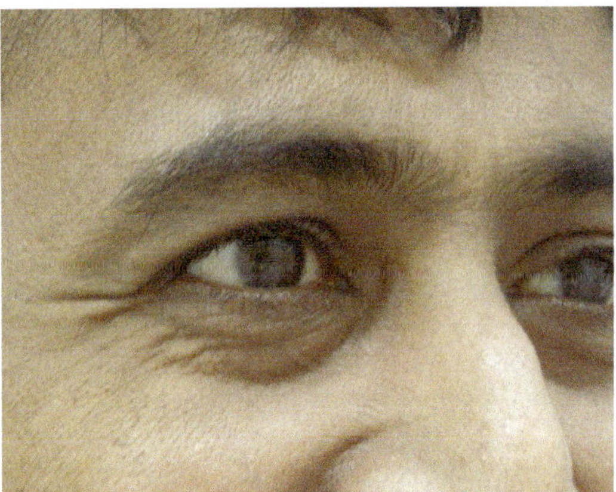

FIG. 20: Lower fan crow's feet.

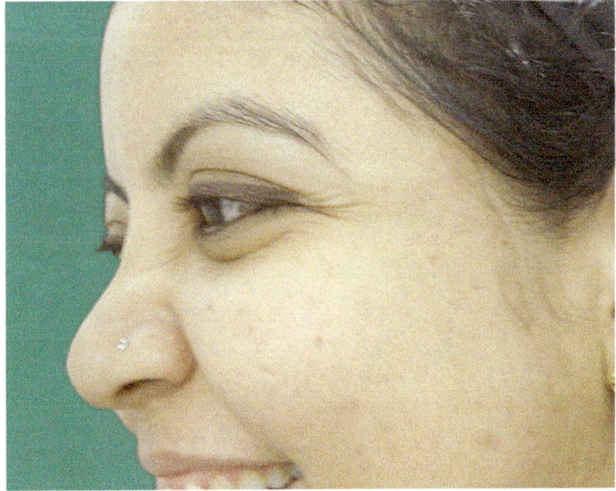

FIG. 21: Central fan.

Ethnic Differences

Asians have fewer wrinkles compared to Caucasians and will need lesser number of units to treat crow's

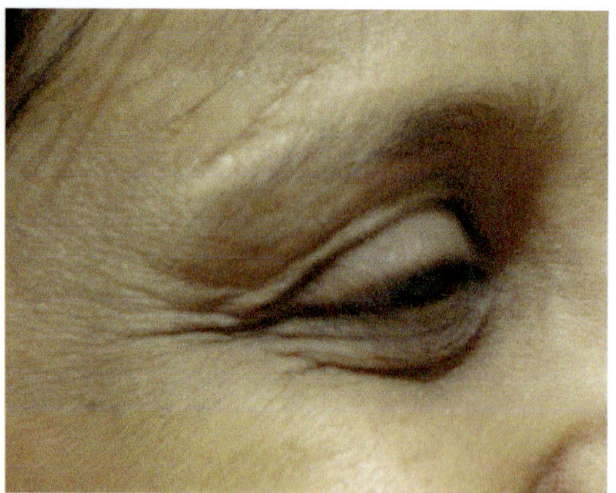

FIG. 22: Upper fan crow's feet.

feet. Sometimes in Caucasians, two rows of injection points may be needed. In Asians, especially Indians, only one row and three points usually suffice.[23]

Gender Differences

Males usually need higher doses than females due to thicker and stronger muscles. However, males prefer to have a rustic look and usually do not prefer all the crow's feet to be removed. Hence, always undercorrect and make the lines appear softer rather than making them disappear.

Complications

- Asymmetric smile or lip ptosis: Lip ptosis can occur if botulinum toxin is injected below the zygoma and deeply into the zygomaticus major. It can also occur if the toxin is injected too low into the orbicularis oculi fibers below the zygomatic arch whereby, it diffuses into the zygomatic major and minor muscles. Zygomaticus major and minor are important elevators of the upper lip and mouth. Paralyzing these muscles can cause an appearance similar to that of Bell's palsy. Resolution may take 8–10 weeks, so one must be extremely cautious not to hit this muscle (Fig. 24)
- Cheek ptosis: Injecting botulinum toxin too medially in order to treat infraorbital lines can cause a cheek drop. Medial fibers of the orbicularis oculi muscle are accessory cheek elevators and on being injected give a flat cheek appearance
- Diplopia and strabismus: It is important to keep at least 1 cm lateral to the lateral canthus while injecting crow's feet. Diffusion of the toxin from the lateral canthus medially into lateral rectus or inferior oblique muscle can result in diplopia or strabismus. An ophthalmologist has to be consulted in such cases. However, it is best to avoid injecting medial to a vertical line through the lateral canthus
- Ectropion and eyelid edema: Patients with lower lid laxity and positive snap test should not be injected in the sub-orbital region because they are predisposed to develop ectropion and lagophthalmos. A higher dosage in this region will also result in lower eyelid edema and incomplete sphincter function.[24]

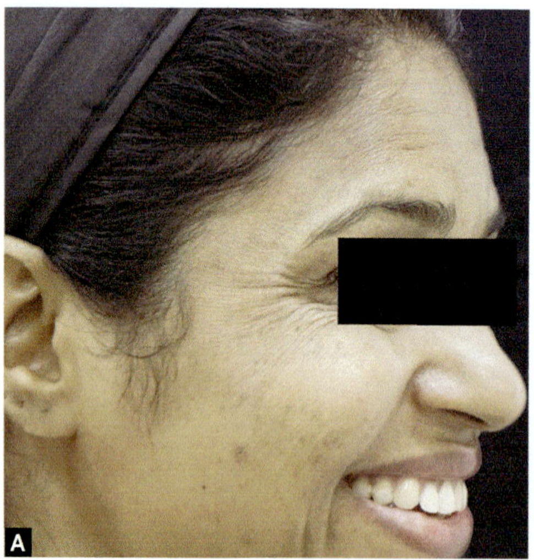

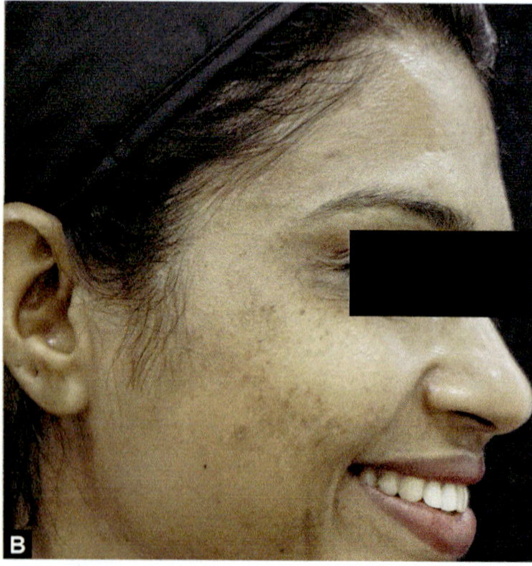

FIG. 23: A, Crow's feet before injecting botulinum toxin and B, disappearance of crow's feet after injecting botulinum toxin.

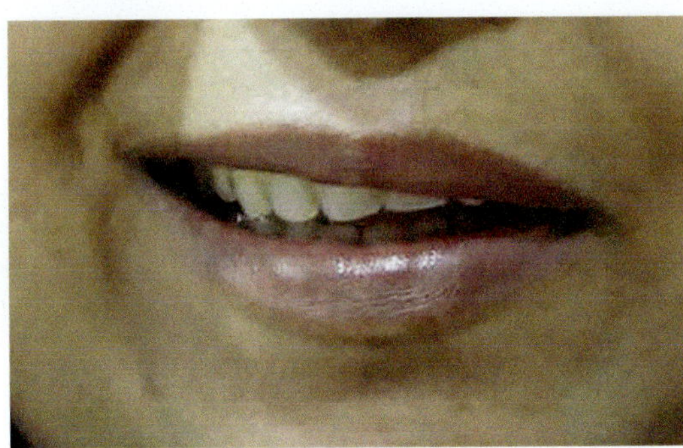

FIG. 24: Asymmetrical smile (complication due to diffusion into zygomaticus major muscle).

- Snap test: To do this test, gently pull the lower lid down for 5 seconds. After you release the lid, it should return to its normal position within 1-2 seconds. Lower eyelid laxity or positive snap test exists when tugging the lid results in a lid separation that lasts for 7 or more seconds
- Bruising and ecchymosis: In order to avoid bruising, one must examine the blood vessels underneath the skin carefully and avoid injecting into them.

Tips to Get Optimum Results

- Always inject at least 1 cm away from the orbital rim.
- Do not inject below the zygomatic arch to prevent lip ptosis.
- Do not inject into medial fibers of orbicularis oculi in order to prevent cheek ptosis.
- The skin is thin and the muscle is superficial in this area. Hence, it is best to raise superficial blebs.
- Watch out for superficial blood vessels in this region and avoid hitting them while injecting.
- Do not inject into the lower lid wrinkles if snap test is positive.
- Injections under the eye must be approached cautiously and should not be attempted if the patient exhibits a significant degree of scleral show before treatment, or if the patient has significant surgery under the eye previously or if the patient has a lot of redundant skin under the eye.
- Inject with caution when treating patients who have a history of dry eyes.[25]

EYEBROW SHAPING

The appearance of the brow is synonymous with an emotional, expressive, and psychological significance that makes it one of the most prominent feature of the face. As the brow naturally descends with aging, its position often imparts undesired characteristics to the face, such as fatigue, sadness, anger, or other qualities that do not represent the individual's state of mind.

Chemical brow shaping can be done with botulinum toxin by treating the corrugators, procerus, depressor supercilii, orbicularis oculi, and frontalis muscles. In males, the brows are usually horizontal (Fig. 25). Females usually desire flared brows or arched brows. Injection points can be seen in the figures 26 and 27.

Pearls

- Assess natural shape of brow and understand the patient's preference for shape.

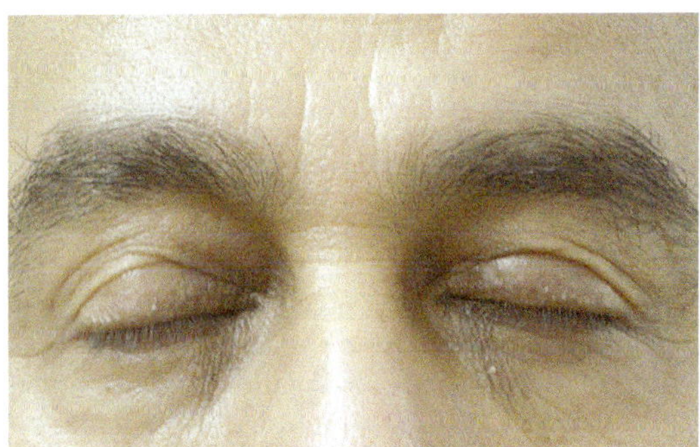

FIG. 25: Horizontal brow seen in males.

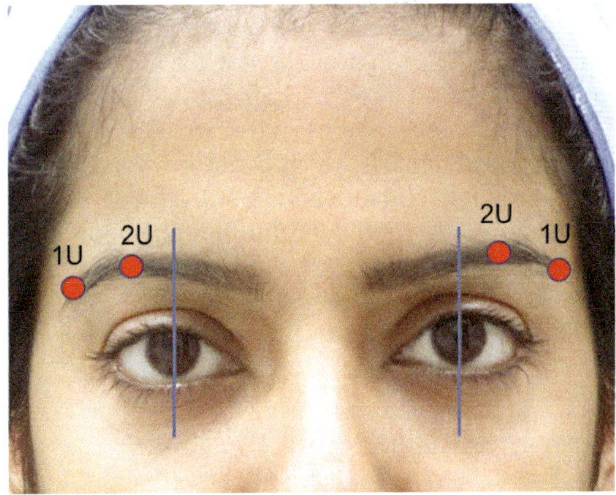

FIG. 26: Flared brow injection points.

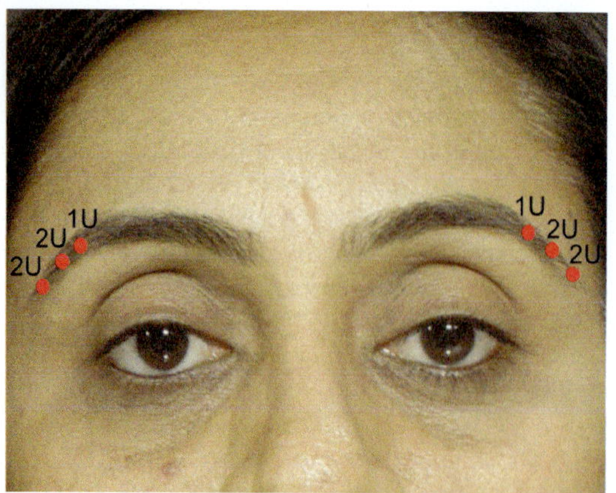

FIG. 27: Arched brow injection points.

- Inject cautiously as overdosing may result in undesirable brow shape or asymmetry.
- Stay away from the orbital rim.
- Look for any preexisting asymmetry to correct.

Complications

- Asymmetry
- Upper lid ptosis
- Bruising
- Swelling.

INFRAORBITAL WRINKLES

Along with crow's feet, many people have excess folds and creases along the lower eyelids, which gives them the appearance of being tired, sleep deprived, or even older than their current age. These under eye creases or infraorbital wrinkles which are known as "festoons" or "jelly rolls" are caused by contraction and hypertrophy of the pretarsal orbicularis oculi. These under eye creases also cause narrowing of the palpebral aperture particularly when smiling. They can be decreased by botulinum toxin.

Older patients may also have extra skin under the brow (pseudoptosis) which could be worsened by botulinum toxin treatment (Fig. 28).

Appropriate candidates for the treatment of the lower eyelids rhytides are those who have normal eyelid elasticity, determined by a normal snap test, and who have not had any previous lower eyelid surgery, including blepharoplasty.

Conventional Injection Technique, Sites and Doses[26,27]

Pull the skin of the lower eyelid down with the nondominant hand so that the skin becomes taut, insert the needle at an angle of 45°, approximately 3 mm below the ciliary margin and inject 1–2 units of botulinum toxin into the subcutaneous layer. Around one to two injection points are recommended for each eye with the total dose not exceeding 2 U. This will relax and flatten the pre-tarsal orbicularis, and improve the appearance of the lower lid (Fig. 29).

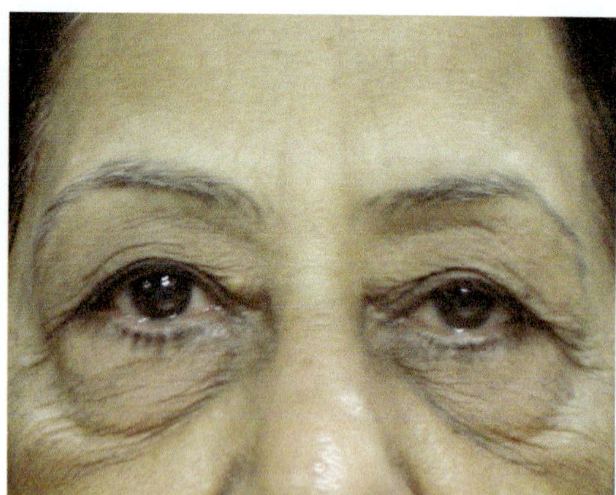

FIG. 28: Infraorbital wrinkles: Avoid injecting if snap test positive.

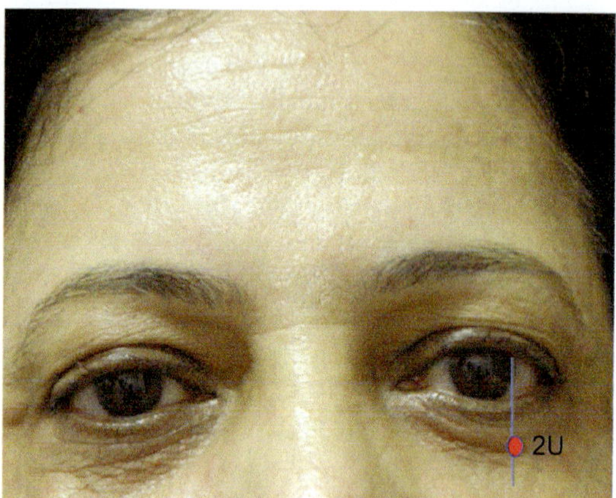

FIG. 29: Infraorbital wrinkles: Injection point

TABLE 1: Doses of botulinum toxin males and females

	Male (dose in units)	Female (dose in units)
Vertical frown lines	16–24	12–20
Horizontal forehead lines	8–12	6–10
Crow's feet	12–18	8–16
Brow shaping	5–8	5–6
Infraorbital wrinkles	2	2

CONCLUSION

Careful examination and selection, planning of accurate doses, and injection of botulinum toxin in the right planes can take away years from the patient and make him or her feel confident. Wrinkles on the upper face become more prominent with muscle use. Hence, when the muscles are resting, the lines disappear. Although the effect lasts only for 4-6 months, it does prevent worsening of the situation. Moreover, patients do not mind repeating the injections once the effect wears away.

REFERENCES

1. Charles Finn J, Cox SE, Earl ML. Social implications of hyperfunctional facial lines. Dermatol Surg. 2003;29(5): 450-5.
2. Sommer B, Sattler G. Botulinum toxin in Aesthetic Medicine. Vienna: Blackwell Science; 2001. p. 31.
3. Carruthers J, Fagien S, Matarasso SL, et al. Consensus recommendations on the use of botulinum toxin type a in facial aesthetics. Plast Reconstr Surg. 2004;114 (6 Suppl):1S-22S.
4. Draelos ZD. The shrinking word: skin considerations in a global community. J Cosmet Dermatol. 2006;5(1).1-2.
5. Porter JP, Lee JI. Facial analysis: maintaining ethnic balance. Facial Plast Surg Clin North Am. 2002;10(4):343-9.
6. Ahn KY, Park MY, Park DH, et al. Botulinum toxin A for the treatment of facial hyperkinetic wrinkle lines in Koreans. Plast Reconstr Surg. 2000;105(2):778-84.
7. Rexbye H, Petersen I, Johansens M, et al. Influence of environmental factors on facial aging. Age Ageing. 2006;35(2):110-5.
8. Shetty MK, IADVL Dermatosurgery Task Force. Guidelines on the use of botulinum toxin type A. Indian J Dermatol Venereol Leprol. 2008;74 Suppl:S13-22.
9. Klein AW. Contraindications and complications with the use of botulinum toxin. Dermatol Clin. 2004;22:197-205.
10. Kim HS, Kim C, Cho H, et al. A study on glabellar wrinkle patterns in Koreans. J Eur Acad Dermatol Venereol. 2014;28(10):1332-9.
11. de Almeida AR, da Costa Marques ER, Banegas R, et al. Glabellar contraction patterns: a tool to optimize botulinum toxin treatment. Dermatol Surg. 2012;38(9):1506-15.
12. Carruthers JD, Lowe NJ, Menter MA, et al. Double-blind, placebo controlled study of the safety and efficacy of botulinum toxin type A for patients with glabellar lines. Plast Reconstr Surg. 2003;112:1089-98.
13. Carruthers A, Carruthers J, Cohen J. A prospective, double-blind, randomized, parallel-group, dose-ranging study of botulinum toxin type A in female subjects with horizontal forehead rhytides. Dermatol Surg. 2003;29:461.
14. Kaminer MS, Hruza GJ. Botulinum A exotoxin injections for photoaging and hyperhidrosis. In: Kaminer MS, Dover JS, Arndt KA (Eds). Atlas of Cosmetic Surgery, 1st edition. Philadelphia: Saunders; 2002. pp. 292-309.
15. Wieder JM, Moy RL. Understanding botulinum toxin: surgical anatomy of the frown, forehead, and periocular region. Dermatol Surg. 1998;24:1172.
16. Nouveau-Richard S, Yang Z, Mac-Mary S, et al. Skin ageing: a comparison between Chinese and European populations. A pilot study. J Dermatol Sci. 2005;40:187-93.
17. Tzou CH, Giovanoli P, Ploner M, et al. Are there ethnic differences of facial movements between Europeans and Asians? Br J Plast Surg. 2005;58:183-95.
18. Wu WT, Liew S, Chan HH, et al. Consensus on Current Injectable Treatment Strategies in the Asian Face. Aesthetic Plast Surg. 2016;40(2):202-14.
19. Jankovic J, Brin MF. Therapeutic uses of botulinum toxin. N Engl J Med. 1991;324:1186-93.
20. Kang SM, Feneran A, Kim JK, et al. Exaggeration of Wrinkles after Botulinum Toxin Injection for Forehead Horizontal Lines. Ann Dermatol. 2011;23(2):217-21.
21. Fraenkel AS, Kamer FM. Chemical brow lift. Arch Otolaryngol Head Neck Surg. 1998;124:321-3.
22. Kane MA, Cox SE, Jones D, et al. Heterogeneity of crow's feet line patterns in clinical trial subjects. Dermatol Surg. 2015;41(4):447-56.
23. Tsukahara K, Fujimura T, Yoshida Y, et al. Comparison of age-related changes in wrinkling and sagging of the skin in Caucasian females and in Japanese females. J Cosmet Sci. 2004;55(4):351-71.
24. Brandt FS, Bellman B. Cosmetic use of botulinum A exotoxin for the aging neck. Dermatol Surg. 1998;24: 1232-4.
25. Cheng CM. Cosmetic use of botulinum toxin type A in the elderly. Clin Intervent Aging. 2007;2(1):81-3.
26. Carruthers J, Fournier N, Kerscher M, et al. The convergence of medicine and neurotoxins: a focus on botulinum toxin type A and its application in aesthetic medicine—a global, evidence-based botulinum toxin consensus education initiative: part II: incorporating botulinum toxin into aesthetic clinical practice. Dermatol Surg. 2013;39:510-25.
27. Gadhia K, Walmsley AD. Facial aesthetics: Is botulinum toxin treatment effective and safe? A systematic review of randomized controlled trials. Br Dent J. 2009; 207(5):E9.

14 CHAPTER

Midface Indications

Rasya Dixit

INTRODUCTION

The midface is an uncommon area to treat with onabotulinum toxin A [botulinum toxin (BoNT)] when compared to the upper face. Since diffusion of toxin and inadvertent injection of adjacent musculature can result in functional deficits and unwanted limited motion, injections in these areas need to be precise in both the injection points as well as the number of units used.

BUNNY LINES (NASAL SCRUNCH LINES)

The bunny lines (scrunch lines) are the lines which appear on the sides or dorsum of the nose bridge. These appear during a wide smile and squinting. They should be differentiated from the transverse lines on the dorsum of the nose, which occur because of contraction of the procerus muscle. The lines are caused predominantly by the contraction of the nasalis. However, the levator labii superioris alaeque nasi (LLSAN) and the medial part of orbicularis oculi also produce bunny lines. Table 1 captures the snapshot of major muscles involved in this indication.

TABLE 1: Bunny lines, muscles involved

Major muscle	Nasalis, transverse part
Minor muscle contributors	Levator labii superioris alaeque nasi few fibers, orbicularis oculi, medial fibers
Nasalis (transverse part) origin	Maxilla, above the incisive fossa
Nasalis (transverse part) insertion	Forms a aponeurosis over the nasal bridge to meet its counterpart from the other side

Bunny lines may become prominent in patients who have been treated with BoNT in the glabella area and crow's feet region, and the nasalis was untreated. In such patients, the nasal scrunch lines stand out prominently during animation such as a wide smile or squinting and have caused many a celebrity's BoNT treatment being discovered by the media. (The appearance of bunny lines on the nose, with no lines over the midbrow or periorbital area is a giveaway for many a celebrity who got BoNT done.)

Anatomy

The nasalis consists of the transverse and alar parts. The transverse part arises from the maxilla, proceeds upward and medially, expanding into a thin aponeurosis that is continuous, the bridge of the nose with that of its counterpart muscle of the opposite side. This aponeurosis is continuous with the procerus muscle over the dorsum of the nose. The alar part is attached to the alar cartilage.[1-3]

Variations in Anatomy

In a Korean study which looked at the anatomy of this region, it was found that the superficial part of the LLSAN gives some muscle fibers to the nasalis in 90% of specimens.[4] The transverse part of the nasalis originated from the maxilla and ascended, passing posterior to the superficial layer of LLSAN in 65% of specimens. However, it originated as two muscle bellies from the maxilla and the upper half of the alar facial crease, respectively, in 35% of the specimens.[4] Injections into the nasalis if positioned inferiorly or laterally, or if product is massaged inferiorly could diffuse into the LLSAN and cause lip ptosis.[5,6]

Injection Technique

Animate the Muscle

Ask the patient to give a wide smile, sniff or squeeze their eyes (as if against a bright light). This brings the muscle into action with oblique lines over the sides and dorsum of the nose.

Mark the Injection Points (Video 5)

The injection points are marked on both the sides on the nose, in the middle of the plicature made by the contraction of the muscle, one point on each side. A third point can be added over the dorsum of the nose, for the procerus muscle. The injections should be superficial (Fig. 1).

Carruthers et al. described the point of injection as a single point 1 cm above the alar grove.[7] Tamura et al. reported that in up to 60% of patients treated with 3 units (U) of BoNT, there were still persistent nasal rhytides. Up to 30% had persistent nasoorbicular, nasoalar, and nasociliary wrinkles. Injection of additional BoNT into the additional locations, according to the variable anatomy of the individual, showed excellent resolution of the rhytides. These patterns of wrinkles that appear within the first 4 weeks of application of BoNT must be treated at the follow-up visit. The nasoalar lines must be treated just over the nasal ala. The nasoorbicular and the nasociliar are produced by the contraction of the orbicularis oculi and must be treated with additional BoNT (Fig. 2).[8]

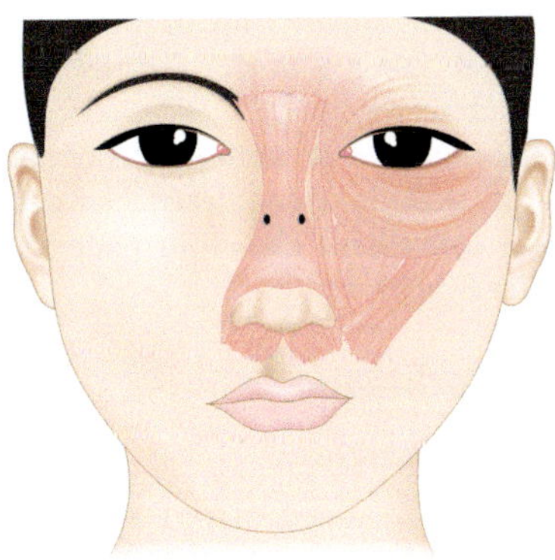

FIG. 1: Points of injection for treatment of bunny lines.

Dosage

Table 2 summarizes the dosage recommendations for various ethnic groups. 2–5 U are injected per side. A additional 3–5 U can be delivered to the procerus muscle.[8,9]

Points to Remember

In some patients who do not respond to injections into nasalis, injecting 2 U into LLSAN may be needed. However, injections should be done symmetrically to avoid asymmetry.

Botulinum toxin should be injected medial to a imaginary line connecting the medial limits of the nasal alae to the medial end of the ipsilateral eyebrow.[7]

Stretch the skin to check for blood vessels to avoid bruises.

Avoid injecting too lateral or too low into the levator labii superioris (LLS) to prevent upper lip drooping. Keep injections superficial to avoid touching the periosteum which is painful for the patient and to avoid bruising in this vascular area.

Transverse nasal lines can be addressed by a midline procerus injection.

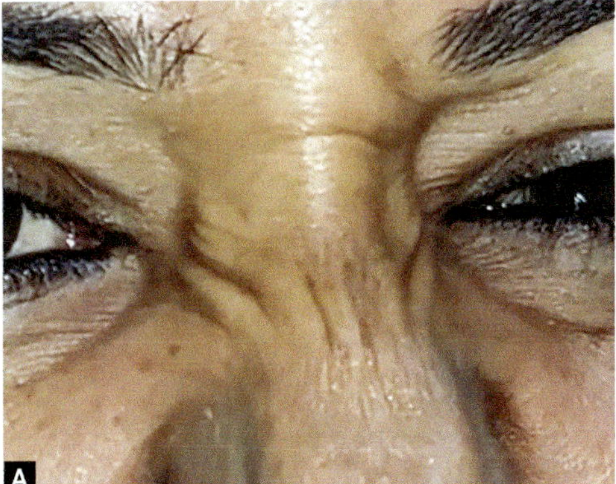

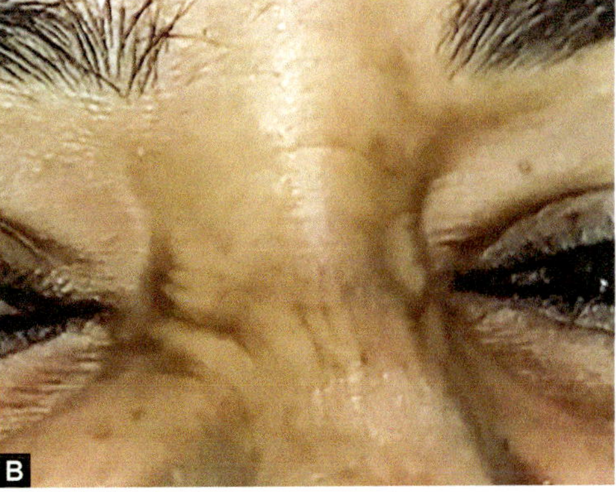

FIG. 2: Bunny lines before and after treatment with botulinum toxin.

TABLE 2: The dosage recommendations for various ethnic groups

Dosage in Asian men	Dosage in Asian women	Dosage in Caucasian men	Dosage in Caucasian women
5 U/side	2–5 U/side	5–7 U/side	6–7 U/side

Massaging vigorously in a downward direction can lead to lip ptosis due to diffusion of toxin. If there is bleeding, use pressure instead.

Inject 1-2 U/side of the upper nasalis when treating the glabellar area, to avoid enhancing the secondary appearance of bunny lines.

Less frequent, but not less important complication is toxin diffusion to the orbicularis oculi, diminishing the pump effect over the lacrimal sac causing tearing. Diffusion to the medial or inferior rectus of the eye has been described, causing blurred vision.[10]

Complications

Injections that are performed too low can result in paresis of levator anguli oris or LLSAN resulting in lip ptosis and an asymmetric smile.

Conversely, over injection at the superior aspect can result in medial rectus paresis and epiphora.[11]

NASAL TIP ELEVATION

The nose is the central focal point of the face. The treatment of the nose with BoNT is a emergent indication with few publications. With its lack of dorsal height, poor tip support, and wide nasal alar base, the Asian nose can often be treated with hyaluronic acid (HA) fillers and botulinum toxin rather than surgery.[12]

The nasal tip tends to turn down due to the action of the depressor septi nasi (DSN) muscle over the lower end of the nasal septum (Table 3). The importance of this muscle in rhinoplasty has been described.[13] Wright et al. have described the smile test to diagnose the hyperactive muscle.[14] Ham et al. have recommended transection of this muscle during rhinoplasty to release the tension in the nasal tip and dorsum.[15]

Both the nasal flare and the dynamic nasal tip ptosis (nasal tip dips during smile) can be addressed by BoNT. Botulinum toxin and fillers can be combined to achieve an atraumatic nasal remodeling or a medical rhinoplasty.[14,15]

TABLE 3: Muscles indicated in dynamic nasal tip depression

Major muscle	Depressor septi nasi
Origin	Maxilla, nasal spine
Insertion	Membranous septum and medial crus of alar cartilages

Anatomy

The DSN originates in the nasal spine of the maxilla inserting in the membranous septum and medial crus of alar cartilages. The contraction of this muscle turns downward the nasal tip. Some of the superficial fibers of this muscle originates in the orbicularis oris and insert in the columella. This cause the elevation of the lip (as in a smile) even as the nose tip turns down.[16-18] Rohrich et al. have described the interdigitation of the DSN with fibers of the dilator naris, the latter muscle originates in the incisor fossa of the maxilla, just below the orbicularis oris, and in the mucosa of the superior lip. In this cases provoke a paradoxical opening of the nostrils when these muscles contract together.[19]

As above, several authors recommend the incision of DSN in rhinoplasty; however, BoNT provides a convenient choice in patients with no need for surgical procedure.[20]

Injection Technique

Animate the Muscle

Botulinum toxin treatment of the DSN will have good results only if the main cause of the drooping nose tip is muscle hyperactivity. The smile test evaluates the muscular strength of the inferior third of the nose during a full smile. This observation has to be documented with frontal and lateral photography. Patients who have a dynamic nose tip ptosis are likely to have good result with toxin.[20]

Mark the Injection Points

Single injection point at the center of the septum at the level of the nasal spine. The direction of injection is perpendicular to the nasal spine, with the toxin being deposited deep into the septum (Fig. 3).[20,21]

Dosage

Two units in the septum will suffice for a tip lift.[21,22]

Benedetto et al. recommend that for a soft elevation 2 UI must be injected in each dilator naris

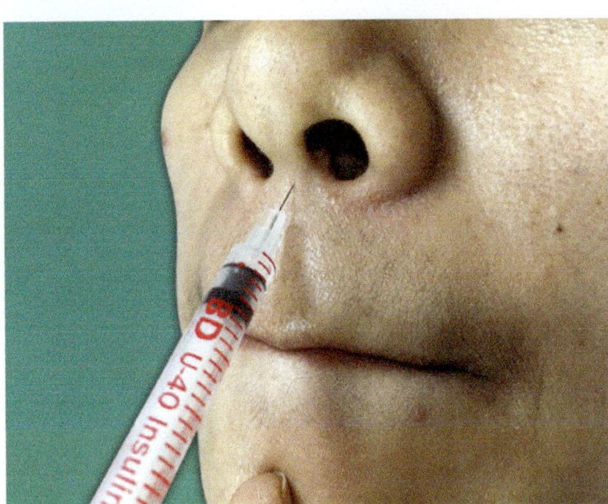

FIG. 3: Injection Points for elevation of the nasal tip.

TABLE 4: Dosage for nasal tip elevation

Dosage in Asian men	Dosage in Asian women	Dosage in Caucasian men	Dosage in Caucasian women
2–4 U	2–4 U	2–4 U	2–4 U

and 2 U in the DSN (total of 6 U).[23] However, both the international and Asian consensus recommends a single point of injection (Table 4).[11,21]

Points to Remember

During injection, ask the patient to pull down the upper lip over the teeth, to open the nasolabial angle. This way the base of the columella, where the needle should be introduced is easily accessible.

The needle should be introduced deep into the columella to avoid diffusion into the orbicularis oris.

Injection of the dilator naris can increase the distance between the columellar base and the vermilion border, creating a lengthier upper lip. So this can be used in a short upper lip to elongate the lip.

The clinical effect in this area usually lasts for a shorter time than other parts of the face.[24]

Complication

If the toxin diffuses laterally in the base of the columella, it can affect the LLS, cause a lip drop.

Diffusion into the orbicularis oris in the mid upper lip can cause flattening of the philtrum and unaesthetic elongation of the upper lip.

Lateral diffusion into orbicularis oris can cause sphincter incompetence during talking or drinking with pooling of saliva.

NASAL FLARE

Nostril reshaping to reduce the nasal flare can be performed by weakening the dilator nasi with small doses of BoNT. The nasal flare is the result of involuntary or sometimes voluntary contraction of the inferior portion of the alar nasalis (dilator naris) muscle (Table 3). The side of the columella and the septum turns visible when the nostrils open exaggeratedly and gives an unaesthetic appearance (Table 5).

Anatomy

The dilator naris originates in the maxilla over the lateral incisors travels through the nasal ala, and inserts in the alar cartilage and skin of the nostrils. The medial fibers can join the depressor septi nasi. The side of the columella and the septum turns visible when the nostrils open exaggeratedly.

Injection Technique

Animate the Muscle

Ask the patient to flare the nostrils.

Mark the Injection Points

Mark the point of injection over the area of greatest contraction of the nasal ala (usually in the middle of the ala). The injection depth is subcutaneous (Figs. 4 and 5).[11,21]

TABLE 5: Muscles involved in nasal flare

Major muscle	Dilator naris
Origin	Maxilla, over the lateral incisors
Insertion	Alar cartilages and skin of nostrils

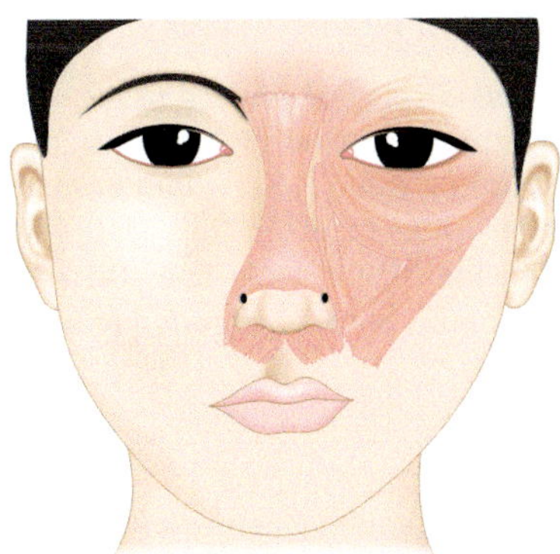

FIG. 4: Points of injection for the reduction of nasal flare.

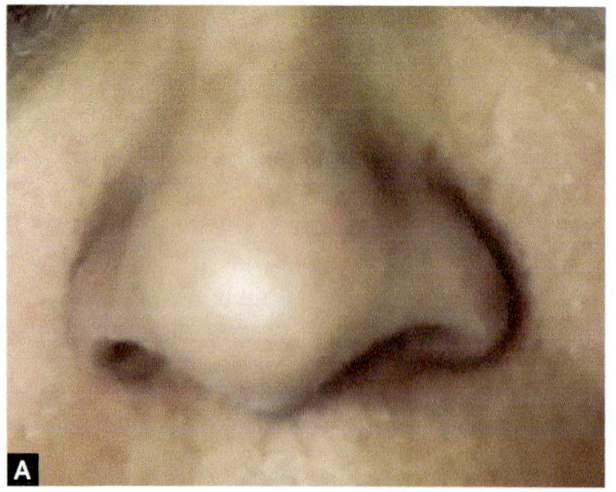
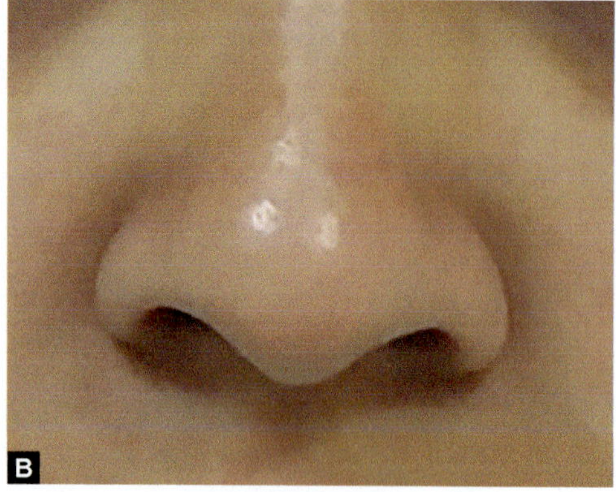

FIG. 5: Nasal flare before and after botulinum toxin.

TABLE 6: Dosage for reduction of nasal flare

Dosage in Asian men	Dosage in Asian women	Dosage in Caucasian men	Dosage in Caucasian women
2–8 U	2–8 U	4–8 U	4–8 U

Dosage

One to two units to be injected per side (Table 6).[11,21]

Points to Remember

The Current Asian Aesthetics Expert Consensus group recommends that one indication (either nasal tip elevation or nasal flare) is addressed at a time.[11]

The same technique can be used to treat nasal flutter, an involuntary and repeated contraction of the alar muscle.

Botulinum toxin can be used as an adjunct to rhinoplasty, postsurgical treatment complements the results of surgery.[25,26]

GUMMY SMILE

An excessive display of gingival tissue exposure of 3 mm of gum or more on smiling is usually referred to as a "gummy smile (GS)".[27] Tjan et al. described the gender differences in the smile line, with women having higher smile lines than men, as a consequence, GS is more common in women than men (Table 7).[28]

TABLE 7: Muscles involved in gummy smile

Major muscle	LLSAN
Accessory muscles	Zygomaticus minor
Origin	Maxilla, frontal process
Insertion	Upper lip, ala of the nose

LLSAN, levator labii superioris alaeque nasi.

Anatomy

The beauty of a smile depends on the relationship between teeth, the lip, and the gingival scaffold. The various facial muscles, such as LLS, LLSAN, and zygomaticus minor (ZMi) determine the amount of lip elevation that occurs during smiling. The LLS originates from the orbital rim of the maxilla and inserts into the upper lip, and the medial most fibers insert into the ala of the nose; the LLSAN originates from the frontal process of the maxilla and inserts into the upper lip and the skin tissue of the ala of the nose. The ZMi originates from the zygomatic bone and inserts into the skin tissue of the upper lip.[29] Therefore, the LLSAN and LLS not only pull the middle of the upper lip upward, but also pull the ala of the nose upward and laterally.[30] These three muscles converge lateral to the ala of the nose, where the LLS is deeper, the LLSAN is superficial, and the ZMi is more lateral. However, during BoNT treatment, all the muscles are not usually weakened as that could cause ptosis of the upper lip and drooping of the angle of the mouth.[31]

Injection Technique (Video 6)

Animate the Muscle

Ask the patient to smile fully with full teeth exposure.

Mark the Injection Points

The classical point of injection is just lateral to the upper margin of the ala, into the LLSAN. The injection is superficial to avoid diffusion into the LLS (Fig. 6).

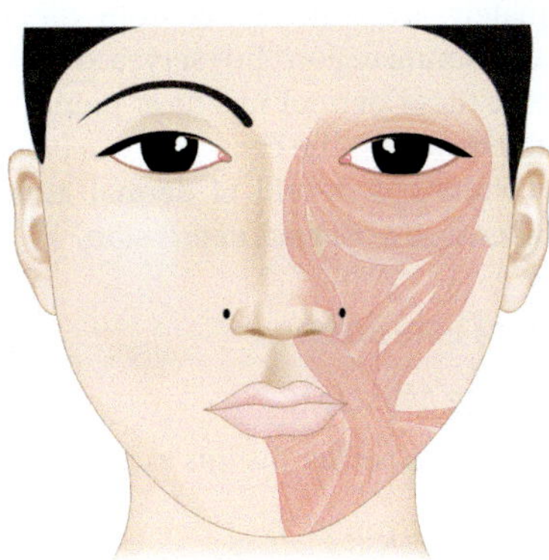

FIG. 6: Points of injection for gummy smile.

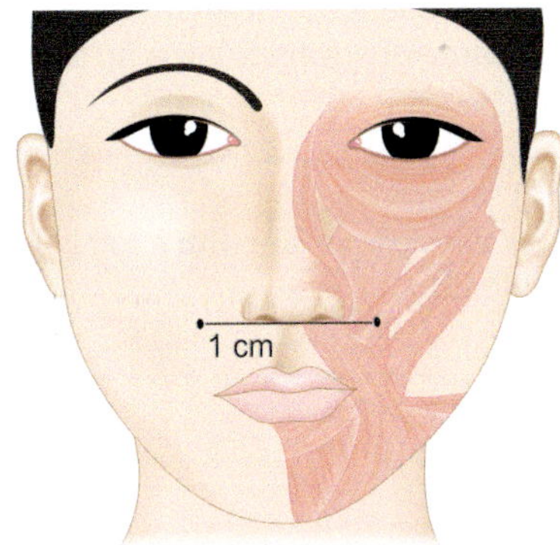

FIG. 7: Additional points of injection for severe gummy smile.

A second point has been described as the Yonsei point, and it targets all the three muscles. This point is 1 cm away from the nasal ala at the level of the nasal base, and is recommended only for the treatment of severe GS (Fig. 7).[32]

TABLE 8: Dosage of treatment of gummy smile

Dosage in Asian men	Dosage in Asian women	Dosage in Caucasian men	Dosage in Caucasian women
2–8 U	2–8 U	4–12 U	4–12 U

Dosage

Two to four units of BoNT is sufficient (Table 8).[10]

Mazzuco et al. have described four different types of GS, based on the area of the excessive gum display. Anterior GS (less than 3 mm of gum exposed anteriorly between canines) due to LLSAN hyperactivity, posterior GS (less than 3 mm of gum exposed posterior to the canines, and normal anteriorly) due to ZMi activity, mixed (with both anterior and posterior GS) and asymmetric GS. The Anterior GS was treated with 2 U of BoNT at the upper alar margin. For the posterior GS, BoNT was delivered in two points, the first point was located in nasolabial fold, at the point of greatest lateral contraction during the smile and the other point was 2 cm lateral to the first point, at the level of the tragus. At each point, 2.5 IU BoNT was injected. The mixed GS was treated with BoNT at all the above three points. In the asymmetric GS, BoNT was injected in both points described in the posterior GS, on the side with greater posterior exposure, and on the contralateral side, only the lower point was injected (Fig. 8).[32]

Sarrabayrouse et al. report that in of 20 patients injected in the middle and lower face, only two patients experienced partial lip ptosis following injection into the upper lip for the treatment of nasolabial fold.[33]

Points to Remember

Inject superficial to avoid diffusion into LLS causing smile asymmetry, lip ptosis.

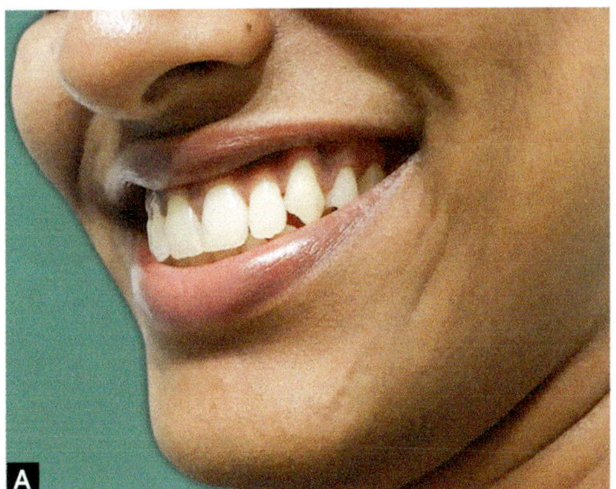

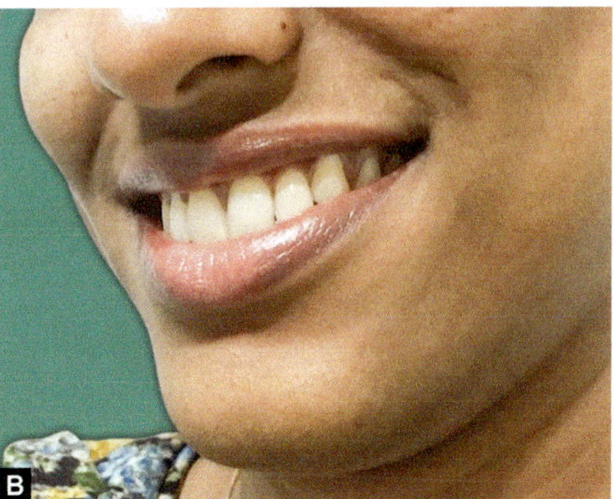

FIG. 8: Gummy smiles before and after botulinum toxin treatment.

Inject on both sides at similar depth to avoid smile asymmetry.

Lower volumes of dilution are preferred in this area, given the proximity to other important functional muscle groups [33]

PERIORAL LINES/LIPSTICK LINES

Vertical rhytids of the upper and lower lip tend to develop from persistent repetitive contraction of the orbicularis oris muscle. These wrinkles, often known as smoker's lines or lipstick lines, are common in smokers, wind-blowing musicians, and patients with chronic sun damage. It is important to take utmost care while treating this area since the muscles in that area are involved in important functions such as smiling, phonation, and mastication as well as in facial expressions (Table 9).[34]

Anatomy

The orbicularis oris forms a sphincter around the mouth. The muscle has superficial and deep parts. The superficial portion intermingles with fibers of several other perioral muscles to produce the fine movements of the lips. The deep orbicularis oris is responsible for the sphincteric action of the lips.

In the upper lip, the orbicularis oris fibers decussate in the midline and have dermal insertions approximately 4–5 mm lateral from the midline, sparing the central region. This serves to pull the skin medially at these dermal insertion points, forming the philtral columns. The central region between the philtral columns is devoid of dermal attachments and is pulled into a concave depression.[34,35]

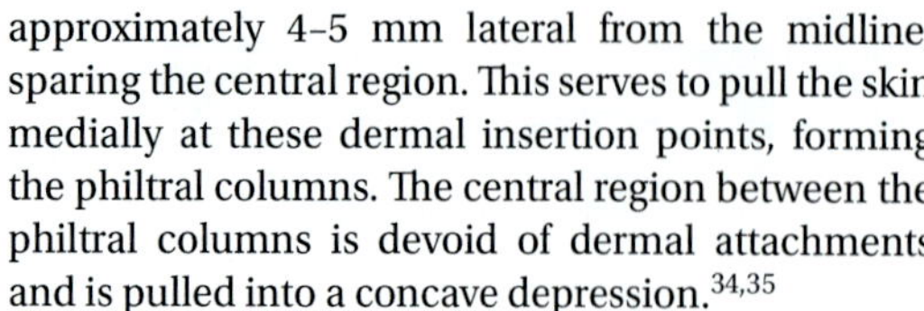

TABLE 9: Muscles involved in perioral lines

Major muscle	Orbicularis oris
Origin	Maxilla and mandible anterior portion and modiolus
Insertion	Dermal insertion into the skin around the lips and forms the lip muscle

Injection Technique

Animate the Muscle

Ask the patient to pucker the lips as if whistling.

Mark the Injection Points

Mark four points on the upper lip, two on each side, in between the plicatures caused by the muscle. Do not mark close to the midline or lip corners. The injection points should be close (within 5 mm) of the vermillion border. Two on the lower lip are sufficient (Figs 9 and 10).[11,21]

Dosage

One unit is injected per site with a total of 4–6 U of BoNT (Table 10).

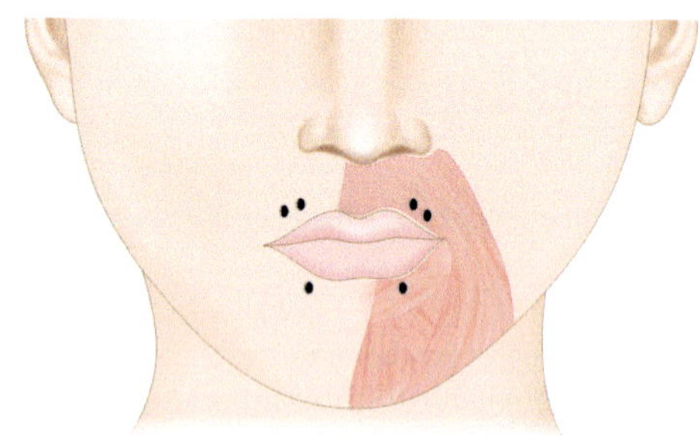

FIG. 9: Injection points for the treatment of perioral lines.

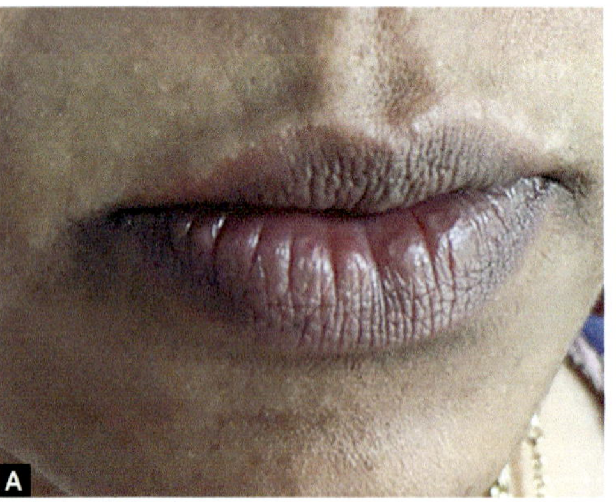

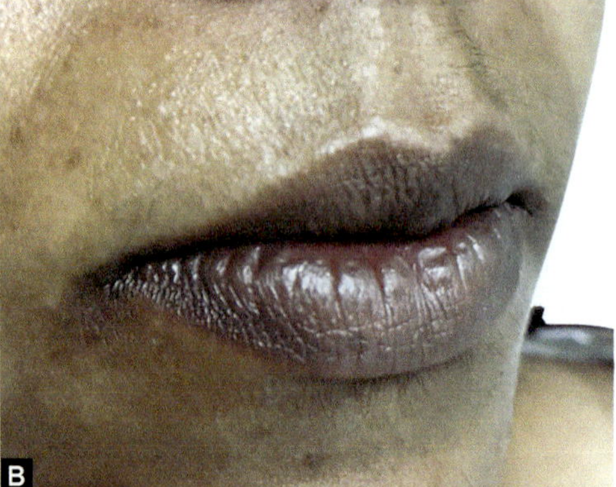

FIG. 10: Perioral lines before and after botulinum toxin injection.

TABLE 10: Dosage of treatment of perioral lines

Dosage in Asian men	Dosage in Asian women	Dosage in Caucasian men	Dosage in Caucasian women
2–8 U	2–8 U	4–8 U	4–8 U

The expert consensus group recommends not more than 4 U of BoNT in the upper lip for the correction of labial rhytides. The BoNT is injected at the vermillion border of the lip. An alternative technique described by the consensus group defines injection points slightly wider distance of about 2 mm from the vermillion border of the upper and lower lips, in the middle of the plicature.[11]

Points to Consider

Treat both the upper and lower part of the orbicularis oris muscle simultaneously. This is to balance the proprioception of decreased muscle contraction, including during reflex contractions.

Treatment of this area should be avoided in patients who make intense use of their perioral muscles such as singers and musicians.

Place and dose in a symmetrical manner and with an extreme precision to avoid weakening of the medial depressor labii (flattened cupid bow, flattened lower lip contour when the mouth attempts to form an "O"), lateral ptosis of the lip, facial and smile asymmetry and jeopardizing of mouth competence, causing difficulties with speech and suction or facial or smile asymmetry.

Placing the BonT within 5 mm of the vermillion is recommended.[10]

An initial minimum dose is recommended and then increased on a case-to-case basis. Trevidic et al. recommend an initial four point treatment (two in the upper lip and two in the lower lip as an initial starting dose), to avoid complications in this area.[30]

Best results in this area are achieved by combing treatments like laser skin rejuvenation and fillers along with BoNT.[36]

Give prophylactic antiherpetic treatment if indicated.

Complications

Lateral ptosis of lip can occur due to injection diffusion into the modiolus. To avoid this, keep the injection at least 1.5 cm away from the corners of the lips.

Injection points too close to the midline can cause flattening of the philtrum.

Smile asymmetry can occur.

Mouth incompetence including difficulty in eating, brushing teeth, and using a straw for drinking; difficulty in pursing the lips; and speech impairments, such as inability to pronounce b and p may be seen.[37]

DIFFERENCE BETWEEN ASIANS AND CAUCASIANS

Optimal doses of BoNT are lower for Asians in comparison to Caucasians, and this holds true for the above indications as well. Intrinsic ethnic factors, facial muscle mass as well as facial expression difference could contribute to the lower doses.[11] Europeans have larger facial movements in the frontal region than Asians.[11] Significantly higher wrinkle scores were seen in Caucasians than in Japanese in areas of lower face like lower eyelid, cheek, and corner of mouth. This could account for the lower doses needed in the Asians in the midface indications as well.[38] A study of the nostril shapes in Asians, revealed a horizontal nostril type with larger dilator naris anterior and posterior muscular components, with a more extensive insertion of the depressor septi muscle in this type. In the Causasians, there is a vertical nostril type.[39] The degree of perioral wrinkling is higher in Caucasians than Asians.[40] All these factors contribute to lesser dose in Asians compared to Caucasians.

CONCLUSION

Botulinum toxin treatment in the midface is evolving with newer indications and recommendations being available. But the complex interplay of muscles in this region makes BoNT treatments in this area an advanced indication. Keeping the doses low and dilutions in lower volumes makes for complication-free treatments. Botulinum toxin in combination with fillers and laser techniques are able to offer nonsurgical improvements for midface indications.

REFERENCES

1. Hur MS, Hu KS, Youn KH, et al. New anatomical profile of the nasal musculature: dilator naris vestibularis, dilator naris anterior, and alar part of the nasalis. Clin Anat. 2011;24(2):162-7.
2. Mythos Anatomy. [online] WebMD Anatomy. Available from http://www.mythos.com/webmd [Accessed June 2004].
3. Gray's Anatomy Online (2005). Available from http://education.yahoo.com/reference/gray/106.htm [Accessed June 2004].

4. Hur MS, Hu KS, Park JT, et al. New anatomical insight of the levator labii superioris alaeque nasi and the transverse part of the nasalis. Surg Radiol Anat. 2010;32(8):753-6.
5. Carruthers J, Fagien S, Matarasso SL, et al. Consensus recommendations on the use of botulinum toxin type a in facial aesthetics. Plast Reconstr Surg. 2004;114(6 Suppl.):1S-22S.
6. Carruthers J, Carruthers A. Aesthetic botulinum A toxin in the mid and lower face and neck. Dermatol Surg. 2003;29(5):468-76
7. Tamura BM, Odo MY, Chang B, et al. Treatment of nasal wrinkles with botulinum toxin. Dermatol Surg. 2005;31(3):271-75.
8. Ahn BK, Kim YS, Kim HJ, et al. Consensus recommendations on the aesthetic usage of botulinum toxin type A in Asians. Dermatol Surg. 2013;39(12):1843-60.
9. Curinga G, Rusciani A (Eds). Chemical peels. In: Minimally Invasive Procedures for Facial Rejuvenation. Foster City. CA: OMICS Group eBooks. 2014. Available from: https://www.esciencecentral.org/ebooks/uploads/chapterfiles/155-ebook-chapterfile-1499323233.pdf.
10. Shetty MK. Cosmetic uses of botulinum toxin. In: Mysore V (Ed). ACS(I) Textbook on Cutaneous and Aesthetic Surgery. New Delhi: Jaypee Brothers Medical Publishers (P) Ltd. 2012. pp. 607-12.
11. Wu WT, Liew S, Chan HH, et al. Consensus on current injectable treatment strategies in the Asian face. Aesthetic Plast Surg. 2016;40(2):202-14.
12. Sinno S, Chang JB, Saadeh PB, et al. Anatomy and surgical treatment of the depressor septi nasi muscle: a systematic review. Plast Reconstr Surg. 2015;135(5): 838e-48e.
13. Wright WK. Symposium: the supra-tip in rhinoplasty-A dilemma: II. Influence of surrounding structure and prevention. Laryngoscope. 1976;86(1):50-2.
14. Ham KS, Chung SC, Lee SH, et al. Complications of Oriental augmentation rhinoplasty. Ann Acad Med Singapore. 1983;12(2 Suppl.):460-2.
15. Wong GR, Chen WP. Phosphatidylcholine/deoxycholate lipolysis and hyaluronic acid augmentation to enhance nonsurgical lower facial contouring using botulinum toxin type A. J Cosmet Dermatol. 2011;10(2):159-62.
16. Braccini F, Dohan Ehrenfest DM. Medical rhinoplasty: rationale for atraumatic nasal modelling using botulinum toxin and fillers. Rev Laryngol Otol Rhinol. 2008;129(4-5): 233-8.
17. Zide BM. Nasal anatomy: the muscles and tip sensation. Aesthetic Plast Surg. 1985;9(3):193-6.
18. Rohrich RJ, Huynh B, Muzaffar AR. Importance of the Depressor Septi Nasi Muscle in Rhinoplasty: Anatomic Study and Clinical Application. Plast Reconstruct Surg. 2000;105(1):376-83.
19. Cigna E, Sorvillo V, Stefanizzi G, et al. The use of botulinum toxin in the treatment of plunging nose: cosmetic results and a functional serendipity. Clin Ter. 2013;164(2):e107-13.
20. Carruthers JD, Glogau RG, Blitzer A, et al. Advances in facial rejuvenation: botulinum toxin type a, hyaluronic acid dermal fillers, and combination therapies--consensus recommendations. Plast Reconstr Surg. 2008;121 (5 Suppl.):5S-30S.
21. De Maio M. The minimal approach: an innovation in facial cosmetic procedures. Aesthetic Plast Surg. 2004;28(5):295-300.
22. Benedetto AV. Botulinum Toxin in Clinical Medicine. Clin Dermatol. 2003;21(6):465-8.
23. Schavelzon D, Blugerman G, Wexler G, et al. Botulinum toxin in the nasal area. In: Serdev N (Ed). Miniinvasive Techniques in Rhinoplasty. Rijeka: InTech; 2016. Available from http://www.intechopen.com/books/miniinvasive-techniques-in-rhinoplasty/botulinum-toxin-in-the-nasal-area
24. Simons RL. Adjunctive measures in rhinoplasty. Clin Plast Surg. 2001;28(1):127-48.
25. Fagien S, Brandt FS. Primary and adjunctive use of botulinum toxin type A (Botox) in facial aesthetic surgery: beyond the glabella. Otolaryngol Clin North Am. 1975;8(3):717-42.
26. Goldstein RE (Ed). Esthetics in dentistry. Philadelphia, PA: JB Lippincott Co.; 1976.
27. Tjan AH, Miller GD, The JG. Some esthetic factors in a smile. J Prosthet Dent. 1984;51:24-8.
28. Hwang HS, Park MK, Lee WJ, et al. Facial soft tissue thickness database for craniofacial reconstruction in Korean adults. J Forensic Sci. 2012. 57(6):1442-47.
29. Trevidic P, Sykes J, Criollo-Lamilla G. Anatomy of the lower face and botulinum toxin injections. Plast Reconstr Surg. 2015;136(5 Suppl.):84S-91S.
30. Hwang WS, Hur MS, Hu KS. Surface anatomy of the lip elevator muscles for the treatment of gummy smile using botulinum toxin. Angle Orthod. 2009;79(1):70-7.
31. Mazzuco R, Hexsel D. Gummy smile and botulinum toxin: a new approach based on the gingival exposure area. J Am Acad Dermatol. 2010;63(6):1042-51.
32. Sarrabayrouse MA. Indications and limitations for the use of botulinum toxin for the treatment of facial wrinkles. Aesthetic Plast Surg. 2002;26(4):233-8.
33. Semchyshyn N, Sengelmann RD. Botulinum toxin A treatment of perioral rhytides. Dermatol Surg. 2003; 29(5):490-95.
34. Mazzuco R. Perioral wrinkles. In: Hexsel D, Almeida AT (Eds). Cosmetic use of botulinum toxin. Porto Alegre: AG Editora; 2002. pp. 158-63.
35. Dorizas A, Krueger N, Sadick NS. Aesthetic uses of the botulinum toxin. Dermatol Clin. 2014;32(1):23-36.
36. Garber DA, Salama MA. The aesthetic smile: diagnosis and treatment. Periodontol 2000. 1996;11:18-28.
37. Kane MA. Asian consensus recommendations on the aesthetic usage of botulinum toxin type A. Dermatol Surg. 2013;39(12):1861-7.
38. Tsukahara K, Fujimura T, Yoshida Y, et al. Comparison of age-related changes in wrinkling and sagging of the skin in Caucasian females and in Japanese females. J Cosmet Sci. 2004;55(4):351-71.
39. Ducut EG, Han SK, Kim SB, et al. Factors affecting nostril shape in Asian noses. Plast Reconstr Surg. 2006; 118(7):1613-21.
40. Nouveau-Richard S, Yang Z, Mac-Mary S, et al. Skin ageing: a comparison between Chinese and European populations. A pilot study. J Dermatol Sci. 2005;40(3): 187-93.

15
CHAPTER

Lower Face and Neck Indications

Jaishree Sharad

INTRODUCTION

As we age, the inverted triangle of beauty with a pointed chin turns into a pyramid of age where the lower face becomes wider. This is due to changes in skin, subcutaneous tissue, superficial musculoaponeurotic system (SMAS), muscle, and bone. In the lower face, marionette lines, popply chin, and vertical neck bands can be addressed with the help of botulinum toxin in adequate doses. The jaw can be contoured with the Nefertiti lift.

MARIONETTE LINES

Also known as the mouth frown, these lines appear as oblique lines from the corner of the lips on either side, running obliquely downward to the mandible. They give an expression of sadness, frustration or even disapproval. The muscle responsible is the depressor anguli oris (DAO) which depresses the angle of the mouth and its hyperactivity causes the mouth frown. Denervation of the DAO with botulinum toxin results in elevation of the angle of mouth.

Muscle Anatomy (Fig. 1)

The DAO originates at the outer surface of the mandible, posterior to the oblique line, and inserts into the modiolus at the angle of the mouth. It is innervated by the mandibular branch of the facial nerve and serves primarily to depress the oral commissure (Table 1).

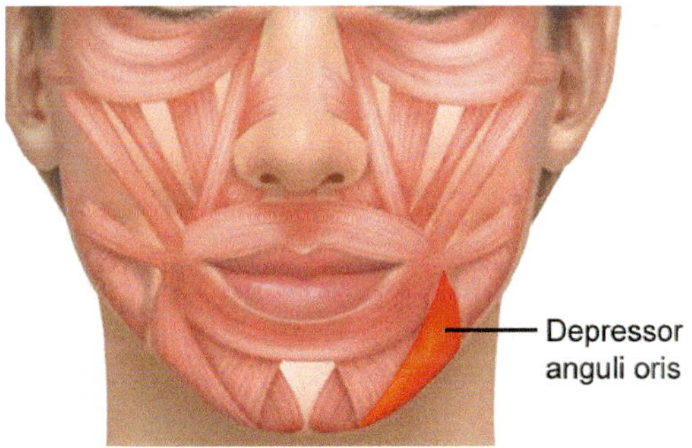

FIG. 1: Depressor anguli oris muscle.

TABLE 1: Muscle anatomy

	Name of the muscle	Origin	Insertion	Action	Indication of botox
1	DAO	Arises from outer surface of the mandible posterior to the oblique line	The modiolus at the angle of the mouth	Depresses the angle of the mouth	Prominent marionette lines
2	Mentalis	Arises from the incisive fossa located on the anterior aspect of the mandible	Skin of the chin	Primary evertor of the lower lip and also, serves to elevate the skin of the chin	Popply chin
3	DLI	Arises from the oblique line of the mandible between the symphysis and mental foramen	Skin of the lower lip, blending with orbicularis oris	Pulls down the corner of the mouth inferiorly	If hit, will cause asymmetrical smile. Should be avoided

Contd...

Contd...

	Name of the muscle	Origin	Insertion	Action	Indication of botox
4	Platysma	Originates in the superficial fascia of the upper portion of the thorax, clavicle, and acromion	• The anterior fibers (pars mandibularis) are inserted into the periosteum of the medial portion of the mandibular border • The pars labialis inserts into the lateral half of the lower lip, passing beneath the DAO muscle fibers • The posterior fibers (pars modiolaris) are inserted into the modiolus	Anchors and depresses the lower facial musculature	Turkey neck (vertical neck bands)
5	Masseter	• The superficial portion arises from the zygomatic process of the maxilla, and from the anterior two-thirds of the lower border of the zygomatic arch • The deep portion arises from the posterior third of the lower border, and from the medial surface of the zygomatic arch	• Superficial fibers pass downward and backward, to be inserted into the angle and lower half of the lateral surface of the ramus of the mandible • Deep fibers pass downward and forward, to be inserted into the upper half of the ramus and the lateral surface of the coronoid process of the mandible	Elevates the mandible	Square jaw

DAO, depressor anguli oris; DLI, depressor labii inferioris.

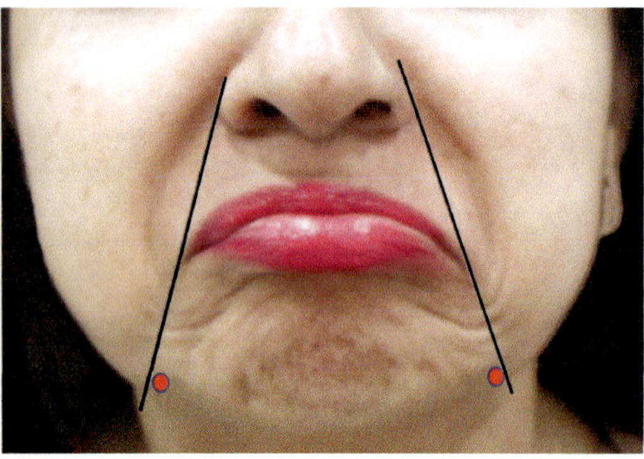

FIG. 2: Injection points.

The Conventional Injection Technique, Sites, and Doses (Figs. 2 to 4) (Video 7)

Ask the patient to make a sad face by actively contracting the corners of the mouth downward. Palpate the DAO as the patient does this manoeuvre and mark the injection site at its origin at the border of the mandible 1 cm lateral to the oral commissure.

A better way to mark the injection point is to follow an imaginary line along the extent of the nasolabial crease until it crosses the mandible. Inject the neurotoxin about 1/2 cm above this junction of the mandibular ramus on either side of the chin. A 2–4 U of botulinum toxin are injected intramuscularly on either side with the patient in the upright sitting or semirecumbent position.

It is important not to inject too high or too medially in order to avoid diffusion into orbicularis oris or depressor labii inferioris (DLI) (Table 2).[1-3]

Gender Difference

Although, men have stronger DAO muscles, they do not prefer to be treated with botulinum toxin. Upturned corner of the lips is considered more of a feminine thing.

Complications

Asymmetrical smile, oral incompetence, and drooling could result if the orbicularis oris is injected while trying to inject DAO too close to the mouth, or if there

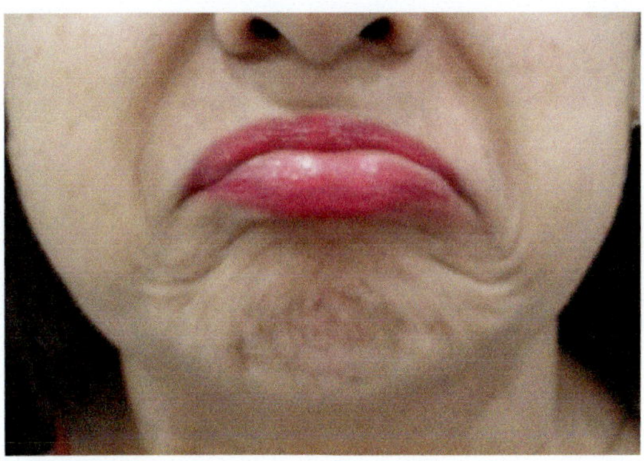

FIG. 3: Before injection of botulinum toxin into depressor anguli oris (DAO) for marionette line.

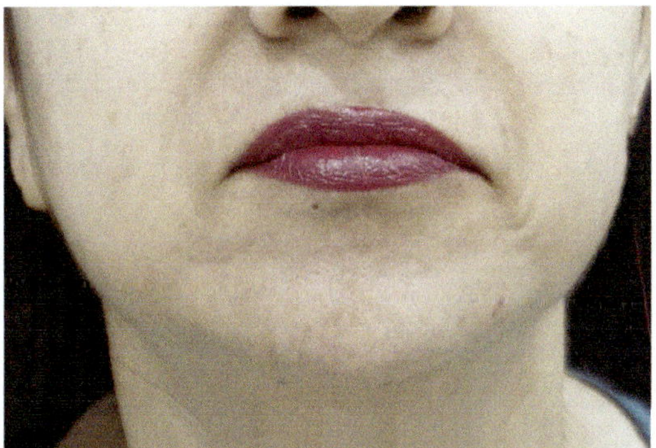

FIG. 4: After injection of botulinum toxin into depressor anguli oris (DAO) for marionette line.

TABLE 2: Botulinum toxin doses in males and females

	Muscle involved	Units in male	Units in female
Marionette lines	Depressor anguli oris (DAO)	2–3 per side	2 units per side
Popply chin	Mentalis	3–4 per side	2–3 per side
Turkey neck	Platysma	Total 40–60 units	Total 30–50 units
Nefertiti lift	Platysma	12–20 units per side	12–15 units per side
Square jaw/ masseter hypertrophy	Masseter	25–30 units per side	15–25 units per side

is diffusion into the orbicularis oris from the DAO. There may also be a flattening of the lower lip contour when the mouth attempts to form an "O" (Fig. 5).

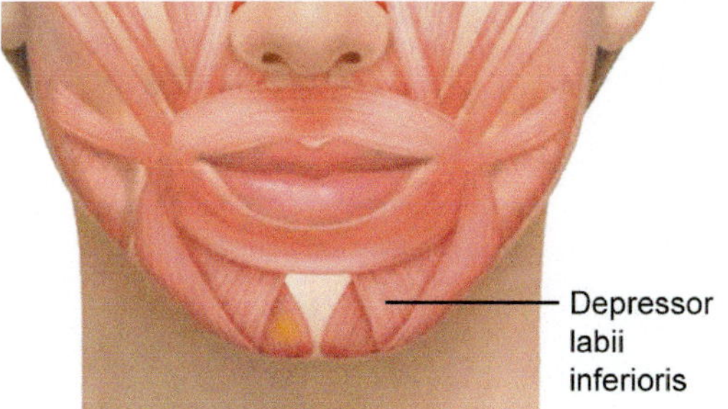

FIG. 5: Asymmetrical smile if the toxin diffuses to the depressor labii inferioris muscle.

Treatment Pearls

Always stick to the oblique line drawn along the naso-labial fold and corner of the mouth down to the mandible. Do not inject medial and higher to this point.

Stay as low and close to the ramus of the mandible as possible. Injecting too high will affect the orbicularis oris muscle. Never go higher than halfway between the lip and the mandible.

Inject botulinum toxin only when the DAO can be precisely palpated and securely identified.

Avoid injecting Botulinum toxin into the marginal mandibular nerve, facial artery, and vein by lifting the soft tissue before injecting.

POPPLY CHIN

A hyperdynamic mentalis muscle can create unwanted wrinkling and creasing, sometimes resembling a peau d'orange, of the mental area. Appreciation of this effect is best noticed when the patient is performing facial expressions. This is also known as popply chin or cobblestone chin. Botulinum toxin A can be used to reduce dimpled effects of the chin and give an appearance of lengthening of the chin.

Muscle Anatomy

The mentalis muscle originates and arises from the incisive fossa located on the anterior aspect of the mandible and inserts into the skin of the chin. Its fibers intermingle with the orbicularis oris and DLI. The mentalis muscle is the primary evertor of the lower lip and also serves to elevate the skin of the chin (Fig. 6).

Injection Sites and Dosage (Video 8)

The mentalis can be injected in two ways depending on the muscle bulge. Four units of botulinum toxin can be injected directly into the insertion point of

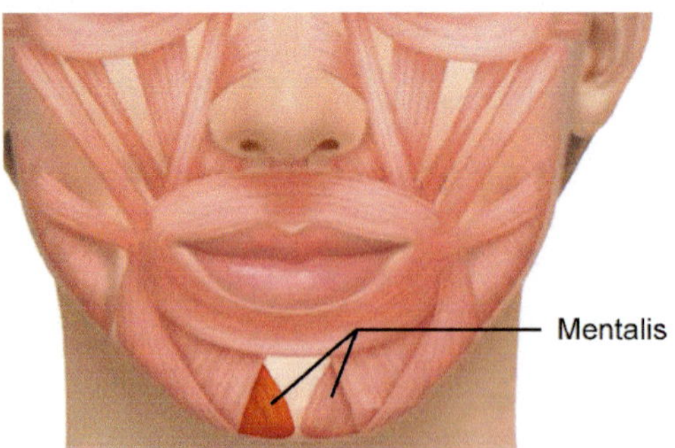

FIG. 6: Mentalis muscle.

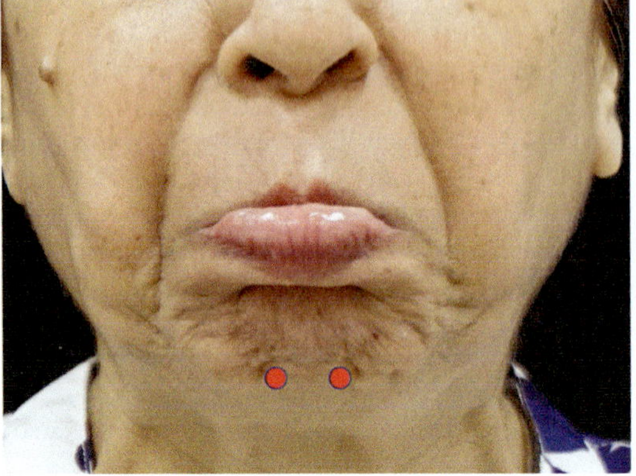

FIG. 7: Injection points for popply chin.

both bellies of the mentalis muscle centrally on the mandible at the apex of the mentum (Fig. 7).

A more common technique is to inject 2 units of botulinum toxin into each belly of the muscle, staying close to the midline, and close to the mandibular ramus to avoid spread to the DLI.[4]

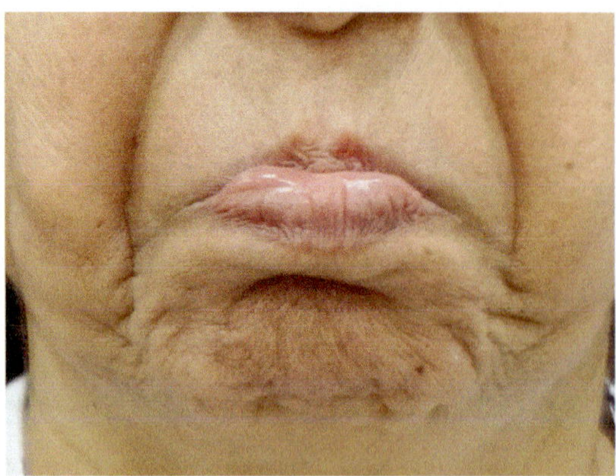

FIG. 8: Before injection of botulinum toxin into mentalis muscle for popply chin.

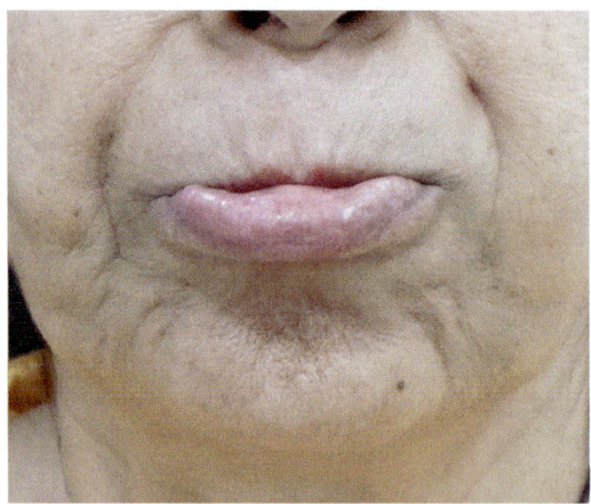

FIG. 9: After injection of botulinum toxin into mentalis muscle for popply chin.

Doses

Depending on the size of the chin and the strength of the mentalis, 4-6 U can be used, either as one shot or split into two shots (Figs 8 and 9).

Asians

A hyperactive mentalis associated with retrogenia and microgenia is very common in Asians. About 5-10 units of botulinum toxin may be required for treating the mentalis in South East Asians.

Treatment Pearls

- Patients are often unaware of their popply chin which appears on animation. They should be given a mirror and made aware of the popply chin and explained what the neurotoxin would do.
- Individuals with a dimpled chin may have hypertrophic mentalis muscles and may indicate a predilection to oral incompetence. In such cases, do not treat with botulinum toxin.
- One should aim at weakening the superficial fibers of the mentalis without affecting the deeper structures.

Complications

Diffusion into DLI muscle or diffusion into orbicularis oris if injected too high can result in asymmetrical smile, drooling, or lip ptosis.

NECK BANDS (PLATYSMAL BANDS)

The platysma depresses the lower jaw, pulls the lower lips, and corners of the mouth laterally and downward, partially opening the mouth.

Vertical platysmal bands develop as the result of a hyperactive platysma attempting to support the ptotic structural changes that occur due to aging and changes in the submental space. The anterior edges of the fibers eventually lose muscle tone, separate over time, and protrude anteriorly, creating bands that are sometimes referred to as the "turkey neck" deformity.

Anatomy

The platysma muscle originates in the superficial fascia of the upper portion of the thorax, clavicle, and acromion. The anterior fibers known as pars mandibularis are inserted into the periosteum of the medial portion of the mandibular border. The pars labialis inserts into the lateral half of the lower lip, passing beneath the DAO muscle fibers. The posterior fibers known as pars modiolaris are inserted into the modiolus (Fig. 10).[5]

Injection Site and Dosage

With the patient sitting upright or in a semi-recumbent position, he/she should be asked to clench his teeth and depress the lateral oral commissure in order to contract his anterior neck. One can also extend the neck, stretch it and say "e" aloud. This will exaggerate the platysmal bands and the injection points can be marked all along the bands 1–1.5 cm apart. Three to five sites per band are usually enough. Grasp the band with the non-dominant hand and inject 1–2 units directly into the belly of the muscle. The needle may be pointed perpendicular to the band but care should be taken not to inject deep. A safer way is to hold the band and inject from medial to lateral side of the band. A total of 30–40 units are usually sufficient for the entire neck the first time. The patient should be called after 2 weeks and more units may be injected if needed (Figs 11 to 13).

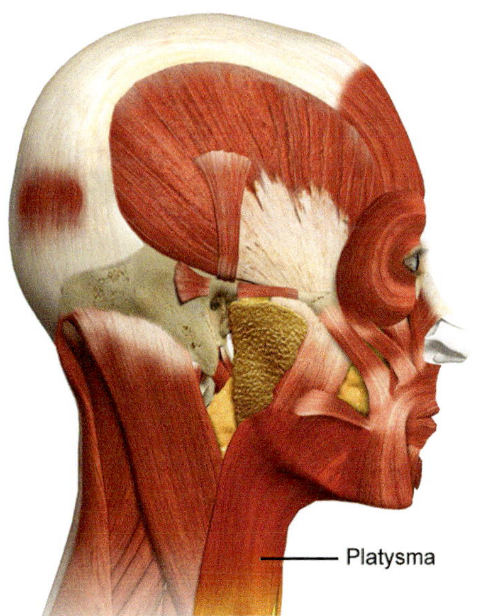

FIG. 10: Platysma muscle.

Complications[6]

- Muscle soreness or neck discomfort may occur for 2–3 days
- Deep injections into the neck or overdosing with botulinum toxin when treating the platysmal bands can result in dysphagia due to diffusion into sternocleidomastoid and other strap muscles of the neck. Diffusion into the cricothyroid muscle can cause dysarthria, hoarseness.

Tips to Get Optimum Results[7]

- This procedure works best on younger patients with good skin elasticity or postoperatively for residual bands
- Platysmal band injection does not substitute for surgical procedures, and it will not correct skin laxity or submental fat deposits
- In patients with extensive cutaneous laxity and flaccid platysmal cords, injections of botulinum toxin can actually cause the neck to appear worse, and therefore, should not be attempted
- Inject multiple sites per band for the most satisfactory results
- The strap muscles should be avoided. Grasping of the bands and direct injection into the band is a safe technique. Raising a visible wheal with each injection attests to the appropriately superficial position of the injected botulinum toxin
- The most posterior limit to the injections should be the anterior edge of the sternocleidomastoid on the lateral sides of the neck
- Older patients are more at risk for complications, because they present with more wrinkling and banding of their necks, and commonly require higher doses of botulinum toxin for satisfactory results. They also have a diminution in the soft tissue support of the neck, making it easier for

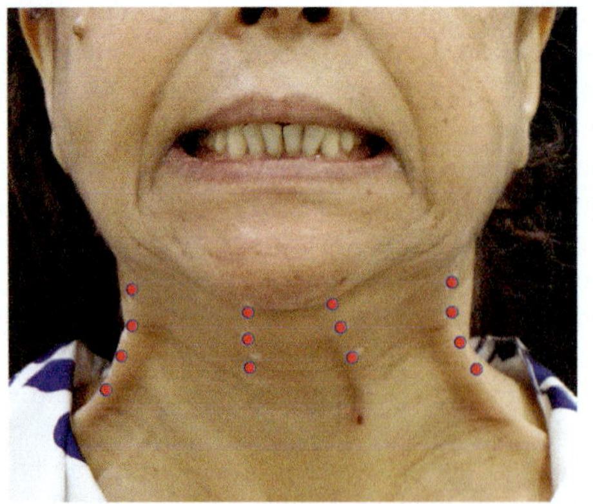

FIG. 11: Injection points for treating the vertical platysmal bands (turkey neck).

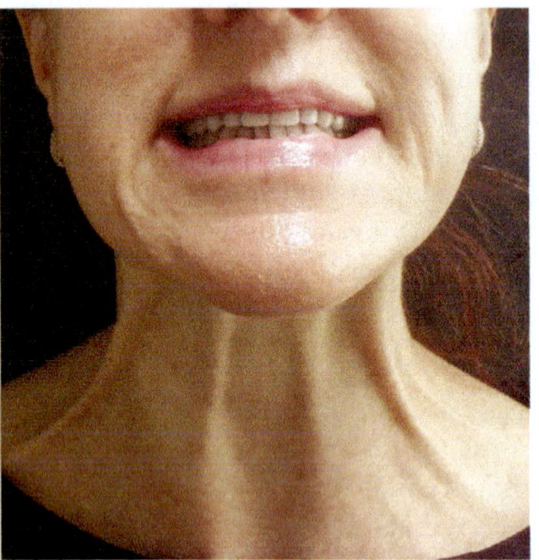

FIG. 12: Vertical neck bands (turkey neck) before injecting botulinum toxin into the platysmal bands.

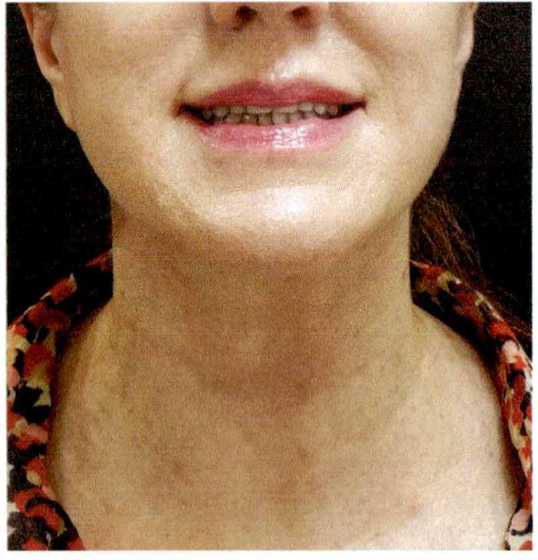

FIG. 13: Disappearance of vertical neck bands (Turkey neck) after injecting botulinum toxin into the platysmal bands.

the neurotoxin to diffuse to other deeper muscles of the neck which will affect deglutition, speech, and the overall strength of the neck in keeping it erect.

HORIZONTAL NECK BANDS

With age, the skin of the neck progressively develops increased laxity, loss of elasticity, and redundancy. There is a diminution of soft tissue support, causing the skin of the neck to be susceptible to continuous horizontal creasing which leads to persistent transverse wrinkles on the neck. These horizontal lines traverse the anterolateral aspect of the neck like multiple parallel rings around the neck.

Injection Technique (Video 9)

Inject 1–2 units each along the linear horizontal line, either above or below the horizontal line. Start at the midline of the neck and proceed laterally. The most posterior limit to the injections should be the anterior edge of the sternocleidomastoid on the lateral sides of the neck. Usually, three or four injection points are required to adequately treat these horizontal lines of the neck. Raise a wheal to make sure injections are superficial. Total dose of 30 units is adequate (Fig. 14).

Complications

Same as that of platysmal bands.

Treatment Pearls

The results of botulinum toxin injected along the horizontal lines on neck are not very satisfactory. Combining with laser resurfacing or skin booster injections would give better results.

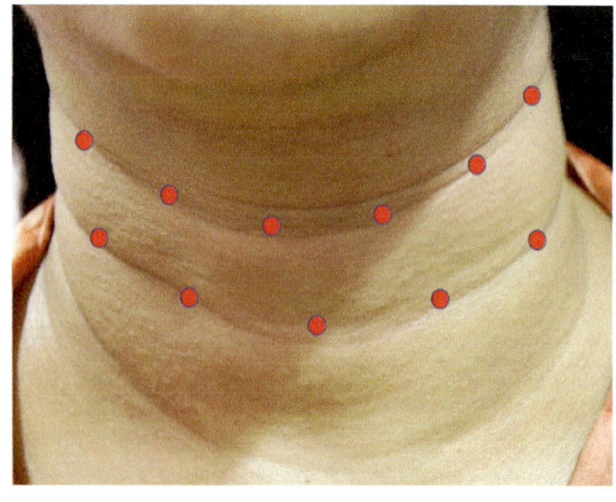

FIG. 14: Horizontal neck bands: Injection points.

NEFERTITI LIFT[8]

Nefertiti was the queen of Egypt during the 14th century BC. The bust of Nefertiti is on display at the Neues Museum in Berlin and is one of the most iconic symbols of Egypt. Nefertiti means "a beautiful woman has arrived". In her book titled, "Nefertiti", Michelle Moran says "the graceful curve of her neck, her thinly arched brows, and cheekbones so rigid they could cut you".

Dr Philip Levy described the Nefertiti lift in 2007.[8] He said the technique aims to lift and improve the definition of the mandibular border and angle, elevate the corners of the mouth, and drape the skin of the jawline contour giving the visual effect of a "mini lift".

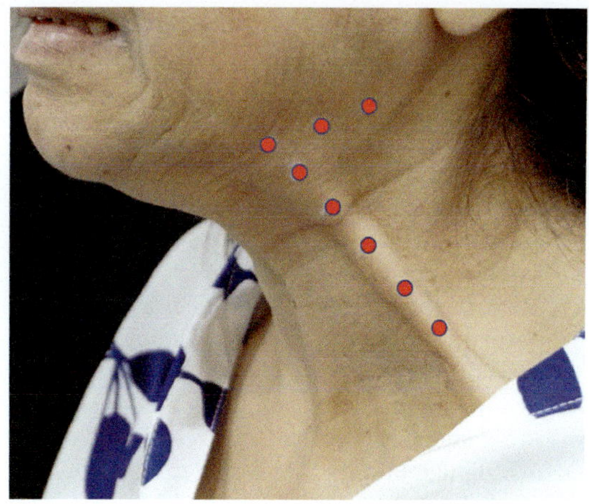

FIG. 15: Injection points for Nefertiti lift.

Muscles Involved

Platysma.

Injection Technique

Ask the patient to elevate the chin and say the letter "e", pulling down hard on the platysma muscle as shown in figure 15. Taking the posterior platysmal band as a reference, mark the injection points along and under each mandible behind the posterior platysmal band, and on the upper part of the posterior platysmal band. One point may be marked ahead of the band, too. Each injection point should be 1-1.5 cm apart. Then ask the patient to contract the platysma muscle, grasp the prominent band, and inject 1-2 units of botulinum toxin at the marked points. A total of 12-16 units are usually enough per side though, Dr Levy suggests 15-20 units per side (Figs 15 to 17).

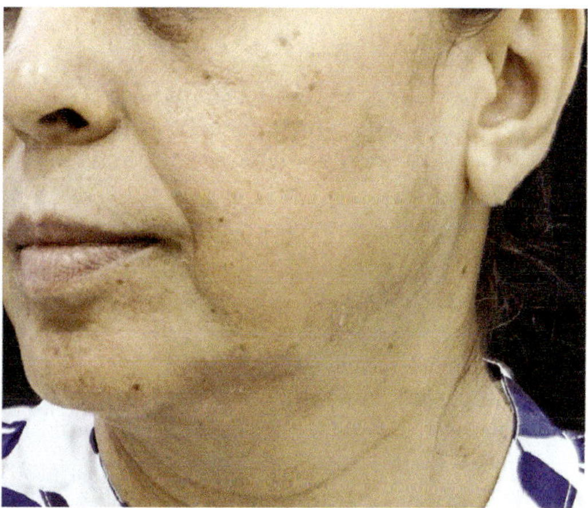

FIG. 16: Jawline before Nefertiti lift.

Mechanism of Action

With age, the platysma muscle contracts and pulls down on the cheeks and jawline (depressor effect). This effect is not precise and creates an ill-defined jawline and angle. Injecting with botulinum toxin releases the downward tension on the jawline and alleviates the depressor effect. This removes the pull-down depressor effect on the cheek and releases the skin to the elevator muscles lifting action.

Complications

Mild dysphagia and excess "lifting" muscular effect were found in the study conducted by Dr Levy but this resolved within 4 weeks. Two patients presented with very slight unilateral, rapidly reversible smile

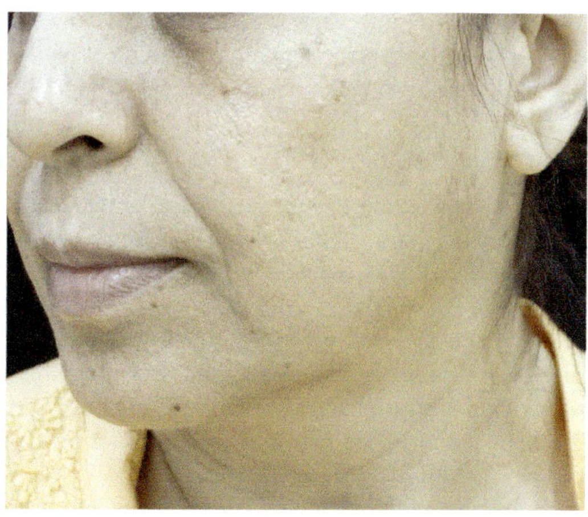

FIG. 17: Jawline after Nefertiti lift.

incontinence due to partial chemodenervation of depressor labii.

Treatment Pearls

- Ask the patient to say "e" loudly contracting their platysma. Disappearance of the mandibular border with this action indicates the potential for successful treatment.
- Avoid injecting anterior to a line drawn from the nasolabial fold down to the mandible. This will prevent diffusion into DLI and thus prevent an asymmetrical smile.
- Avoid injecting patients with excessive fat on the mandibular border. They would not get a desired result and will remain dissatisfied.
- Do not over inject the neck, 20 units is the maximum you can inject per side.

MASSETER HYPERTROPHY

A square jawline seen more commonly in Asians, widens the lower face, and is considered masculine.[9] In most patients, the square lower jawline is created by masseteric muscle hypertrophy.

Masseteric muscle hypertrophy may be unilateral or bilateral. It is most common between the ages of 20–40 years and is not gender specific.[9]

Causes of masseter hypertrophy includes:

- Idiopathically enlarged masseters
- Asymmetric chewing due to dental problems
- Temporomandibular joint dysfunction, bruxism
- Focal dystonia
- Genetics: Asians are predisposed to a wider mandibular and thicker masseter
- Diet: Chewing dried squid, meat, fibrous vegetables, and betel nut, etc. can increase masseter bulk and mandibular size
- Personal habits: Jaw clenching/grinding, bruxism, and gum chewing.

Functional Anatomy[10]

The masseter is one of the muscles of mastication. It is a thick, quadrilateral muscle, consisting of two portions: (i) Superficial, and (ii) Deep. The superficial portion arises from the zygomatic process of the maxilla, and from the anterior two-thirds of the lower border of the zygomatic arch. Its fibers pass downward and backward, to be inserted into the angle, and lower half of the lateral surface of the ramus of the mandible. The deep portion arises from the posterior third of the lower border and from the medial surface of the zygomatic arch. Its fibers pass downward and forward, to be inserted into the upper half of the ramus, and the lateral surface of the coronoid process of the mandible. The fibers of the two heads are continuous at their insertion (Fig. 18).

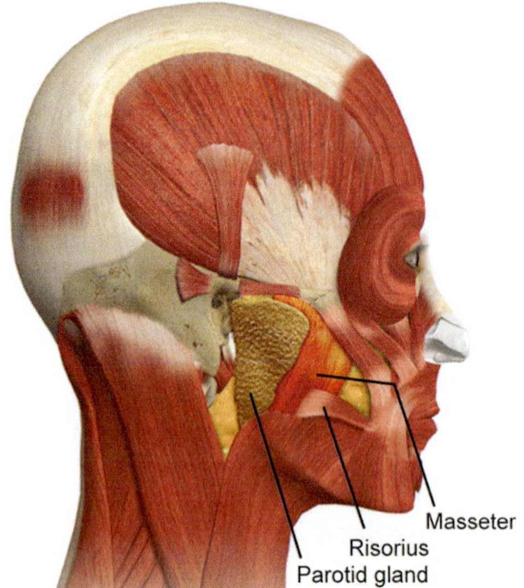

FIG. 18: Masseter muscle.

Intimate knowledge of the surrounding anatomy is very important before injecting the masseter to prevent inadvertent injections into the surrounding tissues. Most at risk are the superficial mimetic muscles of the face. These are located just below the skin overlying the masseter. Above the masseter and just below these muscles lie their motor nerves. Overlying the masseter posteriorly is the parotid gland. The facial artery and vein cross the masseter at its anteroinferior corner and then, course superiorly and anteriorly.

Injection Technique (Video 10)

Draw a line from the corner of the angle of lip to the lower part of the external auditory meatus. Keep all injections below this line. Ask the patient to clench the teeth tightly to accentuate the contours of the masseter muscle at the angle of the jaw. Palpate the masseter muscle and assess its bulkiness. Draw two lines marking the anterior border and posterior border of the muscle. Now palpate the center of the muscle which is also the point of maximum bulge, and mark it as the first point of injection. The second point is marked lower down, 1 cm lateral to the anterior border of the masseter muscle. The third point is marked a centimeter medial to the lateral border of the masseter muscle in the same line as the second point. Depending on the bulk of the muscle, 5-15 units should be injected per injection point and a total of 15-35 units are injected per side. Deep intramuscular injections should be given with the needle perpendicular to the skin surface so that the neurotoxin diffuses into both the superficial head and part of the deep head of the masseter muscle. About 15-30 units per side in females and 25-35 units in males were adequate in Indian patients for desirable results.

Many authors have described four and five point injection technique.[11,12] However, in Indians, the three point injection technique seems to be giving best cosmetic results (Figs 19 to 21).

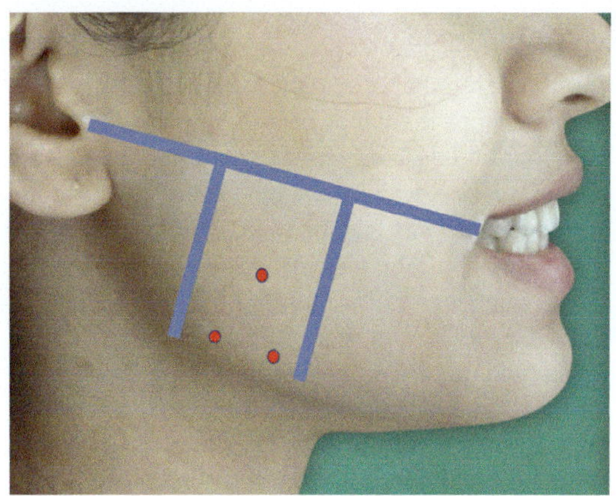

FIG. 19: Injection points for masseter muscle.

Mechanism of Action

The masseter muscle is one of the four muscles involved in mastication. Hypertrophy of the muscle leads to a square face and a broad jaw which is aesthetically not pleasing to most people. Botulinum toxin is injected into the enlarged masseter muscle to reduce its size giving a more oval and slim look to the face. The best results are seen only 6-8 weeks after the neurotoxin is injected unlike the other cosmetic indications where the results may become evident as early as even 24 hours.

By binding to the presynaptic cholinergic nerve terminals, botulinum toxin blocks the release of acetylcholine. This causes atrophy of the masseter muscle. Although, the binding is permanent, muscle contraction usually recovers over 3-4 months as new nerve terminal axon sprouts form, restoring neuromuscular transmission. The muscle thus, begins to increase in size after 4-6 months.[13]

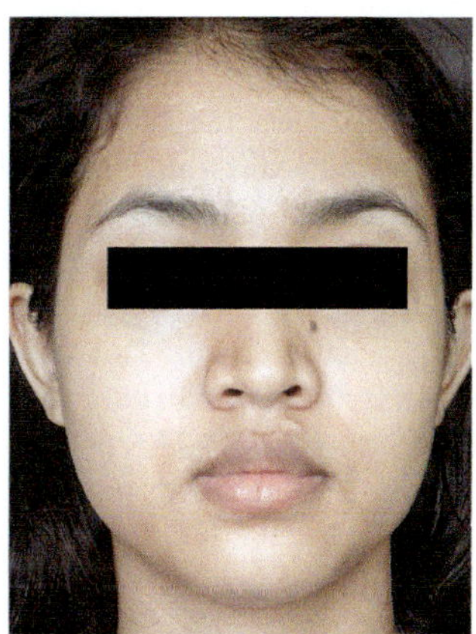

FIG. 20: Masseter hypertrophy.

Ethnic Variations

A square jawline seen more commonly in Asians, widens the lower face, and is considered masculine.[9] In most patients, the square lower jawline is created by masseteric muscle hypertrophy. This is more common in Koreans, Chinese, and other South East Asians as opposed to Caucasians. Caucasians have long, narrow faces, while Asians typically have short, wider faces. A dose of 25-30 units of botulinum toxin was found to be sufficient for each masseter muscle in Caucasians in a study by Lieu et al. In Southeast Asian patients, the initial dose was 40-45 units on each side. Patients who showed a minimum response on week 8 were offered additional injection of 10-20 units on each side.[12]

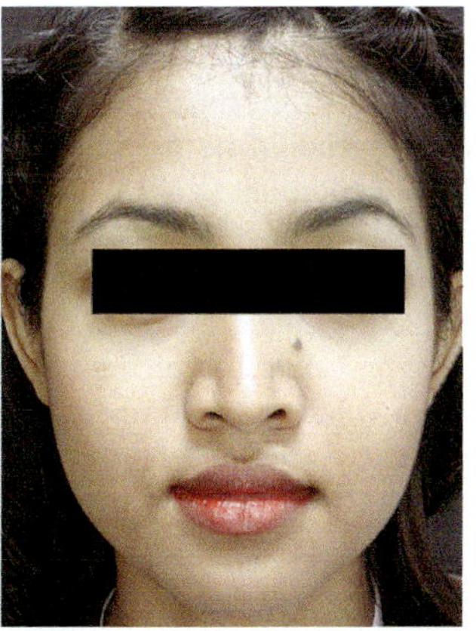

FIG. 21: Improvement of masseter hypertrophy after injecting botulinum toxin.

Complications[9]

Based on a number of studies, it has been seen that in some patients, there may be a temporary inability to chew hard foods from 1 week post-injection, lasting up to 6 weeks. Localized swelling at the injection site due to hematomas may be seen but they resolve on their own within a week. Muscle ache and pain at site of injection is also reported. Minor changes in facial expression can occur. This is due to accidental weakening of the zygomaticus major or risorius muscle. Smile asymmetry and difficulty in smiling from diffusion into zygomaticus major or levator anguli is a temporary complication if botulinum toxin is injected too high into the masseter.

It has also been seen that the cheeks appear sunken following injection. This is because of atrophy of the superior portion of the masseter in these patients. The superior portion of the masseter lies just below the bony prominence of the cheekbone, thus, thinning the masseter may result in a sharp drop-off between the zygomatic arch and cheek causing the sunken cheek appearance.[14] Sometimes, a minor skin "sagging" has been seen post-injection. This is because the muscle shrinks faster than skin contracts. It usually resolves in 6–12 weeks.[15] There have been no permanent complications reported.[16,17]

Treatment Pearls

- The injection points, two and three are kept as low as possible, closer to the mandibular margin.[10]
- Make sure the needle used for injection is at least 1 inch long so that both the superficial and deep part of the muscle are injected. In case the deep part is left unattended, it bulges out like a chipmunk every time the patient speaks.
- The patients should be asked to follow-up in 6 weeks and additional units of botulinum toxin can be injected if the masseter is still palpable.
- Avoid injecting those with a bony enlargement of the mandibular angle.
- In order to prevent diffusion into the buccinators or risorius which can lead to smile asymmetry, one must remember to keep the injection point at least 1 cm away from the anterior border of the masseter muscle.
- Injection points should also be kept below the sigmoid notch of the mandible in order to prevent inadvertent paralysis of other muscle of mastication, namely the pterygoid muscles.[12] This can be done by staying below an imaginary line from the auditory meatus to mid philtrum while injecting.
- Always keep injections below the line drawn from lip corner to ear tragus.
- Mark and delineate the muscle with the patient's teeth clenched. Always inject at least 1 cm away from muscle borders.
- Lastly, do not be in a hurry to do a touch-up before 6 weeks of the first injection.

CONCLUSION

Botulinum toxin injected into lower face muscles can take away signs of aging by getting rid of the jowls, the popply chin, the marionette lines, and the neck bands. Adequate knowledge of anatomy is a must. A combination of injectables, lasers radiofrequency tightening, etc. gives good aesthetic results.

REFERENCES

1. Choi YJ, Kim JS, Gil YC, et al. Anatomical considerations regarding the location and boundary of the depressor anguli oris muscle with reference to botulinum toxin injection. Plast Reconstr Surg. 2014;134(5):917-21.
2. Atamoros FP. Botulinum toxin in the lower one third of the face. Clin Dermatol. 2003;21(6):505-12.
3. Carruthers J, Carruthers A. BOTOX use in the mid and lower face and neck. Semin Cutan Med Surg. 2001; 20(2):85-92.
4. Wu DC, Fabi SG, Goldman MP. Neurotoxins: Current Concepts in Cosmetic Use on the Face and Neck—Lower Face. Plast Reconstr Surg. 2015;136(5 Suppl):76S-79.
5. Loos BM, Maas CS. Relevant anatomy for botulinum toxin facial rejuvenation. Facial Plast Surg Clin North Am. 2003;11(4):439-43.
6. Shetty MK. Cosmetic uses of botulinum toxin. In: Mysore V (Ed). ACS(I) Textbook on Cutaneous and Aesthetic Surgery. New Delhi: Jaypee Brothers Medical Publishers (P) Ltd; 2012. pp. 607-12.
7. Sharad J. Botulinum toxin. In: Viswanath V (Ed). Cosmetic Dermatology: A Practical and Evidence-Based Approach, 1st edition. New Delhi: CBS Publishers and Distributors; 2016.
8. Levy PM. The 'Nefertiti lift': a new technique for specific re-contouring of the jawline. J Cosmet Laser Ther. 2007;9(4):249-52.
9. Park MY, Ahn KY, Jung DS. Botulinum toxin type A treatment for contouring of the lower face. Dermatol Surg. 2003;29(5):477-83.
10. Raspaldo H, Niforos FR, Gassia V, et al. Lower-face and neck antiaging treatment and prevention using onabotulinumtoxin A: the 2010 multidisciplinary French consensus—part 2. J Cosmet Dermatol. 2011;10(2):131-49.

11. Ahn J, Horn C, Blitzer A. Botulinum toxin for masseter reduction in Asian patients. Arch Facial Plast Surg. 2004;6(3):188-91.
12. Liew S, Dart A. Nonsurgical reshaping of the lower face. Aesthet Surg J. 2008;28(3):251-7.
13. Yu CC, Chen PK, Chen YR. Botulinum toxin a for lower facial contouring: a prospective study. Aesthetic Plast Surg. 2007;31(5):445-51.
14. Kim HJ, Yum KW, Lee SS, et al. Effects of botulinum toxin type A on bilateral masseteric hypertrophy evaluated with computed tomographic measurement. Dermatol Surg. 2003;29(5):484-9.
15. Wu WT. Botox facial slimming/facial sculpting: the role of botulinum toxin-A in the treatment of hypertrophic masseteric muscle and parotid enlargement to narrow the lower facial width. Facial Plast Surg Clin North Am. 2010;18(1):133-40.
16. Sharad J, Contouring of lower face with injection of botulinum toxin into the masseter muscle, Cosmetic Medicine, Issue 15-1.
17. Sharad J. Botulinum toxin. In: Savant S, editor. Textbook of Dermatosurgery and Cosmetology. Mumbai: Bhalani Publishing House; 2018.

16

CHAPTER

Botulinum Toxin for Hyperhidrosis

Renita Lourdhurajan

INTRODUCTION

Hyperhidrosis is a chronic, socially debilitating condition, characterized by sweating beyond the physiological levels considered appropriate for temperature regulation.[1] It can be primary and idiopathic, or secondary, attributable to any of the following: infections, poisoning, endocrine, neurological, psychiatric, metabolic and cardiac disorders, or drug reactions.

MAGNITUDE OF THE PROBLEM

An estimated 200 million people worldwide, are considered to be suffering from hyperhidrosis,[1] with a prevalence of 1–3%.[1-4] To add to this magnitude, one in two patients have a positive family history, underscoring a genetic predisposition,[1] with a likely autosomal dominant inheritance.[5,6]

The problem of primary hyperhidrosis seems to have its onset at between 14 and 25 years of age.[7] Symptoms were first noticed in adolescents, but medical help was sought only after 1–2 decades,[2] possibly only after professional functioning was affected.[8] Axillae are most commonly involved,[9,10] followed by the hands, feet, craniofacial region, and the groins.[1,11] Stress and anxiety both exaggerated and were exaggerated by the sweating.[1,12]

ASSESSMENT OF DISEASE BURDEN

The social and psychological impact of hyperhidrosis has been evaluated on various scales.

The Hyperhidrosis Disease Severity Scale (HDSS) has been used in many studies, to measure the impairment in quality of life (QOL).[7,12] It evaluates subject's perspective of his/her sweating over a four point scale, and correlates positively with gravimetric sweat production measurements, and with other indices such as the Dermatology Life Quality Index and the Hyperhidrosis Impact Questionnaire (Table 1).[13]

TABLE 1: Hyperhidrosis Disease Severity Scale for the measurement of quality of life

Patient complaints	Grades	Scores
My sweating is never noticeable and never interferes with my daily activities	Grade 1 (dry)	Score 1
My sweating is tolerable but sometimes interferes with my daily activities	Grade 2 (moist)	Score 2
My sweating is barely tolerable and frequently interferes with my daily activities	Grade 3 (wet)	Score 3
My sweating is intolerable and always interferes with my daily activities	Grade 4 (dripping wet)	Score 4

Being a qualitative index, the HDSS can also be considered a tool on which to base treatment recommendations based on severity.[4,7]

PATHOPHYSIOLOGY AND DIAGNOSIS

Overstimulation of the eccrine sweat glands by sympathetic postganglionic cholinergic fibers is considered the underlying cause of primary hyperhidrosis. Botulinum toxin targets these unmyelinated class C fibers, causing chemical denervation of the sweat glands, with a gravimetric reduction in sweat output.[5,14] On the palms and soles, sweat glands are activated by emotional stimuli, probably mediated by frontal and premotor projections to the hypothalamus. A hypothalamic sweat center, distinct from other centers which responds to thermosensitive triggers, functioning exclusively under cortical control, is said to control sweating of the palms, soles, and sometimes, the axilla. Abnormal central control, independent of thermoregulatory signals, is likely implicated in primary hyperhidrosis. Supporting this, is the fact that sleep abolishes primary hyperhidrosis, its regulation being under cortical control. This interesting clinical feature is one of the criteria for the diagnosis of primary hyperhidrosis, listed here:

- Sweating that is bilaterally symmetrical
- Focal sweating that ceases with sleep
- Frequency of more than one episode per week
- Impairment of daily activities
- Onset of symptoms before age 25 years, and
- A positive family history.

A diagnosis of idiopathic focal hyperhidrosis is made[4,5,8,15] if the subject has two or more of the earlier criteria, with a history of over 6 months of visibly excessive sweating, without any obvious underlying reason.

TREATMENT OF PRIMARY HYPERHIDROSIS

The spectrum of treatment options for hyperhidrosis, extends from topical through minimally invasive to surgical. At the lower most rung, are topical antiperspirants containing aluminum salts, 20% aluminum chloride hexahydrate, or 1% aluminum acetate, the former being more effective.[16] They form a plug in the acrosyringium by precipitating the mucopolysaccharides, and causing damage to the epithelial cells along the duct lumen.[8] This forms a physical blockade and may be of some use in focal sweating. Irritation occurring in about 1% of users can be reduced with the use of a low potency steroid cream, the morning after.[3] Another topical agent is glycopyrrolate, typically used for craniofacial hyperhidrosis.[3] Topical astringents like formaldehyde, tannic acid, trichloroacetic acid, and glutaraldehyde, act by denaturing the keratin of the stratum corneum, which temporarily blocks the sweat pore. This is an outdated mode of treatment, though small quantities of astringents may be found in commercial antisweat agents.[8]

Another noninvasive, though tedious treatment option is iontophoresis,[17] useful, especially in the pediatric population.[18] Tap water, normal saline with or without added glycopyrrolate have all been tried, with variable results, but almost always thwarted by poor compliance.[19]

Oral anticholinergic agents have been found to be useful for hyperhidrosis for over 7 decades.[3] The agent used initially was methantheline, followed by its longer acting analog propantheline, preferred for its more favorable side effect profile. Glycopyrrolate and oxybutynin are newer options.[1,3,8] Glycopyrrolate can be used in oral and topical forms, as also with iontophoresis, and provides good relief. Oxybutynin is favored in postmenopausal hyperhidrosis.[3] The limiting side effects of oral agents are dryness of the mouth and constipation, with more significant side effects like blurred vision, tachycardia, dizziness, and urinary retention, noted at higher doses.[1]

Surgical management for hyperhidrosis, namely, sympathectomy, is now close to a 100 years old. The open thoracotomy approach was first performed in 1919, with the endoscopic approach following in 1951. However, procedure and anesthesia associated morbidity, particularly, the highly distressing problem of compensatory hyperhidrosis, coupled with availability of less invasive options, has led to the declining popularity of sympathectomy as an option for hyperhidrosis.[1,3] Tumescent liposuction with or without curettage has been found to be useful in hyperhidrosis,[20-22] with reasonable durability of results.[23] Bipolar radiofrequency, microwave devices can be used to cause reasonably selective thermolysis of the sweat glands at the dermis–subcutaneous tissue level, with encouraging results.[22,24-26] Other emerging therapies include the 808 nm diode and the 1,064 nm neodymium-doped yttrium aluminum garnet lasers, and ultrasound energy-based devices.[27,28]

Botulinum Toxin for the Treatment of Hyperhidrosis

The use of botulinum toxin for treating hyperhidrosis was first established in 1996 by Bushara et al. Since then, this modality of treatment has come to be well established,[14] with the use of onabotulinum toxin A receiving Food and Drug Administration (FDA) approval for primary axillary hyperhidrosis in 2004.[1]

The common indications for the use of botulinum toxin in hyperhidrosis are as follows:

- Axillary hyperhidrosis
- Palmar hyperhidrosis
- Plantar hyperhidrosis
- Craniofacial hyperhidrosis.

Less common indications include submammary, inguinal and anal fold hyperhidrosis, eccrine sweat gland nevi, prosthesis-related hyperhidrosis, and compensatory hyperhidrosis.[11] Botulinum toxin has also been used successfully in managing Frey's syndrome and sialorrhea.[29,30]

Studies have found over 94% reduction in sweating post onabotulinum A toxin injection for the axillae at 4 weeks, with the reduction sustaining at 82% at the 16 weeks, compared to only 21% in the placebo group.[1] The fact that a better QOL is afforded by botulinum toxin treatment to patients with focal hyperhidrosis, is well established.[31]

Research has also established the durability of botulinum toxin treatment in axillary hyperhidrosis. Several physiological factors influence the longevity of results, namely, the choice of the toxin, area treated, dosing protocols, time to axonal sprouting, and SNARE protein synthesis and toxin degradation. A return of symptoms occurs between 3 months and 12 months, with the maximum being 24 months.[1,32] However, with longer disease duration, the results may be less durable.[33] On the other hand, the durability was not affected by age, sex, site, extent, QOL impairment, or with the number of previous therapies. The last factor is significant, in view of the significant psychosocial morbidity of the disease which must be traded off against the development of antitoxin antibodies.[34]

Botulinum toxin treatment compares quite favorably with the other treatments discussed earlier. In a crossover control study, comparing botulinum toxin to a combination of iontophoresis and topical antiperspirant, it was found that the neurotoxin arm provided better relief for a longer duration.[4]

The introduction of botulinum toxin into the treatment algorithm, can be done based on disease severity as per the HDSS.[7] The HDSS also allows for monitoring of treatment results, and for identifying the suitable time for a follow-up session.[7]

INDICATIONS

Axillary Hyperhidrosis

For axillary hyperhidrosis, botulinum toxin injections are recommended as the treatment of choice, if antiperspirants fail, either on count of inadequate efficacy or poor tolerability.[1,7] Thus far, only onabotulinum toxin A injections are FDA cleared for the treatment of primary axillary hyperhidrosis.

Choice of Toxin

As of now, only the onabotulinum toxin A (Botox, Allergan) has been licensed for use in primary axillary hyperhidrosis. The others, namely abobotulinum toxin A, incobotulinum toxin A, and rimabotulinum toxin B, have all been used off-label in the treatment of hyperhidrosis, and are considered safe. However, these different preparations are not interchangeable, and conversion values between them are not universally consistent or absolutely reliable.[1]

Lakraj et al., analyzed the data available for the four toxins, and summarize that while onabotulinum toxin is established for the treatment of axillary hyperhidrosis, abobotulinum is probably effective.[5] An et al., have demonstrated the comparability of rimabotulinum to onabotulinum at a ratio of 30:1.[35] Onabotulinum toxin and abobotulinum toxins were found to be comparable,[36] as was incobotulinum toxin.[5] This is beneficial from the point of view of repetitive treatments, as incobotulinum toxin is free of complexing proteins, and is therefore considered less immunogenic.[1] Botulinum toxin B has been said to have more impact in indications with autonomic involvement, and is favored in conditions like hyperhidrosis and sialorrhea.[37]

Since most clinical experience in the Indian subcontinent is currently limited to onabotulinum toxin A, the clinical usage described here pertains to onabotulinum toxin A only.

Dosage

The recommended dosage is about 50–100 units of onabotulinum toxin per side, calculating for 1 unit for an area of about 1 sq. cm.[7]

Comparison of efficacy across doses has been studied, and suggests a starting dose of 50 units per axilla. Dressler et al. found that the therapeutic efficacy of the treatment saturated at higher doses.[38] Higher doses did not offer longer relief, either.[39]

It is recommended to consider a dosing of about 3–4 units, for every 1.5–2 sq. cm or as above, 1 unit/sq. cm,[7] trying, always, to administer the lowest effective dose.[1] A dose reduction may be possible with better diffusion of toxin aided by the addition of hyaluronidase.[40]

Technique of Injection

After cleansing the area to be treated using an alcohol swab, the injection points are marked out in a grid (Fig. 1), spaced around 1.5 cm apart. The recommended dilution is 50 units in 1.25 mL of saline, i.e., 1 unit for every 0.025 mL, corresponding to one division on the swaged insulin syringe. Dilutions of 50 units in 2 mL of saline yielding 2.5 units for every 0.1 mL may also be considered, but

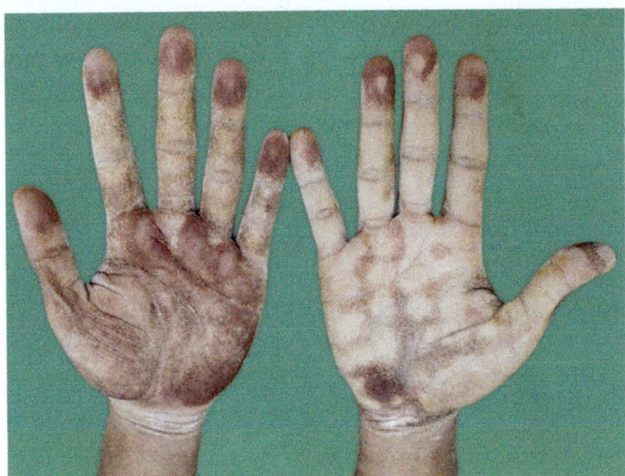

FIG. 1: Starch iodine testing to identify skip areas on the right palm, untreated left palm for comparison.

it must be remembered that the more the dilution, the greater the diffusion into surrounding tissue.[1,11]

The 31-G needle is introduced at angle of 45° to a depth of 2–3 bevels, and the toxin deposited in the dermis. An oblique introduction of the needle prevents wastage and helps ease the needle point more comfortably into the skin.[11] Injections are done at an intradermal level, keeping in mind that the sweat glands lie at the deep reticular dermis and the dermis-subcutis junction[41] at a depth of 2–5 mm from the skin surface, depending on the thickness of the skin. This helps in preventing diffusion of toxin to more deeply located muscles. At each injection point about 1.5–2 units are deposited. Regardless of the anesthesia used, icing the area prior to injections helps to reduce minor injection-related side effects like bruising.

Frequency of Treatments

The treatment can be repeated at 4–7 months intervals. Symptom relief can be followed up with either the Minor's starch iodine test, the HDSS or, where facilities exist, a gravimetric quantification of sweat production.

Pearls

The author recommends starting out with a dosage of 50 units per axilla, and reviewing the results at 2 weeks, using a modified starch iodine test, to treat any skip areas. The area to be evaluated is painted with povidone-iodine solution, and once dry, cornflour is sieved on to the painted area, to reveal bluish discoloration over areas of sweating (Fig. 1). Alternatively, a thin soft tissue paper can be placed directly on the skin and left on for a few minutes to soak up any emergent sweat droplets. Alternatively, simply touching the skin may help to identify the sweating, though less objectively so. USB dermatoscopes are now available, which can help to visualize the sweat duct openings and aid in identification of missed areas.

Efficacy of treatment increases with repetition of treatment at regular intervals.[10,42] This must always be addressed at the initial counseling session, and reinforced at every visit thereafter.

Palmoplantar Hyperhidrosis

The off-label use of botulinum toxin in the treatment of palmoplantar hyperhidrosis is recommended where topical treatments have failed, with iontophoresis as an alternative option for HDSS of 2 or less. For HDSS more than 2, the employment of botulinum is recommended as a first-line therapy.[1,7] Weinberg et al. compared available studies on the efficacy of botulinum toxin for hyperhidrosis of the palms and soles to their own practice's efficacy rates of about 50%,[43] which is quite less than the efficacy rates observed for axillary hyperhidrosis.[1] More encouraging results were, however, obtained in other studies. Symptom relief was evident in a month and lasted between 5 months and 9 months.[44,45] Better results were noted for the nondominant hand where both hands were treated.[1]

Plantar hyperhidrosis has relatively lesser volume of published data, but onabotulinum toxin treatment has been found to be efficacious for a period of 3–6 months postinjection.[1] Other indications like epidermolysis bullosa simplex, pachyonychia congenita, and pitted keratolysis were found to respond favorably.[46,47]

Choice of Toxin

Abobotulinum was found to fare slightly better than onabotulinum toxin in a study comparing the two at dose equivalency of 2.5:1 for palmar hyperhidrosis.[33] Transient muscle weakness, after palmar treatment, was found to be less with incobotulinum as compared to onabotulinum and more with abobotulinum over onabotulinum. Together with the lesser propensity of autoantibody formation, incobotulinum has a good scope, considering the repetitive treatment protocol,[1] and has also been demonstrated to be comparable to onabotulinum toxin in the treatment of primary palmar hyperhidrosis.[48] From the point of comfort, rimabotulinum toxin is felt to be more painful than the other preparations.[1]

As with other indications, the doses discussed here are in terms of onabotulinum only.

Dosage

Comparing 100 and 50 units per palm, the higher treatment dose offered a longer symptom relief by a month.[44] The recommended dose is around 100 units per palm, going up to 150 units as required,[1,4,7] though lesser doses may be used as depending on the area.[43]

For the soles, recommended dosages vary from 50 to 250 units per side.[1]

Technique of Injection

As significant pain is experienced particularly during the treatment of the palms with botulinum toxin, adequate anesthesia is crucial. After ensuring asepsis, the toxin is injected at 2–2.5 units for every 1 sq. cm, evenly spaced out over the palms and the fingers. Care should be taken to treat the fingertips, and the sides of the palms. The recommended dilution is 100 units in 2.5 mL of saline, giving about 1 unit in 0.025 mL. This helps to limit deeper diffusion and resultant muscle weakness.

For the soles, it is suggested that a dilution of 100 units in 4 mL be considered, given the larger area to be covered, and the lesser likelihood of muscle weakness.[1,43] Injection technique is as earlier, with care taken to include the tips of the toes and the sides of the soles. Icing is done in the area during and after treatment to reduce pain (Fig. 2).

Frequency of Treatments

As the treatment results are noted to last on average for about 5–6 months across various studies, two treatments per year may be considered.[43] It is also fine to wait for recurrence of symptoms along with evaluation of the palm sweating area (PSA), and the HDSS scores, to guide the frequency of treatment.

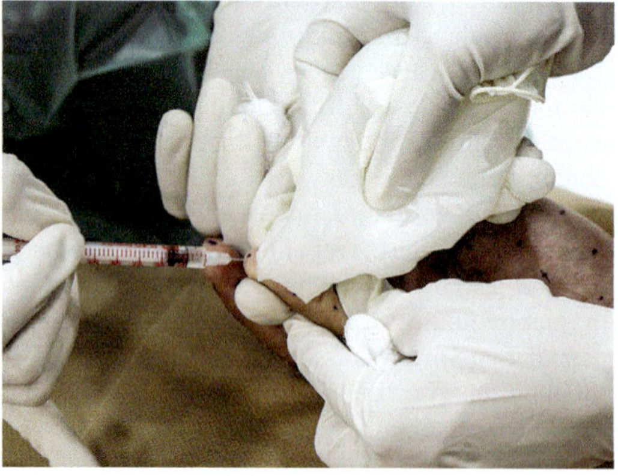

FIG. 2: Use of ice cubes in sterile gloves for pain relief.

Scoring the PSA is done with the starch-iodine test, with 0 being no change in the color of the painted iodine and 4 indicating a color change to blue in over 75% of the target area. Scores 1, 2, and 3 correspond to color changes in less than 25%, 25–50%, and 50–75%, respectively.[33]

Pearls

Needles tend to get blunt sooner when injecting the thick palmar skin. Loading the reconstituted solution in multiple needles, helps to increase patient comfort and pain tolerance,[43] as well as preventing wastage.

The point of the needle is gently inserted past the thick stratum corneum, to where the tissue "gives away". This is the optimum plane for injection.[4] If the point of the needle has advanced beyond the level where the resistance "gives", then the needle should be withdrawn till the resistance is felt again just behind the bevel, and the toxin deposited thereafter.

A keratolytic applied for a few days prior to the procedure, can ease the injection process over the soles.

Craniofacial Hyperhidrosis

More commonly seen in men, craniofacial hyperhidrosis seen in up to 20% of patients with any form of focal hyperhidrosis.[1,49] Sweating in the craniofacial region can occur in one of four patterns[11]—forehead pattern, ophiasis pattern in the shape of a band around the scalp, a combination of these two to give the third pattern, and the fourth pattern involving the entire scalp and forehead. A unilateral distribution is very unusual, and calls for a neurological evaluation. Secondary causes of craniofacial hyperhidrosis include Frey's syndrome and diabetic neuropathy.[7]

Other areas of involvement include the nose, upper lip, cheeks, and chin. It is desirable to do a starch-iodine test to examine the extent of involvement in these lesser known areas, which however, could be very distressing to the patient.[11]

Studies have shown encouraging results for botulinum toxin in craniofacial hyperhidrosis, with 87% being satisfied with the outcome and 74% returning for the follow-up treatment after a median 5 months.[50] Botulinum toxin is recommended as first line for HDSS of 2 or more.[7]

Choice of Toxin

Comparing onabotulinum and abobotulinum toxins, it was found that the latter had a larger area of diffusion.[49,51] This may be troublesome, in view of adverse events, however, a wider diffusion of toxin also means a larger area of response to treatment.[1] A newer toxin, claims to provide the ideal area of diffusion with efficacy comparable to onabotulinum toxin, but further studies are lacking.[49] However, this study discussed the diffusion pattern with placement of injections at the intramuscular level, which is not an ideal location for evaluating a hyperhidrosis outcome.[41] Rimabotulinum toxin is considered to have lesser adverse outcomes on muscle strength, however, it was found to cause eyebrow ptosis and stiffness of the forehead.[50]

Dosage

For the forehead, the recommended dose is 40 units, ranging between 33 and 100 units of onabotulinum toxin,[7,11] depending on the affected area. For the other three patterns, a larger dose is required, even up to 300 units for the entire scalp and face. The physician should exercise his/her discretion when faced with the need to inject such larger doses.

For nasal, labial, and chin hyperhidrosis, smaller dosages of 2–10 units are sufficient.[11]

Technique of Injection

Injections have to be kept strictly intradermal, to avoid as deeper diffusion and unwanted complications.[1] The injections are made at an oblique angle, with the bevel up, and to a depth of 2–3 mm into the skin. A dose of 2–3 units per injection site is recommended, with sites spaced 1–2 cm apart. The injections may need to be carried for about 2–3 cm, or more, into the hairline. This provides a good clinical outcome, and is also an area where the margin for error is lesser. Injections should be avoided in the area about 1–2 cm above the eyebrows to prevent ptosis.[1,11] Smaller, limited areas of involvement may be treated with smaller doses of about 0.5 units/sq. cm.[7]

Nasal hyperhidrosis is treated with small doses of 1–2 units, placed at intervals of 0.5–1 cm. One should avoid the lacrimal system, and keep the injections more medial to prevent involving the nasal muscles. Upper lip hyperhidrosis can be treated with 0.5–1 units per 1–2 cm. It is recommended to use 2 units per injection spot for chin hyperhidrosis.[11]

Frequency of Treatments

Results are expected to last for a lesser duration for hyperhidrosis in this area, when compared to elsewhere. Studies report remission of symptoms for a median 5 months,[1,50] accordingly, treatment sessions may be required twice to thrice yearly.[11]

Pearls

Treating an area fraught with the possibilities of muscle weakness, requires a very careful and cautious approach, especially where a higher dose is required. It is better to start with smaller doses and gradually completes the area to be treated in 3–4 sessions.

Adverse events can occur even in patients who had tolerated the higher doses in earlier sessions,[52] so each session must be planned with caution.

OTHER AREAS

Frey's Syndrome

Frey's syndrome, also called gustatory hyperhidrosis, is characterized by sweating along the distribution of the greater auricular and the auriculotemporal nerves. A history of injury to the parotid gland, as with parotid surgery or face lift procedures, can often be elicited. Treating the affected area with 1.5–3 units/sq. cm of botulinum toxin, provides lasting relief from sweating.[1,11] The symptom free period can stretch to as long as a year, sometimes even up to 3 years[11]—which is the longest reported for any site treated with botulinum toxin for focal hyperhidrosis. Asymmetry and unwanted muscle paralysis should be considered ahead, and injection points planned accordingly. Onabotulinum, abobotulinum, and rimabotulinum have all been used for this indication with fairly comparable efficacy.[1]

Submammary Hyperhidrosis

Starch-iodine testing to map the area becomes mandatory here, because of the often ill-defined limits of the area to be treated. If this is difficult or not feasible, it is advised to treat an area 2 cm above and below and the inframammary crease, extending from the midline to the outer border of the breast, or even up to the midaxillary line. It is expected that 50–150 units of onabotulinum may be required for covering this area adequately, using 2–2.5 units spaced 1.5–2 cm apart.[11]

Perianal and Groin Hyperhidrosis

Excessive sweating in these areas can be very distressing to the patient, and may be associated with significant social stigma due to the visibility of the sweating in severe cases. If mapping using a starch-iodine test is not feasible, a 2 cm area on either side of the inguinal crease is treated, with 2–3 units of onabotulinum toxin per injection site, spaced 1–2 cm apart, to a total of 50 units per inguinal fold.[11] One unit per injection point, spaced at intervals of 1 cm, to a total dose of 30 units, is recommended for the perianal region.[1] Treatment of the inguinal region should cautiously avoid the labia, and that of the perianal region should stay 1–2 cm away from the anal verge, to reduce the possibility of fecal incontinence.[11]

Compensatory Hyperhidrosis

Postsympathectomy compensatory hyperhidrosis can be much worse and more debilitating than the primary hyperhidrosis itself, and has a reported prevalence of 30–100%.[53] The areas affected in order of decreasing frequency are the back, abdomen, lower limbs, and chest.[1] Botulinum toxin has been used to effectively treat this condition with durable remissions,[5] with a significant improvement in QOL.[53]

PRACTICAL CONSIDERATIONS

Before embarking on treatment, it is very important to look for secondary causes such as diabetes mellitus, hyperpituitarism, thyroid dysfunction, neurological causes like myasthenia gravis, nerve injuries and Parkinson's disease, cardiorespiratory conditions, and psychiatric ailments.[8] A systematic history of elicitation, for allergies, and intake of drugs such as aminoglycosides, macrolides and blood thinners, and a thorough clinical evaluation for infections and bleeding or clotting disorders should be done.[5]

Though relatively contraindicated in children and adolescents, studies in children as young as 12 years demonstrate good outcomes, and treatment of this group should be considered after duly evaluating the risks and benefits.[10,54]

As symptoms may arise even within 3 months, though more commonly after 6 months, the timing of the second treatment must be considered in advance.[1,27] It is recommended that a second treatment be avoided until at least 16 weeks have elapsed after the first treatment, and definitely not before 8 weeks are up.[1] Though the significance of antitoxin antibodies on efficacy of hyperhidrosis treatment with botulinum is not fully understood, higher doses and frequent injections are not to be preferred.[1] It may be necessary to treat different areas in separate sessions, to keep the dosing safe and optimal.[52]

Depth of injection is paramount in reaching the toxin to the sweat glands, both for efficacy as well as for safety. The injector should be aware of the position of the needle at all times. Using a needle bent at the desired depths can be useful to some.[55]

SIDE EFFECTS AND COMPLICATIONS

Pain

This is the most common and troublesome issue with botulinum for hyperhidrosis. This leads to noncompliance, and apprehension over what is really a very useful treatment. As topical analgesia is often inadequate, many attempts have been made to alleviate the pain during injections, with reasonable success.

Injectors have successfully tried reconstituting the onabotulinum toxin with lidocaine, without compromising efficacy.[5,56] However, there has been a fatality, attributed to anaphylaxis, after injecting onabotulinum toxin mixed with lidocaine, used for chronic neck and back pain.[1]

Median and ulnar nerve blocks have been tried, but their long-term use comes with some risk of permanent nerve damage.[1] Precooling the area with ice packs, followed by ethyl chloride spray has been reported to be very useful.[57] Bier blocks, and modified Bier blocks have all been tried, but are not always feasible in the outpatient setup, as is general anesthesia or intravenous sedation.[58]

The use of nitrous oxide, oxygen mixture inhalation, started 5 minutes prior to the procedure and stopped as soon as the injections were done, was pioneered by Paracka et al.[59] This provides a safe, effective, readily reversible, and nonsedative mode of analgesia.

The use of jet nebulization for needleless delivery of botulinum for palmar, plantar, and axillary hyperhidrosis has been found to be effective, though less durable, as are the options of iontophoresis and phonophoresis.[60] In a comparison between injections and iontophoresis for abobotulinum delivery, the injected axilla was found to have better outcomes than its counterpart.[61] Still, iontophoresis of onabotulinum toxin provided a symptom relief of 34% at 2 weeks follow-up, compared to the placebo iontophoresis arm where sweat production actually increased.[62] Needleless injection of anesthesia, called "jet anesthesia" has been tried before injecting botulinum.[58] The delivery of botulinum toxin in the skin through pocketed microneedles, with an anticipated better tolerance, is yet to become a clinical reality.[63] The influence of needle size and spacing of injection points have also been studied with no conclusive consensus.[64]

Injections with rimabotulinum toxin are said to be more painful,[1] due to the acidic nature of the product.

Injection-related Side Effects

These include bruising, mild edema, and rarely, a hematoma formation—all of which usually resolve spontaneously. Icing the treated area immediately before the procedure helps in vasoconstriction, and helps to avoid the injection-related troubles to some extent.

Muscle Weakness and Asymmetry

This is more common and most noticeable when treating craniofacial hyperhidrosis. It is not always possible to avoid muscle weakness especially when attempting to treat the lower forehead, nose, upper lip, and chin.[11] With palmar hyperhidrosis, patients often complain of difficulty in texting and typing,[65] which usually resolves over 4–8 weeks.[1]

Headache

This is common in treatments involving the face and/or head.[11] It usually resolves with basic pain relief medications like paracetamol.

Rare Complications

Generalized muscle weakness has been reported following the injection of botulinum toxin for localized hyperhidrosis. Though more common with higher doses, or simultaneous treatment of many areas at the same session, this has also been reported with doses as low as 30 units.[52] Botulinum toxin-induced motor neuron disorder, mimicking amyotrophic lateral sclerosis (ALS), has been described following treatment of axillary hyperhidrosis with abobotulinum toxin. In contrast to ALS, the botulinum toxin-induced symptoms, had a remitting-relapsing course, and may have unmasked an existing, though latent, neurological condition.[66] Also, rare occurrences of a prolonged flu-like syndrome, with dryness of the mouth, difficulties in accommodation, and ocular irritation, have all been reported with rimabotulinum toxin.[1,67,68]

CONCLUSION

As with many other conditions, the treatment of hyperhidrosis has greatly evolved from a few surgical options to many minimally invasive possibilities, botulinum toxin, among the most promising choices.[1,27] Despite the significant disease burden, the level of awareness about the problem and its solutions is low, both among patients and physicians. Given the large amount of psychosocial disadvantage brought on by hyperhidrosis, it is imperative that effective treatment is initiated early,[1] more so since disease duration correlates negatively with treatment outcome.[32,33]

REFERENCES

1. Hosp C, Naumann MK, Hamm H. Botulinum Toxin Treatment of Autonomic Disorders: Focal Hyperhidrosis and Sialorrhea. Semin Neurol. 2016;36(1):20-8.
2. Park EJ, Han KR, Choi H, et al. An Epidemiological Study of Hyperhidrosis Patients Visiting the Ajou University Hospital Hyperhidrosis Center in Korea. J Korean Med Sci. 2010;25(5):772-5.
3. Lee KY, Levell NJ. Turning the tide: A history and review of hyperhidrosis. JRSM Open. 2014;5(1): 2042533313505511.
4. Rajagopal R, Mallya NB. Comparative evaluation of botulinum toxin versus iontophoresis with topical aluminium chloride hexahydrate in treatment of palmar hyperhidrosis. Med J Armed Forces India. 2014;70(3):247-52.
5. Lakraj AA, Moghimi N, Jabbari B. Hyperhidrosis: Anatomy, Pathophysiology and Treatment with Emphasis on the Role of Botulinum Toxins. Toxins (Basel). 2013;5(4):821-40.
6. Kaufmann H, Saadia D, Polin C, et al. Primary hyperhidrosis—evidence for autosomal dominant inheritance. Clin Auton Res. 2003;13(2):96-8.
7. Solish N, Bertucci V, Dansereau A, et al. A comprehensive approach to the recognition, diagnosis, and severity-based treatment of focal hyperhidrosis: recommendations of the Canadian Hyperhidrosis Advisory Committee. Dermatol Surg. 2007;33(8):908-23.
8. Campanati A, Gregoriou S, Kontochristopoulos G, et al. Oxybutynin for the Treatment of Primary Hyperhidrosis: Current State of the Art. Skin Appendage Disord. 2015;1(1):6-13.
9. Gelbard CM, Epstein H, Hebert A. Primary pediatric hyperhidrosis: A review of current treatment options. Pediatr Dermatol. 2008;25(6):591-8.
10. Glaser DA, Pariser DM, Hebert AA, et al. A Prospective, Nonrandomized, Open-Label Study of the Efficacy and Safety of OnabotulinumtoxinA in Adolescents with Primary Axillary Hyperhidrosis. Pediatr Dermatol. 2015;32(5):609-17.
11. Glaser DA, Galperin TA. Botulinum toxin for hyperhidrosis of areas other than the axillae and palms/soles. Dermatol Clin. 2014;32(4):517-25.
12. Bragança GM, Lima SO, Pinto Neto AF, et al. Evaluation of anxiety and depression prevalence in patients with primary severe hyperhidrosis. An Bras Dermatol. 2014;89(2):230-5.
13. Hamm H. Impact of hyperhidrosis on quality of life and its assessment. Dermatol Clin. 2014;32(4):467-76.

14. Bushara KO, Park DM, Jones JC, et al. Botulinum toxin—a possible new treatment for axillary hyperhidrosis. Clin Exp Dermatol. 1996;21(4):276-8.
15. Perera E, Sinclair R. Hyperhidrosis and bromhidrosis—a guide to assessment and management. Aust Fam Physician. 2013;42(5):266-9.
16. Swary JH, West DP, Kakar R, et al. Quantitative comparison of topical aluminum salt solution efficacy for management of sweating: A randomized, controlled trial. J Cosmet Dermatol. 2015;14(4):E1-6.
17. Pariser DM, Ballard A. Iontophoresis for palmar and plantar hyperhidrosis. Dermatol Clin. 2014;32(4):491-4.
18. Dogruk Kacar S, Ozuguz P, Eroglu S, et al. Treatment of primary hyperhidrosis with tap water iontophoresis in paediatric patients: A retrospective analysis. Cutan Ocul Toxicol. 2014;33(4):313-6.
19. Özcan D, Güleç AT. Compliance with tap water iontophoresis in patients with palmoplantar hyperhidrosis. J Cutan Med Surg. 2014;18(2):109-13.
20. Rezende RM, Luz FB. Surgical treatment of axillary hyperhidrosis by suction-curettage of sweat glands. An Bras Dermatol. 2014;89(6):940-54.
21. Tronstad C, Helsing P, Tønseth KA, et al. Tumescent suction curettage vs. curettage only for treatment of axillary hyperhidrosis evaluated by subjective and new objective methods. Acta Derm Venereol. 2014; 94(2):215-20.
22. Glaser DA, Galperin TA. Local procedural approaches for axillary hyperhidrosis. Dermatol Clin. 2014;32(4):533-40.
23. Feldmeyer L, Bogdan I, Moser A, et al. Short- and long-term efficacy and mechanism of action of tumescent suction curettage for axillary hyperhidrosis. J Eur Acad Dermatol Venereol. 2015;29(10):1933-7.
24. Abtahi-Naeini B, Naeini FF, Saffaei A, et al. Treatment of Primary Axillary Hyperhidrosis by Fractional Microneedle Radiofrequency: Is it Still Effective after Long-term Follow-up? Indian J Dermatol. 2016;61(2):234.
25. Hong HC, Lupin M, O'Shaughnessy KF. Clinical evaluation of a microwave device for treating axillary hyperhidrosis. Dermatol Surg. 2012;38(5):728-35.
26. Glaser DA, Coleman WP, Fan LK, et al. A randomized, blinded clinical evaluation of a novel microwave device for treating axillary hyperhidrosis: The dermatologic reduction in underarm perspiration study. Dermatol Surg. 2012;38(2):185-91.
27. Glaser DA, Galperin TA. Managing hyperhidrosis: emerging therapies. Dermatol Clin. 2014;32(4):549-53.
28. Stashak AB, Brewer JD. Management of hyperhidrosis. Clin Cosmet Investig Dermatol. 2014;7:285-99.
29. Mazlan M, Rajasegaran S, Engkasan JP, et al. A Double-Blind Randomized Controlled Trial Investigating the Most Efficacious Dose of Botulinum Toxin-A for Sialorrhea Treatment in Asian Adults with Neurological Diseases. Toxins (Basel). 2015;7(9):3758-70.
30. Møller E, Pedersen SA, Vinicoff PG, et al. Onabotulinumtoxin A Treatment of Drooling in Children with Cerebral Palsy: A Prospective, Longitudinal Open-Label Study. Toxins (Basel). 2015;7(7):2481-93.
31. Kouris A, Armyra K, Christodoulou C, et al. Quality of Life in Patients with Focal Hyperhidrosis before and after Treatment with Botulinum Toxin A. ISRN Dermatol. 2014;2014:308650.
32. Moffat CE, Hayes WG, Nyamekye IK. Durability of botulinum toxin treatment for axillary hyperhidrosis. Eur J Vasc Endovasc Surg. 2009;38(2):188-91.
33. El Kahky HM, Diab HM, Aly DG, et al. Efficacy of Onabotulinum Toxin A (Botox) versus Abobotulinum Toxin A (Dysport) Using a Conversion Factor (1:2.5) in Treatment of Primary Palmar Hyperhidrosis. Dermatol Res Pract. 2013;2013:686329.
34. Campanati A, Sandroni L, Gesuita R, et al. Treatment of focal idiopathic hyperhidrosis with Botulinum Toxin Type A: clinical predictive factors of relapse-free survival. J Eur Acad Dermatol Venereol. 2011;25(8):917-21.
35. An JS, Hyun Won C, Si Han J, et al. Comparison of onabotulinumtoxinA and rimabotulinumtoxinB for the treatment of axillary hyperhidrosis. Dermatol Surg. 2015;41(8):960-7.
36. Talarico-Filho S, Mendonça DO Nascimento M, Sperandeo DE Macedo F, et al. A double-blind, randomized, comparative study of two type A botulinum toxins in the treatment of primary axillary hyperhidrosis. Dermatol Surg. 2007;33(1 Spec No.):S44-50.
37. Bentivoglio AR, Del Grande A, Petracca M, et al. Clinical differences between botulinum neurotoxin type A and B. Toxicon. 2015;107(Pt A):77-84.
38. Dressler D, Adib Saberi F. Towards a dose optimisation of botulinum toxin therapy for axillary hyperhidrosis: Comparison of different Botox(®) doses. J Neural Transm (Vienna). 2013;120(11):1565-7.
39. Lowe NJ, Glaser DA, Eadie N, et al. Botulinum toxin type A in the treatment of primary axillary hyperhidrosis: A 52-week multicenter double-blind, randomized, placebo-controlled study of efficacy and safety. J Am Acad Dermatol. 2007;56(4):604-11.
40. Goodman G. Diffusion and short-term efficacy of botulinum toxin A after the addition of hyaluronidase and its possible application for the treatment of axillary hyperhidrosis. Dermatol Surg. 2003;29(5):533-8.
41. Hussain AB, Kavanagh GM. Site of botulinum toxin type A administration in craniofacial hyperhidrosis. Clin Exp Dermatol. 2015;40(5):570-1.
42. Lecouflet M, Leux C, Fenot M, et al. Duration of efficacy increases with the repetition of botulinum toxin A injections in primary axillary hyperhidrosis: A study in 83 patients. J Am Acad Dermatol. 2013;69(6):960-4.
43. Weinberg T, Solish N, Murray C. Botulinum neurotoxin treatment of palmar and plantar hyperhidrosis. Dermatol Clin. 2014;32(4):505-15.
44. Saadia D, Voustianiouk A, Wang AK, et al. Botulinum toxin type A in primary palmar hyperhidrosis: randomized, single-blind, two-dose study. Neurology. 2001;57(11):2095-9.

45. Doft MA, Hardy KL, Ascherman JA. Treatment of hyperhidrosis with botulinum toxin. Aesthet Surg J. 2012;32(2):238-44.
46. Swartling C, Karlqvist M, Hymnelius K, et al. Botulinum toxin in the treatment of sweat-worsened foot problems in patients with epidermolysis bullosa simplex and pachyonychia congenita. Br J Dermatol. 2010;163(5):1072-6.
47. Tamura BM, Cucé LC, Souza RL, et al. Plantar hyperhidrosis and pitted keratolysis treated with botulinum toxin injection. Dermatol Surg. 2004;30(12 Pt 2):1510-4.
48. Campanati A, Giuliodori K, Martina E, et al. Onabotulinumtoxin type A (Botox(®)) versus Incobotulinumtoxin type A (Xeomin(®)) in the treatment of focal idiopathic palmar hyperhidrosis: Results of a comparative double-blind clinical trial. J Neural Transm (Vienna). 2014;121(1):21-6.
49. Ko EJ, Mun SK, Oh IY, et al. Comparison of efficacy and diffusion of three formulations of botulinum toxin type A in two patients with forehead hyperhidrosis. Clin Exp Dermatol. 2014;39(5):673-5.
50. Karlqvist M, Rosell K, Rystedt A, et al. Botulinum toxin B in the treatment of craniofacial hyperhidrosis. J Eur Acad Dermatol Venereol. 2014;28(10):1313-7.
51. Trindade de Almeida AR, Marques E, de Almeida J, et al. Pilot study comparing the diffusion of two formulations of botulinum toxin type A in patients with forehead hyperhidrosis. Dermatol Surg. 2007;33(1 Spec No.):S37-43.
52. Kouris A, Agiasofitou E, Gregoriou S, et al. Generalized neurological symptoms following treatment of focal hyperhidrosis with botulinum toxin A. Int J Dermatol. 2014;53(11):e544-7.
53. Karlsson-Groth A, Rystedt A, Swartling C. Treatment of compensatory hyperhidrosis after sympathectomy with botulinum toxin and anticholinergics. Clin Auton Res. 2015;25(3):161-7.
54. Boharty BR, Hebert AA. Special considerations for children with hyperhidrosis. Dermatol Clin. 2014;32(4):477-84.
55. Blugerman G, Schavelzon D, Labaronnie H, et al. Our Trick to Control the Depth of Injection of the Botulinum Toxin in the Treatment of Hyperhidrosis. Plast Reconstr Surg. 2011;127(6):e165-6.
56. Chen S. Clinical uses of botulinum neurotoxins: current indications, limitations and future developments. Toxins (Basel). 2012;4(10):913-39.
57. Richards RN. Ethyl chloride spray for sensory relief for botulinum toxin injections of the hands and feet. J Cutan Med Surg. 2009;13(5):253-6.
58. Benohanian A. What stands in the way of treating palmar hyperhidrosis as effectively as axillary hyperhidrosis with botulinum toxin type A. Dermatol Online J. 2009;15(4):12.
59. Paracka L, Kollewe K, Dengler R, et al. Botulinum toxin therapy for hyperhidrosis: Reduction of injection site pain by nitrous oxide/oxygen mixtures. J Neural Transm (Vienna). 2015;122(9):1279-82.
60. Andrade PC, Flores GP, Uscello Jde F, et al. Use of iontophoresis or phonophoresis for delivering onabotulinumtoxinA in the treatment of palmar hyperidrosis: a report on four cases. An Bras Dermatol. 2011;86(6):1243-6.
61. Montaser-Kouhsari L, Zartab H, Fanian F, et al. Comparison of intradermal injection with iontophoresis of abobotulinum toxin A for the treatment of primary axillary hyperhidrosis: a randomized, controlled trial. J Dermatolog Treat. 2014;25(4):337-41.
62. Kavanagh GM, Shams K. Botulinum toxin type A by iontophoresis for primary palmar hyperhidrosis. J Am Acad Dermatol. 2006;55(5 Suppl):S115-7.
63. Torrisi BM, Zarnitsyn V, Prausnitz MR, et al. Pocketed microneedles for rapid delivery of a liquid-state botulinum toxin A formulation into human skin. J Control Release. 2013;165(2):146-52.
64. Skiveren J, Nordahl Larsen H, Kjaerby E, et al. The influence of needle size on pain perception in patients treated with botulinum toxin A injections for axillary hyperhidrosis. Acta Derm Venereol. 2011;91(1):72-4.
65. Lehman JS. Writer's block: "texting" impairment as a complication of botulinum toxin type A therapy for palmar hyperhidrosis. Arch Dermatol. 2011;147(6):752.
66. Chiarello D, Piombo M, Corbetto M, et al. Relapsing-remitting severe generalized muscular weakness after botulinum toxin treatment for hyperhidrosis. Muscle Nerve. 2014;50(3):456-7.
67. del Boz J, Padilla-Espana L, Segura-Palacios J. Botulinum Toxin Injection Technique for Axillary Hyperhidrosis. Actas Dermosifiliogr. 2014;105(5):517-8.
68. Iannitti T, Palmieri B, Aspiro A, et al. A preliminary study of painless and effective transdermal botulinum toxin A delivery by jet nebulization for treatment of primary hyperhidrosis. Drug Des Devel Ther. 2014;8:931-5.

17

CHAPTER

Complications of Botulinum Toxin in Aesthetic Procedures

Mansi S Mukherjee

INTRODUCTION

Botulinum toxin (BTX) has been in use for more than 20 years to treat a variety of therapeutic conditions. These include blepharospasm, strabismus, cervical dystonia, migraine, hyperhidrosis, and muscle spasticity. It was first approved for cosmetic use as Botox in 2002 by the U Food and Drug Administration (FDA), for frown lines and in 2013 to treat lateral orbicularis oculi muscles for crow's feet.[1] It has been in use off-label for all other cosmetic facial indications and has become the treatment of choice for wrinkles in the upper one-third of the face (i.e., frown lines, horizontal forehead lines, and crow's feet). Use of BTX in the lower two-third of the face is becoming more popular but this is more technically challenging and should be performed by experienced injectors.[2-7]

In 2014, the American Society for Aesthetic Plastic Surgery reported more than 3.5 million[8] aesthetic procedures. The International Society of Aesthetic Plastic Surgery survey reported more than 4.8 million procedures worldwide in 2014[9] and the 2013 American Society for Dermatologic Surgery survey found a 20% increase in the procedures as compared with 2012.[10] Similar trends are reported in Europe and Asia.[11]

Based on clinical experiences, retrospective reviews, and meta-analysis, botulinum toxin type A (BTX A) has excellent safety and tolerability across a spectrum of therapeutic and aesthetic applications.[12-14]

SAFETY PROFILE

Numerous studies have documented the safety and efficacy of neurotoxins for aesthetic purposes, especially for the reduction of glabellar, forehead, periocular and perioral lines.[2] The excellent safety profile of BTX is illustrated by the paucity of reported medical complications in aesthetic use. The amount of neurotoxin used is small and most of the side effects are transient, mild, and reversible. There are no reports of life-threatening allergic or urticarial reactions with facial BTX injections.[15]

A systematic review of 31 randomized or open-label clinical studies of BTX type A in aesthetic treatments quantified the incidence of treatment related with blepharoptosis (2.5%), brow ptosis (3.1%), eye sensory disorders (3%), lip asymmetries, and imbalances of lower face (6.9%).[12]

Complications related to BTX can be grouped in the following categories:

- Serious adverse events
- Nonserious adverse events
  - Injection related complications
  - Diffusion/dose-related/improper placement
- Improper patient selection and alignment
- Immunologic/no response to BTX.

Serious Adverse Events

As practitioners, we should be aware of these. They have been more commonly reported after the therapeutic use of BTX, but may also be seen with use in aesthetics.[16] Serious adverse events (SAEs) like thyroid eye disease in a patient with Graves' hyperthyroidism, sarcoidal granuloma, pseudoaneurysm of the frontal branch of the superior temporal artery, and severe respiratory failure[17-20] have been reported after the cosmetic use of BTX. Botulism-like generalized weakness was reported in a patient treated with BTX for axillary and palmar hyperhidrosis.[21]

An extensive review analysed SAEs reported to the FDA of BTX A for both therapeutic and cosmetic uses over a 13.5-year time period and non-SAEs over a 1-year time period. There were no reported deaths from cosmetic use of BTX A. Of the 36 reported SAEs, 6 reports were unrelated to the drug treatment while 30 were possible complications of the FDA-approved label.[22]

Serious adverse events, including 28 deaths, were reported with therapeutic uses. This was most likely due to the larger doses required for therapeutic use and the underlying disease state of patients requiring treatment. All neuromodulators, despite the lack of reported SAEs for dermatological use, have an FDA-mandated black box warning indicating the potential for distant spread resulting in swallowing or breathing difficulties and the risk of death.

A recent case report of vasculitis with panniculitis has been reported recently postinjection of an unlicensed Chinese brand of BTX for glabellar and perorbital rhytids.[23] She responded to treatment with oral prednisolone and hydroxyzine.

The dose of BTX is expressed in mouse units. One unit is described as the amount required, when injected intraperitoneally, to kill 50% of a group of 18 to 22 gram of Swiss Webster mice. The human lethal dose (LD) for BTX A purified neurotoxin complex is estimated at approximately 3000 units. Botulinum toxin type A usage in aesthetics allows a wide safety margin as the use is usually less than 100 units and between 300–600 units for other purposes. It is important to understand that doses are not interchangeable among different formulations of BoT (BOTOX®, Dysport, Myobloc) and different doses are used to achieve similar clinical results.[24]

Pseudoaneurysm of the Superficial Temporal Artery[19,25]

Pseudoaneurysm can arise in the forehead and scalp due to blunt traumatic impingement of the superficial temporal artery against the calvarium. A recent report described it after forehead injections of BoT. The anterior branch of the artery in the lateral forehead is most vulnerable as it courses over the frontal osseous ridge in the galea aponeurotica formed by the fusion line of the deep and superficial temporalis muscle fascia. Arterial wall is injured during trauma, or subsequent wall necrosis occurs post the contusion. Extravasation of blood from the injured artery leads to the formation of a hematoma and a pseudocapsule around it. The hematoma capsule possibly expands, and the clot reabsorbs, resulting in a cavity leading to pseudoaneurysm formation. A history of recent blunt trauma or surgery to the forehead with swelling and a pulsatile bruit on physical examination should aid the physician to this diagnosis.

Nonserious Adverse Events

Injection Site Reactions

Pain: Injection site pain is usually minimal and is dependent on sensitivity of the patient. It can be minimised through pretreatment with topical anesthetic (lidocaine/prilocaine or tetracaine/lidocaine), use of small-gauge needles (e.g., 30 or 31), changing needles after every 3 injections, cold gauze or ice compresses before and after the injection. However reactions to the local anesthetic are common and one should be vigilant about the same. Pinching the skin before injection have also been described to reduce the pain.[26]

Various distraction techniques like talking to the patient, a distraction device such as a massager, "stress ball" to squeeze, can be used.[2] Using the gate theory of pain, tapping with the non-injection hand/index finger on the patient's skin near the injection site, can distract them into feeling the vibration rather than the injection.

In a post approval double-blind, randomized, controlled study demonstrated less procedural pain with benzoic acid (bacteriostatic) preserved with 0.9% saline.[27] This reduction of injection pain may be due to the higher pH of the preservative-enhanced saline solution.[15]

Hypesthesia: Reports of injection site with temporary hypesthesia are not well-documented in most of the studies. Cases may have occurred due to localized edema and trauma or may be related to the localized antinociceptive properties of BoT.[15]

Bruising: Ecchymosis at the injection site has been reported to occur in less than 1% of injections. Patients on certain medications (Box 1) are at a higher risk of ecchymosis. Avoiding these for 7–10 days before the procedure can mitigate the risk.[26]

BOX 1 Medications that may increase risk of bruising

- Anticoagulants
- Aspirin and nonsteroidal anti-inflammatory drugs
- Vitamins (vitamin E or omega fatty acids)
- Herbal supplements (e.g., vitamin E, ginkgo, ginseng, garlic), St John's wort, Kava Kava, fish oils, celery root
- Alcohol

Certain areas like periocular area, perioral area, and lid margins have thin skin and superficial vessels and are more prone to ecchymosis. In one study, up to 25% of patients had bruising after onabotulinum toxin A (BTX A-ONA) for crow's feet (periocular) and similar rates also occurred in the placebo group, thereby implying that ecchymosis results from the injection rather than the toxin itself.[26]

A well-lit room, sidelight to highlight blue vessels, well-cleansed skin to avoid camouflage of vessels can avoid bruising in most of the cases. Direct firm pressure, immediately after injection and the use of cold compression can help reduce the risk of postinjection ecchymosis. Magnifying loops, or an infrared device (VeinVeiwer® Flex, Christie Digital Systems USA, Inc.), which shows vessels within 2–3 mm of the skin surface, can be used for visualising small vessels within the injection site.

Anecdotal and reports of small clinical trials have shown that certain herbal remedies like Arnica Montana and/or Bromelain, when started preoperatively reduces bruising and swelling. Another study showed an accelerated resolution of laser-induced bruising with topical 20% arnica ointment.[28,29] Topical preparations of vitamin K and C have been reported to be useful.[26] Most postprocedure bruising is benign and will resolve spontaneously. Pulsed dye laser or intense pulsed light can be used for a speedy recovery for distressed patients.

Headache: Headaches were the most frequently reported adverse events in the initial trials of BoNTA-ONA for the treatment of glabellar lines. The Botox glabellar lines II study group found that 11% of BTX and 20% placebo patients reported postinjection headache. Thus it was postulated that the micro trauma of needle penetration into the periosteum rather than action of the neurotoxin may be responsible for the same.[30]

One case report of five patients who received cosmetic BTX A reported severe and debilitating headaches that resolved with appropriate therapy. Microtrauma of needle penetration or toxin-induced muscle spasm were the postulated causes.[27] Fortunately, headaches are usually mild and require no specific treatment. Severe headaches or migraines can be treated with stronger analgesics or short courses of oral corticosteroids, although it is unclear if corticosteroids are helpful in mitigating headache symptoms.[27]

Skin reactions:[15] In the event where the skin barrier is violated, infection can be a potential complication. This can be avoided with proper injection, asepsis, and site selection. Psoriasiform eruption was described in a case report, which resolved spontaneously 5 months posttreatment.[31] Localized skin dryness and flakiness, was described in 3.8% (2 out of 52) patients who received Botox for upper face rejuvenation, in a prospective study by Bulstrode and Grobelaar. Both patients were men and their symptoms resolved with the application of skin moisturizers.[32] It has been hypothesized that localized skin dryness may be due to decreased sweat gland activity. This localized side effect may be underreported as more women than men received Botox injections; women are more likely to use skin moisturizers on a regular basis which masks skin dryness.

Unwanted Diffusion of Botulinum Toxin

Muscle paralysis/weakness is the required goal of cosmetic use of BTX A. However, local diffusion of up to 3 cm in diameter from the injection point can also lead to an unintended effect on neighbouring muscles.[33] This can present with localized functional or aesthetic deficits. Nearby spread of BTX is influenced by:[34]

- Diffusion of unbound toxin through the extracellular matrix
- The concentration gradient in this space
- The physical and anatomic boundaries in the injected area
- Volume injected
- The mechanics of injection.

A good knowledge of facial anatomy, good injection technique, and appropriate dosing of toxin can help minimize the complications. Most of the complications are reversible and short-lived. Proper patient education, emotional support, and appropriate medical intervention can help minimize the impact of the complication on the patient.[15]

EYELID PTOSIS

True eyelid ptosis is a rare complication, usually seen with novice injectors. The BTX A-ONA package insert reported that blepharoptosis occurred in 3% of 405 individuals, while another large multicenter study reported that 5.4% of 264 patients experienced this complication when treated for glabellar lines with 20 units.[2,35]

Eyelid opening is controlled by levator palpabrae superioris muscle which in turn inserts into the levator aponeurosis of the upper eyelid. Local diffusion of the toxin from the procerus and corrugator supercilii muscles to the superior tarsal muscle (Muller's muscle) and levator palpebrae superioris through the orbital septum can result in lid ptosis and diplopia. BoNTA induced lid ptosis can manifest within 48 hours or as late as a week after injections, and can last for weeks. It usually resolves within 2 to 6 weeks, with the cosmetic benefits of Botox outlasting the negative eyelid effects. [36]

Injections of the orbicularis oculi, corrugator supercilii, and procerus muscles have the highest likelihood of producing lid ptosis, especially in elderly patients and those with preexisting lid ptosis or levator function weakness. In the older patients, a combination of loose skin and attenuated orbital septum can further facilitate the dissection of injected Botox.[15]

Prevention

- It is important to look for excess skin on upper eyelid or a minimal ptosis especially in older patients. These patients maybe compensating by contracting the frontalis to open the eye and the treatment may result in an apparent lid ptosis. This is not due to true paralysis of the superior tarsal muscle, but rather the effect of neurotoxin on the frontalis in a patient who is reliant on the muscle to lift the brow and upper eyelid. One can assess for recompensation by pressing a finger above the brow, without moving the skin, and asking the patient to open the eye normally. This will demonstrate an otherwise subtle lid ptosis. The degree of ptosis can also be assessed by measuring levator excursion or the distance, the upper lid margin moves from full downgaze to full top gaze without brow movement. Levator function can be classified as excellent (>10 mm), good (8–10 mm), fair (5–7 mm), or poor (1–4 mm)[37]
- Avoid injecting corrugators with needle angled towards the orbit and keep all injections 1 cm above the bony orbital rim
- In individuals with a thin eyelid and associated hollow upper eyelid sulcus, avoid injecting low and deep along the eyebrow.[38] Inject superficially into lateral tail of corrugator
- Look for preexisting lid ptosis or levator function weakness especially in the elderly.

Treatment

Reassurance. Ptosis can be partially alleviated (up to 2 mm of eyelid elevation) with Apraclonidine drops administered two to three times daily.

DRY EYE SYNDROME

Dry eye syndrome of varying severity may develop with repeated neurotoxin injection into the lateral canthal region. These complications may occur in two ways:

1. Direct diffusion of Botulinum exotoxin A into the lacrimal gland which inhibits its normal secretory function
2. Paralytic lagophthalmos due to a partial paralysis of the orbicularis oculi muscles. This can lead to corneal exposure, decreased blink strength and decreased tonic orbicularis contraction.

Prevention

Early symptoms of this condition are subtle eye irritation, foreign body sensation, and epiphora. These manifestations seem to be due to orbicularis oculi muscle weakness and may become worse and possibly persistent if BoNTA injection is not delayed or discontinued. It is important to take history and recognize the presence of any dry eye symptoms as well as routine snap-back and distraction tests prior to BoNTA injections to help early detection of this condition.[39]

Treatment

It can usually be managed by lubricant eye drops, however in unresponsive cases, surgical treatment like lateral musculoplasty may be considered.

DIPLOPIA/DOUBLE VISION

Diplopia can occur during the treatment of crow's feet, due to diffusion of BTX into the extraocular muscles, usually the lateral rectus muscle.

Prevention

- Inject 1 cm outside the bony orbital rim.

Treatment

The patient should be referred to an ophthalmologist for the management. It may be treated with an eye patch, with prismatic lenses or with the injection of the neurotoxin in the opposing medial rectus.[40] Improvement is usually seen in approximately 7–10 weeks.[41]

ECTROPION

Botulinum toxin, when injected around the lower eyelid can compromise orbicularis oculi function, especially in older patients, patients who have had lower eyelid surgery, or in any individual with preexisting lower lid laxity or ectropion. It is important to remember that periorbital injections are usually well-tolerated in a younger patient and may result in ectropion in the older patient.[15]

Prevention

Assess lower lid tone by performing the "snap test" or "lower lid retraction test" in any patient who receives periorbital injections.

Treatment

Immediate attention is needed to prevent exposure keratitis and corneal damage. Lid taping, topical lubricating drops, and ocular moisture chambers may be helpful.

PSEUDOHERNIATION OF INFRAORBITAL FAT PADS[15]

The appearance of orbital fat pseudoherniation is prevented by orbicularis oculi muscle, along with the orbital septum which together provides the requisite sling-like support to the periocular area. In the patient who has lax septal support, compromise of orbicularis oculi tone can cause a temporary herniation of infraorbital fat.[42]

Prevention

Avoid injecting the inferior orbital, inferolateral canthal, and high malar regions in patients who have existing fat herniation or lower orbicularis oculi muscle tone.

LAGOPHTHALMOS[15]

Lagophthalmos is rarely seen following aesthetic Botox treatments. Some cases were reported in patients who received BTX injection for blepharospasm. Orbicularis oculi function may be compromised following injections of larger quantities of Botox into the lateral canthal area, resulting in lagophthalmos and secondary dry eyes.

FLAT CHEEK/FLACCID CHEEK[43]

Inadvertent paresis of the zygomaticus major muscle while injecting the inferior orbicularis oculi muscle (Crow's feet) can lead to a flat cheek. The zygomaticus major arises from the posterior portion of the lateral surface of the zygomaticus bone, where it is covered by the orbicularis oculi muscle, and travels diagonally to insert into the lateral aspect of the orbicularis oris muscle. It is the primary muscle responsible for smiling; therefore significant paresis can result in lip ptosis.

Prevention

Stay 1 cm above the zygomatic notch when treating the crow's feet.

FOREHEAD INJECTIONS

Eyebrow Ptosis

The frontalis muscle, being the only brow elevator, needs to be treated conservatively. Excessive treatment of this muscle (high doses of neurotoxin in the frontalis) can be associated with eyebrow ptosis. It can also occur due to inappropriate selection of patients, incorrect injection sites or very high dosage of toxin.[44] It can also be seen as a complication of glabellar treatment, from an injection placed too low in the corrugator or frontalis or diffusion of the drug into the frontalis muscle while treating the glabella. Occasionally, lateral brow elevation and central eyebrow ptosis may occur from muscle recruitment.

Prevention

- Pretreatment evaluation and discussion to determine the existing brow position and asymmetry. Choose appropriate placement of BTX on the basis of the size of forehead and the width and depth of the furrows The ultimate goal of the treatment is to achieve a natural result.[45,46]Pre-screen patients who unconsciously use the frontalis to lift excess of the upper eyelid skin. With the overtreatment of frontalis in such patients, they are no longer able to lift the brows after treatment
- Avoid isolated frontalis injections as unopposed action of brow depressors may lead to brow ptosis. Use smaller doses of neurotoxin in the frontalis in such patients. It is advisable to treat the brow depressors (corrugators and orbicularis oculi) first and treat the frontalis after 2 weeks in first time patients
- When injecting the glabella, inject deep into the corrugators
- Avoid overlapping the frontalis and glabellar injection points/treating the lower 2 cm of the forehead when injecting the frontalis.

GLABELLAR PROTRUSION

The medial fibers of frontalis intersect with the procerus at the glabellar region, whereas its central and lateral fibers intermingle with the corrugators in the central and lateral parts.[7] Another recently described complication that injectors must be aware of is glabellar protrusion.[47] This occurs due to the relative hyperactivity of the lower part of the muscle when the upper half part of the muscle is weakened with BTX for treatment of forehead wrinkles. Kang et al. reported that the mild hyperactivity of corrugators nearly disappeared without treatment by week 4; however, a severe case showed only slight improvement and persisted beyond 4 week.[48]

Treatment

Review at 1–2 weeks to treat the hyperactive muscles proactively. It is important to inform the patient of side effects such as eyelid ptosis that can occur with repeated injections of the corrugators. These can usually be avoided with proper injection technique.

EXAGGERATION OF LOWER FOREHEAD RHYTIDS

Several publications with consensus recommendations for BoNTA treatment of the forehead [7,45,46,49] suggest treating only the upper half or two-thirds of the forehead (measured between the orbital rim and the hairline) and staying 1–2 cm above the orbital rim. This is because the risk of brow and eyelid ptosis is greatest with treatment of the lower forehead. However, it is also important to know that, particularly in patients with a high forehead, treating only the upper two-thirds of the forehead may leave visible rhytides in the lower one-third of the forehead. This can be handled with proper alignment and follow up of the patient at 2 weeks for treating lower forehead.

THE 'SPOCK' (MEPHISTO SIGN)[15]

Excessive doses of BTX in the eyebrow depressors (orbicularis oculi, depressor supercilii, procerus and corrugator muscles) with concurrent treatment of the mid-frontalis may cause lowering of the midbrow and subsequent elevation of the lateral eyebrow, giving the patients a quizzical or surprised appearance (Spock brow). This occurs because of unopposed action of lateral fibres of frontalis which causes an elevation of the lateral aspect of the eyebrow.

Prevention

Injections of small amount of the neurotoxin lateral to the temporal fusion lines above the lateral eyebrow.

Treatment

It can be treated using 1–2 units of ONA or INO or 2.5 to 5 units of ABO, in the lateral frontalis fibres that have not been adequately treated.

FROZEN FACE APPEARANCE [50]

Over treated patients may lead to an expressionless, mask-like face or unnatural animation which patients most often don't like. It is important to balance the need of rhytid effacement with the patient's need for facial expression.[36] The contemporary treatment goals are softening and relaxing the muscle movement and the "frozen face" appearance is disdained by patients. It is important to make patients understand that any aesthetic treatment is a sculpting process and a follow up of 1 to 2 weeks after the injection is a good thing so that they can be precision treated.

LIP COMPLICATIONS

Injections of BTX into the chin, oral commissure, perioral area, and rarely orbicularis oculi can cause perioral complications.

INCOMPETENT MOUTH

Overtreatment of the orbicularis oris can lead to difficulty in speaking, eating, drinking out of a straw, and whistling.[49]

Prevention

Appropriate minimal dosing and proper alignment of the patient regarding potential complications when treating the lower face with BTX is must.

LIP ASYMMETRY/LIP PTOSIS[27]

With Botulinum injections into or around the lip, lip ptosis can be a potential complication as many muscles of the face are involved in the movement and positioning of the lips.

- Unintentional injection/unwanted spread into the depressor labii inferioris during injections of the mentalis, depressor anguli oris or orbicularis oris, may cause an abnormal/asymmetrical smile, difficulty in depressing the lower lip, and/or difficulty while eating

- Inadvertent spread /injection of the zygomaticus major can occur while treating the lower orbicularis oculi or due to overtreatment of the levator labii superioris alaeque nasi when treating "gummy smile". This can also cause an abnormal smile. Botulinum toxin in this muscle when used to reduce the appearance of nasolabial fold also has the potential side effect of lip ptosis.

One study described partial lip ptosis in 3 cases in over 1000 patients following injection of 7.5 units of BTX A to the lateral canthal rhytides (crow's feet). All these patients had undergone previous blepharoplasties, which suggest that altered anatomical planes may have resulted in toxin diffusion.[51]

Prevention

A detailed knowledge on anatomy, appropriate dosing and depth of injection will avoid these side effects.

- Treatment of orbicularis oris muscle should be performed conservatively (4-6 injection points of no more than 1 unit each of ONA and INO, or 2.5 units of ABO, split over the upper and lower cutaneous lip/vermillion border) with extensive patient education regarding these potential complications[52]
- If injections into the mentalis for the treatment of dimpling are too lateral or superficial, the toxin may spread to the depressor labii inferioris (DLI), causing an incompetent mouth or asymmetrical smile
- Neurotoxin injections into the depressor anguli oris should be made at the posterior aspect of the muscle, below the midway point between the vermillion and the mandible. If the toxin is placed medial to the melomental fold, it can diffuse to denervate the DLI and cause slurred speech. If it is placed above the midway point between the vermillion and the mandible, it can result in asymmetry of the mouth[48]

PLATYSMAL BANDS

Dysphagia/Voice changes/ Neck weakness

Diffusion of neuromodulator into the parapharyngeal muscles while treating the platysmal bands or horizontal neck lines can lead to these complications. In a study by Matarasso and colleagues[5], platysmal bands were treated with BTX injections in 1500 patients. Ten percent of the patients reported a mild and transient cervical discomfort 2 to 5 days after toxin injections. Neck weakness upon head elevation was observed by 1% of the patients. One patient (0.067%) experienced clinically significant dysphagia. This resolved spontaneously within 2 weeks. Another similar study of 26 patients[53] did not report any cases of dysphagia with lower dose of the toxin.

Prevention

Consensus recommendations 2016[54] suggests injection of 6-12 units per band with a maximum dose of 60 Units (ONA) when treating the neck. Injections must be intracutaneous or intramuscular and above the level of the thyroid cartilage.

Treatment

Dysphagia is mild and transient in most cases. Emotional support, soft diet or pureed foods may be helpful in cases of severe dysphagia until full recovery occurs. This may be potentially life-threatening complication, and such patients should be monitored for airway compromise.[46]

Hyperhidrosis[26,55]

The most significant complication is a varying degree of temporary hand weakness as the result of BTX A diffusion to lumbrical muscles and other unintended targets. As many as two thirds of patients experience a temporary minor weakening of finger grip strength that is noted a week after treatment and may last for 3-5 weeks. Patients may have difficulty with fine motor tasks, such as pushing a button through a buttonhole or using chop sticks. Patients can usually write and type without difficulty but may find that opening a tight jar is difficult for few weeks. Dentists, surgeons, musicians, and others in profession that require precise hand control should be alerted prior to injection to the possibility of transient functional impediment. Lehman recently reported the inability to type on a cellular phone following BTX A injection in a 17-year-old girl. [56]

Prevention

- Doses should be tailored according to the size of the palm with appropriate dosing spaced every 1-2 cm
- Injections should be intradermal.

Masseter[57-59]

Injections of the masseter with BTX have been used in facial reshaping to reduce the appearance of hypertrophic masseters. Some studies have shown that there may be a temporary inability to chew hard food 1 week postinjection, lasting up to 6 weeks. Minor changes in facial expression can occur. This is due to accidental weakening of the zygomaticus major or risorius. Smile asymmetry & difficulty in smiling from diffusion into zygomaticus major or levator anguli is a temporary complication if BTX is injected too high into the masseter.

It has also been seen that the cheeks appear sunken following injection. Atrophy of the superior portion which lies just below the bony prominence of the cheek bone may result in a sharp drop-off between the zygomatic arch and cheek causing the sunken cheek appearance.[60] Localized swelling at the injection site due to hematomas may be seen but they resolve on their own within a week. Muscle ache and pain at site of injection is also reported. Sometimes, a minor skin 'sagging' has been seen postinjection. This is because the muscle shrinks faster than skin contracts. It usually resolves in 6–12 weeks.[61]

Prevention of Lip Asymmetry

- Keep injections below the line drawn from lip corner to ear tragus
- Mark and delineate the muscle with the patient's teeth clenched. Always inject at least 1 cm away from muscle borders
- Do not do a touch up before 6 weeks of the first injection.

IMPROPER PATIENT SELECTION AND ALIGNMENT[62]

In 2003 patient satisfaction survey conducted by the American Academy of Dermatology, 78% of respondents did not know how long cosmetic procedures take or how long they last, 67% were uncertain about what procedures would work best for them, and only 35% believed that cosmetic procedures were safe.[62] This data highlights an important need to ensure adequate patient understanding and knowledge about procedures before starting a treatment.

- When treating a patient with BoT, choose your patient carefully, understand patient expectations and discuss treatment goals. Ensure that the patient understands the progressive nature of the aging process
- Aligning the patient that BTX, will only soften static lines and does not erase them is important. Combination with lasers and light therapy, dermal fillers can be discussed and an individualized treatment plan should be formulated in each patient to focus on treating areas that will have the greatest impact
- Take a proper informed consent and pretreatment photographs at rest and in animation. Pretreatment assessment should be performed in repose and in animation. Assessment when the patient is engaged in routine activities such as speaking (informal assessment) is frequently of more value than assessment during animation on command (formal assessment)[54]
- Avoid overtreatment and unnatural results or, conversely, undertreatment and suboptimal results
- Avoid treating patients with suspected or diagnosed with body dysmorphic disorder.

NO RESPONSE

Primary nonresponders are those who do not respond to injections or/and have never previously responded to BTX injections. There can be many reasons for a lack of response.

- Static rhytids with no dynamic component (e.g., photodamage, age-related changes) do not respond to toxin
- Therapeutic failure may also occur due to improper injection technique or the denatured toxin
- Individual variations in docking proteins may exist or some patients may have neutralizing antibodies from prior to subclinical exposure.[63]

Secondary nonresponders respond initially but lose the response on subsequent injections. These patients may have developed neutralizing antibodies. There is a potential for immunogenicity, as with any therapeutic proteins. The effectiveness of BTX may reduce due to the formation of neutralizing antibodies to BTX A which inactivates the biological action of the toxin.

An open-label study, long-term study evaluated 326 cervical dystonia patients. These patients were treated for an average of 9 times with the current formulation of BTX. A total of 4 (1.2%) patients had positive antibody tests. However all of these 4 patients responded to BTX therapy at the time of the positive antibody test. Three of these patients developed clinical resistance after a subsequent treatment, while the fourth patient continued to respond to BTX.[64] It has been reported that 5-15% of patients, who were injected serially with earlier preparations of Botox® (batch 79-11) developed secondary nonresponsiveness due to neutralizing antibodies.[65] The major risk factors postulated with the development of neutralizing antibodies are:

- Injection of more than 200 units per session
- Repeat or booster injections given within one month of treatment.

The new formulation of Botox® (BCB 2024) has decreased protein load[66] and appears to have reduced immunogenicity and a lower potential for neutralizing antibody production. Dressler et al., in their studies have reported that the rate of developing neutralizing antibodies is substantially reduced with BCB 2024.[63] In rabbit studies, no antibody formation occurred with new (BCB 2024) Botox® after six months of treatment, while old (batch 79-11) Botox® caused antibody formation in all rabbits by five months.

Prevention

- Use the lowest dose of toxin necessary to achieve the clinical result
- Avoid reinjection within one month as this may keep antibody formation as low and unlikely as possible.[68]

CONTRAINDICATIONS TO BOTULINUM TOXIN INJECTION[68]

Some of the contraindications to BTX injections are listed in box 2.

DRUG INTERACTIONS[15]

The quantities of BTX used in aesthetic cases are usually small and clinically significant drug-drug interactions have not been reported. However drugs that interfere with neuromuscular transmission could potentially interact with BTX. Drugs that may alter the effects of BTX are given in box 3.

Drugs have an intrinsic inhibitory effect on neuromuscular transmission that may potentiate the effect of BTX.

BOX 2 Contraindications to Botulinum toxin injection

- Body dysmorphic disorder
- Dependency on facial expression for livelihood (e.g., actors, singers)
- Dermatoses in the treatment area (e.g., psoriasis, eczema)
- Gross motor weakness in the treatment area (e.g., Bell's palsy)
- Immunocompromised
- Infection in the treatment area
- Keloidal scarring
- Neuromuscular disorder (e.g., amyotrophic lateral sclerosis, myasthenia gravis, Lambert-Eaton syndrome, myopathies)
- Pregnancy or breastfeeding
- Sensitivity or allergy to constituents of the botulinum toxin product [e.g., cow's milk protein allergy with abobotulinumtoxin A (Dysport)]
- Unrealistic expectations

BOX 3 List of drugs that alter the effect of Botulinum toxin injection

- Aminoglycosides (gentamicin)
- Cyclosporine
- D-penicillamine
- Muscle relaxants (curare type nondepolarizing blockers, succinylcholine)
- Aminoquinolines
- Quinidine
- Magnesium sulfate
- Lincosamide

CONCLUSION

The key to successful treatment is to follow an individualized approach, detailed assessment meticulous treatment planning. Certain patients may have specific preferences regarding the magnitude and nature of results. A thorough knowledge of anatomy, contraindications, drug-interactions, and complications is a must for all injectors. Analyze target muscles in the context of adjacent muscles and associated anatomical landmarks. It is advisable to for new injectors to gain adequate experience with treating upper face with BTX before treating lower face. Appropriate doses and injection techniques can go a long way in preventing most of the side effects.

REFERENCES

1. FDA approves Botox Cosmetic to improve the appearance of crow's feet lines [news release]. Silver Springs, MD: U.S. Food and Drug Administration. [online] Accessed from: http://www.fda.gov/newsevents/newsroom/pressannouncements/ucm367662.htm. Accessed in, 2014].
2. Carruthers JA, Lowe NJ, Menter MA, et al.; BOTOX Glabellar Lines I Study Group. A multicenter, double-blind, randomized, placebo-controlled study of the efficacy and safety of botulinum toxin type A in the treatment of glabellar lines. J Am Acad Dermatol. 2002;46(6):840-9.
3. Carruthers A, Carruthers J, Cohen JL. A prospective, double-blind, randomized, parallel- group, dose-ranging study of botulinum toxin type A in female subjects with horizontal forehead rhytides. Dermatol Surg. 2003;29(5):461-7.

4. Lowe NJ, Lask GP, Yamauchi PS, et al. Bilateral, double-blind, randomized comparison of 3 doses of botulinum toxin type A and placebo in patients with crow's feet. J Am Acad Dermatol. 2002;47(6):834-40.
5. Michaels BM, Csank GA, Ryb GE, et al. Prospective randomized comparison of onabotulinumtoxinA (Botox) and abobotulinumtoxinA (Dysport) in the treatment of forehead, glabellar, and periorbital wrinkles. Aesthet Surg J. 2012;32(1):96-102.
6. Sattler G, Callander MJ, Grablowitz D, et al. Noninferiority of incobotulinumtoxin A, free from complexing proteins, compared with another botulinum toxin type A in the treatment of glabellar frown lines. Dermatol Surg. 2010;36(4):2146-54.
7. Ascher B, Talarico S, Cassuto D, et al. International consensus recommendations on the aesthetic usage of botulinum toxin type A (Speywood Unit)–Part I: Upper facial wrinkles. J Eur Acad Dermatol Venereol. 2010;24(11):1278-84.
8. American Society for Aesthetic Plastic Surgery (ASAPS). Cosmetic surgery national data bank statistics. [online] Accessed from: http://www.surgery.org/sites/default/files/2014-Stats.pdf [Accessed in 2015].
9. International Society of Aesthetic Plastic Surgery (ISAPS). International survey on aesthetic/cosmetic procedures. American Society of Plastic Surgeons. 528e Plastic and Reconstructive Surgery. [online] Accessed from: http://www.isaps.org/Media/Default/global-statistics/2015%20ISAPS%20Results.pdf [Accessed in 2015].
10. American Society for Dermatologic Surgery (ASDS). ASDS survey: Skin cancer, cosmetic procedures jump 22 percent in 2013. ASDS survey on dermatologic procedures. [online] Accessed from: https://www.asds.net/_Media.aspx?id=7744 [Accessed in 2014]
11. Italian Association of Aesthetic Plastic Surgery (AICPE). Press Releases: Beauty, AICPE data: Almost one million cosmetic medicine and surgery treatments performed in 2013. [online] Available from: http://www.medicitalia.it/news/chirurgia-plastica-e-ricostruttiva/4829-dates-2013-surgery-medicine-aesthetics.html [Accessed in 2015].
12. Brin MF, Boodhoo TI, Pogoda JM, et al. Safety and tolerability of onabotulinumtoxin A in the treatment of facial lines: A meta-analysis of individual patient data from global clinical registration studies in 1678 participants. J Am Acad Dermatol. 2009;61:961-70.
13. Naumann M, Jankovic J. Safety of botulinum toxin type A: A systematic review and meta-analysis. Curr Med Res Opin. 2004;20:981-90.
14. Cavallini M, Cirillo P, Fundarò SP, et al. Safety of botulinum toxin A in aesthetic treatments: A systematic review of clinical studies. Dermatol Surg. 2014;40:52536.
15. Vartanian AJ, Dayan SH. Complications of botulinum toxin A use in facial rejuvenation. Facial Plast Surg Clin North Am. 2003;11(4):483-92.
16. Yiannakopoulou E. Serious and Long-Term Adverse Events Associated with the Therapeutic and Cosmetic Use of Botulinum Toxin. Pharmacology. 2015;95(1-2):65-69.
17. Ahbib S, Lachapelle JM, Marot L: Sarcoidal granulomas following injections of botulinum toxin A (Botox) for corrections of wrinkles. Ann Dermatol Venereol. 2006;133(1):43-45.
18. Harrison A, Erickson J: Thyroid eye disease presenting after cosmetic botulinum toxin injections Ophtal Plast Reconstr Surg. 2006;22(5):397-8.
19. Prado A, Fuentes P, Guerra C, et al: Pseudoaneurysm of the frontal branch of the superficial temporal artery: an unusual complication after the injection of Botox. Plast Reconstr Surg. 2007;119(7):2334-5.
20. Nong LB, He WQ, Xu YH, et al: Severe respiratory failure after injection of botulinum toxin: Case report and review of the literature. Zhonghua Jie He He Hu Xi Za Zhi. 2008;31(5):369-71.
21. Tugnoli R, Eleopra R, Quatrale R, et al. Botulism-like syndrome after botulinum toxin type A injections for focal hyperhidrosis. Br J Dermatol. 2002;147:808-809.
22. Coté TR, Mohan AK, Polder JA, et al. Botulinum toxin type A injections: Adverse events reported to the US Food and Drug Administration in therapeutic and cosmetic cases. J Am Acad Dermatol. 2005;53(3):407-15.
23. Namazi N, Robati RM, Dadkhahfar S, et al. Vasculitis with panniculitis following botulinum toxin A injection for cosmetic use. Dermatology Practical & Conceptual. 2016;6(1):19-21.
24. Sternick I, Pitanguy I. Botulinum toxin dosage template for frontal wrinkle effacement. Aesthet Surg J. 2011;31(7):814-20.
25. Skaf GS, Domloj NT, Salameh JA, et al. Pseudoaneurysm of the superficial temporal artery: A complication of botulinum toxin injection. Aesth Plast Surg. 2012;36:982-5.
26. Levy LL, Emer JJ. Complications of Minimally Invasive Cosmetic Procedures: Prevention and Management. Journal of Cutaneous and Aesthetic Surgery. 2012;5(2):121-132.
27. Alam M, Arndt KA, Dover JS. Severe, intractable headache after injection with botulinum a exotoxin: Report of 5 cases. J Am Acad Dermatol. 2002;46(1):62-5.
28. MacKay D, Miller AL. Nutritional support for wound healing. Altern Med Rev. 2003;8(4):359-77.
29. Leu S, Havey J, White LE, et al. Accelerated resolution of laser-induced bruising with topical 20% arnica: A rater-blinded randomized controlled trial. Br J Dermatol. 2010;163(3):557-63.
30. Carruthers JD, Lowe NJ, Menter MA, et al. Botox Glabellar Lines II Study Group. Double-blind, placebo-controlled study of the safety and efficacy of botulinum toxin type A for patients with glabellar lines. Plast Reconstr Surg. 2003;112(4):1089-98.
31. Bowden JB, Rapini RP. Psoriasiform eruption from intramuscular botulinum A toxin. Cutis. 1992;50:415-6.
32. Bulstrode NW, Grobelaar AO. Long-term prospective follow-up of botulinum toxin treatment for facial rhytids. Aesthetic Plast Surg. 2002;26(5):356-9.
33. Huang W, Foster JA, Rogachefsky AS. Pharmacology of botulinum toxin. J Am Acad Dermatol. 2000;43(2):249-59.
34. Borodic GE, Ferrante RJ, Pearce LB, et al. Pharmacology and histology of the therapeutic application of botulinum toxin. In: Jankovic J, Hallet M. Eds. Therapy with Botulinium toxin. New York: Marcel Dekker, Inc., 1994:119-157.

35. Botox Cosmetic. FDA approved labeling. [online] Accessed from: https://www.accessdata.fda.gov/drugsatfda_docs/label/2009/103000s5109s5210lbl.pdf
36. Matarasso SL. Complications of botulinum A exotoxin for hyperfunctional lines. Dermatol Surg. 1998;24(11): 1249-54.
37. Finsterer J. Ptosis: Causes, presentation, and management. Aesthetic Plast Surg. 2003;27(3):193-204.
38. Steinsapir KD, Groth MJ, Boxrud CA. Persistence of Upper Blepharoptosis After Cosmetic Botulinum Toxin Type A. Dermatol Sur. 2015;41(7):833-40.
39. Ozgur O, Murariu D, Parsa AA, et al. Dry Eye Syndrome Due to Botulinum Toxin Type-A Injection: Guideline for Prevention. Hawai'i Journal of Medicine & Public Health. 2012;71(5):120-3.
40. Isaac CR, Chalita MR, Pinto LD. Botox® after Botox® - a new approach to treat diplopia secondary to cosmetic botulinic toxin use: Case reports. Arq Bras Oftalmol. 2012;75(3):213-4.
41. Aristodemou P, Watt L, Baldwin C. Diplopia associated with the cosmetic use of botulinum toxin A for facial rejuvenation. Ophthal Plast Reconstr Surg. 2006;22(2): 134-6.
42. Paloma V, Samper A. A complication with aesthetic use of Botox: herniation of the orbital fat. Plast Reconstr Surg. 2001;107(5):1315-6.
43. Vanaman M, Fabi SG, Carruthers J. Complications in the Cosmetic Dermatology Patient: A review and our experiences. Dermatol Surg. 2016;42(1):1-11.
44. Redaelli A, Forte RJ. How to avoid brow ptosis after forehead treatment with botulinum toxin. Cosmet Laser Ther. 2003;5(3-4):220-2.
45. Carruthers JD, Glogau RG, Blitzer A. Advances in facial rejuvenation: Botulinum toxin type A, hyaluronic acid dermal fillers, and combination therapies: consensus recommendations. Plast Reconstr Surg. 2008;121(5): 5S-30S.
46. Kane M, Donofrio L, Ascher B, et al. Expanding the use of neurotoxins in facial aesthetics: a consensus panel's assessment and recommendations. J Drugs Dermatol. 2010;9(1):7-22.
47. Kim MW, Jang S, Yoon H, et al. Correction of glabellar protrusion after botulinum toxin injection for forehead wrinkles. J Surg Dermatol. 2016;1(1):2-3.
48. Kang SM, Feneran A, Kim JK, et al. Exaggeration of wrinkles after botulinum toxin injection for forehead horizontal lines. Ann Dermatol. 2011;23(2):217-21.
49. Carruthers J, Fagien S, Matarasso SL. Consensus recommendations on the use of botulinum toxin type A in facial aesthetics. Plast Reconstr Surg. 2004;114(6): 1S-22S.
50. Niamtu J. Complications in Fillers and Botox. Oral and Maxillofacial Surg Clin North Am. 2009;21(1):13-21.
51. Matarasso SL, Matarasso A. Treatment guidelines for botulinum toxin type A for the periocular region and a report on partial upper lip ptosis following injections to the lateral canthal rhytids. Plast Reconstr Surg. 2001;108(1):208-14.
52. Matarasso A, Matarasso SL, Brandt FS, et al. Botulinum toxin for the management of platysmal bands. Plast Reconstr Surg. 1999;103(2):645-52.
53. Kane MAC. Nonsurgical treatment of platysmal bands with injection of botulinum toxin A. Plast Reconstr Surg. 1999;103(2):656-63.
54. Sundaram H, Signorini M, Liew S, et al. Global Aesthetics Consensus: Botulinum Toxin Type A--Evidence-Based Review, Emerging Concepts, and Consensus Recommendations for Aesthetic Use, Including Updates on Complications. Plast Reconstr Surg. 2016;137(3):518e-529e.
55. Klein AW. Complications with the use of botulinum toxin. Dermatol Clin. 2004;22(2):197-205.
56. Lehman JS. Writer's block: "Texting" impairment as a complication of botulinum toxin type A therapy for palmar hyperhidrosis. Arch Dermatol. 2011;147(6):752.
57. Ahn J, Horn C, Blitzer A. Botulinum toxin for masseter reduction in Asian patients. Arch Facial Plast Surg. 2004;6(3):188-91.
58. Liew S, Dart A. Nonsurgical reshaping of the lower face. Aesthet Surg J. 2008;28(3):251-7.
59. Kim HJ, Yum KW, Lee SS, et al. Effects of botulinum toxin type A on bilateral masseteric hypertrophy evaluated with computed tomographic measurement. Dermatol Surg. 2003;29(5):484-9.
60. Wu WT. Botox facial slimming/facial sculpting: The role of botulinum toxin-A in the treatment of hypertrophic masseteric muscle and parotid enlargement to narrow the lower facial width. Facial Plast Surg Clin North Am. 2010;18(1):133-40.
61. Carruthers J1, Burgess C, Day D, et al. Consensus Recommendations for Combined Aesthetic Interventions in the Face Using Botulinum Toxin, Fillers, and Energy-Based Devices. Dermatol Surg. 2016;42(5):586-97.
62. American Academy of Dermatology. Facing the age old question...how to turn back the hands of time. New Academy of Dermatology survey finds women overwhelmed by anti-aging treatment options [Press Release]. [online] Accessed from: www.aad.org [Accessed in 2003].
63. Dressler D, Saberi A. New formulations od botox: Complete antibody-induced treatment failure in cervical dystonia. J Neurol Neurosurg Psychiatry. 2007;78:108-9.
64. Botox package insert. Allergan Pharmaceuticals Ireland. Pp. 1-34. Available from: http://www.vidyya.com/6pdfs/BotoxPI.pdf
65. Göschel H, Wohlfarth K, Frevert J, et al. Botulinum A toxin therapy: Neutralizing and nonneutralizing antibodies and therapeutic consequences. Exp Neurol. 1997;147(1):96-102.
66. Benedetto AV. The cosmetic uses of Botulinum toxin type A. Int J Dermatol. 1999;38(9):641-55.
67. Nigam PK, Nigam A. Botulinum Toxin. Indian J Derm. 2010;55(1):8-14.
68. Small R. Botulinum toxin injection for facial wrinkles. Am Fam Physician. 2014;90(3):168-75.

18

CHAPTER

Intradermal Botulinum Toxin: Uses and Techniques

Abhay Talathi

INTRODUCTION

Botulinum toxin (BTX) is an exotoxin obtained from an anaerobic bacteria *Clostridium botulinum.* Botulinum toxin type A (BTX A) is the most potent among all subtypes of BTXs (eight subtypes). Botulinum toxin A has been effectively used in multiple cosmetic and therapeutic indications for more than two decades now. Most common of all cosmetic indications is the treatment of dynamic upper facial rhytids. Commonly used commercial BTX A preparations include Botox Cosmetic (onabotulinum toxin by Allergan), Dysport (abobotulinum toxin by Galderma), Xeomin (incobotulinum toxin by Merz Aesthetics), and Neuronox (Medy-Tox).

SKIN REJUVENATION AND BOTULINUM TOXIN

With progression of science of cosmetology there has been a plethora of procedures aimed at skin rejuvenation. The term skin rejuvenation in the author's opinion relates to improvement in skin texture, skin firmness, reduction in pore size and seborrhea, and achievement of an even skin tone. Alongside other procedures like chemical peels, microneedling and energy-based devices, BTX A has also been studied to achieve skin rejuvenation. Intradermal BTX A (mesotherapy with BTX A) can be effectively used in improving skin texture, skin firmness, and reducing pore size.

Mechanism of Action

When used in the treatment of dynamic facial rhytids BTX A acts by inhibiting the release of acetylcholine at neuromuscular junction. As no acetylcholine is released the neuromuscular signaling is interrupted and muscle fails to contract thus relaxing hyper-dynamic wrinkles.

However, mechanism of action of microbotox is majorly by its action on the skin adnexa and the superficial muscle fibers as it is inserted into the dermis.[1] Botulinum toxin A has shown to reduce sebum production after intradermal injection. Exact mechanism involved in this is not clearly understood, however, intradermal BTX may reduce sebum production through its neuromodulatory effects on the arrector pili muscles and the local muscarinic receptors in the sebaceous gland. The highest concentration of acetylcholine receptors is at the infundibulum of the pilosebaceous unit. It is plausible that blockade of local acetylcholine receptors in the pilosebaceous unit with BTX could result in altered rates of sebum production.[3]

Overall effect of intradermal BTX A on superficial muscle fibers and skin adnexa results in lifting, tightening, and a smoother skin appearance with reduced pore size.

Indications for Intradermal Botulinum Toxin Type A

- Skin rejuvenation on face and neck (improve skin surface, turgor, firmness, and reduces pore size)
- To achieve firming (mild lifting) of midface
- To improve horizontal neck wrinkles and cervico-mental angle (jaw line definition).

Contraindications

- Myasthenia gravis, Lambert-Eaton syndrome
- Pregnancy and lactation
- Acute infection at the site of injection.

Dosages and Injection Technique

Variable dosages have been tried to achieve improvement in skin surface, skin turgor, and firmness with good results. The use of BTX A for skin rejuvenation, however, is not US Food and Drug Administration approved.

- Skin rejuvenation: Four to five units/side of onabotulinum toxin in 0.5 mL of normal saline is injected intradermally over 10 points in midface to improve the quality of skin of the midface (Fig. 1).[1]

  Five units/side of BTX A in 0.5 mL of normal saline is used in lowerface.[1] It is important to understand that BTX A is hyperdiluted when it is used for intradermal injection and small volumes are placed per point of injection so as to avoid diffusion to deeply placed muscles.
- Midface firming: Botulinum toxin type A is not the treatment of choice for midface lifting; however, there has been a mention in literature about a technique with intradermal BTX in midface lift (Fig. 2).

  Injections are placed intradermally targeting orbicularis oculi and the platysma muscles. For the platysma the injections are performed in two parallel rows, the lateral row starting from about the temporomandibular joint, down along the mandibular line, at about 1 cm intervals. The medial row was about 1 cm from the lateral row, with the injection points between those of the lateral ones. Lateral part of orbicularis oculi in the temporal area is injected as a part of treatment of the orbicularis oculi (Table 1).

  This technique was extensively studied by Dr. Chariya Petchngaovilai with satisfactory results. For this technique 50–70 units of abobotulinum toxin (approximately equivalent to 20–30 units of onabotulinum toxin) were used.[3]
- To improve cervicomental angle and neck creases: In a technique published by Dr. Woffles Wu, 56 units of onabotulinum toxin were used over 240 injection points in the lower face and neck. The results were better demonstrated in subjects with less subcutaneous fat in the neck.[1,4]

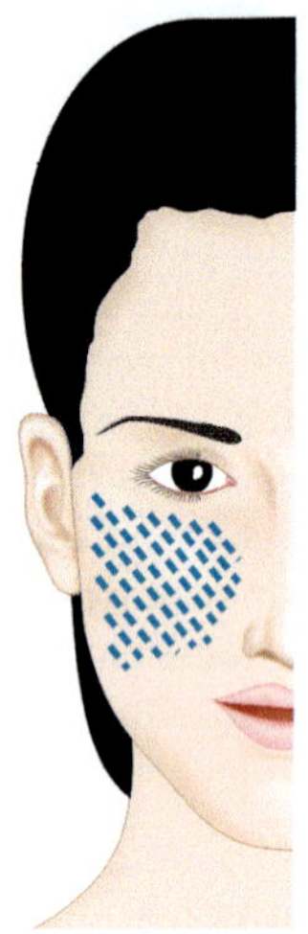

FIG. 1: Skin rejuvenation technique: 5 Units/side onabotulinum toxin, intradermal injections, under topical anesthesia.

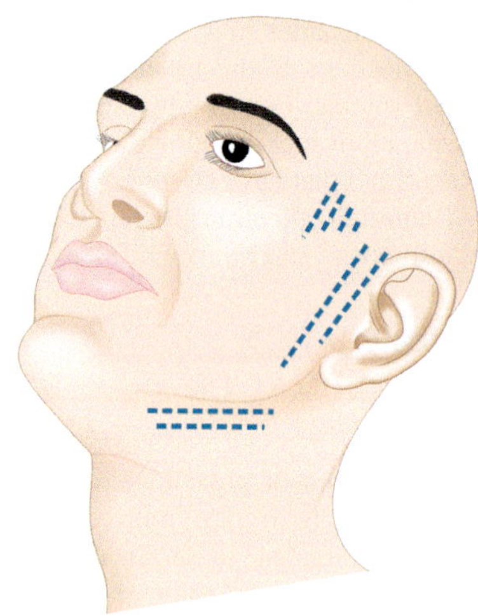

FIG. 2: Midface lifting and jaw line definition with intradermal botulinum toxin.

TABLE 1: Dilution chart for intradermal onabotulinum toxin

Indication	Units	Dilution amount	Approximate number of pricks
Skin rejuvenation	10 units (5 units/side)	Hyperdilution (5 units/0.4 mL)	20–30 pricks per side
Midface firming[2]	20–30 units (10–15 units/side)	Hyperdilution (20–30 units/0.8 mL)	20–30 pricks/side
Lower face and neck tightening[4]	56 units (20–28 units/side)	Hyperdilution (20–28 units/1 mL)	100–120 pricks/side

Note: Standard dilution considered is 100 units/2.5 mL of normal saline.

Author's Technique (Unpublished Data)

Author recommends the use of BTX A in midface rejuvenation where 5 units (onabotulinum toxin) in 0.4 mL of normal saline/side are used over 20–30 sites. Wheals of BTX are created while injecting area is not to be massaged by the injector or the patient on the same day so as to avoid diffusion in the wrong plane. The procedure comfort is increased by performing it under topical anesthesia. The results are established in 7–14 days and are usually short-lived lasting about 10–12 weeks postprocedure (Figs 3 and 4).

Side Effects

- Temporary paralysis of deeply placed muscles by diffusion of toxin shall result in facial asymmetry. It is the most common complication which may arise from a wrong injection technique. The injections in the area of the lower face are more complicated and carry higher risks of complications as small muscles are joined together in that area and they are difficult to distinguish from one another. The risk is even higher when the injection is performed with more diluted toxin. Higher dilutions of BTX result in greater areas of diffusion and, therefore, a greater incidence of adverse effects.[5] If the toxin diffuses to the nontargeted muscles, it may cause an asymmetrical smile, difficulty in smiling, or drooping of the angle of the mouth.[6]

  This can be prevented by careful intradermal placement and raising a wheal while injecting. If these complications accidentally occur, they are temporary and reversible.
- Bruising: This is very common with intradermal BTX A as number of pricks given per treatment area are more. It can be reduced with a careful and slow injection technique. Most of the bruises completely resolve in 8–10 days
- Pain and mild discomfort during and after the treatment may be experienced by a few patients.

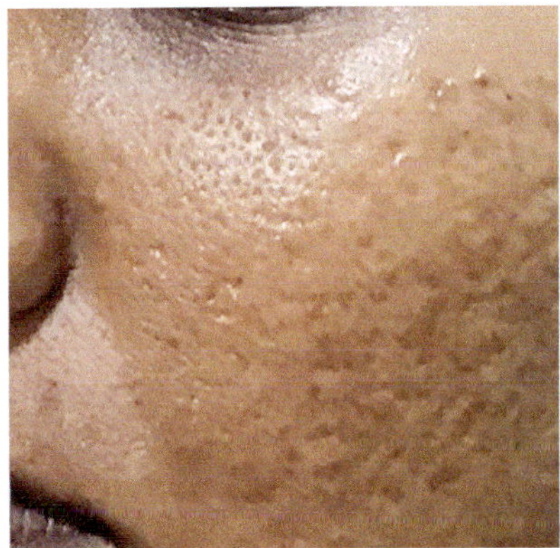

FIG. 3: Before intradermal botulinum toxin injection.

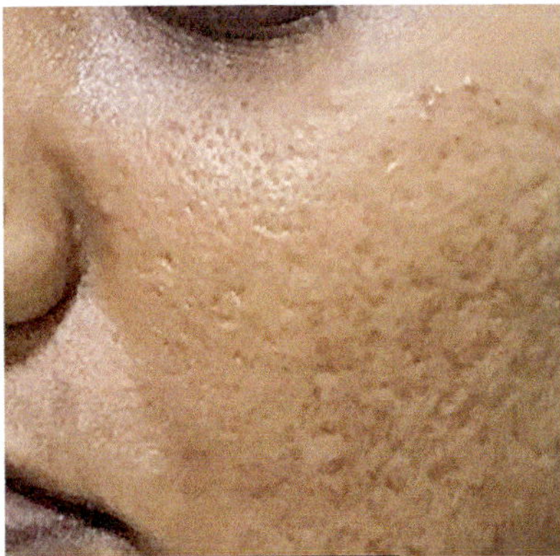

FIG. 4: After intradermal botulinum toxin injection.

CONCLUSION

Botulinum toxin type A can be effectively and safely used for skin rejuvenation. The results are usually short lived than conventional BTX A. The technique of injection is simple and easy to master.

REFERENCES

1. Liew S. Discussion: Microbotox of the lower face and neck: Evolution of a personal technique and its clinical effects. Plast Reconstr Surg. 2015;136(5 Suppl):101S-3S.
2. Petchngaovilai C. Midface lifting with botulinum toxin: intradermal technique. J Cosmet Dermatol. 2009;8(4): 312-16.
3. Rose AE, Goldberg DJ. Safety and efficacy of intradermal injection of botulinum toxin for the treatment of oily skin. Dermatol Surg. 2013;39:443-48.
4. Wu WTL. Microbotox of the lower face and neck: evolution of a personal technique and its clinical effects. Plast Reconstr Surg. 2015;136:92S-100S.
5. Carruthers A, Carruthers J, Cohens J. Dilution volume of botulinum toxin type A for the treatment of glabellar rhytides: does it matter? Dermatol Surg. 2007;33:S97-104.
6. Benedetto AV. Asymmetrical smiles corrected by botulinum toxin serotype A. Dermatol Surg. 2007;33(1 Spec No.):S32-6.

19
CHAPTER

Nonesthetic Dermatological Uses of Botulinum Toxin

Jaishree Sharad, Aditi Bhagat-Patil

INTRODUCTION

Botulinum toxin was first Food and Drug Administration (FDA) approved in 1989 for nondermatological indications, which were strabismus and blepharospasm. It has been used in a wide range of specialities since then. The first FDA approval for botulinum toxin in dermatology and dermatological surgery was in 2002 for cosmetic treatment of moderate to severe glabellar lines, and in 2004 it was approved to treat severe primary axillary hyperhidrosis. Botulinum toxin has also been used for various off-label indications in dermatology based on its mechanism of action.

INDICATIONS

- Sweating-related disorders:
  - Palmoplantar hyperhidrosis
  - Frontal hyperhidrosis
  - Gustatory hyperhidrosis
  - Hidradenitis suppurativa
  - Pachyonychia congenita and epidermolysis bullosa simplex (worsened with sweat)
  - Hailey-Hailey disease
  - Dyshidrotic hand eczema (pompholyx)
  - Granulosis rubra nasi
  - Pitted keratolysis
  - Chromhidrosis
  - Inverse psoriasis
  - Eccrine hidrocystoma
  - Eccrine angiomatous hamartoma
  - Aquagenic syringeal acrokeratoderma
- Pain and itch-related disorders:
  - Postherpetic neuralgia
  - Dystonia
  - Migraine
  - Painful scars
  - Leiomyoma-related pain
  - Lichen simplex chronicus
  - Raynaud syndrome
  - Notalgia paresthetica
  - Thelalgia
  - Brachioradial pruritus
  - Vulvodynia
  - Chronic anal fissure
- Others:
  - Hypertrophic scars and keloids
  - Facial scars
  - Breast lift
  - Ophthalmology
  - Urology.

Hyperhidrosis

Refer to chapter 16, section 2, "Botulinum Toxin for Hyperhidrosis."

Hailey–Hailey Disease

Hailey-Hailey disease is an extremely rare intraepidermal, blistering disorder with an autosomal dominant inheritance. It has a prevalence of around 1 in 50,000. It was described by the Hailey brothers in 1939 and is characterized by recurrent vesicles and erosions, affecting the neck, axillae, and groins (Fig. 1).

Many case reports showed the beneficial effect of botulinum toxin as one of the treatment options for Hailey-Hailey disease.[1-7] The dosage and injection technique is similar to that for the treatment of flexural hyperhidrosis. According to Giancarlo Bessa et al., 50 units of botulinum toxin A (BTXA), given per side of the axilla and groin, gave good results in two cases of Hailey-Hailey disease, who have been treated earlier with oral antibiotics and oral and topical corticosteroids (Figs 2 and 3).[6]

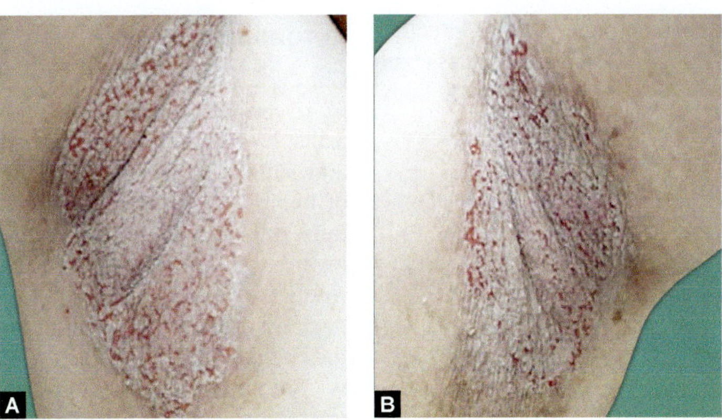

FIG. 1: Oozing, erythema, and crusting in bilateral axillae in a known case of Hailey–Hailey disease.

Source: Bessa GR, Grazziotin TC, Manzoni AP, et al. Hailey-Hailey disease treatment with Botulinum toxin type A. An Bras Dermatol. 2010;85(5):717-22.

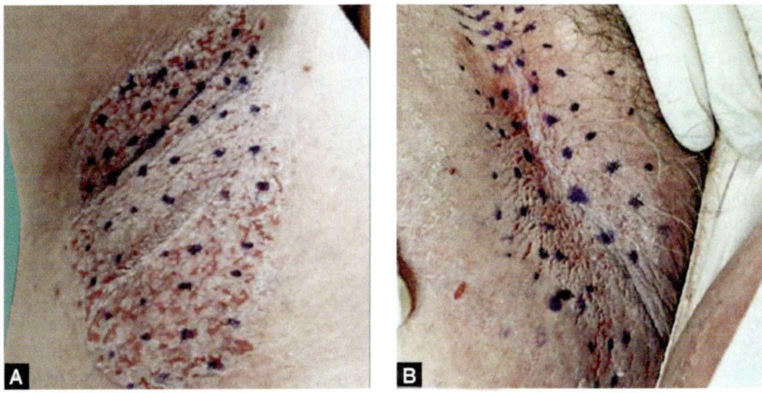

FIG. 2: Markings for botulinum toxin injection spaced 1 cm apart on axilla and groin region.

Source: Bessa GR, Grazziotin TC, Manzoni AP, et al. Hailey-Hailey disease treatment with Botulinum toxin type A. An Bras Dermatol. 2010;85(5):717-22.

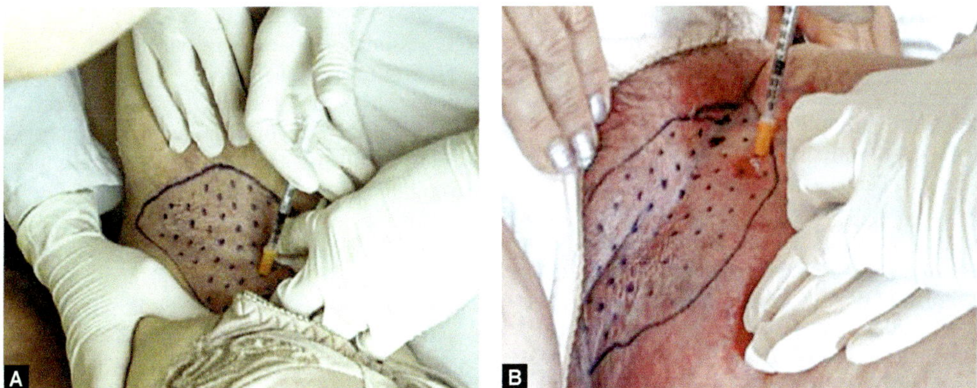

FIG. 3: Botulinum toxin injection being given in each of the markings at a dose of 2.5 U per marking up to a total of 125 units per site.

Source: Bessa GR, Grazziotin TC, Manzoni AP, et al. Hailey-Hailey disease treatment with Botulinum toxin type A. An Bras Dermatol. 2010;85(5):717-22.

Thus, botulinum toxin appears to be an effective nonsurgical alternative for the treatment of resistant cases of Hailey-Hailey disease, involving large body surface areas.

Dyshidrotic Hand Eczema (Pompholyx)

Pompholyx is a common and recurring vesiculobullous eczema which occurs on the palms and soles. It is also known as dyshidrotic hand dermatitis and palmoplantar eczema. Botulinum toxin A has been used to treat hyperhidrosis with success. Besides its effect on reducing the sweating associated with pompholyx, botulinum toxin is also useful for decreasing the itching by blocking the action of substance P and glutamate. In a study of 10 patients with pompholyx, onabotulinum toxin A (average of 162 U) was injected intradermally in one hand and the untreated hand served as a control. At follow up 5–6 weeks after injection showed that seven of 10 patients experienced good or very good effect.[8]

It was shown in a study that BTXA was effective as an adjuvant treatment not as single agent.[9] Thus, botulinum toxin can be used in the treatment of pompholyx, especially in those cases with a summer exacerbation of the disease.

Eccrine Hidrocystoma

It is a benign cystic lesion produced by mature, deformed eccrine sweat units. They could be either solitary (also known as the Smith type) or multiple (or Robinson type). The condition is exacerbated in summers and with sweating.

Many studies have found an excellent outcome of BTXA in the treatment of multiple facial eccrine hidrocystomas.

About 2 units of BTXA are injected intradermally in the perilesional skin. In one case report, two female patients with multiple facial eccrine hidrocystomas, were injected with BTXA (onabotulinum toxin A) and got excellent results within 1 week of injection. The effect was maintained for 6 months in both the patients.[10] A total of 10 units of Botox were injected intradermally on the cheeks perilesionally. In another case report of a 56-years-old female with recurrent eccrine hidrocystomas treated with multiple medical and surgical lines of treatment was treated with BTXA injected perilesionally in the superficial dermis as 1 unit per 40 mm of the region up to a total of 60 units.[11]

Adverse effects can be due to deeper diffusion of the toxin affecting the muscles and causing facial asymmetry, especially if injected in areas not in the midline.

Chromhidrosis

Chromhidrosis is the presence of colored secretion from the apocrine glands present on the face, axilla, or areolar region. It usually starts at puberty and subsides with age. It occurs due to secretion of lipofuscins in the apocrine sweat. It should be differentiated from pseudochromhidrosis, which involves discoloration of normal sweat after it reaches the skin surface due to external factors like bacteria present on skin surface or colored dyes in the clothes.

Botulinum toxin is found to be very useful to treat this condition.[12,13] Botulinum toxin A is thought to suppress apocrine secretion through different mechanisms. Although apocrine glands are said to be unresponsive to cholinergic stimulation, some researchers have proved otherwise and found them to respond to cholinergic compounds injected locally.[14] Some researchers have also demonstrated cholinergic nerve fibers around the secretory coils of apocrine sweat glands, although at a lower density as compared to the adjacent eccrine glands.[15,16] Therefore, it is possible that BTXA suppresses apocrine secretion by its anticholinergic action. In addition, it also suppresses the apocrine glands by inhibiting the substance P release.[17]

Many case reports showed the effectiveness of BTXA in treating chromhidrosis. Perez et al. used a dose of 1 unit of Botox per injection site intradermally for a case of facial chromhidrosis.[18] A maximum of 10 units were used per side of the face. The effect of BTXA in all reports was noted within 7 days and the effect was maintained for up to 4 months.

Bromhidrosis

It is a condition characterized by foul smelling sweat which is to a large extent of apocrine origin. The other causes of bromhidrosis include sebaceous gland secretion, decomposition of products of keratinization, and the eccrine sweat secreted after consumption of substances such as garlic.

The underlying principal behind the use of botulinum toxin for bromhidrosis is that the reduction of sweating in the axillary region results in lesser amount of the foul smelling by products of sweat. Also some amount of apocrine secretion is also reduced. Same dosage of botulinum toxin is used as for hyperhidrosis.

Postherpetic Neuralgia

This is an extremely painful condition defined variably as any pain persisting after complete healing of the zoster lesions or 30–120 days after the onset of lesions. It is rare in younger individuals and incidence increases with age. Only 16% of those younger than 60 years are affected while 47% of those above 60 years of age develop herpes zoster. The pain in postherpetic neuralgia (PHN) may be a continuous throbbing or aching type of pain or an intermittent stabbing, shooting pain. There may also be allodynia with innocuous stimuli like touching of clothes cause severe pain leading to depression and even suicidal tendencies in the affected individuals.

The pathophysiology of PHN involves the peripheral nervous system, autonomic nerves, and the central nervous system (CNS). Whenever there is damage at one of the components of the peripheral nervous system such as afferent neuron, dorsal root ganglion or the spinal cord, there is ectopic impulse generation at the site of damage. Also, it is found that nociceptors in painful skin of PHN patients have enhanced adrenergic sensitivity. Lastly, in cases of damage of the dorsal root ganglion causing peripheral sensory deficits, the pain is caused by processes in the CNS known as the deafferentation pain.[19]

Based on the earlier pathophysiology of PHN and herpetic pain, there are various therapeutic modalities used in the treatment of PHN like early institution of antivirals for an episode of herpes zoster to decrease the duration of PHN, antidepressants, gabapentin, anticonvulsants like carbamazepine, valproate, etc., opioid analgesics, topical analgesics like 5% lidocaine patches, and surgical modalities like tractotomy. The drawbacks of using strong pharmacological agents for the treatment of PHN are the systemic side effects of these agents in the elderly with multiple comorbidities.

Thus, BTXA has been used in this condition. It can be administered as follows: It is diluted by adding 4 mL of normal saline to 100 units of BTXA containing vial, resulting in a concentration of 25 U/mL. The volume that can be injected at each site is 0.2 mL (i.e., 5 units of botulinum toxin) up to a maximum total of 200 units for the entire area.[20]

The mechanism of action of botulinum toxin in herpetic neuralgia is mainly due to its effect on acetylcholine release. In addition, the local peripheral BTXA injection reduces the various substances that sensitize nociceptors. This is associated with the inhibition of formalin-induced glutamate release. It also reduces the peripheral nociceptive input by inhibiting the release of substance P and calcitonin gene-related peptide, which play a significant role in neurogenic inflammation. The beneficial effect of Botulinum toxin A in treating neuropathic pain is also attributed to a blocking action on the parasympathetic nervous system. The retrograde uptake of BTXA into the CNS influences the substance P and enkephalin levels in the spinal cord and nucleus raphe. In addition, there is a blockade of the autonomic pathways due to the inhibition potential on the sensory system, since BTXA has been shown to have a direct effect on afferent fibers.[21]

Hypertrophic Scar and Keloid

Reduction of the muscular tensile force during scar formation as well as restoration of the balance between fibroblast proliferation and cellular apoptosis may represent a novel therapeutic option for the aesthetic improvement of postsurgical scars.[22] Botulinum toxin A paralyzes local muscles and reduces skin tension caused by muscle pull, thereby decreasing scar tension and subsequent inflammation in wound edges. Xiao et al. reported that BTXA may exert its beneficial effects on excessive scar appearance by inhibiting the proliferation of fibroblasts and by decreasing the levels of transforming growth factor beta-1 (TGF-β1). Xiao et al. studied 19 patients with hypertrophic scars who received intralesional injections of BTXA (2.5 units/cm^3 of lesion at 1-month intervals) for 3 months. At 6-months follow up, all of the patients showed acceptable improvement of the scars and the therapeutic satisfaction was very high. The erythema, pruritus, and pliability score after the BTXA injections were significantly lower than before the injections.[23] In study done by Gauglitz et al., BTXA (125 Speywood units diluted in 0.5 mL saline) a total dose varying from 70 Speywood units to 140 per session was injected directly into the keloid tissue every 2 months using a 24-gauge needle for a maximum of 6 months did not change the macroscopic appearance, morphology, or size of keloid scars in four patients. Hence, more in-depth studies on the *in vitro* and *in vivo* effects are required for this use of botulinum toxin.[24]

Dystonia

Management of most focal dystonia with botulinum toxin injections has replaced surgical alternatives. The most common type of dystonia is cervical dystonia. A substantial improvement in neck movement and decrease in pain can be obtained with BoNT.[25] Botulinum toxin is also very useful in oromandibular dystonia, pharyngolaryngeal dystonias, occupational cramps, limb, and axial dystonias.

Headache/Migraine[26]

Botulinum toxin has also been studied as a potential treatment option for headache and migraine. It is given as multiple injections around the head and neck at 3 monthly intervals and over a span of 15 months.

Ophthalmological Uses

Botulinum toxin has been used in ophthalmology for the treatment of blepharospasm strabismus, dysthyroid ophthalmopathy, medical tarsorrhaphy, and nystagmus. In a study by Costa et al., 90% of patients benefited with the use of botulinum toxin in blepharospasm.[27]

Urology Uses[28]

Botulinum toxin injections have been used in the treatment of idiopathic overactive bladder where it acts by weakening the activity of the neurogenic detrusor muscle and by reducing afferent stimulation signals. It is also considered to be useful for benign prostatic hyperplasia.

CONCLUSION

A lot of research has been going on for other indications of botulinum toxin. It is emerging as a revolutionary treatment for many indications. Topical botulinum toxin is also undergoing clinical trials and its efficacy remains to be seen.

REFERENCES

1. Kang NG, Yoon TJ, Kim TH. Botulinum toxin type A as an effective adjuvant therapy for Hailey-Hailey disease. Dermatol Surg. 2002;28(6):543.
2. Wollina U, Konrad H, Petersen S. Botulinum toxin in dermatology–beyond wrinkles and sweat. J Cosmet Dermatol. 2005;4(4):223-7.
3. Lapiere JC, Hirsch A, Gordon KB, et al. Botulinum toxin type A for the treatment of axillary Hailey-Hailey disease. Dermatol Surg. 2000;26(4):371-4.
4. Koeyers WJ, Van der Geer S, Krekels G. Botulinum toxin type A as an adjuvant treatment modality for extensive Hailey-Hailey disease. J Dermatolog Treat. 2008;19(4):251-4.
5. Konrad H, Karamfilov T, Wollina U. Intracutaneous botulinum toxin A versus ablative therapy of Hailey-Hailey disease–a case report. J Cosmet Laser Ther. 2001;3(4):181-4.
6. Bessa GR, Grazziotin TC, Manzoni AP, et al. Hailey-Hailey disease treatment with Botulinum toxin type A. An Bras Dermatol. 2010;85(5):717-22.
7. Messikh R, Atallah L, Aubin F, et al. Botulinum toxin in disabling dermatological diseases. Ann Dermatol Venereol. 2009;136 Suppl 4:S129-36.
8. Swartling C, Naver H, Lindberg M, et al. Treatment of dyshidrotic hand dermatitis with intradermal botulinum toxin. J Am Acad Dermatol. 2002;47(5):667-71.
9. Wollina U, Karamfilov T. Adjuvant botulinum toxin A in dyshidrotic hand eczema: a controlled prospective pilot study with left-right comparison. J Eur Acad Dermatol Venereol. 2002;16(1):40-2.
10. Blugerman G, Schavelzon D, D'Angelo S. Multiple eccrine hidrocystomas: a new therapeutic option with botulinum toxin. Dermatol Surg. 2003;29(5):557-9.
11. Kontochristopoulos G, Markantoni V, Stefanaki C, et al. Multiple eccrine hidrocystomas treated with botulinum toxin A. Clin Exp Dermatol. 2011;36(1):95-6.
12. Matarasso SL. Treatment of facial chromhidrosis with botulinum toxin type A. J Am Acad Dermatol. 2005;52(1):89-91.
13. Wu JM, Mamelak AJ, Nussbaum R, et al. Botulinum toxin a in the treatment of chromhidrosis. Dermatol Surg. 2005;31(8 Pt 1):963-5.
14. Aoki T. Stimulation of human axillary apocrine sweat glands by cholinergic agents. J Invest Dermatol. 1962;38:41-4.
15. Uno H. Sympathetic innervations of the sweat glands and piloarrector muscles of macaques and human beings. J Invest Dermatol. 1977;69(1):112-20.
16. Aoki T, Narita T. Morphological evidence for the innervation of apocrine sweat glands in the general hairy skin of the goat. Cell Tissue Res. 1981;221(1):221-6.
17. Aoki KR. Evidence for antinociceptive activity of botulinum toxin type A in pain management. Headache. 2003;43 Suppl 1:S9-15.
18. Pérez Tato B, Zamora Martínez E, Sánchez Albisua B, et al. Facial and axillary apocrine chromhidrosis. Dermatol Online J. 2012;18(3):13.
19. Bonezzi C, Demartini L. Treatment options in postherpetic neuralgia. Acta Neurol Scand Suppl. 1999;173:25-35.
20. Sotiriou E, Apalla Z, Panagiotidou D, et al. Severe post-herpetic neuralgia successfully treated with botulinum toxin A: three case reports. Acta Derm Venereol. 2009;89(2):214-5.
21. Klein AW. The therapeutic potential of botulinum toxin. Dermatol Surg. 2004;30(3):452-5.
22. Lee BJ, Jeong JH, Wang SG, et al. Effect of botulinum toxin type a on a rat surgical wound model. Clin Exp Otorhinolaryngol. 2009;2(1):20-7.
23. Xiao Z, Zhang F, Cui Z. Treatment of hypertrophic scars with intralesional botulinum toxin type A injections: a preliminary report. Aesthetic Plast Surg. 2009;33(3):409-12.
24. Gauglitz GG, Bureik D, Dombrowski Y, et al. Botulinum toxin A for the treatment of keloids. Skin Pharmacol Physiol. 2012;25(6):313-8.
25. Jankovic J, Schwartz K. Botulinum toxin injections for cervical dystonia. Neurology. 1990;40(2):277-80.
26. Aurora SK, Dodick DW, Turkel CC, et al. Onabotulinum-toxinA for treatment of chronic migraine: results from the double-blind, randomized, placebo-controlled phase of the PREEMPT 1 trial. Cephalalgia. 2010;30(7):793-803.
27. Costa J, Espirito-Santo C, Borges A, et al. Botulinum toxin type A therapy for blepharospasm. Cochrane Database Syst Rev. 2005;(1):CD004900.
28. Chung E. Botulinum toxin in urology: a review of clinical potential in the treatment of urologic and sexual conditions. Expert Opin Biol Ther. 2015;15(1):95-102.

3

SECTION

SOFT TISSUE AUGMENTATION

20 CHAPTER

Evaluation of the Aging Face

Stephen H Mandy

INTRODUCTION

Assessment of the aging face must begin with an appreciation of the aesthetics of beauty and an intimate knowledge of facial anatomy. One must know the skin, muscles, skeletal support, facial fat distribution, nerves, vessels, and their three-dimensional relationship to each other (Fig. 1). Further, understanding of the pathophysiology of the aging process as it affects the face and those components of its structure are essential for proper evaluation. Only after such an in-depth evaluation can one begin an appropriate restoration.

BEAUTY

Appearance evokes a primal emotional response within 100 milliseconds. This is part of our genetic survival instinct, and we are born with an image of "humanness" to which we respond within the first few months of life. Infants respond positively to a beautiful face even if racially diverse from their parents, by 2 months of age. Beauty evokes universal as well as a personal pleasure, a form of subconscious communication that sends a message of health and fertility. Beauty is best perceived when it is subtle and is rejected when it is excessive (too much makeup or extreme plastic surgery). Symmetry is a universal and essential element in beauty. It implies good genetics, and asymmetry evokes discomfort. Averageness is also a feature of beauty, as nature favors averages—it is safer to blend than to stand out. Average is familiar and comfortable. Beauty is timeless through the ages and transcends ethnicity. It is essential as part of our reproductive agenda.

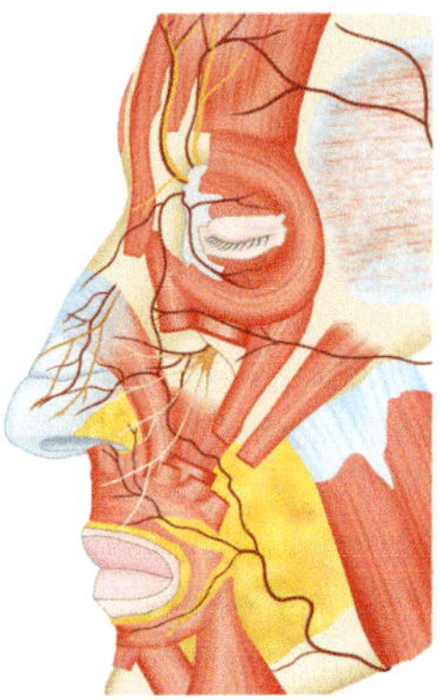

FIG. 1: Critical facial anatomy for the injector.

Studies of female beauty find women most attractive around age 24. A youthful beautiful female face has smooth skin, large eyes, full lips, high cheek bones, and a small chin and is in the shape of an inverted triangle—widest at the cheeks and pointing to the chin. It is symmetrical, shadowless, and the skin is wrinkle and blemish-free, and translucent. Male attractiveness mostly reflects the appearance of the stereotypical "alpha" male—a strong brow, chiseled appearance, and strong jaw with a broad projecting chin. Here too, symmetry is essential and if male features are too strong or exaggerated, they may be perceived as frightening. Sexual dimorphisms are features which differ greatly between the sexes. Generally, the more these are expressed, the more attractive the person of the opposite sex appears unless, however, they are extreme, in which case they may be foreboding.[1]

The literature has many mathematical formulas containing the ideal proportions of beauty. The simplest divides the face horizontally into equal thirds, the upper one-third from the brow to the hairline, the middle one-third from the brow to the tip of the nose, and the lower one-third from the

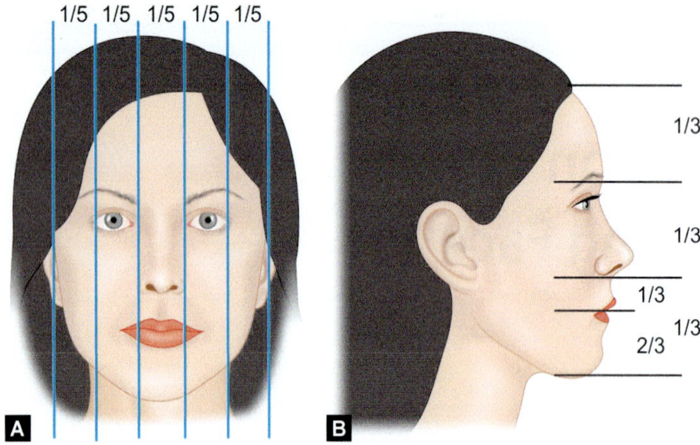

FIG. 2: Vertical and horizontal facial proportions.

nose to the bottom of the chin. The lower one-third is further divided into the upper one-third from the nasal tip through the oral aperture, and the lower two-thirds from the mouth to the chin. Vertically, the face is divided into five equal parts; the middle, a line through the medial brow and inner canthus, the next is through the lateral canthus, and lastly, through the lateral cheek at the zygoma (Fig. 2). Many authors refer to the Phi formula or the Fibonacci ratio as the mathematical formulae for beauty. That magical ratio is 1 to 1.61821 and it is repeated throughout nature, art, and architecture in many beautiful things. It has been applied to masks which may be superimposed on the face and is mostly valuable for those practicing reconstructive facial surgery. For those who seek this information, which has limited application and regenerative aesthetics, may find a great wealth of information online (www.beautyanalysis.com) (Fig 3).[1,2]

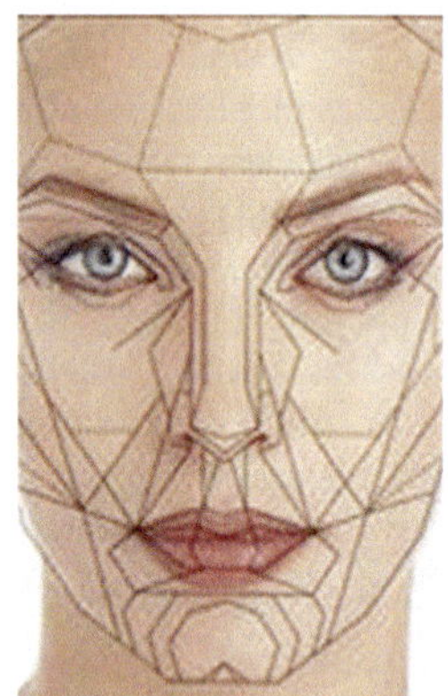

FIG. 3: The beauty mask (based on Phi).

ANATOMY AND PHYSIOLOGY OF FACIAL AGING

In an adult, the classical triangle of beauty is an inverted triangle with its base through the midface at its widest breadth, and its apex at the chin. As we age, this triangle gradually reverses, and the base is at the lower face with the apex towards the brow. The reason for this shift is volume loss, with skeletal loss the single greatest contributor. The skull enlarges as we grow reaching its full development in late adolescence. From that point, it begins to slowly reabsorb. This process begins in females after age 20 and peaks between ages 40 and 60. In men, it occurs somewhat later. There is reabsorption of the mandible, decreasing its height and length causing posterior recession of the chin, and leading to the development of the prejowl sulcus (marionette line), so called "jowls", and redundant skin in the neck. The maxilla reabsorbs along the zygoma both inferiorly and posteriorly, which enlarges the orbit in the lower and lateral area. The enlargement of the orbit unmasks the orbital fat pads and contributes to the descent of the brow. Further, the reabsorption and narrowing of the maxillary bone in the central area supporting the teeth deepens the canine fossa. This contributes to the formation of the nasolabial fold and tear trough. Reabsorption of the frontal bones lead to brow ptosis, a hollowing of the temporal fossa, and periorbital, glabellar, and horizontal forehead wrinkles. It has been said that as we age, our noses and ears enlarge which is, in fact, not true; they are simply adorning a smaller face.[3]

Skin and Fat

Genomic studies have recently revealed that both photodamaged and unexposed aging skin share an upregulation of genes regulating collagen and elastic tissue destruction (collagenase and elastase), and there is also an upregulation of inflammatory mediators. There is downregulation of collagen and elastin production as well as of lipid synthesis and epidermal cell differentiation.[4] These changes lead to cutaneous laxity and an inability of the skin to conform to the skeletal and fat loss. Additionally, it leads to the loss of the skin's barrier function causing cutaneous roughness and loss of tone. Pigmentation, especially in many Asian and Mediterranean populations, tends to increase substantially with aging, and this poses a vexing cosmetic problem.

Fat atrophy is another major contributor to facial volume loss. Facial fat compartments, elegantly described by Rohrich and Pessa, surround the face and are individually compartmentalized by retaining ligaments and facial planes.[5] Each of these is integrated into the large contiguous subdermal fat. The anatomy of these compartments is essential knowledge for the aesthetic specialist, as restoring volume by injecting these fat pads give anatomically correct restoration to the facial contours and provide superior and lateral lifting to the midface. The fat pads of greatest importance are the deep medial, suborbicularis oculi and oris, lateral, subtemporal, buccal, submental, and submaxillary. The fat and bone loss leads to elongation of the upper lip, thinning of the upper lips, and loss of projection of the chin (Figs 4 and 5).

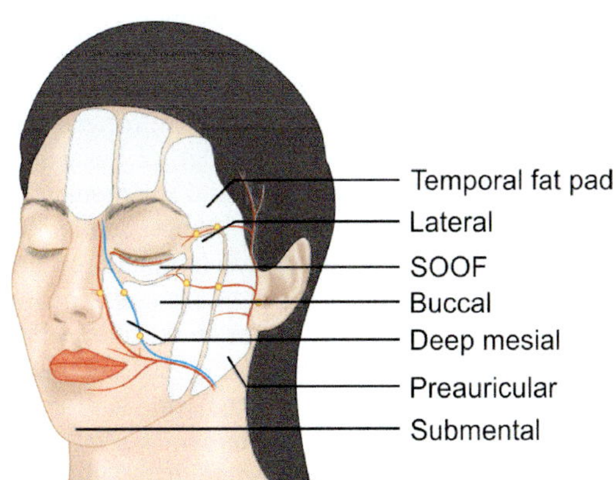

SOOF, suborbicularis fat pad.

FIG. 4: Important fat pads for injection.

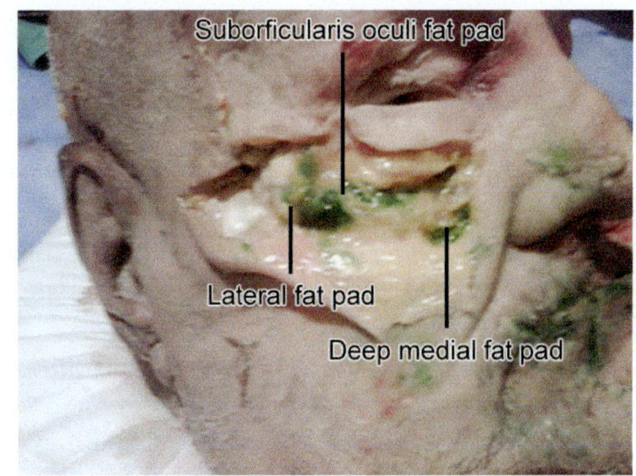

FIG. 5: Cadaver injected with dye to inflate fat pads, then dissected to demonstrate location.

EVALUATING THE PATIENT

Prior to seeing a new patient, your evaluation begins with the image in your mind of the symmetrical, properly-proportioned face of beauty that will stand as a backdrop behind each patient as a standard of comparison. Within seconds of your seeing the patient, you will arrive at many conclusions on symmetry, on proportion, and on each of the many facets of the aging face. As they explain their concerns, it is critical to watch the face animate to make sure there are no neurologic deficits. It is, of course, good medical practice to make certain that the patient's purpose for the consultation is expressed, as often it may not be for facial rejuvenation but simply a matter of removal of a mole or some other specific concern. Often, patients will have vague complaints such as looking tired and it is best when they are uncertain to ask them to specifically describe what they see that makes them feel that way. Assessing the degree of photodamage, bone, and fat loss, presence of dominating or distracting features are all part of the evaluation. Once you have considered the patient's concerns and the areas you feel intervention will improve, it is important to explain to the patient the nature of their defects, what you anticipate from correction, and the methods you suggest.

As we age, there are changes in the bone, soft tissue, ligaments, septii and skin (Described in section 3, chapter 2)

Assessment of the Upper Face

The ideal forehead in a female should have a gentle convex curve and a smooth contour in the glabellar region. The temple should be convex or flat and there should be no hollowing or concavity. The ideal female eyebrow should be over the supraorbital margin. The lateral part of the brow ie the tail should be slightly higher than the medial part of the brow ie the head.

The brow must peak in a vertical line along the lateral limbus of the iris in the centre. There there should be no hooding in the upper eyelid. The upper eyelid should have fullness that follows the natural arc of the upper lid margin.

The male brow is more horizontal and thick. It obscures the sharp bony edges of the orbit.

Aging results in loss of subcutaneous fullness to the forehead, brow, temple, and upper eyelid areas causing a less curved or more flat forehead & hollow temples.

Brow ptosis may be seen due to loss of fullness in the upper eyelid & loss of temporal support to the lateral brow.

Assessment of the Midface

In a youthful midface, the infra-orbital region is smooth, without any shadows or bulges.

The ideal female cheek mound is ovoid and does not extend higher than the limbus of the lower eyelid. The malar prominence is located high on the midface, below and lateral to the lateral canthus, and eccentrically located within the cheek oval and has a defined apex. Lips are full and well defined.

In the aging midface, the infra-orbital region appears hollow with the prominence of tear trough. Sometimes, there is orbital prolapse seen as puffy eyes. Loss of deep fat pads and downward displacement of superficial fat pads results in a flat cheeks, prominence of infra-orbital hollows and prominence of nasolabial folds.The nose appears to curve downwards due to changes in the cartilage and bone. Lips become thinner and perioral rhytids appear.

Assesment of the Lower Face

A sweeping jawline, well defined chin and a firm neck characterize attractive features of the lower third part of a young face. In the aging face, with loss of malar and buccal fat and loss of fat in the peri-oral region as well as resorption of the alveolar bone, there is loss of definition of the jawline. Jowls form due to loss of masseteric ligament support which lead to descent of facial fat to the mandibular border. Loss of bone and fat also results in a wide, small chin which often appears retruded. Skin laxity, loss of chin fat pad and downward pull of platysma muscle leads to the "turkey neck" deformity.

STRATEGIES FOR REJUVENATION

There are an increasing number of preventive and remedial solutions to the aging face. New technology and understanding will, no doubt, lead to better solutions going forward. Currently, maintaining the integrity of the skin at an early age is essential. Sun protection is at the forefront of preventing rhytides an dyspigmentation as well as malignant changes. Early adoption of topical retinoids and maintaining an adequate moisture barrier are beneficial to forestalling deterioration of the skin. Verification of the value of antioxidants, growth factors, and stem cell extracts are yet to be conclusive. Knowledge of cosmetically oriented dentists, hair stylists, and makeup artists can be of great assistance, and enhance even your best efforts.

At this time, revolumizing of the critical areas of skeletal and fat loss are the most effective corrective measures to solve the effects of facial aging. Revolumizing and lifting through the use of subdermal fillers is the current paradigm. There are an ever-increasing number of excellence of dermal fillers which, when injected into the correct anatomic compartments, have remarkable effect on appearance. It is important that their placement and the amounts, used approach anatomic normalcy. Small changes have a remarkably big impact, and overcorrection is immediately obvious to even the casual observer. Regional volumetric replacement to areas such as the maxilla obscures the enlarged orbit and tear trough, and simultaneously lifts the cheek, softening the nasolabial fold. Injecting the submental fat pad restores projection to the chin, elongates the face, and effaces the marionette line. This paradigm has replaced line filling in modern facial restoration (Figs 6 and 7).

Botulinum-derived neuromodulators are quick, efficient, and effective at reducing dynamic wrinkling particularly of the forehead and periorbital area. These are most frequently used in concert with dermal fillers. Intimate knowledge of facial musculature, dosing of the agent, and maintenance of some facial movement yields the best results. Skin tightening devices, whether radiofrequency or ultrasonic-based, are valuable adjuncts to structural filling as they help to compensate for loss of facial tone due to collagen and elastic tissue depletion. They also are usually associated with little risk or hyperpigmentation, or morbidity. Various light devices assist in facial rejuvenation by addressing pigmentation, vascular lesions, and rhytides. As new technology evolves, there may be further pharmacologic or implant capability to restore the aging face.

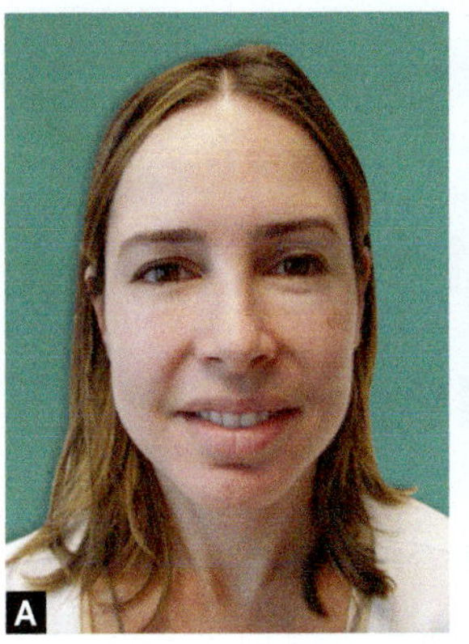

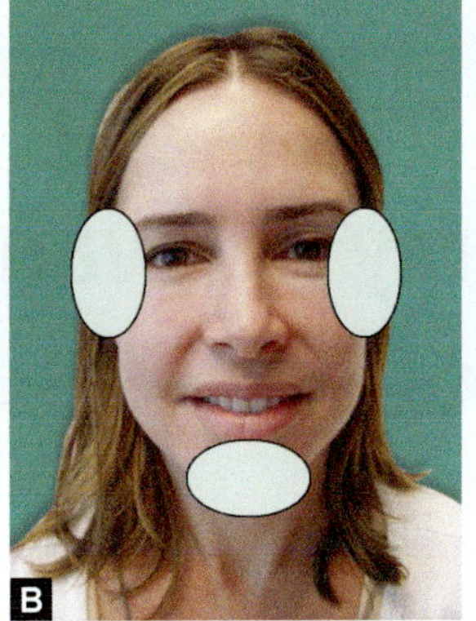

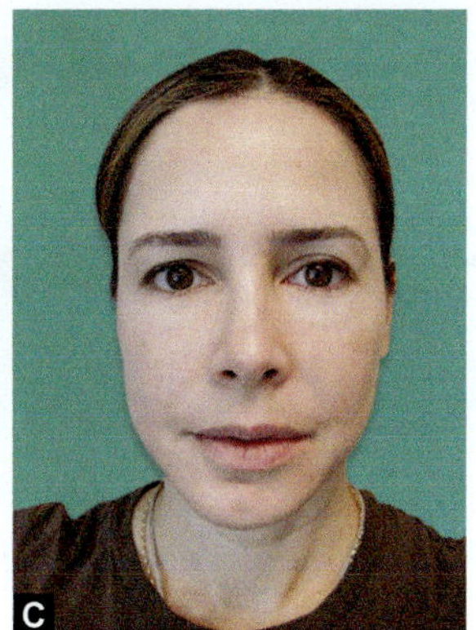

FIG. 6: Before and after injection of lateral fat pads and submental fat pad to reshape the face, restoring the triangle of beauty.

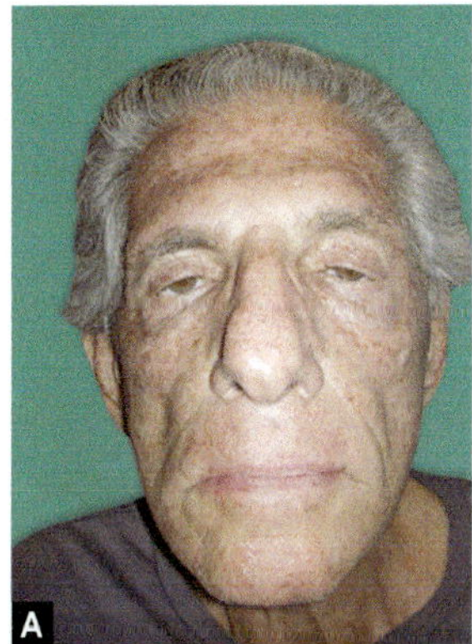

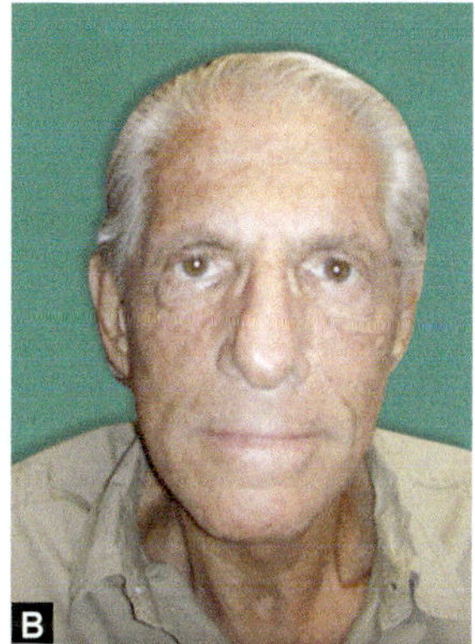

FIG. 7: Before and after of facial restoration using poly-L-lactic acid injected into the temporal, buccal, lateral, medial, and suborbicular fat pads to lift and restore volume.

CONCLUSION

Beauty matters. It promotes pleasure. It rivets the attention. It compels us to action, and it ensures the survival of our genes.[6] As an aesthetic physician, it is essential to carry with them the image as they evaluate and endeavor to restore a face to approximate that ideal. People consult us because the face is their image to the world. It is their brand, and no matter what age they are, their appearance matters to them. We are genetically programmed to reproduce, and even after our capability to do so has declined, the genes that direct our behavior persist. If patients look good, they feel good. Small changes in facial appearance have a big impact on the first impressions people make. As an aesthetic physician, you must first finely tune your esthetic sensitivities, know your anatomy, and be an expert at the tools of your trade.

REFERENCES

1. Dayan S. Subliminally Exposed: Shocking Truths about your Hidden Desires in Mating, Dating and Communicating, 1st edition. New York: Morgan James Publishing; 2013.
2. Marquardt S. (2017). Introduction. [online] Available from www.beautyanalysis.com. [Accessed September, 2017].
3. Shaw RB, Katzel EB, Koltz PF, et al. Aging of the facial skeleton: aesthetic implications and rejuvenation strategies. Plast Reconstr Surg. 2011;127(1):374-83.
4. McGrath JA, Robinson MK, Binder RL. Skin differences based on age and chronicity of ultraviolet exposure: results from a gene expression profiling study. Br J Dermatol. 2012;166 Suppl 2:9-15.
5. Rohrich RJ, Pessa JE, Ristow B. The youthful cheek and the deep medial fat compartment. Plast Reconstr Surg. 2008;121(6):2107-12.
6. Etcoff N. Survival of the Prettiest: The Science of Beauty. New York: Anchor Books; 2000.

21

CHAPTER

Facial Anatomy Relevant for the Application of Soft Tissue Fillers

Sebastian Cotofana, Mansi S Mukherjee, Harish Kasetty

INTRODUCTION

A clear understanding and complete knowledge of the facial anatomy is necessary for a safe and effective aesthetic practice. Cadaveric dissections, imaging, and staining both intraoperatively and in the research laboratory have helped in improving the existing techniques in the field of antiaging as well as inventing newer methods to contour and augment the face.[1]

In this chapter, the anatomy of the face is described with relevance to the importance of different structures while injecting fillers.

General Arrangement

The Layers of the Face

The new understanding of the facial anatomy is based on the new concept that the facial structures are arranged in layers. Each specific layer has its unique characteristics and each specific layer contains important structures like muscles, nerves, and vessels. Starting from superficial to deep, the facial layers can be best summarized as follows:[2]

1. Skin
2. Subcutaneous fat
3. Superficial musculoaponeurotic system
4. Deep fat
5. Deep fascia or periosteum.

However, this classical five-layered arrangement can be found in the middle face, i.e., between the zygomatic arch and the mandible but there are regions of the face where 10 layers are present (temporal region) or just 3 layers (medial part of the infraorbital region, i.e., the tear trough) (Fig. 1). These differences have to be respected when aiming to fight the signs of aging.

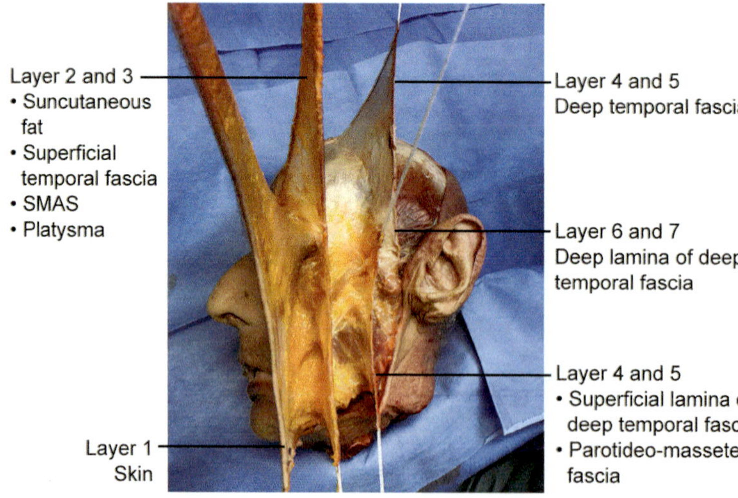

FIG. 1: The layers of the face.

FACIAL SKELETON

The human skull can be classified into the neurocranium (containing the brain) and the viscerocranium (providing support for all facial structures). Both parts influence the facial appearance and are involved in the process of facial aging. The neurocranium contributes the appearance of the frontal and the temporal region, whereas the viscerocranium influences the shape of the periorbital, middle facial, nasal, perioral region, and the neck (Fig. 2).

The contours of the facial bones play an important role in determining the facial appearance of an individual. High cheekbones due to a zygomatic convexity are considered an attractive facial feature. In comparison to women, men have more prominent brow ridges, differently shaped orbital rims, and have a larger pyriform aperture and a larger jaw.[3] As the age advances, the rate and extent of facial bony structural changes also differ in men and women.[4,5] This is being universally seen as the new hallmark in facial rejuvenation, and any rejuvenation procedure becomes limited if these changes in the skeletal foundation are not addressed.

Computed tomography studies have shown that the adult skull begins to gradually decrease in size by 50s and starts to take on similar features of the infant skull.[6,7]

In the adult facial bone, variable resorption and remodeling of different areas of the facial skeleton

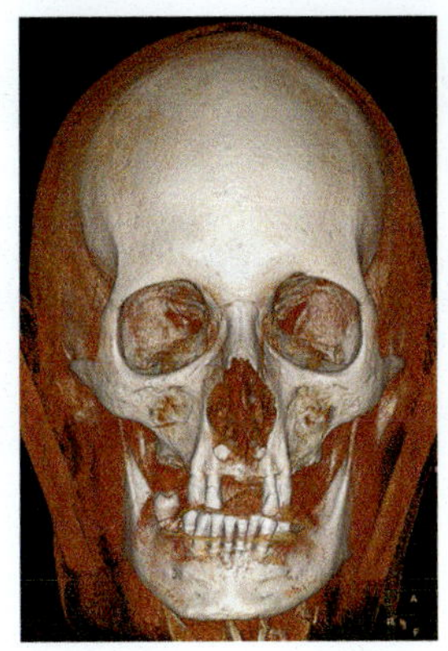

FIG. 2: Computed tomography scan of the face with superimposed soft tissues and skeletal features.

occur with age. In addition, there is an accelerated bony resorption of the mandible and maxillary bone due to loss of dentition.[8] The enlargement of the bony orbits occurs due to the changes in the rate of bone resorption and deposition.[6] There occurs a reduction in height and slight increase in width and depth of an elderly human skull.[9]

The visible signs of aging like hollowing of the temples and periorbital area, exaggeration of the nasolabial folds, and jowling are due to the skeletal aging. This gradual loss of support to the soft tissues leads to changes in the subcutaneous adipose tissue distribution.[10] An overview of bony changes with

TABLE 1: Overview of bony changes with aging and their effects

Name of bone	Changes with aging	Effects due to bony changes with age
Temple	• Significant reduction in volume of temporal fossa • Loss of temporal fascia	• Temporal fossa becomes more apparent and concave • Occurring of brow ptosis due to a descent of remaining soft tissue and loss of support to the eyebrows • Lowering and flattening of the lateral brow formation of forehead rhytides
Periorbital	• Increase in area and width of orbital aperture • Resorption and recession of superomedial and inferolateral aspects of the orbital rim; the changes in the inferolateral orbital rim manifest by middle age, whereas the recession in the superomedial quadrant may be seen only in old age • Loss of bony volume and the projection of the supraorbital rim • Glabellar angle becomes more acute with aging	• Increased prominence of the medial fat pad and lengthening of the lid cheek junction • Appearance of ptosis of the brow and lateral orbital hooding • Descent of the medial brow and glabellar skin creases formation

Contd...

Contd...

Name of bone	Changes with aging	Effects due to bony changes with age
Midface (formed by the body and arch of the zygoma in the lateral third and the maxilla in the medial and middle third)	• Retrusion of maxilla and pyriform angle with aging decrease in the maxillary angle by about 10 degrees between young (<30 years) and old (>60 years)	• Increased prominence of the medial fat pad and nasolabial folds
Perinasal	• Edges of the nasal bones recede with age, causing enlargement of the pyriform aperture • Increased bone loss in the lower part of the pyriform aperture • Recession of anterior nasal spine	• Posterior positioning of the naso-labial fold and adjacent upper lip • Deepening of nasolabial fold • Reduced skeletal support due to aging leads to retraction of the columella and downward nasal tip rotation with apparent lengthening of the nose
Mandible	• Increase in mandibular angle, decrease in ramus height and mandibular body height and length due to bony resorption • Resorption of the bone just below the mental foramen	• Increased labiomental fold and the appearance of a "witch's chin" • Appearance of jowls

aging and their effects have been summarized in the table 1.[11]

FAT COMPARTMENTS

Facial fat can be divided into superficial and deep layers by the superficial musculoaponeurotic system or mimetic muscles. Both fat layers are not continuous but separated by septae into distinct compartments. These septae are forming boundaries for the content of each respective compartment and provide sheltered passages for vessels, nerves, and lymphatic tissues. The enclosed compartments can be understood as fat filled "cushions" which undergo age-related loss of volume and thus a change in position. The change is position, however, is a dual process caused both by the fat redistribution, which is normal and well understood process during aging and the changes of bone, as described above.

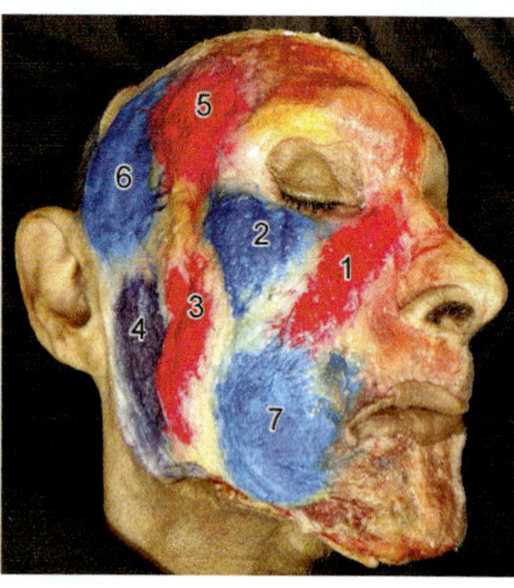

1, superficial nasolabial; 2, medial cheek (also called malar fat pad); 3, middle cheek; 4, lateral cheek; 5, superficial inferior temporal; 6, superficial superior temporal; 7, superficial buccal.

FIG. 3: The subcutaneous facial fat compartments of the face. Note: forehead compartments absent in this dissection.

Superficial Fat Compartments

The superficial facial fat compartments span the entire face and can be subdivided into the following subcutaneous fat compartments (Fig. 3):

- Superficial central forehead
- Superficial lateral forehead left and right
- Superficial superior temporal
- Superficial inferior temporal
- Superficial nasolabial
- Medial cheek (also called malar fat pad)
- Middle cheek
- Lateral cheek
- Superficial buccal.

Forehead[12]

- Central compartment: The central compartment is located in the middle, extending inferiorly to the nasal dorsum and laterally to the temporal septum

- Middle fat compartment: The middle fat pad is bounded medially by the central forehead fat compartment and inferiorly by the orbicularis retaining ligament
- Lateral temporal fat compartment: It lies adjacent to the superior temporal septum and is confluent and contiguous with the lateral subcutaneous cheek fat and subcutaneous cervical fat. The lateral temporal-cheek fat pads span the entire face from the forehead to the cervical area. Its anterior boundary is formed by the lateral cheek septum. In the forehead, its upper and lower boundaries are identifiable as the superior and inferior temporal septa.[13]

Cheek

- Nasolabial fat (NLF) compartment: The compartment, responsible for the overhang of nasolabial fold, is located laterally to the nasolabial groove, which forms the medial border. This is laterally bounded by the cheek fat pad compartments
- Medial cheek compartment: The medial cheek compartment is a triangular compartment with its apex downwards and lies lateral to the NLF compartment. It is bounded by orbital retaining ligament (orbitomalar septum) superiorly and jowl fat inferiorly
- Middle cheek compartment: The middle cheek fat compartment lies between the medial and lateral temporal-cheek fat compartments, and anterior and superficial to the parotid gland
- Lateral cheek compartment: This is confluent with the lateral temporal compartment and lies immediately over the parotid gland. The platysma-auricular ligaments delimit the lateral-temporal compartment posteriorly.

Formation of the Nasolabial and the Labiomandibular Sulcus

According to Ghassemi et al., the subcutaneous arrangement of the subcutaneous fatty layer varies between different areas of the face. In the lateral midface, a clear separation is given between the skin (layer 1), the subcutaneous fat (layer 2), and the superficial musculoaponeurotic system (SMAS; layer 3). This clear separation allows the layers to glide and to provide space for movement which occur in these areas most during talking, chewing, and various facial expressions. Here, this layered arrangement was identified to be different and was termed type 1 subcutaneous arrangement. On the contrary, in the perioral region and in the medial eyebrow, this subcutaneous arrangement is different and was termed type 2; here a strong connection is given between the skin (layer 1) and the underlying muscles of facial expression (layer 3) with having the subcutaneous fat encapsulated between and within fibrous connective tissue. This strong interaction allows the skin to be moved in accurate concordance to the movement of the deeper muscles as no gliding space is needed in these regions. The change in subcutaneous arrangement between type 1 and type 2 is represented by the nasolabial and the labiomandibular sulcus. With increasing age, the fat superior (subcutaneous NLF compartment) or lateral (superficial buccal) to these sulcus is prone to inferior/anterior displacement following gravity leading to a relative deepening and thus to an aggravation of the clinical appearance of these sulcus. The theory of a ligament contributing to the formation of these sulcus is not supported by the current data in literature.

Deep Fat Compartments of the Cheek (Fig. 4)

The deep fat compartments lie deep to the SMAS and provide volume and shape to the face. They act as gliding planes allowing free movement to the muscles of facial expression.

Suborbicularis Oculi Fat

The suborbicularis oculi fat (SOOF) protrudes from the inferior margin of the orbicularis oculi muscle. It lies on the zygomaticus major and the levator labii superioris muscle and has two components, medial and lateral.[14] The medial SOOF is adherent to the

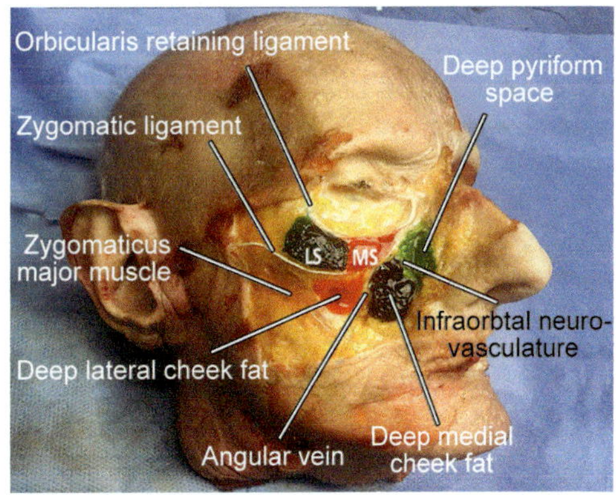

FIG. 4: The deep facial fat compartments and their boundaries. Note the forehead compartment.

periosteum along the orbital rim and lies inferior to the orbicularis retaining ligament, under the orbicularis oculi muscle.[14] It extends from the medial limbus to the outer canthus.

Medial SOOF is separated from the deep lateral cheek fat by the zygomatico cutaneous ligament.[15] Lateral SOOF extends from the lateral canthus to the inferior temporal fat pad and is bounded superiorly by the lateral orbital thickening.

The space named prezygomatic is a gliding space that lies between the SOOF and the periosteum of the zygomatic process of maxilla.[16] This space is bounded superiorly by the orbicularis retaining ligament and inferiorly by the zygomatico cutaneous ligament.

Malar Fat Pad

Deep to the SOOF, lies the malar fat pad, between the levator labii superioris and the levator anguli oris muscle.

Deep Medial Cheek Fat

The deep medial cheek (DMC) fat is located between the levator labii superiors alaeque nasi and the levator anguli oris. The infraorbital neurovascular structures form the medial boundary, whereas the angular vein forms the lateral boundary. The DMC fat lies medial to the deep pyriform space (previously called Ristow's space).[17,18]

Augmentation of deep medial fat has been described by Rohrich et al. to produce following effects. It increases anterior projection, diminishes the nasolabial fold, corrects the V-deformity, and creates a youthful cheek with natural boundaries.[19]

Buccal Fat Pad

The buccal fat pad lies on the posterolateral part of the maxilla, superficial to the buccinator muscle and deep to the anterior part of masseter. It has its own capsule and is aesthetically a very important structure. The main body of this fat pad is located medial to the mandible and has four extensions—buccal, pterygoid, pterygopalatine, and temporal. The latter one is also known as the deep temporal fat pad of the temporal region and is found between the deep lamina of the deep temporal fascia and the temporalis muscle.[20,21] It facilitates a free gliding movement for the surrounding muscles of mastication. The buccal fat is uniquely present in humans and absent in most of the ape species.

The buccal extension of this fat compartment influences the aesthetic appearance of cheeks. Mainly affected by hypotrophic aging, loss of volume of this fat pad leads to a lack of support for the medial cheek and middle cheek fat, consequently accelerating the descent of these compartments.[15]

Perioral Suborbicularis Oris Fat Pad

Deep to the orbicularis oris and mentalis muscles, lies the perioral SOOF pad. The wet-dry border of the lip is anterior boundary of the submuscular lip fat. It is bounded laterally by the zygomaticus muscle. This fat is distinct from the more superficial fat of the cutaneous lip.

Chin

The superficial chin fat is a superficial fat compartment that is delineated laterally by the labiomandibular fat, superiorly reaches up to the mentolabial sulcus and inferiorly, the superficial portion of the submentalis fat.

The submentalis fat, as the name suggests, lies under the mentalis muscle. It has a superficial and a deep portion. The superficial, inferior portion of this fat compartment is located directly under the skin and accentuates the shape of the mentum.[22] The deep portion is located above the periosteum, topographically below the mentolabial sulcus.

Importance of Fat Pads while Injecting Fillers

An even distribution of superficial and deep fat gives a well-rounded, three-dimensional topography of the face. This is delineated by a series of arcs and convexities which are the important attributes of a youthful face. With increasing age, there is loss of subcutaneous fat particularly around the orbit, forehead, glabella, and mandible, and in malar, mental, and perioral areas. Also, there is hypertrophy along the infraorbital, malar fat pads, later nasolabial fold, labiomental crease, submental, and jowls areas.[20] The dynamic wrinkles become prominent and become static lines due to the contraction of the underlying muscle.

Many studies have described changes in fat compartments with aging. It has been seen that deep fat compartments tend to atrophy with age, while the superficial compartments may be more prone to hypertrophy.[18] Donofrio[22] proposed that the periorbital, buccal, and perioral fat tend to atrophy while the submental, jowl, nasolabial, and lateral malar regions tend to hypertrophy.

Rohrich et al.[19] noted excess fat in superficial compartments such as the infraorbital fat pad, lateral temporal cheek fat, and submental fat, and a deflation of deep cheek fat in older patients. This selective deflation of the deep fat pads with age leads to loss of support and descent of the overlying superficial fat, thereby contributing to the ptotic appearance of the aging face. This differential behavior of deep versus superficial fat pads has also been shown in imaging and histologic studies.[18]

Gierloff[23] proposed that deflation of the deep fat pads, DMC, and buccal fat pad leads to a lack of support and thus contributes to the inferior volume shift or ptosis in the overlying superficial fat pads, NLF, and superficial medial cheek (SMC).

In the lateral and medial SOOF, the DMC compartment, and the chin fat compartments, most of the volume loss takes place in the deep supraperiosteal layer.

The volume loss in the superficial subcutaneous layer is seen in the lateral compartments, both in the temporal and preauricular areas, and to a lesser extent, in the middle and medial fat compartments of the superficial cheek fat pad.[12,24]

The compartments that are not greatly affected by volume loss are the superficial nasolabial compartment and the superior and inferior jowl compartments. They tend to move medially due to the lack of fibrous fixation points and the lack of lateral support due to volume depletion in the lateral fat areas.[25]

Suborbicularis oculi fat lies superficial to the facial mimetic muscles and deeper to the orbicularis muscle. The malar fat pad which is located in the subcutaneous plane, superficial to the SMAS descends with increasing age, unmasking the orbital fat pads and increasing prominence of nasolabial folds. With pseudoherniation of the orbital septum, the orbital fat pads become more visible. The descent of the buccal fat makes the marionette fold and the jowls more prominent. The medial fat pad in the upper lid is a separate structure and has a ligamentous attenuation and it protrudes as one age. The medial, middle, and lateral compartments come together in the lower lid and with age, the unified sausage shaped protrusion defines their prominence.[11]

As one age, a relative concavity occurs between the thin medial eyelid skin and thicker cheek skin due to the deflation of the deep periorbital fat, in the form of a nasojugal groove or tear-trough deformity. This leads to a harsh transition between the lid-cheek junction as the smooth contour between the medial SOOF and the superior edge of the malar fat pad is lost. Deep augmentation of the medial SOOF or DMC just superficial to the underlying periosteum has thus been shown to improve the tear-trough deformity. The DMC fat also undergoes concomitant deflation which leads to ptosis of the overlying superficial malar fat including the NLF and SMC, further elongating the tear-trough deformity. With the inferior orbital rim becoming more visible, a "V" deformity results in the form of a centromedial cheek hollow below the tear-trough. Augmentation of the DLC and medial SOOF has been shown to not only improve this "V" deformity, but to also smooth the transition between the anterior and lateral cheek and improve anterior cheek projection.

Lastly, as the DMC compartments deflate with age, the nasolabial fold is harshened. Volume augmentation of the DMC and Ristow's space is shown to soften this crease.[18]

Fillers with high elastic and viscous moduli have a volumizing effect. When injected in specific anatomical regions within specific deep fat compartments, they can have a lifting action that helps in regaining the lost volume, leading to the lifting action of the superficial fat compartments.

Supraperiosteal bolus technique allows for a precise injection into the fat pad and it is the most effective and least traumatic and guarantees an anatomically correct volumetric correction.[15]

Changes in the deep fat pads of the cheek and the resulting topographical changes have been highlighted in the table 2.

Superficial Musculoaponeurotic System (Fig. 5)

Mitz et al., described a fibrofatty superficial facial system called SMAS.[26] It is a sheet of connective tissue which is formed by a network of collagen fibers, elastic fibers, and fat cells, and connects the mimetic muscles to the overlying dermis and plays an important functional role in facial expression. In most of the current facelift techniques, the SMAS is very essential, where it is usually dissected, mobilized, and redraped.

It is located between the superficial and the deep facial fat compartments and can be classified as layer 3 in the 5-layered arrangement of the face. It extends from the neck (platysma) into the face (SMAS proper), temporal area (superficial temporal fascia), and medially beyond the temporal crest into the forehead (galea aponeurotica). With regards to the precise anatomy, regional variations, and even its existence, SMAS still remains debatable.[27] In the

TABLE 2: Changes in the deep fat pads of the cheek and the resulting topographical changes

Medial suborbicularis oculi fat	• Atrophy/hypotrophy	• Hollowing in the infraorbital region • Tear trough deformity • Increases the orbital cheek crease and the 'V' deformity of the lower-lid • The medial suborbicularis oculi fat supports the palpebral tissues of the inferior eyelid; so its volume reduction increases the relaxation of the tissue of the inferior eyelid and causes herniation of the infraorbital fat
Lateral suborbicularis oculi fat	• Atrophy/hypotrophy	• Decreases the projection of the malar area and cheekbone, facilitating the ptosis of superficial fat compartments of the cheek • Appearance of orbitomalar groove
Deep medial cheek fat	• Atrophy in upper two-thirds mainly, ptosis and mild atrophy of lower one-third	• Decreases support to the superficial fat compartments, decreased anterior projection • Prominent nasolabial fold • V-deformity of the lower lid
Buccal extension of buccal fat pad	• Deflation • Anteroinferior protrusion of buccal fat responsible for the increase in the convexity of the cheeks and jowl ptosis	• Lack of support for the medial cheek and middle cheek fat, aggravating the descent of these compartments

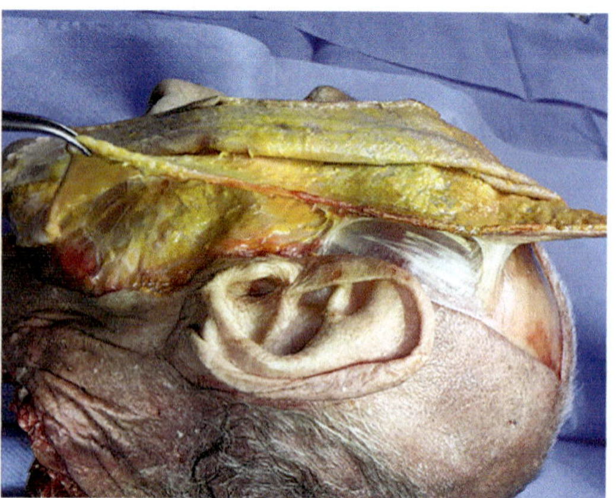

FIG. 5: Elevation of the superficial musculoaponeurotic system.

anterior cheek region, it comes in contact with the superficial facial muscles, which are enveloped by the SMAS. In this region, the SMAS no longer forms a continuous layer of connective tissue but splits and disperses into the surrounding tissue.

Two variations of SMAS architecture have been described by Ghassemi et al.[28] as follows:

1. Type I SMAS is seen in the forehead, parotid, zygomatic, and infraorbital areas. It consists of a network of small fibrous septae that traverse perpendicularly between fat lobules to the dermis down to the facial muscles or periosteum
2. Type II SMAS is found medial to the nasolabial fold, in the upper and lower lips, and consists of a dense mesh of collagen, elastic, and muscle fibers. Type II SMAS despite being extremely thin, binds the facial muscles around the mouth to the overlying skin. It thus has an important role in transmitting complex movements during animation.

The SMAS is relatively thick in the parotid-masseteric region, where it is attached to the parotid sheath. Further medially, it thins considerably making it difficult to dissect. In the lower face, the SMAS covers the facial nerve branches as well as the sensory nerves. Dissection superficial to the SMAS in this region protects facial nerve branches.[29] Above the zygomatic arch, the SMAS exists as the superficial temporal fascia, which splits to enclose the temporal branch of the facial nerve and the intermediate temporal fat pad.

Facial Retaining Ligaments

The anatomy of retaining ligaments of the face is of prime importance in understanding concepts of facial aging. They are located in constant anatomic locations over the facial skeleton to stabilize the soft tissue planes. The retaining ligaments basically bind all the concentric layers together in fixed immobile points. The spaces and compartments are the areas in between the ligaments where facial movements take place.[20,30-32] The ligaments connect the superficial fascia (SMAS or its equivalent) to the dermis and enable the movement of these layers as a single unit during facial expression.[33,34]

Surgical release of these ligaments is needed to achieve the desired aesthetic outcome. Furthermore, they have a sentinel role in their anatomic relationship to facial nerve branches.[35]

They can be classified into true and false retaining ligaments.[36,37] Both types of ligaments insert into the dermis.

True Retaining Ligaments (Fig. 6)

These structures are found especially in the region of sutures, and originate from the periosteum. They connect the dermis to the underlying periosteum and are easily identifiable.

1. Temporal ligamentous adhesion
2. Lateral orbital thickening
3. Zygomatic ligament: This originates from the temporozygomatic suture and the zygomatic arch.[39] The inferior border of the zygomatic arch is connected to the dermis by the zygomatic ligament (McGregor's patch). It is found just posterior to the origin of the zygomaticus minor muscle
4. Orbicularis retaining ligaments: The orbital retaining ligaments (orbitomalar septum) arise from the infraorbital and supraorbital margin and penetrate the orbicularis oculi muscle. They are very strong in the region of the frontozygomatic suture. The lateral orbital thickening on the superolateral orbital rim arises as a thickening of the orbicularis retaining ligament
5. Mandibular retaining ligament: This ligament connects the periosteum of the mandible just medial to the origin of depressor anguli oris to the overlying dermis. This attachment gives rise to the labiomandibular sulcus just anterior to the jowl.

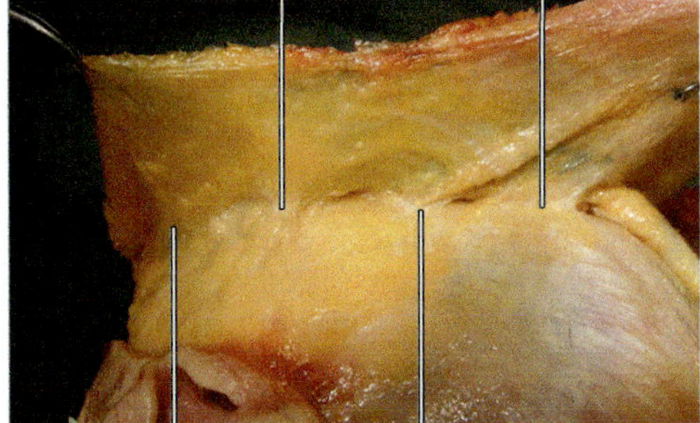

FIG. 6: Ligaments of the face when view from posterior during a subsuperficial musculoaponeurotic system flap.

False Retaining Ligaments

False retaining ligaments arise from the SMAS or the superficial fascia. They are diffuse condensations of fibrous tissue that connect superficial and deep facial fasciae.[38]

1. Zygomaticocutaneous ligament: This ligament arises from the zygomatic bone and has an identical course as the zygomaticus minor muscle. It forms the inferior boundary of the SOOF and incorporates the angular vein in its medial portion. Medial to the mid-pupillary line, it fuses with the orbicularis retaining ligament and gives thus shape to malar mounds, i.e., the banana like shaped swelling in the lateral infraorbital region
2. Masseteric ligaments: These ligaments are a long band of connections between the buccinator muscle and the mid-facial SMAS located anterior to the masseter muscle. These ligaments have no connection with the masseter muscle but provide sheltered pathways for the branches of the facial nerve which changes planes from deep to the parotidomasseteric fascia to reach the more superficially located muscles of facial expression. With advancing age, these ligaments attenuate and the SMAS over the masseter becomes ptotic, leading to the formation of jowls.[32]

Importance

A clear definition to the role of retaining ligaments in the process of aging has not been defined. However, some authors believe that attenuation and laxity of the retaining ligaments causes laxity and descent of the soft tissue that they support.[17,40] Some authors have also suggested that the ligaments remain relatively strong while the unsupported soft tissue in between (in the spaces and compartments) descends with time. This manifests as bulges and grooves and is classically the "stigmata" of facial aging.[39]

Usually, the volume deflation is identified by the grooves on the skin surface and these areas of fat reabsorption are confined in between the ligaments.[12,41] The tear trough and the palpebromalar groove lie in between the tear trough ligament and orbital retaining ligaments, the mid-cheek groove lies in between the zygomaticocutaneous ligament, the nasolabial fold between the nasolabial ligament, the buccal fat groove between the parotidomasseteric ligament, and the marionette line within the labio-mandibular ligament.[41-43] The strength of the ligaments lie in the central area of the face where a strong fixation exists, and later they become loose laterally.

There is a better aesthetic outcome, when the fillers are injected below and anterior to these ligaments to support them.

ARTERIES OF THE FACE

Vascular occlusion is the most concerning complication regarding filler injections. It can be a localized occlusion, resulting in skin necrosis, or a distant occlusion causing blindness or cerebral ischemic events.[44,45] Localized vascular occlusion results from either direct intravascular injection or the compression of the vessels by the injected filler material.[46]

A thorough knowledge of the vascular anatomy of the face is important to avoid and reduce the risk of the rare but serious adverse events due to arterial occlusion or compression.[47]

Understanding the depth of needle tip is very important. The anatomy of the face is too complex and varied and there could be minor variations, however, depth of the vessel in specific zones is fairly predictable and injecting at the right depth the risk of intravascular accidents.[48]

Necrosis due to arterial occlusion is not frequently reported, but there have been many reports of alar necrosis after augmenting the nasolabial fold. Further, several cases of retinal artery occlusion has been reported after augmentation in the glabellar and cheek area. Facial artery occlusion due to filler can explain these adverse events, as it runs in the depth near the nasolabial fold.

The face is supplied by both the internal and the external carotid arterial system with having a plethora of anastomoses between them. The facial, maxillary, and superficial temporal arteries and their branches arise from the external carotid artery and supply the skin and soft tissue of the face. The central forehead, eyelids, and upper part of the nose are supplied through the internal carotid system by the ophthalmic arteries.

Important Vessels When Injecting Important Areas of the Face[13]

Cheeks:
- Facial artery
- Transverse facial artery
- Buccal branch of the maxillary artery
- Infra-orbital artery
- Zygomatic branch of the lacrimal artery

Glabella:
- Supratroclear artery
- Supraorbital artery

These vessels are small and do not have a good source of collateral circulation, hence glabella is a high risk area.[49]

Nasal Ala:
- Dorsal nasal artery
- Angular artery: Is an extension of the facial artery, supplies to the medial cheek, nasal ala, and sidewall and dorsum of the nose. Proper care needs to be taken while injecting at the alar grove because excessive amount here can cause compression or direct injection into the vessel can lead to the necrosis of nasal ala, nasal tip, nasolabial fold, and upper lip.[50]

Perioral:
- Superior labial artery
- Inferior labial artery.

Temples:
- Superficial temporal artery[51]
- Zygomatico-orbital branch of the superficial temporal artery
- Deep temporal arteries.

Supraorbital and the Supratrochlear Arteries

The supraorbital and the supratrochlear arteries are an important part of arterial anastomoses, which supply terminal arteries namely, the ophthalmic and retinal arteries. It is advisable to inject fillers in the glabella with extreme caution as arterial embolism can lead to an immediate and irreversible amaurosis, which can even be bilateral.[52]

FACIAL ARTERY

Facial artery arises from the external carotid in the region of the carotid triangle, just anterior to the masseter and runs across the inferior and anterior borders of the mandible to the insertion of the masseter muscle where it pierces the masseteric fascia and ascends upwards and medially towards the eye. It lies there anterior to the vein, posterior to the mandibular ligament, deep to the marginal mandibular nerve, and deep to the platysma. The pulse can be felt at the anterior edge of the masseter muscle. Along its course towards the angle of mouth, the artery lies superficial to the buccinator and levator anguli oris but deep to the zygomaticus and risorius muscles.[53] At the level of the mouth, the facial artery divides into inferior and superior labial arteries and then continues to run across to end in the medial canthus as the angular artery. The surface marking can be drawn as an imaginary line from the anterior margin of the masseter muscle to the medial canthus. The facial vein, running behind, accompanies the facial artery.

Variations in the course and branching pattern of the facial artery have been described by Yang et al. In their dissection on 60 cadavers, branches of the facial artery were observed at the vicinity of the nasolabial fold in 56 cases. The facial artery was located 13.5 ± 5.4 mm lateral to the oral commissure and 3.2 ± 4.5 mm (mean ± standard deviation) lateral to the ala of the nose. In 42.9% cases, it ascended within 5 mm of the nasolabial fold and in 33.9% of cases, it crossed the nasolabial fold. In 18 cases with detoured branches, the facial artery turned medially over the infraorbital area at 39.2 ± 5.8 mm lateral to the facial mid-sagittal line and 35.2 ± 8.2 mm inferior to the plane connecting the medial epicanthi of both sides. The nasojugal portion of the detoured branch traveled along the inferior border of the orbicularis oculi and then ascended toward the forehead, forming the angular artery[54,55] (Fig 7).

Furukawa and Anzai classified the facial artery into four patterns after dissecting 94 cadavers with 187 facial arteries:

- Type 1: Short course, terminate proximal to the superior labial artery
- Type 2: Terminate distal to the superior labial artery near nasolabial fold

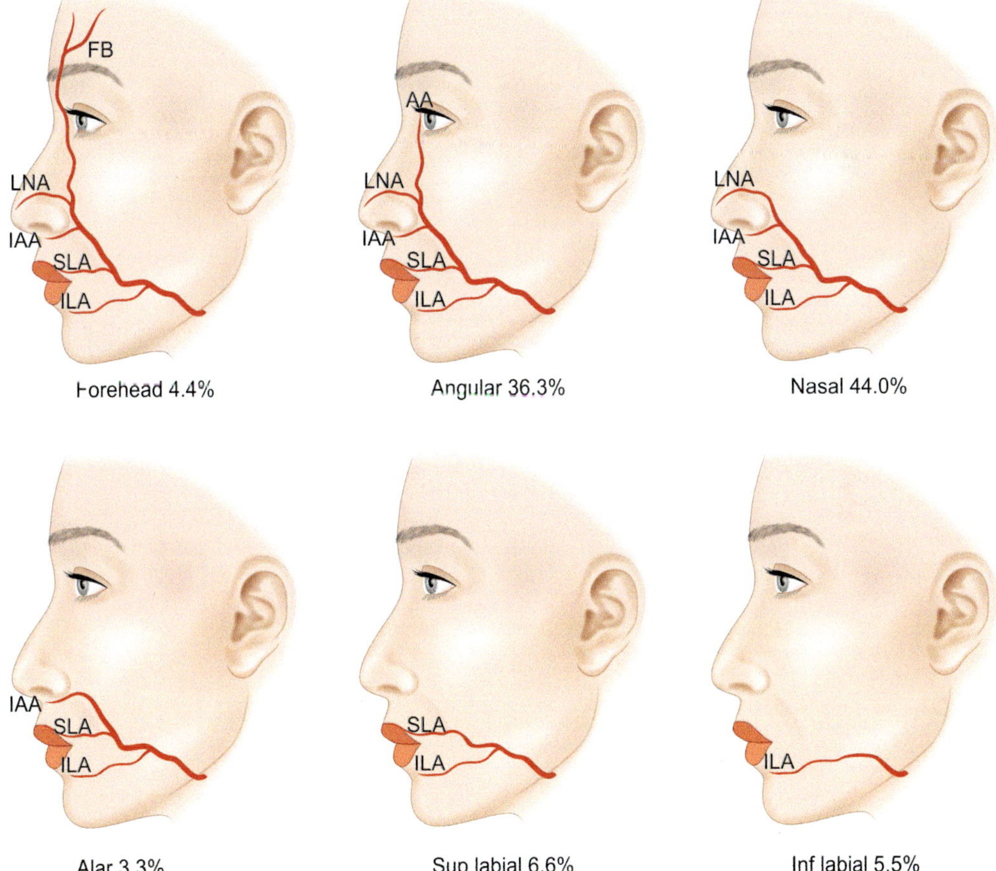

ILA, inferior labial artery; SLA, superior labial artery; IAA, inferior alar artery; LNA, lateral nasal artery; AA, angular artery; FB, forehead branch; INF, inferior; sup, superior.

FIG. 7: Variations in the branching pattern of the facial artery.[55] Branching patterns of facial artery according to its termination.

- Type 3: Classic course, extends to lateral nasal-superior alar or angular branch
- Type 4: Duplex with dominant lateral angular branch[56] (Fig. 8).

In another study by Kim et al., 26 hemi faces from 13 Thai cadavers and 31 hemi faces from 17 Korean cadavers were dissected to find the course of the angular artery.

The topography of the AA was classified into four types according to its course (Fig. 9):

- Type I (persistent pattern: The AA traverses the lateral side of the nose (11%)
- Type II (detouring pattern): The AA traverses the cheek and tear trough area (18%)
- Type III (alternative pattern): The AA traverses the medial canthal area through a branch of the ophthalmic artery (22.8%)
- Type IV (latent pattern): The AA is absent (26.3%)[57] (Fig. 9).

In a study involving 14 Thai soft embalmed cadavers, the distance, depth, and diameter of the facial artery were measured at the level of the oral commissure and the nasal ala. It was seen that the maximum risk of arterial complication from dermal filler injection is approximately 15 mm lateral to the oral commissure at the depth of 11 and 7 mm from lateral nasal ala at a depth of 12 mm.[58]

It is advisable to stay medial to the nasolabial fold and inject deep on the bone in the canine fossa. The main blood vessels which may also be compromised depending on the portion of the nasolabial fold where the filler is injected are the angular arteries and part of the superior labial artery.

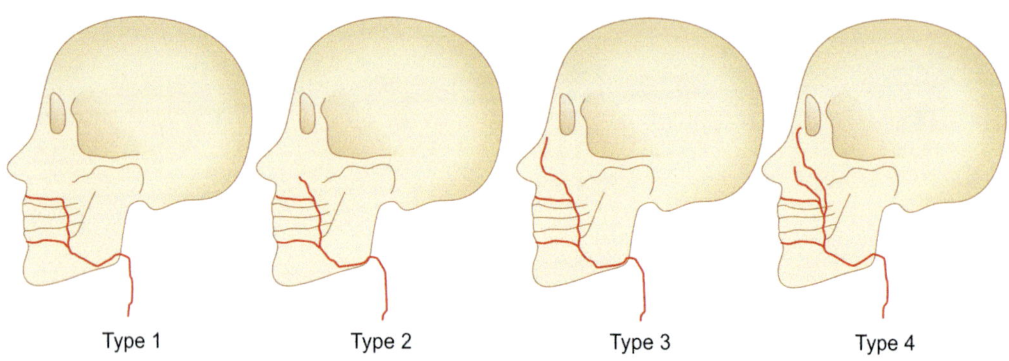

FIG. 8: Four patterns of facial artery.

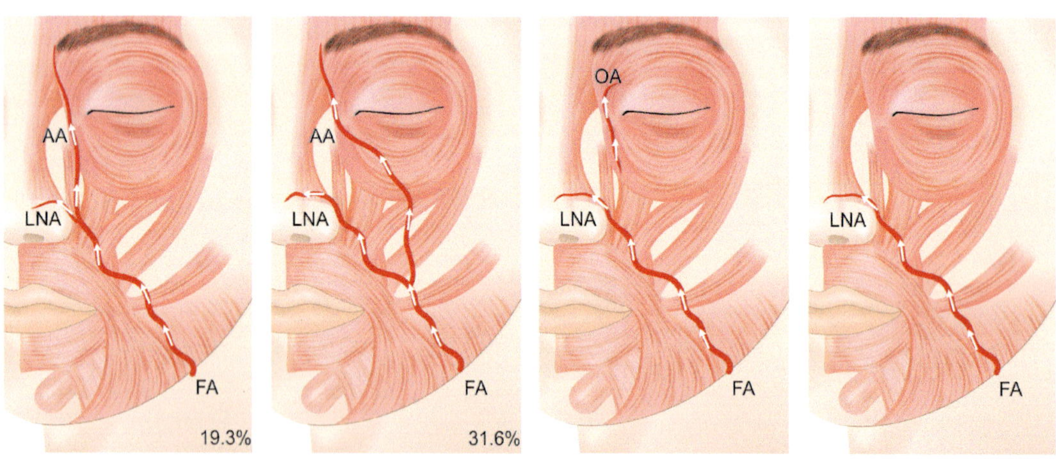

FIG. 9: Variations in angular artery.

MAXILLARY ARTERY

This is a terminal branch of the external carotid artery. It gives three main branches:

1. Mental: Terminal branch of the inferior alveolar artery. It passes through the mental foramen to supply the chin and lower lip
2. Buccal: Supplies the cheek tissue after crossing the buccinator
3. Infraorbital: Runs through the infraorbital canal below the orbit and enters the face through the infraorbital foramen. Here, it anastomoses with the branches of the transverse facial, ophthalmic, buccal, and facial arteries, thereby supplying the lower eyelid, cheek, and lateral nose.

Caution needs to be exercised while injecting the infraorbital hollow, especially in the medial limbal line as these vessels can be severed with sharp needles, leading to hematomas.

SUPERFICIAL TEMPORAL ARTERY

Superficial temporal artery is the terminal branch of the external carotid artery. It emerges from the depth behind the parotid gland and penetrates the superficial temporal fascia 1 cm anterior and 1 cm superior to the tragus. On the temporal fascia, it branches into its terminal vessels.

The superficial temporal artery gives two branches for the cheek:

- Transverse facial artery: In the substance of the parotid, just before reaching the zygomatic arch, it gives off the transverse facial artery which runs inferior and parallel to the arch and supplies the parotid, parotid duct, masseter, and skin of the lateral canthus
- Zygomatico-orbital artery: This is found superior to the zygomatic arch, parallel to the transverse facial artery and runs over the temporal fascia to the orbicularis oculi muscle.

The superficial temporal artery crosses the zygomatic arch superficially within the superficial temporal fascia and gives off a middle temporal artery above the arch. This pierces the deep temporal fascia and supplies the temporalis muscle. About 2 cm above the zygomatic arch, the superficial temporal artery divides into anterior and posterior branches. The anterior branch supplies the forehead and anastomoses with the supraorbital and supratrochlear vessels. The posterior part supplies the parietal scalp and periosteum.

Knowledge of the surface anatomy and depth of these vessels is important while treating injecting the temporal fossa.

OPHTHALMIC ARTERY

This is a branch of the internal carotid artery. It branches into lacrimal, supraorbital, supratrochlear, infratrochlear, and external nasal arteries. There is significant communication between the external and internal carotid artery systems around the eye through several anastomoses. Inadvertent intra-arterial injection of fillers for soft tissue augmentation around the eye can cause blindness due to occlusion of the central retinal vessels.[59,60] Such complications can be avoided by slowly injecting small aliquots of fillers, using blunt cannulas and a careful retrograde injection technique.[61]

NERVE SUPPLY

A good understanding of the nerve supply helps us to minimize pain and nerve injury and identify precise injection points. It also allows us to give a nerve block when a large or sensitive area is treated.

Sensory Innervation: Trigeminal Nerve

Facial sensory innervation is via ophthalmic nerve, maxillary nerve, and mandibular nerves, the three branches of the trigeminal nerve (Table 3).

Special Anatomic Considerations (Fig. 10)

- Supraorbital
  - Emerges from the orbit at the supraorbital foramen, however, sometimes it exit from separate foramina[62]
  - Superficial and deep branches straddle the corrugator muscle. The deep branch is usually lateral to the superficial one. It runs superiorly between the galea and the periosteum of the forehead, medial to the superior temporal crest line
- Supratrochlear nerve
  - Exits the orbit about 1 cm medial to the supraorbital nerve
  - Runs close to the periosteum under the corrugator and frontalis
  - Branches supply the skin over the lower medial forehead and the medial eyelid
- Infratrochlear nerve
  - Terminal branch of the nasociliary nerve
  - Supplies a small area on the medial aspect of the upper eyelid and bridge of the nose

TABLE 3: Facial sensory innervation via ophthalmic nerve, maxillary nerve, and mandibular nerves

Name	Branches	Innervation
Ophthalmic nerve	• Supraorbital • Supratrochlear • Infratrochlear • Lacrimal • External nasal	• Forehead, upper eyelid, and dorsum of the nose
Maxillary nerve	• Infraorbital • Zygomaticofacial • Zygomaticotemporal • Alveolar nerves • Pterygopalatine nerves	• Lower eyelid, cheek, upper lip, ala of the nose, and part of the temple • Maxillary teeth • Nasal cavity
Mandibular nerve (motor and sensory)	• Inferior alveolar nerve • Lingual nerve • Buccal nerve • Auriculotemporal nerve	• Skin over the mandible • Lower cheek • Part of the temple and ear • The lower teeth • Gingival mucosa • Lower lip
Mandibular nerve (sensory)	• Auriculotemporal • Mental • Buccal	• Cheek • Skin of the ear and temple (auriculotemporal)

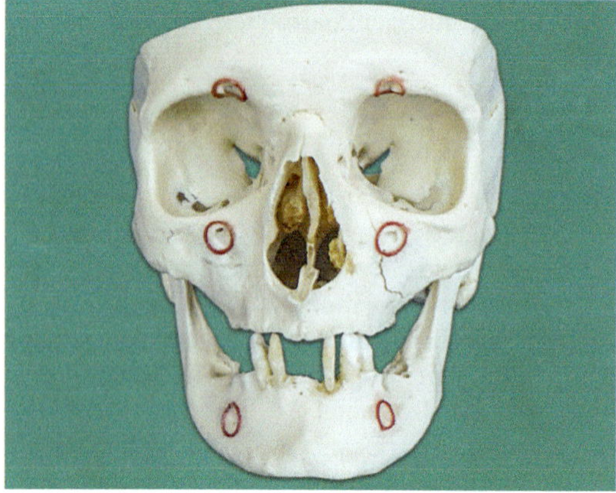

FIG. 10: Location of the supraorbital, infraorbital, and mental foramen on the human skull.

- Infraorbital nerve
  - Largest cutaneous branch of the maxillary nerve
  - Only branch of the maxillary nerve for the cheek
  - Runs in the infraorbital canal below the orbit and reaches the skin of the anterior cheek through the infraorbital foramen
  - It can be palpated through the skin, the superficial fat, the inferior extension of the orbicularis oculi muscle, the SOOF, and the levator labii superioris muscle and lies usually in the medial limbal line, 8 mm below the orbital margin
  - It supplies the lower eyelid, ala of the nose, and upper lip
- External nasal nerve
  - Supplies the skin of the nose below the nasal bone, except the skin over the external nares
- Lacrimal nerve supplies the skin over the lateral part of the upper eyelid
- Zygomaticofacial nerve
  - Arises from the zygomaticofacial foramen below and lateral to the orbital rim
  - Supplies skin of the malar eminence
- Zygomaticotemporal nerve
  - Emerges on the deep surface of the zygomatic bone
  - Supplies the anterior temple
- Auriculotemporal nerve
  - Located at the posterior border of the cheek
  - Runs laterally behind the neck of the mandible
  - Then it runs along with the superficial temporal artery to innervate the skin of the ear and the temple

- Mental nerve
  - Terminal part of the inferior alveolar nerve
  - Travels through the mandibular canal and ends as the mental nerve
  - Mental nerve exits the mental foramen at the level of the second premolar, to supply the skin of the lower lip and chin
- Buccal nerve
  - Innervates the skin of the cheek
  - Present at the anterior border of the masseter muscle and runs superficial to the buccinator muscle
- Greater auricular nerve
  - Innervates the skin over the angle of the mandible.

Motor Innervation—Facial Nerve[13]

The branches of the facial nerve provide motor innervation to the muscles of facial expression. It emerges from the stylomastoid foramen and gives off the posterior auricular nerve, nerves to the posterior belly of digastric, and stylohyoid branch before entering the substance of the parotid gland. The facial nerve divides into its main branches within the parotid gland (Fig. 11):

- Temporal
- Zygomatic
- Buccal
- Marginal mandibular
- Cervical.

These branches emerge at the anterior border of the parotid gland and run transverse to the sensory nerves, superficial to the arteries, and are located between the superficial and deep layers of the mimetic muscles.

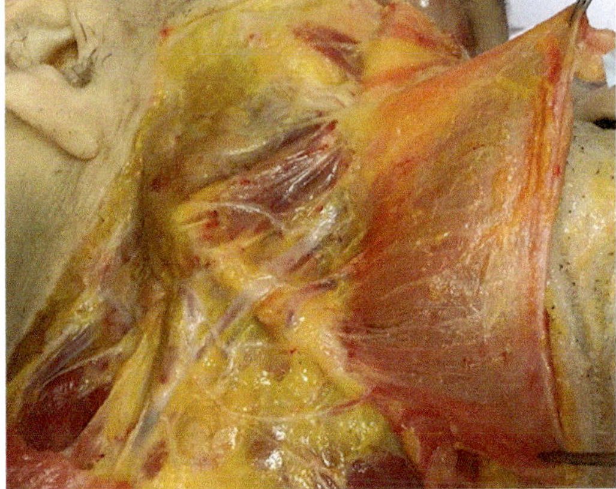

FIG. 11: Branches of the facial nerve deep to the platysma after their emergence from the parotid gland.

Temporal branches:

- Leaves the superior border of the parotid gland as three or four rami that cross the zygomatic arch anterior to the external acoustic meatus, and at the level of the zygomatic arch, posterior to the lateral orbital rim
- The branches pass between the superficial temporal fascia with the intermediate fat pad, and the deep temporal fascia and enter frontalis above the brow, just below the anterior branch of the superficial temporal artery

Zygomatic branches:

- Run upward obliquely to the muscles between the palpebral fissure and the oral fissure
  - Up to three zygomatic branches may be present
  - Upper branch passes above the eye to supply frontalis and orbicularis oculi. The lower branch always passes under the origin of zygomaticus major and supplies this muscle, other lip elevators, and the lower orbicularis oculi. Smaller branches continue around the medial aspect of the eye to supply depressor supercilii and the superomedial orbicularis oculi.

The buccal branches:

- Exits the parotid and is tightly bound to the anterior surface of masseter within the parotido-masseteric fascia
- Runs horizontal, anteriorly over the buccal fat pad, below and parallel to the parotid duct to supply the buccinator muscle and to the muscles of the upper lip and nose

The marginal mandibular branch:

- Runs above the inferior border of the mandible, posterior to the angle of the mouth
- Passes upward and more superficially to innervate the mentalis, depressor labii inferioris and platysma

The cervical branch:

- Passes into the neck at the level of the hyoid bone to innervate platysma.

CONCLUSION

A thorough knowledge of anatomy helps one avoid complications and achieve natural results with the least amount of dermal fillers. With the growing demand of aesthetic procedures and injectors worldwide, complications are also on the rise. Most of these can be avoided by a little care and thorough knowledge of anatomy of the area treated.

REFERENCES

1. Gassner HG, Rafii A, Young A, et al. Surgical anatomy of the face. Implications for modern face-lift techniques. Arch Facial Plast Surg. 2008;10(1):9-19.
2. Cotofana S, Schenck TL, Trevidic P, et al. Midface: Clinical anatomy and regional approaches with injectable fillers. Plast Reconstr Surg. 2015;136(5, Suppl):219S-34S.
3. Rosas A, Bastir M. Thin plate spline analysis of allometry and sexual dimorphism in the human craniofacial complex. Am J Phys Anthropol. 2002;117:236.
4. Jacobson AL. Radiographic cephalometry. Quintessence Publishing Co.: Chicago; 1995.
5. Ferrario VF, Sforza C, Poggio CE, et al. Effects of growth and development on cephalometrics shapes in orthodontic patients: A Fourier analysis. Eur J Orthod. 1997;19:669.
6. Mendelson B, Wong CH. Changes in the facial skeleton with aging: Implications and clinical applications for facial rejuvenation. Aesthetic Plast Surg. 2012;36:753-60.
7. Albert AM, Ricanek K Jr, Patterson E. A review of the literature on the aging adult skull and face: Implications for forensic science research and applications. Forensic Sci Int. 2007;172(1):1-9.
8. Bolin A. Proximal alveolar bone loss in a longitudinal radiographic investigation. Swed Dent J. 1986;Suppl 35:1.
9. Coleman SR, Grover R. The anatomy of the aging face: Volume loss and changes in 3-dimensional topography. Aesthetic Surg J. 2006;26(1S):S4-9.
10. Kaur M, Garg RK, Singla S. Analysis of facial soft tissue changes with aging and their effects on facial morphology: A forensic perspective. Egypt J Forensic Sci. 2015;5:45-56.
11. Ilankovan V. Anatomy of ageing face. Br J Oral Maxillofac Surg. 2014;52(3):195-202.
12. Rohrich RJ, Pessa JE. The fat compartments of the face: Anatomy and clinical implications for cosmetic surgery. Plast Reconstr Surg. 2007;119(7):2219-27.
13. Prendergast PM. Anatomy of the face and neck. In: Shiffman M, Di Giuseppe A, editors. Cosmetic surgery. Springer, Berlin, Heidelberg; 2013.
14. Rohrich R, Arbique GM, Wong C, et al. The anatomy of suborbicularis fat: Implications for periorbital rejuvenation. Plast Reconstr Surg. 2009;124(3):946-51.
15. Fundarò S. Treatment of the midface with fillers. Prime Journal. Available from: https://www.prime-journal.com/treatment-of-the-midface-with-fillers/.
16. Mendelson BC, Muzaffar AR, Adams WP Jr. Surgical anatomy of the midcheek and malar mounds. Plast Reconstr Surg. 2002;110:885-911.
17. Muzaffar AR, Mendelson BC, Adams WP. Surgical anatomy of the ligamentous Attachments of the lower lid and lateral canthus. Plast Reconstr Surg. 2002;110:873.
18. Wan D, Amirlak B, Rohrich R, et al. The clinical importance of the fat compartments in midfacial aging. Plast Reconstr Surg Glob Open. 2013;1(9):e92.
19. Rohrich RJ, Pessa JE, Ristow B. The youthful cheek and the deep medial fat compartment. Plast Reconstr Surg. 2008;121(6):2107-12.
20. Larrabee WF, Makielski KH, Henderson JL. Cheeks and neck. In: Larrabee WF, Makielski KH, Henderson JL, editors. Surgical anatomy of the face. Lippincott Williams & Wilkins: Philadelphia; 2004. p. 178.
21. O'Brien JX, Ashton MW, Rozen WM, et al. New perspectives on the surgical anatomy and nomenclature of the temporal region: Literature review and dissection study. Plast Reconstr Surg. 2013;131(3):510-22.
22. Donofrio LM. Fat distribution: A morphologic study of the aging face. Dermatol Surg. 2000;26:1107-12.
23. Gierloff M, Stöhring C, Buder T, et al. Aging changes of the midfacial fat compartments: A computed tomographic study. Plast Reconstr Surg. 2012;129:263-73.
24. Sandoval SE, Cox JA, Koshy JC, et al. Facial fat compartments: A guide for filler placement. Semin Plast Surg. 2009;23:283-7.
25. Ozdemir R, Kilinç H, Unlü RE, et al. Anatomicohistologic study of the retaining ligaments of the face and use in face lift: Retaining ligament correction and SMAS plication. Plast Reconstr Surg. 2002;110:1134-49.
26. Mitz V, Peyronie M. The superficial musculo-aponeurotic system in the parotid and cheek area. Plast Reconstr Surg. 1976;58(1):80-8.
27. Gardetto A, Dabernig J, Rainer C, et al. Does a superficial musculoaponeurotic system exist in the face and neck? An anatomical study by the tissue plastination technique. Plast Reconstr Surg. 2003;111(2):664-72.
28. Ghassemi A, Prescher A, Riediger D, et al. Anatomy of the SMAS revisited. Aesthetic Plast Surg. 2003;27(4):258-64.
29. Wobig JL, Dailey RA. Facial anatomy. In: Wobig JL, Dailey RA, editors. Oculofacial plastic surgery. Thieme Medical Publishers, New York; 2004. p. 5.
30. Moss CJ, Mendelson BC, Taylor GI. Surgical anatomy of the ligamentous attachments in the temple and periorbital regions. Plast Reconstr Surg. 2000;105:1475-98.
31. Warren RJ, Aston SJ, Mendelson BC. Face lift. Plast Reconstr Surg. 2011;128(6):747e-64e.
32. Mendelson BC, Freeman ME, Wu W, et al. Surgical anatomy of the lower face: The premasseter space, the jowl, and the labiomandibular fold. Aesthetic Plast Surg. 2008;32(2):185-95.
33. Gosain AK, Yousif NJ, Madiedo G, et al. Surgical anatomy of the SMAS: A reinvestigation. Plast Reconstr Surg. 1993;92:1254-65.
34. Mendelson BC. Extended sub-SMAS dissection and cheek elevation. Clin Plast Surg. 1995;22:325-39.
35. Alghoul M, Codner MA. Retaining ligaments of the face: Review of anatomy and clinical applications. Aesthet Surg J. 2013:33(6) 769-82.
36. Thaller SR, Kim S, Patterson H, et al. The submuscular aponeurotic system (SMAS): A histologic and comparative anatomy evaluation. Plast Reconstr Surg. 1990;86: 690-6.
37. Pensler JM, Ward JW, Parry SW. The superficial musculo-aponeurotic system in the upper lip: An anatomic study in cadavers. Plast Reconstr Surg. 1985;75:488-94.
38. Jones BM, Grover R. Anatomical considerations. In: Jones BM, Grover R, editors. Facial rejuvenation surgery. Mosby Press: London; 2008. pp. 18-22.

39. Furnas DW. The retaining ligaments of the cheek. Plast Reconstr Surg. 1989;83(1):11-6.
40. Stuzin JM, Baker TJ, Gordon HL, et al. Extended SMAS dissection as an approach to midface rejuvenation. Clin Plast Surg. 1995;22:295-311.
41. Russo PR, Fundarò PS. The invisible lifting. Florence: OEO; 2014. p. 109-57.
42. Haddock NT, Saadeh PB, Boutros S, et al. The tear trough and lid-cheek junction: Anatomy and implications for surgical correction. Plast Reconstr Surg. 2009;123:1332-42.
43. Salti G, Rauso R. Facial rejuvenation with fillers: The dual plane technique. J Cutan Aesthet Surg. 2015;8(3):127-133.
44. Carle MV, Roe RH, Novack RL. Occlusion caused by cosmetic facial filler injection – reply JAMA Ophthalmol. 2015;133(2):225.
45. DeLorenzi C. Complications of injectable fillers, part 2: Vascular complications. Aesthet Surg J. 2014;34(4):584-600.
46. Cox SE, Adigun CG. Complications of injectable fillers and neurotoxins. Dermatol Ther. 2011;24(6):524-36.
47. Bachmann F, Erdmann R, Hartmann V, et al. The spectrum of adverse reactions after treatment with injectable fillers in the glabellar region: Results from the injectable filler safety study. Dermatol Surg. 2009;35(Suppl 2):1629-34.
48. Swift A. Cosmetic surgery times Injection savvy: Using anatomy to your advantage. 2015.
49. Glaich AS, Cohen JL, Goldberg LH. Injection necrosis of the glabella: Protocol for prevention and treatment after use of dermal fillers. Dermatol Surg. 2006;32(2):276-81.
50. Emer J, Waldorf H. Injectable neurotoxins and fillers: There is no free lunch. Clin Dermatol. 2011;29(6):678-90.
51. Brennan C. Avoiding the "danger zones" when injecting dermal fillers and volume enhancers. Plast Surg Nurs. 2014;34(3):108-11.
52. Tamura BM. Facial topography of the injection areas for dermal fillers, and associated risks. Surg Cosmet Dermatol. 2013;5(3):234-8.
53. Berkovitz BK, Moxham BJ. Head and neck anatomy. In: Dunitz M, editor. A clinical reference. London; 2002. P. 118
54. Yang HM, Lee JG, Hu KS, et al. New anatomical insights on the course and branching patterns of the facial artery: Clinical implications of injectable treatments to the nasolabial fold and nasojugal groove. Plast Reconstr Surg. 2014;133(5):1077-82.
55. Yang HM, Lee YI, Lee JG, et al. Topography of superficial arteries on the face. Korean J Phys Anthropol. 2013;26(4): 131-40.
56. Anzai F. Evaluation of facial artery with CT angiography using 64 slice MDCT: Implications for facial reconstruction in plastic surgery. 91st Annual meeting of American Association of Plastic Surgeons. 2012.
57. Kim YS, Choi DY, Gil YC, et al. The anatomical origin and course of the angular artery regarding its clinical implications. Dermatol Surg. 2014;40(10):1070-6.
58. Phumyoo T, Tansatit T, Rachkeaw N. The soft tissue landmarks to avoid injury to the facial artery during filler and neurotoxin injection at the nasolabial region. J Craniofac Surg. 2014;25(5):1885-9.
59. McCleve D, Goldstein JC. Blindness secondary to injections in the nose, mouth, and face: Cause and prevention. Ear Nose Throat J. 1995;74:182-8.
60. Dreizen NG, Framm L. Sudden unilateral visual loss after autologous fat injection into the glabellar area. Am J Ophthalmol. 1989;107:85-7.
61. Coleman SR. Avoidance of arterial occlusion from injection of soft tissue fillers. Aesthet Surg J. 2002; 22(6):555-7.
62. Defatta RJ, Williams EF. Evolution of midface rejuvenation. Arch Facial Plast Surg. 2009;11:6-12.

22
CHAPTER

Soft Tissue Augmentation: Dermal Fillers

Maya Vedamurthy

INTRODUCTION

Soft tissue augmentation has entered a period of Renaissance with the aging of the baby boomers.[1] Dermal fillers are gaining more importance in aesthetic practice as majority of the patients wishing to restore a youthful appearance are opting for procedures with less downtime. With surgical face lifts there is a two-dimensional improvement whereas with soft tissue augmentation there is a three-dimensional enhancement in the appearance of the face.

History of soft tissue augmentation dates back to use of autologous fat by Neuber in 1893 and subsequent modification by Lexer in 1910.[2]

Use of silicone and liquid paraffin for soft tissue augmentation fell into disrepute because of their side effects. The emergence of use of collagen by Knapp, Luck, and Daniels in 1977 turned out to be a successful technique and was considered as the 'gold standards' against which all newer injectable or implantable fillers were measured. In the world of dermal fillers that emerged subsequently for soft tissue augmentation, hyaluronic acid (HA) fillers has withstood the test of time and continues to be one of the most wanted fillers in cosmetic practice. The HAs are now the traditional volume filling products where the final result is approximately obtained soon after the injection and remains so until complete degradation.[3]

PROPERTIES OF HYALURONIC ACID

Hyaluronic acid also called hyaluronan is present in abundance in all living species as a component of connective tissue. It is a linear polysaccharide consisting of glucuronic acid and *N*-acetylglucosamine that provides a fluid lattice on which collagen and elastic fibers may develop.[4] The identical structure of HA in all species and tissues makes it an ideal substance for use as a biomaterial in medicine.

Hyaluronic acid is hydrophilic and is responsible for maintaining adequate internal hydration, lubrication, and moisture retention.

Hyaluronic acid plays an important role for both mechanical and transport purposes. It gives volume to the skin, shape to the eyes, and elasticity to the joints. In the skin, HA molecules bind to water and create volume. With aging the amount of HA decreases and there is resultant loss of water leading to tissue dehydration and volume loss. Refilling the lost volume with natural HA would be ideal, but it lasts only 1–2 days in the natural form and this challenge has been overcome with the development of nonanimal stabilized hyaluronic acid. Nonanimal stabilized HA is produced by bacterial fermentation; scientists have carefully designed a method of stabilizing the nonanimal HA to meet the demand for prolonged residence time in the human tissues without affecting its biocompatibility.

The physical properties of HA that determine its behavior in tissues include (Table 1):

- Gel hardness which determines the structure and stiffness

TABLE 1: Physical characteristics of HA-based fillers

Characteristic	Clinical importance
Gel Hardness	Structure and stiffness
Particle size	Degree of volume replacement
HA Concentration	Durability and stability
Swelling	Degree of inflammation and induration

- Particle size within the gel which influences the degree of correction and volume restoration
- Concentration of HA measured as mg/mL which determines the longevity and stability
- The ratio of soluble to insoluble HA which determines the time for degradation.

The variables among the different commercial preparation of HA fillers are the concentration per milliliter and the method and degree of cross linking that has a significant impact on the physical properties.[5]

BASIC INDICATIONS FOR HYALURONIC ACID FILLERS

- Photoaging wrinkles
- Nasolabial folds
- Glabellar lines
- Marionette lines
- Lip augmentation (filling and contouring).

EVALUATION OF A PATIENT FOR TREATMENT WITH HYALURONIC ACID FILLERS

A careful history and examination is essential for optimizing the results with HA fillers. A history of allergies to poultry is to be excluded for HA fillers with avian source. As most HA fillers are from a streptococci source, a history of streptococcal disease has to be elicited as these are not good candidates for such fillers. The site to be treated has to be examined for infection or diseases that are likely to be exacerbated by the procedure and appropriate precautions need to be carried out such as antivirals in case of herpes simplex infection. Pain tolerance and downtime need to be addressed appropriately. Any preexisting asymmetry needs to be explained and documented. The skin type, thickness and the defect needs to be evaluated to choose the correct filler.

INJECTION TECHNIQUES

There are several techniques of injection to deposit the filler substance at the desired depth. Four of these techniques are commonly used for the basic indications.

Linear Threading Technique

This technique is commonly used to treat superficial wrinkles or folds. Here, the full length of the needle is inserted in the middle of the wrinkle or fold and the substance is slowly injected as the needle is pulled backward so that the threads of the gel are placed lengthwise in the middle of the wrinkle (Fig. 1).

Serial Puncture Technique

This technique is used to inject wrinkles, lines, or folds. Here, multiple injections are placed serially along the length of the treated wrinkle or fold. The product is injected closely together so that it merges into a smooth continuous line which lifts the wrinkle or fold (Fig. 2).

Fan Technique

This technique is used to inject a relatively larger area using minimum entry points. Here, the needle is inserted at the periphery of the area to be treated as when using the linear threading technique. After injecting one line of the product, the direction of the needle is changed and injected as before along a new line (Fig. 3).

Cross Hatching Technique

This technique is used to cover large areas uniformly using multiple entry points. Here, the needle is inserted at the periphery of the area intended to be augmented and injected as when using the linear threading technique. The needle is withdrawn from the skin and reinserted 5–10 mm adjacent to the first puncture site and injected in the same way. This procedure is then repeated at right angles to the original lines till target areas are covered (Fig. 4).

Whatever the technique may be the final choice of angle, depth and product depends on the indication for which dermal filler is used.

Placement depth based on indication is given in table 2.[6]

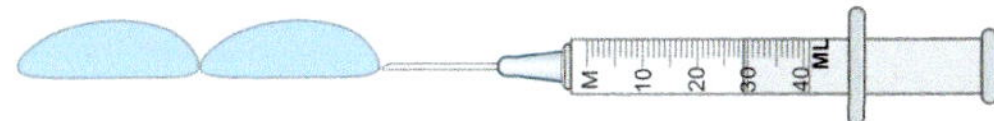

FIG. 1: Linear threading technique.

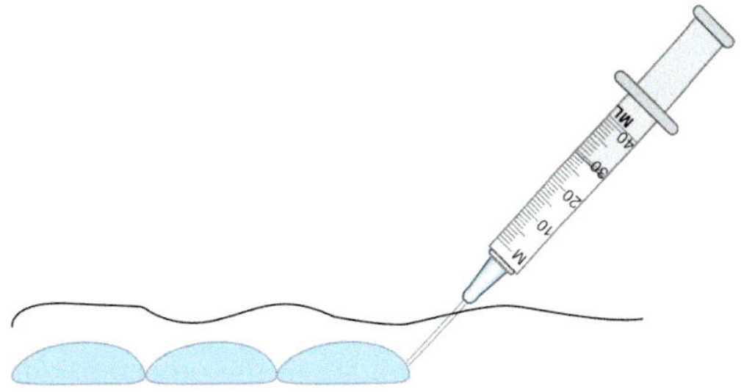

FIG. 2: Serial puncture technique.

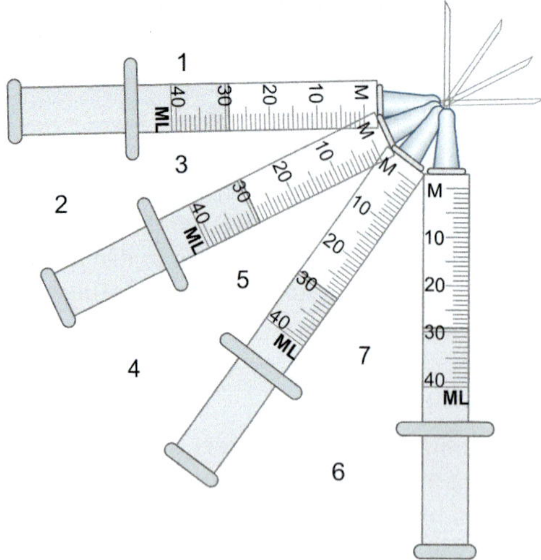

FIG. 3: Fan technique.

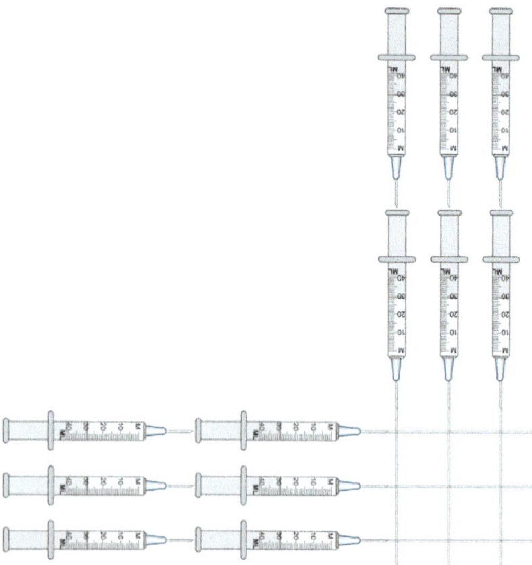
FIG. 4: Cross hatching technique.

PROCEDURE

The two major steps involved in the procedure are: (1) selection of candidate and (2) choice of filler.

Candidate Selection

The first step to success is choosing the right patient. Patients should have realistic expectations and should be aware of the limitations. The patients should be counseled well about the procedure and its outcome. Special information should be provided in terms of side effects, costs, efficacy and duration of correction.

TABLE 2: Indication and depth of placement[6]

Indication	Depth	Angle
Fine lines and rhytides	Superficial dermis	10–30°
Moderate to deep folds	Mid dermis	30–40°
Deeper folds	Deep dermis supraperiosteal	45–90°

Choice of Filler

The choice of a perfect filler for cosmetic indication is an ongoing effort. The most important quality of the filler material is the safety profile. It should be nonimmunogenic, noncarcinogenic, nonteratogenic, noninfectious and nontoxic. It should be stable after injection and preferably nonmigratory. It should be long lasting but resorbable. It should look natural and feel natural after injection into the tissues. Most important is the ease of administration, availability and affordability to the patients. It should have a high end use potential and a low abuse potential.

PREPARATION

Proper counseling regarding the use of the selected product, its limitations, longevity and adverse effects, if any should be carried out. A written informed consent should be obtained for medicolegal purposes.[7]

Clinical Photography

Pre- and post photographs are powerful tools to record images for ourselves and to communicate with the patients and our peers.[8,9]

Practical photography for dermal fillers in basic indications includes the following views:

- Full frontal view
- 30° oblique right and left showing ipsilateral and contralateral cheek
- While injecting perioral and periorbital region close-up shots would be more useful
- Shots for all basic indications should be taken at rest and at full contraction.

Procedure

The patients need for anesthesia should be assessed. Usually no anesthesia is necessary when injecting for basic indications. If the patient requires anesthesia, a topical anesthetic gel can be used or alternatively HA products containing xylocaine may be chosen for areas such as the lips, regional nerve block may be done. For the upper lip 2% lignocaine is injected using a 30 G needle into the mucosal fold in the canine fossa. For the lower lip, the injection is given into the mucosal fold below first premolar.

The area needs to be cleaned with suitable antiseptic solution. The needle supplied with the syringe is fixed to the syringe and the product is injected into the skin.

Tips for Successful Outcomes

Reduce patients discomfort by minimizing pain through following methods:[10]

- Introduce the needle gently and slowly
- Inject the product steadily and slowly
- Use the recommended needle gage
- Ice and long needles will minimize pain[11]
- Use anesthesia as applicable.

Observing certain rules for specific areas will help to optimize the use of fillers in basic indications.

Forehead

When treating glabellar lines and forehead wrinkles, it is desirable to inject in small boluses using linear threading technique. For the glabella folds, a tunneling effect is done with the needle to create space for relative ease of depositing the material in the glabellar area. A relatively superficial injection under moderate pressure is safer to avoid complications (Fig. 5).

Periorbital Area

A depot technique is advised where droplets are preferably placed in small amounts supraperiosteally. The needle is inserted perpendicularly until it reaches the periosteum and the product is injected. Overcorrection and choice of inappropriate filler may lead to unacceptable aesthetic results. Superficial injections in this area will lead to a Tyndall effect (Fig. 6).

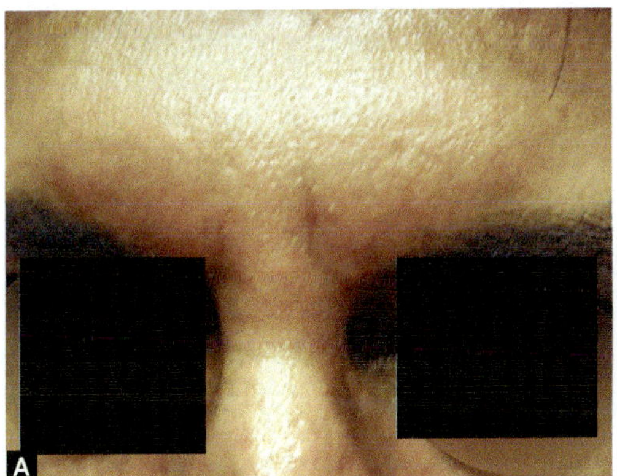

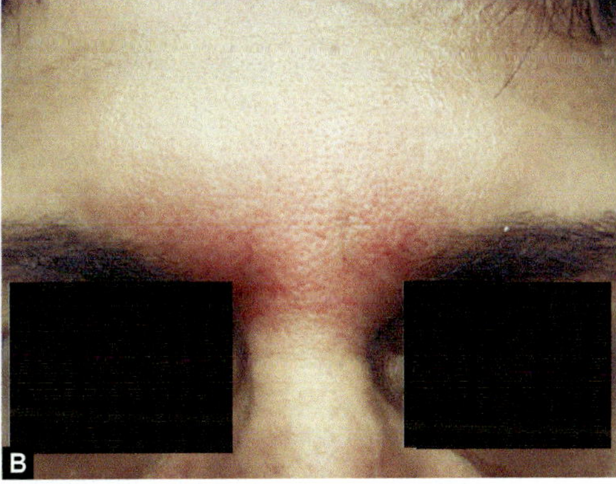

FIG. 5: Glabella: Frown line. **A,** Pretreatment and **B,** after injection.

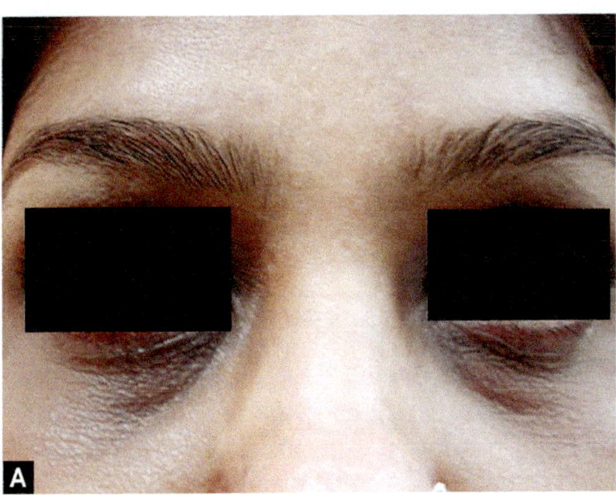

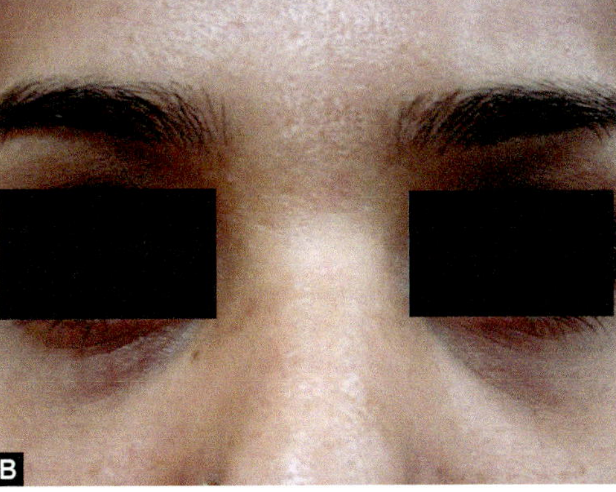

FIG. 6: Periorbital area: **A,** Pretreatment and **B,** after injection.

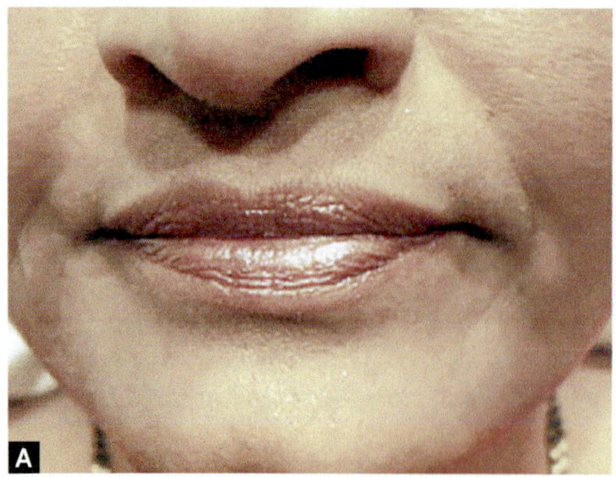

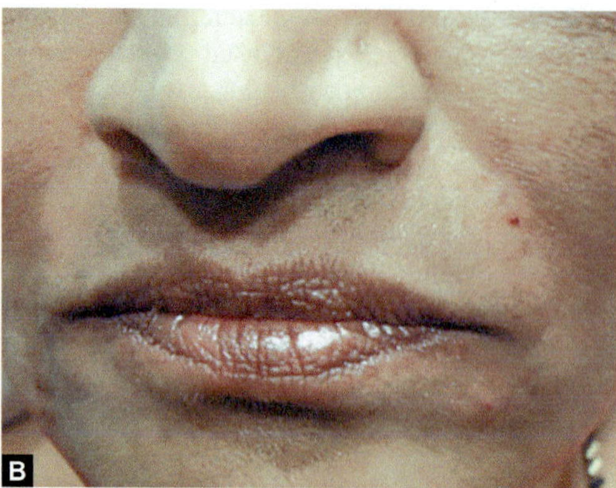

FIG. 7: Nasolabial folds: A, Pretreatment and B, after injection.

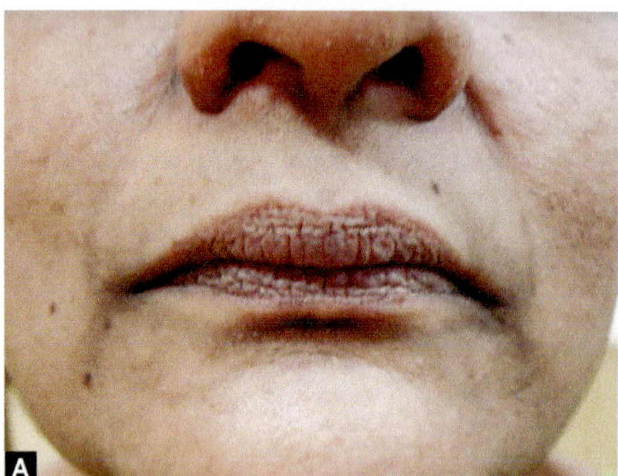

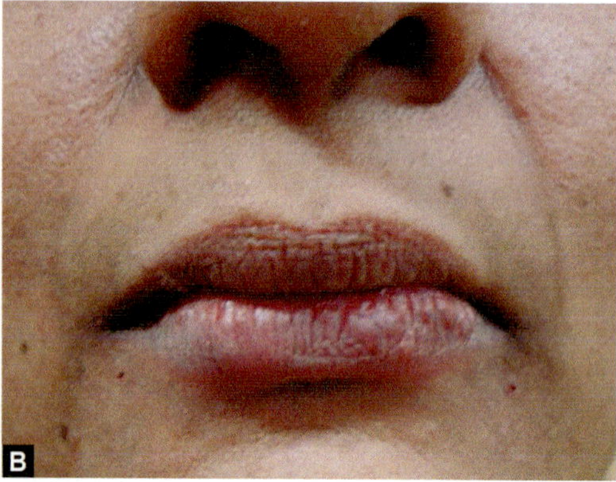

FIG. 8: Lip augmentation: **A,** Pretreatment and **B,** after injection.

Nasolabial Folds

It is good for the clinician to mark the area to be treated with an eyebrow pencil while the patient is smiling. One has to visualize the fold during the injection for better results. Injections to be done medial to the fold to avoid cheek ptosis. At the paranasal area, a fanning technique is useful to fill the depression adequately followed by a linear threading technique along the entire length of the fold to give good results. The number of puncture sites can be minimized by using long needles (Fig. 7).

Lips

Anesthesia is usually recommended when treating the lips. A 25 G, 1 inch long needle is preferable to reduce the number of puncture sites and bruising. The length of the lips are approached from the corners of the mouth and injected in a tunneling fashion to cover the entire length of the upper and lower lips. The proportion of the upper lip to lower lip to be maintained as overcorrection can lead to duck bill appearance. A short course of oral steroids can be administered to avoid excessive swelling in the postprocedure period (Fig. 8).

Marionette Lines

The depressed area near the corner of the mouth may be filled using a fanning technique, if the depression is more and also to give a lift effect to corners of the mouth. The rest of the marionette lines can be filled using a series of parallel linear threads. The area has to be then massaged to mold the area to suit the natural contours (Fig. 9).

COMBINING FILLERS

Combining different HAs can be used to optimize patient's expectations. Different hyalurons may be layered on one another to maximize volumization and thereby the results. Usually thicker products are injected more deeply and thinner products more

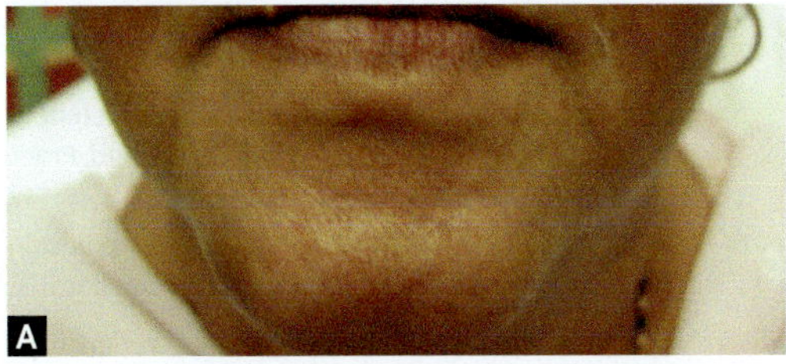

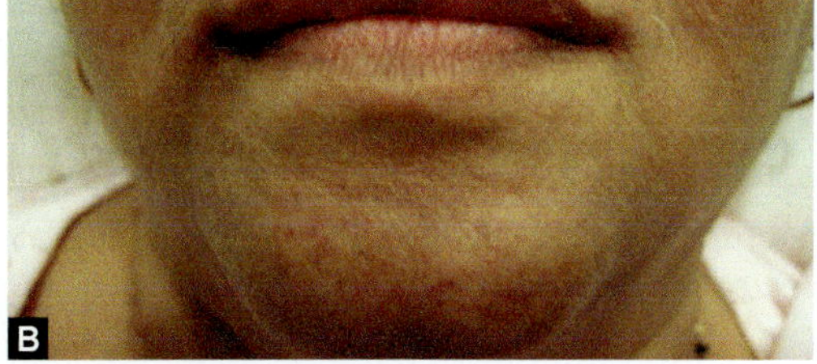

FIG. 9: Marionette lines: **A,** Pretreatment and **B,** after injection.

superficially in the same session or sequentially to achieve results.[12]

Post Treatment Care

The treated area should not be manipulated by the patient for the next 48 hours. Strict instructions should be given to avoid touching the area for first 6 hours. The treated area should not be exposed to extreme heat or cold for the first 48 hours as this may lead to an inflammatory response. A touch up treatment may be recommended after 2–4 weeks, if necessary. Bruising and pain in the injected area can be treated conservatively.

COMPLICATIONS

Complications with temporary fillers like HA are relatively rare and complications are less severe compared to permanent fillers (Table 3).

Onset may be early occurring few hours to days after the treatment or may be delayed occurring from weeks to years following treatment.

Erythema or Redness after Dermal Fillers

Erythema may be transient or persistent lasting for days to months. Transient erythema can be managed by appropriate makeup. Permanent erythema can be managed by using topical corticosteroid or tacrolimus. Redness can also be reduced by propranolol 20 mg or ibuprofen 200 mg BID. Procedures such as intense pulsed light, intralesional steroids, or dermabrasion may also be helpful.

Infections

Infections may occur due to reactivation of herpes simplex or due to improper antiseptic measures. To avoid reactivation in a suspected individual, antivirals may be given for 5 days starting 2 days prior to procedure. Topical application of polidocanol 10% cream may also be useful in prevention.[13,14] Antibacterials such as azithromycin may be given 2 days prior to the procedure and 3 days postoperatively.[15]

TABLE 3: Common complications after filler injections

Early	Late
	Site of injection
Erythema, edema, itching and bruising	Nodule
Injection-reactivation/*de novo*	Erythema persistent
Hypersensitivity	Infection: Atypical mycobacteria
Lumping and clumping	Granulomas
Discoloration: Red and hyperpigmentation	
Tissue necrosis	

Lumping and Clumping

Beading due to lumping or clumping can occur if too much product is placed too superficially due to incorrect technique. Usually this dissipates with time but if it persists after 6–8 weeks, intralesional hyaluronidase may be given or excess material can be removed through a small stab incision made with a no. 11 scalpel blade, if necessary.

Skin Necrosis

Skin necrosis following injection is a rare but a clinically important potential complication which needs early recognition and effective management. Necrosis is known to occur in the glabellar area (supratrochlear artery), nasolabial fold (angular artery), and lips (labial artery). It is caused for interruption of the vascular supply and occlusion of the vessels in that area by compression, injury and/or obstruction of the vessels.[12]

Blindness

Blindness after dermal filler is rare as with all types of injectables like autologous fat, collagen injections and occurs due to injection in the supratrochlear artery.[16]

Granulomas

Hypersensitivity and granuloma formation is less common with HA fillers compared to permanent fillers. Intralesional steroids with or without 5-fluoruracil may be injected into the granuloma at repeated intervals until resolution. In resistant cases, a course of oral steroids, minocycline, colchicine, or cyclosporine may be tried in view of their anti-inflammatory, immunomodulatory, and anti-granulomatous properties.

Lipoatrophy

Facial atrophy has been described in cheeks after injection of resorbable fillers. This complication can arise several months after the injection of the dermal fillers.[17]

CONCLUSION

Soft tissue augmentation with HA as dermal fillers last longer than bovine and human collagen with better patient satisfaction and lesser incidence of complications when compared to semipermanent and permanent fillers. In addition, they look natural and feel natural resulting in a more beautiful appearance.

REFERENCES

1. Hanke CW. Filler materials. In: Thiers B, Lang PG Jr. (Eds). Year Book of Dermatology and Dermatologic Surgery. Philadelphia, PA: Mosby; 2004. pp. 1-15.
2. Klein AW, Elson ML. The history of substances for soft tissue augmentation. Dermatol Surg. 2000;26(12);1096-105.
3. Hurza GJ. Rejuvenating the aging face, editorial. Arch Dermatol. 2004;140(11):1383-6.
4. Monheit GD, Coleman KM. Hyaluronic acid fillers. Dermatol Ther. 2006;19(3):141-50.
5. Solish N, Beer K. Hyaluronic acids: basic science. In: Jones D (Ed). Injectable Fillers Principles and Practice. Oxford: Wiley Blackwell; 2010. pp.19-26.
6. Murray CA, Zloty D, Warshawski L. The evolution of soft tissue fillers in clinical practice. Dermatol Clin. 2005;23(2):343-63.
7. Vedamurthy M. Soft tissue augmentation: use of hyaluronic acid as dermal filler. Indian J Dermatol Venereol Leprol. 2004;70(6):383-7.
8. Bhatia AC. The clinical image: archiving clinical processes and an entire specialty. Arch Dermatol. 2006;142(1):96-98.
9. Monheit GD, Coleman KM. Hyaluronic acid fillers. Dermatol Ther. 2006;19(3):141-50.
10. Busso M. Guidelines for local anaesthesia in use of injectable fillers. In: Jones D (Ed). Injectable Fillers: Principles and Practice. Oxford: Wiley Blackwell; 2010. pp. 8-18.
11. Smith KC. Ice anesthesia for injection of dermal fillers. Dermatol Surg. 2010;36(s1):812-4.
12. Kenneth B. Fillers for facial rejuvenation. Dermatol Clin. 2009;27(41):427-32.
13. Habbema L, De Boulle K, Rodgers GA, et al. n-Docosanol 10% cream in the treatment of recurrent herpes labialis: a randomised, double-blind, placedo-controlled study. Acta Derm Venereol. 1996;76:479-81.
14. Glaich AS, Cohen JL, Goldberg LH. Injection necrosis of the glabella. Dermatol Surg. 2006;32(2):276-81.
15. DeBoulle K. Management of complications after implantation of fillers. J Cosmet Dermatol. 2004;3(1):2-15.
16. Mc Cleve DE, Goldstein JC. Blindness secondary to injections in the nose, mouth and face: cause and prevention. Ear Nose Throat J. 1995;74(3):182-8.
17. Lemperle G, Rullan PP, Gauthier-Hazan N. Dermal filler complications. Plastic Reconstr Surg. 2006;118(3S):92S-107S.

23 CHAPTER

Soft Tissue Augmentation of the Upper Face

Amit Luthra

INTRODUCTION

Fillers for upper face rejuvenation is a recent phenomenon with facial aesthetics undergoing a sea change in author's understanding with the newer concept of volume replacement and structural support replacing the older concept of dynamic and static lines. A decade ago, filler treatments of the face were more focused on elimination or effacement of facial lines and grooves, and more of line chasing.[1] The current trend revolves around the paradigm shift from focal to global corrections.[1] The distinction between the usage of botulinum toxin A (BoNT-A) and the so-called dermal fillers is getting blurred. The use of fillers is on rising trend especially for eyebrows, forehead and temples thereby changing the course of holistic facial rejuvenation. Hyaluronic acid (HA) and fat are the preferred fillers with HA being more widely used.

HISTORY

It has long been acknowledged that facial aging is the result of deterioration and descent of cutaneous structures due to downward gravitational pull, hormonal changes, photodamage and smoking among others.[2] However, skeletal remodeling and subcutaneous fat redistribution and loss are now recognized as key elements responsible for the appearance of age.[2]

Two decades ago, fillers for the face were used for augmentation of nasolabial folds which gradually shifted its focus to midface in the past ten years. The current concept is to look at a global volumization which includes augmentation of the temples and forehead besides the midface and the lower face. These areas are potential mines of complications as it is evident by an increase in number of blindness following filler and fat injections in these locations. Cases of blindness mostly irreversible, from aesthetic filler injections have been reported from Asia, Europe, and NorthAmerica.[3] Autologous fat appears to be the most frequent filler causing blindness. Some cases of partial visual recovery have been reported with HA and calcium hydroxylapatite fillers.[3]

ANATOMY

Key aspects of safe and successful injection of fillers in the upper face include a thorough knowledge of the location of fat compartments and neurovascular structures.[4] Knowing the ideal place and the correct level to inject the filler along with an understanding of the antomy, specially the location of the vessels ought to be the key factor in these risky areas. The subcutaneous fat of the face is divided into two fat compartments- superficial and deep. Facial aging is, in part characterized by how these compartments change with age. The concept of separate compartments of fat suggests that the face does not age as a confluent or composite mass.[5] While treating the upper face, one needs to be aware of depletion of the forehead and lateral-temporal cheek fat pad so as to target the specific areas. This knowledge has created a topographical map allowing for the direct and precise augmentation of those compartments that are deflated prefertially.[6]

Eyebrows

When shaping the eyebrows, one needs to inject the lateral eyebrow in the deep dermis and has to be careful of the supraorbital foramen while injecting medially. Inferiorly one needs to avoid the infraorbital cavity (Fig. 1).

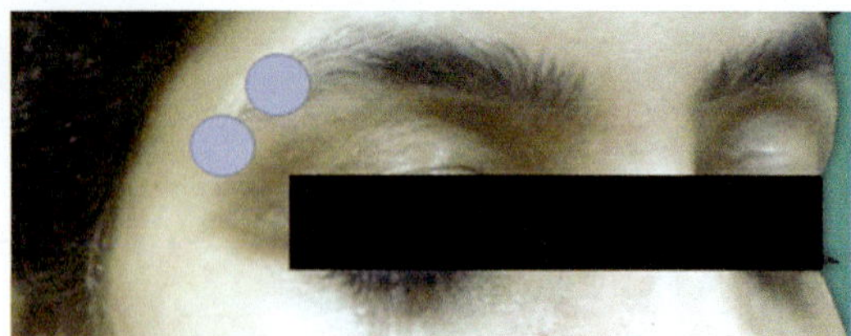

FIG. 1: Injection points for the eyebrows.

Forehead

For males, an ideal forehead shape is straight while in case of females, it is a smooth convex. When injecting the forehead, one needs to inject supra-periosteally in the forehead between the two temporal crests staying at least 1 cm above the eyebrow. The goal is to correct the hollow in the lower two-thirds of the forehead. One can use the needle or the cannula but need to avoid the supratrochlear, supraorbital, and the superficial temporal vessels.

Temples

Identification of the superficial temporal artery and vein is of paramount importance before injecting the temples. One has to demarcate the temporal crest, lateral orbital rim, and the zygomatic arch. Two points can be injected deep on the bone, the first (shown in black in Fig. 2) can be visualized by drawing a circle of 2 cm diameter superior to the zygomatic arch and posterior to the lateral orbital rim. The second point (shown in white in Fig. 2) used is at the intersection,1 cm perpendicular to the temporal crest and the lateral orbital rim.

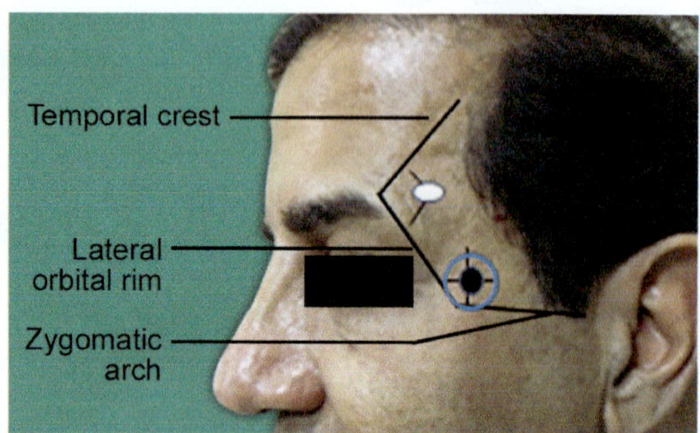

FIG. 2: Temple injection points (two-point technique).

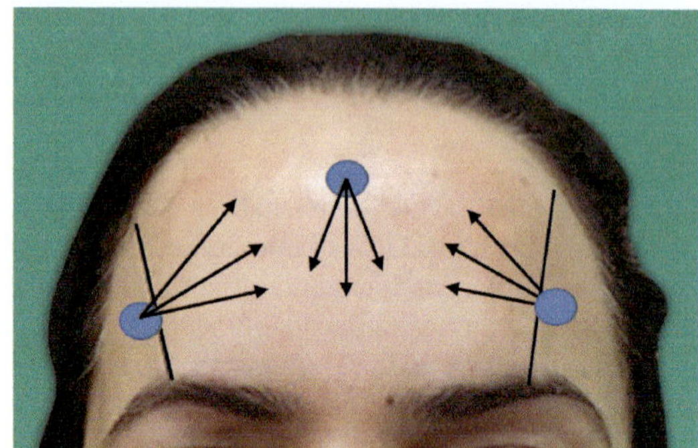

FIG. 3: Injection of the forehead with a cannula.

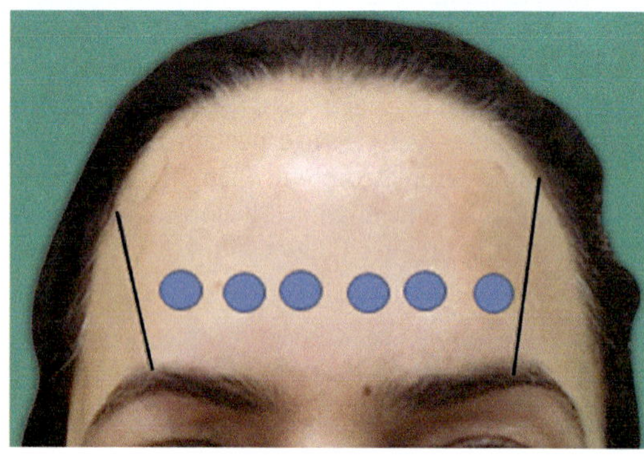

FIG. 4: Injection of the forehead with boluses with a needle.

PROCEDURE

Eyebrow

Either a needle or a cannula is used to deposit a soft filler in the lateral one-third of the eyebrows. When using the needle, the two-point technique as shown in figure 1,should be utilized for optimal results. Care should be taken in preventing the filler from traveling to the infraorbital cavity by the use of the non dominant hand. Overfilling needs to be avoided. In males, generally this area should be avoided for fear of feminizing the male face.

Forehead

Injections can be given using both needle and cannula,with special emphasis on avoiding the superficial temporal, supratrochlear, andsupraorbital vessels. Important point to remember when using a cannula,as shown in figure 3, is to make the opening of the cannula lateral to thetemporal crest, 1 cm above the supraorbital rim for the lateral forehead filling and in the upper one-third of the forehead for the mid forehead filling. Multiple fannings are done across the forehead. Whileinjecting with the needle,one needs to inject between the two temporal crests using small five to six boluses, 1 cm superior to the eyebrows (Fig. 4). Massaging is essential to get a smooth surface. It should be smooth convex in females and straight in males. Recommended volumes are 2 mL across the forehead for females and 0.5 mL across the middle forehead in males.

Temples

Using a needle is preferred and involves deep supraperiosteal injections as illustrated in figure 2. Point 1 is the temporal area within a 2 cm diameter (blackened area in Fig. 2) and the second point is at the intersection of the lines 1 cm perpendicular to the lateral orbital rim and the temporal crest (white area in Fig. 2). Volumizing fillers are used to fill the concavity of the temples so as to achieve a convex contour in females and a straight contour in males. The recommendation for females is to inject 0.7 mL and 0.3 mL at point 1 and 2 respectively, whereas for males it is 0.5 mL at both the points.

Feeling the pulsation of the superficial temporal artery and marking it out cannot be overemphasized. It is highly recommended to slowly aspirate before injecting to rule out intravascular injections. Care needs to be taken to avoid displacement of the product into the uppereyelid by applying finger pressure.

When using a cannula one can use a soft filler and deposit it subcutaneously on top of the temporalis muscle (Fig. 5). Though this appears to be safer in preventing intravascular injections, it can cause an uneven surface and venous congestion.

POSTOPERATIVE INSTRUCTIONS

Patients needs to be informed and made aware of the possible signs of vascular compromise like blanching and severe pain. Pain may be absent, if HA is used with an anesthetic (Figs 6 and 7) or can be delayed, if

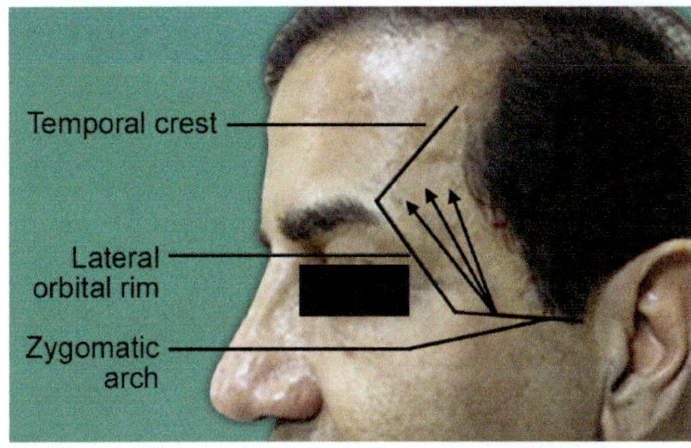

FIG. 5: Injecting the temples with a cannula.

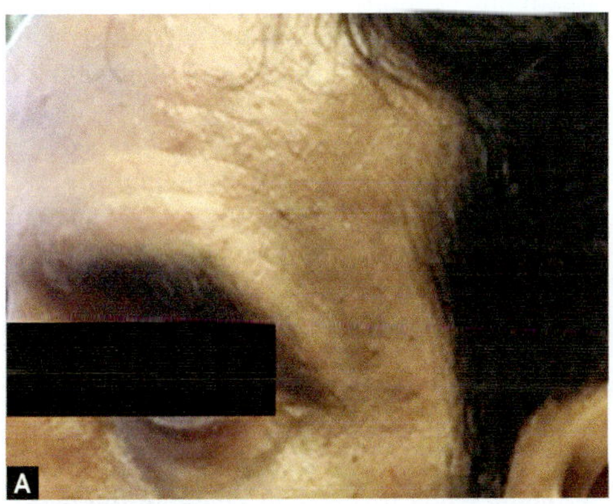

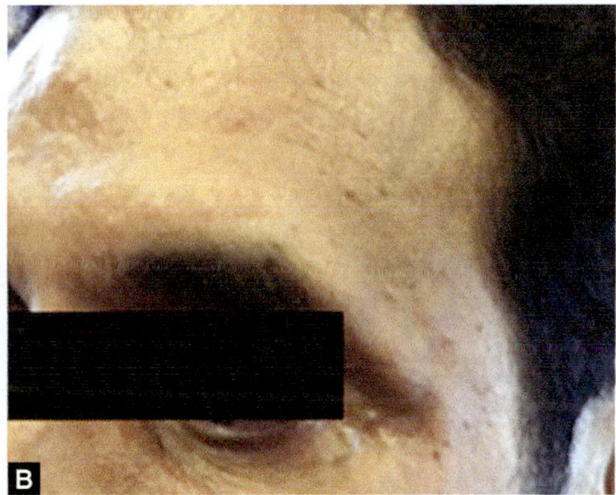

FIG. 6: Temples before and after fillers (0.5 mL of soft filler each side with a cannula).

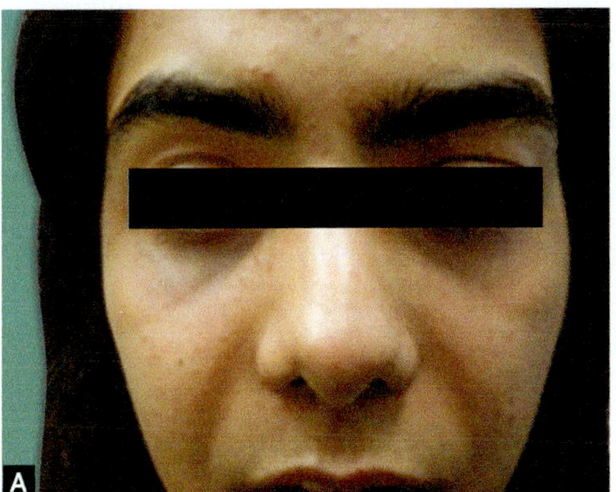

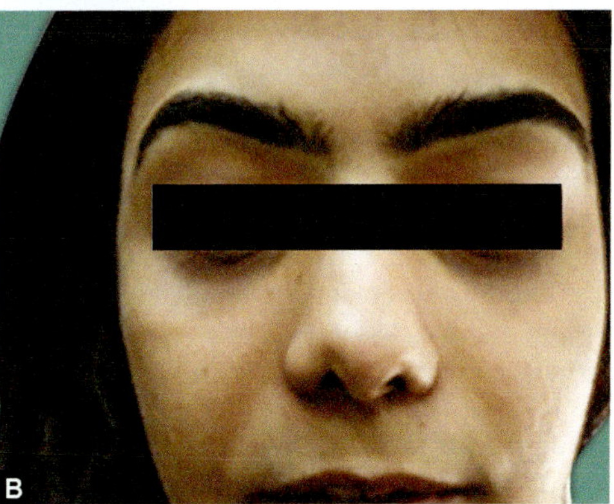

FIG. 7: Eyebrows shaped with hyaluronic acid. **A,** Before and **B,** after.

caused by external compression of a vessel. Avoiding nonsteroidal anti-inflammatory drug (NSAIDs) in the first 6 hours after the procedure can also prevent the masking of pain.

Manipulation of the filler, exercising, alcohol and parlor services should be avoided for a minimum period of 48 hours post procedure. Other aesthetic procedures like lasers and peels are better done at a gap of 15–30 days.

COMPLICATIONS

The adverse effects can be divided into early and late and range from bruising to necrosis. Understanding the anatomy, limitations of the filler and proper technique can reduce the risk of adverse effects.[7]

The most dreaded complication in these areas is that of vascular compromise which refers to direct intravascular injection or rarely extravascular compression of a vessel by a filler. Intravascular injection of the filler into the supratrochlear, supraorbital, and the anterior branch of the superficial temporal arteries can result in the formation of emboli, which may impede the blood supply of the smaller anastomosing vessels. Embolization of the cerebral and ocular arteries may lead to strokes and blindness.

Glabellar area is the most prone area to necrosis because it has the supratrochlear artery giving off small-sized arterial branches with a poor collateral circulation. There is need to exercise caution while injecting the forehead and the use of a thicker bore blunt cannula like a 25 G cannula is highly recommended.

For injecting the temples, supraperiosteal injections with a sharp needle or subcutaneous injections with a blunt cannula are recommended to avoid the superficial temporal artery. Injecting in the subcutaneous plane with a cannula can lead to an uneven surface in the temples and visible vein congestion after the treatment. Massaging the filler post procedure helps in overcoming this problem.

When injecting with a sharp needle, aspiration before injecting (for a reasonable period of time) can be a helpful exercise to prevent intravascular injections.

Superficial placement of the filler in the forehead can also lead to uneven and an undulated forehead, which may require dissolution with hyaluronidase. Hyaluronidase can dissolve subcutaneous nodules or correct excessive quantities of injected filler. Knowledge of the use, methods of application, and adverse effects of hyaluronidase is essential for the aesthetic practitioner.[8]

BOX 1 Patient alignment checklist for upper face fillers

- Synchronization of patient and physician expectations
- Information on immediate and late post procedure outcomes
- Number of syringes and cost
- Longevity of product used
- Repetitive and temporary nature of treatment
- Adverse events
- Post procedure instructions (for signs of vascular compromise)

Bruising is a common procedural concern. Patients need to stop NSAIDs, vitamin E, green tea, and Ginkgo biloba containing vitamins at least a week prior to the procedure. Infections are rare with proper asepsis.

Tips

Knowledge of the facial anatomy is key to successful treatment. One should have adequate injection experience in other areas of the face before venturing into this difficult terrain. Aspiration and slowly injecting small boluses are the keys to success.

For best results and minimal adverse events, a checklist like the one in box 1 is helpful.[9]

CONCLUSION

Fillers in the upper face areas like eyebrows, forehead, and temples are challenging but gratifying. They add the “icing on the cake” post midface and lower face filler injections. Using a cannula or a needle may be a personal choice but cannula definitely scores over a needle when it comes to safety. In the temples, it is recommended to use a needle for better results. Vascular compromise because of embolization of filler intravascularly can be disasterous and can cause blindness and strokes. A good understanding of the anatomy will be helpful in preventing these complications.In fact, Sandoval et al.[10] in their review offacial fat compartments and the placement of fillers have called these fat compartments as the “GPS” for the injection of facial fillers.

REFERENCES

1. Arsiwala SZ. Current trends in facial rejuvenation with fillers. J Cutan Aesthet Surg. 2015;8(3):125-6.
2. Coleman SR, Grover R. The anatomy of the aging face: volume loss and changes in 3-dimensional topography. Aesthet Surg J. 2006;26(1S):S4-9.

3. Carruthers JD, Fagien S, Rohrich RJ, et al. Blindness caused by cosmetic filler injection: a review of cause and therapy. Plast Reconstr Surg. 2014;134(6):1197-201.
4. Sykes JM, Cotofana S, Trevidic P, et al. Upper face: clinical anatomy and regional approaches with injectable fillers. Plast Reconstr Surg. 2015;136(5 Suppl):204S-18S.
5. Rohrich RJ, Pessa JE. The fat compartments of the face: anatomy and clinical implications for cosmetic surgery. Plast Reconstr Surg. 2007;119(7):2219-27.
6. Ramanadham SR, Rohrich RJ. Newer understanding of specific anatomic targets in the aging face as applied to injectables: superficial and deep facial fat compartments–An evolving target for site-specific facial augmentation. Plast Reconstr Surg. 2015;136(5 Suppl):49S-55S.
7. Gladstone HB, Cohen JL. Adverse effects when injecting facial fillers. Semin Cutan Med Surg. 2007;26(1):34-9.
8. Cavallini M, Gazzola R, Metalla M, et al. The role of hyaluronidase in the treatment of complications from hyaluronic acid dermal fillers. Aesthet Surg J. 2013;33(8): 1167-74
9. Luthra A. Shaping lips with fillers. J Cutan Aesthet Surg. 2015;8(3):139-42.
10. Sandoval SE, Cox JA, Koshy JC, et al. Facial fat compartments: a guide to filler placement. Semin Plast Surg. 2009;23(4):283-87.

24

CHAPTER

Soft Tissue Augmentation of the Midface

Jaishree Sharad

INTRODUCTION

Midface comprises of the middle one-third of the face, lying between two parallel lines drawn through the nasion and subnasale (Fig. 1).

When we assess the midface, the primary areas we look at are the infraorbital hollow, the tear trough, the submalar triangle, the nasolabial fold, and the nose. The submalar triangle is an inverted triangle bounded superiorly by the zygomatic prominence, medially by nasolabial fold, and laterally by the body of the masseter muscle.

Midface is considered the support system of a youthful face. A youthful midface in a female comprises of no shadows under the eyes, high cheek bones, and full cheeks. Normally, the cheek mound should not extend higher than the limbus of the lower eyelid and should be ovoid. The cheek axis is angled from the lateral commissure to the base of the ear helix. Each malar prominence has a defined apex, eccentrically located within the cheek oval, below and lateral to the lateral canthus (Fig. 2).[1]

Another mark of beauty is the double ogee curve which is visible if you look at the face from the side such that both medial canthi can be seen. There is a characteristic convexity of the tail of the brow that flows into a concavity of the lateral orbital wall (the upper ogee). This is joined by the convexity of the upper midface that flows into the concavity of the lower midface (the lower ogee).[2]

FIG. 1: Midface—Nasion to subnasale.

According to Dr Arthur Swift, the ideal facial width for most ethnicities falls approximately Phi (1.618) times the intercanthal distance from the medial canthus to the ipsilateral cheek (Fig. 3).[3]

CHEEK AUGMENTATION AND MIDFACE LIFT

The cheek is framed superiorly by the malar complex and inferiorly by the mandible. The size and shape of cheek are determined by the musculature (masseter), the size of parotid gland, and the buccal fat.

ANATOMY OF MIDFACE

The midface skeleton is formed by the maxilla in the medial and middle thirds and by the body and arch

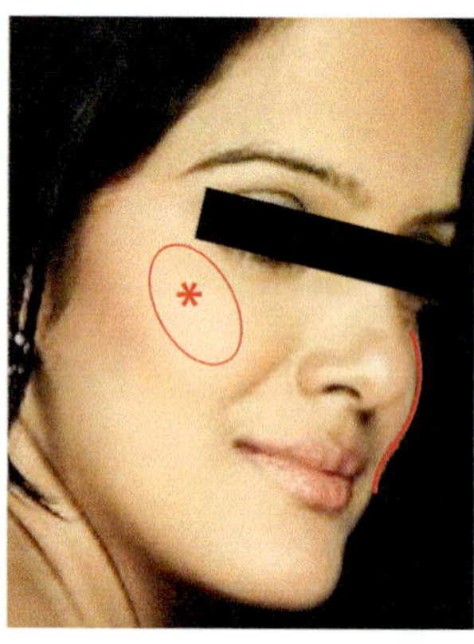

FIG. 2: Ogee curves and an ovoid, angular cheek mound with eccentric apex.

of the zygoma in the lateral third. Studies have shown that aging results in significant bone resorption with loss of projection of the maxilla.[4,5]

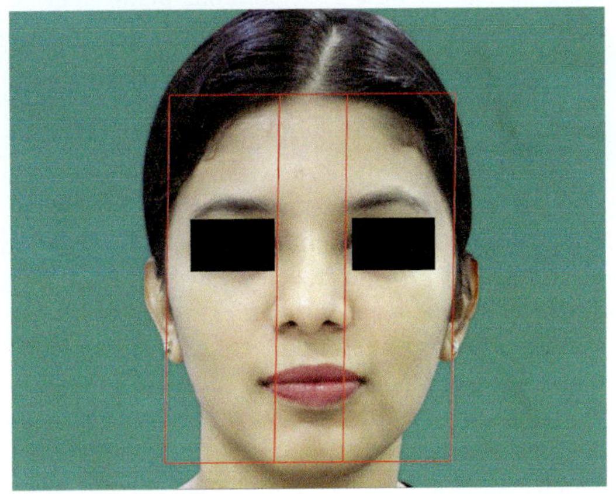

FIG. 3: Phi facial width proportion (i.e., medial canthus to medial canthus measures X; medial canthus to ipsilateral cheek apex measures 1.618X).

The superficial and deep fat compartments have been described in chapter 21. The superficial fat pads of the midface namely the infraorbital fat, the nasolabial fat, and the medial fat pad together form the malar fat pad. The deep fat pads of midface comprise of the deep medial cheek fat pad, the medial and lateral suborbicularis oculi fat (SOOF), and buccal extension of the deep buccal fat (Fig. 4).[6]

Rohrich et al. documented that with aging there is a hypertrophy of the superficial fat pads such as infraorbital fat, lateral temporal cheek fat and submental fat, and a concomitant atrophy of the deep cheek fat.[7]

AGING MIDFACE

As one ages, bone resorption and soft tissue atrophy leads to deflation and ptosis of midface leading to sagging and a haggard look (Fig. 5).

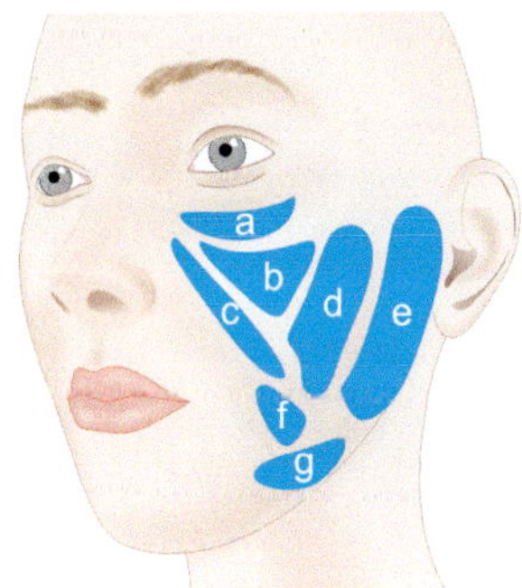

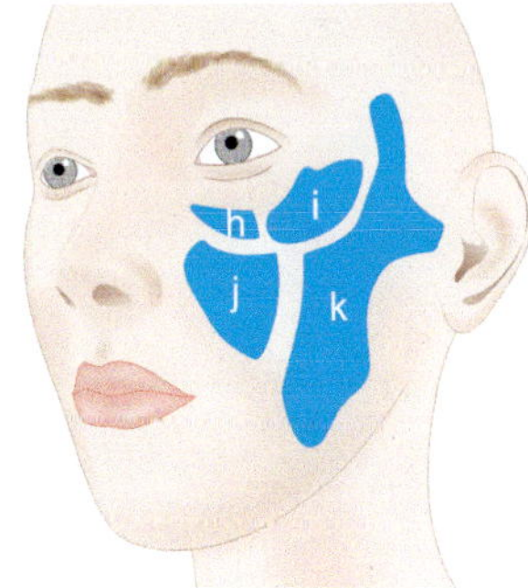

FIG. 4: Fat compartments of midface.

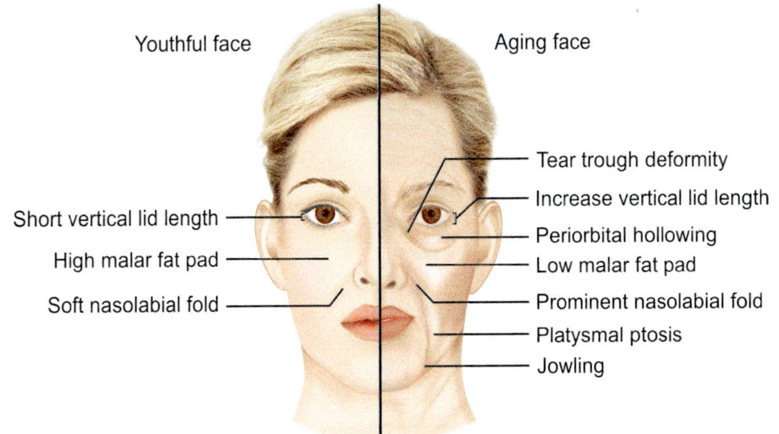

FIG. 5: Aging midface.

VOLUMIZATION OF THE MIDFACE

The midface can be divided into three regions by the Hinderer's lines, namely: (i) The anteromedial, (ii) The zygomaticomalar, and (iii) The submalar.[8]

Hinderer's lines comprise of two intersecting lines: (i) One from the ala to the tragus, and (ii) One from the lateral canthus to the commissure of the ipsilateral lip. Volumization and lifting of the midface will involve injecting a filler into any of the quadrants made by Hinderer's lines depending on the patient's requirement.

Injecting filler into the lateral zygoma (zygomaticomalar region) will increase width of the midface and shift the focal point laterally. This is usually done in Caucasians while treating midface.[9]

Injecting filler into the anteromedial region will result in anterior projection of the midface and may shift the focal point medially.[10] Injections into both lateral zygoma and anteromedial region are done in the supraperiosteal plane.

Injecting filler into the submalar region and preauricular region will help to support and complete the frame of the cheek. Injections into both these areas are done in the subcutaneous plane to avoid deeper structures such as the superficial temporal vessels and parotid gland (Fig. 6).

Small boluses or linear retrograde injections may be given.

The deep medial cheek fat compartment is said to be the key space for injection in order to get an optimal midface augmentation. This was proven by Rohrich et al. who injected normal saline into the deep medial cheek fat compartment of a male cadaver which resulted in effacement of nasolabial folds (NLFs) and tear trough.[11,12]

Some authors prefer to use the MD codes as their injection points. Others prefer to inject in areas which appear hollow (Fig. 7 and Table 1).[13,14]

To create a lifting effect, a filler with high "G" or high cohesivity is selected. The product is placed

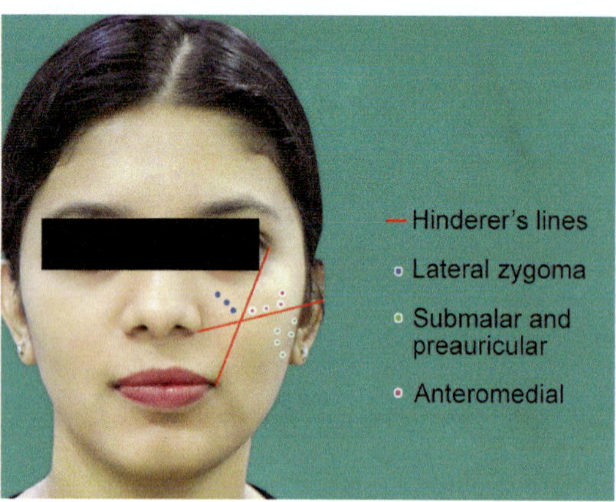

FIG. 6: Hinderer's lines and various injection points for midface filler injection.

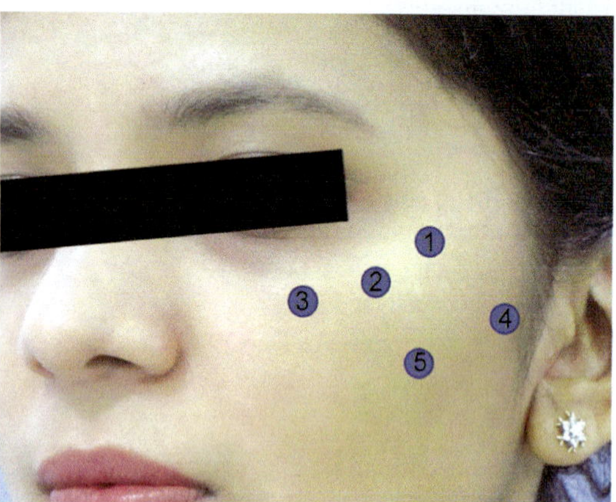

FIG. 7: MD codes for cheek and midface augmentation.

TABLE 1: MD codes for cheek augmentation.

Points in Fig. 7	Code	Injection area	Structures affected	Result
1	Ck1	Zygomatic arch	Bone structure and lateral suborbicularis oculi fat (SOOF)	Lifts the cheek and gives support to eyebrow and lower eyelid
2	Ck2	Zygomatic eminence	Bone structure and lateral SOOF	Provides projection of the cheek and shortening of palpebral-malar sulcus
3	Ck3	Anteromedial cheek	Bone structure; deep malar fat pad; medial SOOF	Improves the medial lid-cheek junction and softens the tear trough
4	Ck4	Lateral lower cheek/parotid area	Subcutaneous	Addresses the sunken area at the parotid level and preauricular volume loss; lifts the jawline
5	Ck5	Submalar	Subcutaneous	Addresses the sunken area and improves volume loss in the submalar area

vertically in the supraperiosteal plane to create two to three pillars. As the needle is withdrawn, the product is placed to create a tent pole effect and a visible lift can be seen. Thirty gauge needles or 25 gauge cannulas are preferred to prevent bruising. Small aliquots of 0.5 mL or less are preferred per injection site. In addition, a filler with low "G" prime may be used superficially in the mid-dermis to create feathering of the cheek contour.

The key in females is to highlight the cheek apex and maintain ogee curve. Avoid sausage like folds in the cheeks. Swift and Remington define cheek apex by a point at the intersection of a line drawn from the nasal alar groove to the upper tragus and a line drawn vertically down from the midpoint of the lateral orbital rim (Figs 8 to 10).[3]

Males prefer correction of hollows and improvement of jowls (Fig. 11).

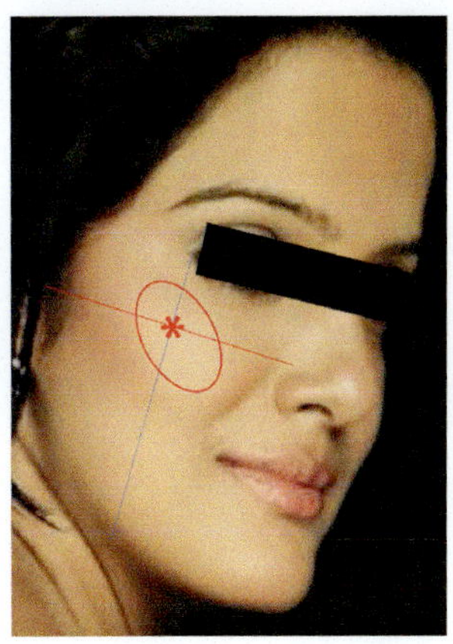

FIG. 8: Cheek apex (star) defined by the intersection of a line drawn from the nasal alar groove to the upper tragus and a line drawn vertically down from the midpoint of the lateral orbital rim.

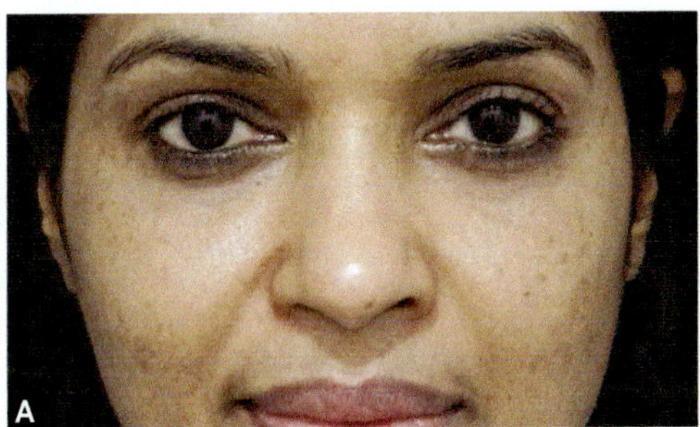

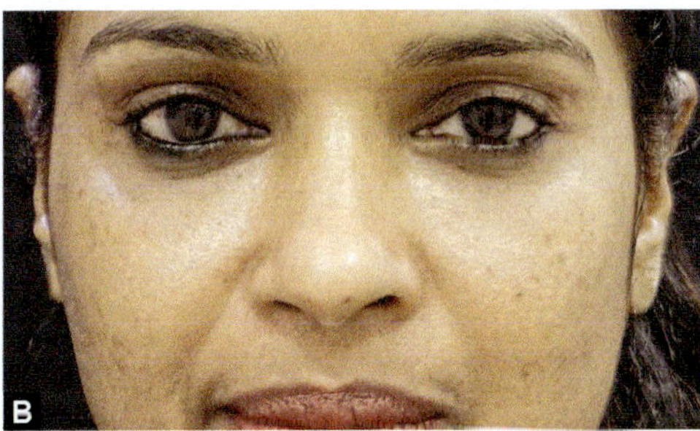

FIG. 9: A, Before injecting midface with 1 mL of Juvederm Voluma; and **B,** After injecting midface, note the improvement of the tear trough, nasolabial folds, and the lifting effect.

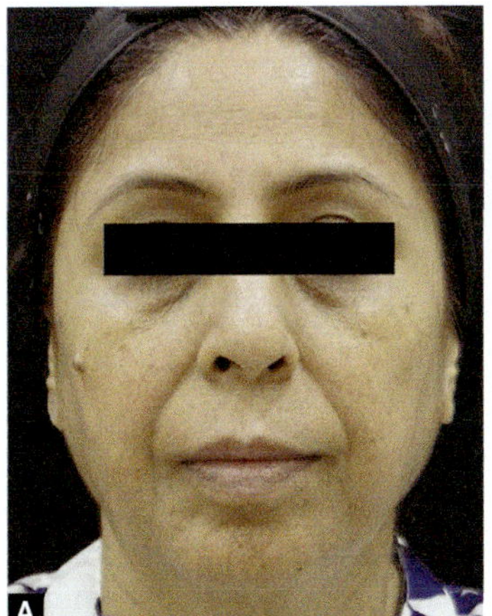

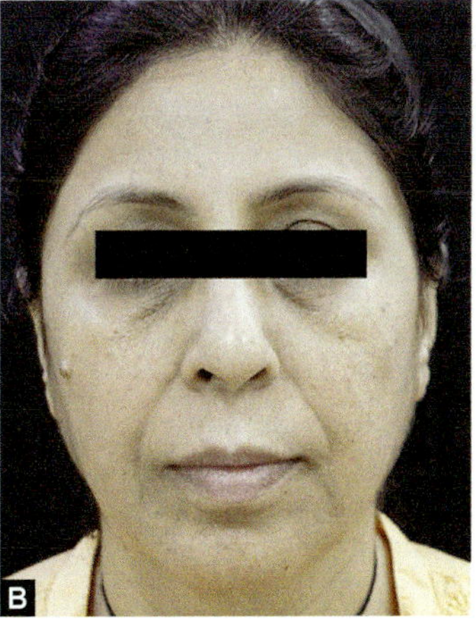

FIG. 10: A, Before injecting the midface and lower face with 2 mL of Juvederm Voluma; and **B,** After injecting the midface and lower face with 2 mL of Juvederm Voluma.

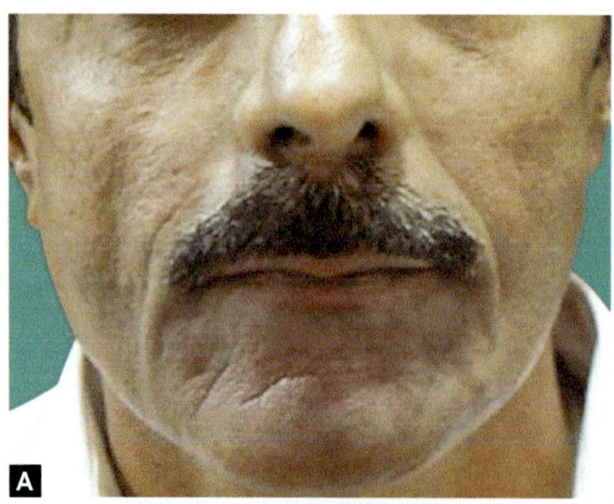
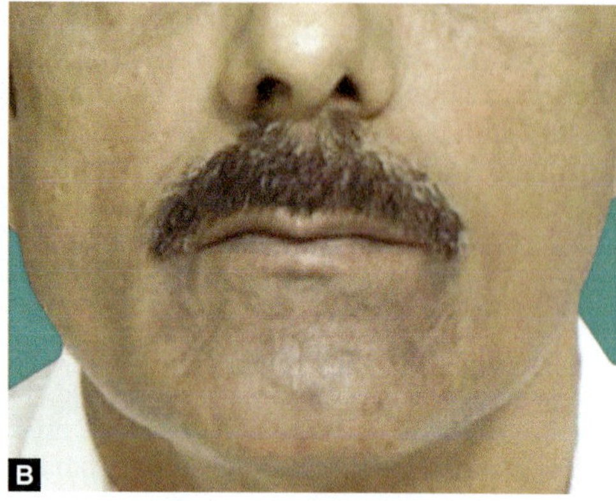

FIG. 11: A, Male face before injecting with 2 mL of Perlane **B,** after injecting with 2 mL of Perlane.

TABLE 2: Consensus recommendations for optimal augmentation of the Asian midface

	Augmentation of the anteromedial cheek	Augmentation of the midzygoma region	Preauricular and submalar contouring
Technique	Vertical depot with needle or fanning with cannula	Vertical depot with needle or linear threading or fanning	Multiple puncture with needle or fanning with cannula
Plane	Deep supraperiosteal	Deep supraperiosteal	Subdermal
Product	High-viscosity HA or CaHA	High-viscosity HA or CaHA	High-viscosity HA or CaHA
Volume	0.3–1.5 mL per side	0.25–1 mL per side	0.5–2 mL per side

HA, hyaluronic acid; CaHA, calcium hydroxylapatite.

ETHNIC DIFFERENCES

Asians have a wide face with a more flat medial and central portion due to a structurally deficient medial maxilla and nasal spine. This is also responsible for a prominent tear trough at a younger age. Hence, it is important to fill the medial part of the midface to provide projection of the midface, improvement of tear trough, and in older patients restoration of volume too. Filling the lateral part will only end up in a wider midface which looks disproportionate (Table 2).[15]

Caucasians on the other hand have narrower faces and prefer a lateral cheek projection.[9]

GENDER DIFFERENCES[16]

Midface in males has less anterior projection both in the lateral part and in the anteromedial cheek area. The nasolabial angle is 90–95° in men as opposed to 95–100° in women. The nose is wider and longer in males. Lambros's theory suggests that as one ages, the cheek rotates from up to down, and lateral to medial producing a pronounced hollowing. The tip of the nose begins to droop too.[17]

Fillers are usually used to correct the tear trough, NLFs, and the lateral part of the cheek to give support. It is important not to feminize the male face by giving too much lateral projection or excessive fullness. The injection sites in male patients along the zygomatic arch are usually lower and with less volume.

TEAR TROUGH DEFORMITY

Tear trough deformity is characterized by a sunken appearance of the under eye region resulting in a dark shadow over the lower eyelid, causing the person to look tired all the time in spite of adequate sleep. It cannot be concealed with makeup and becomes a cause of concern.

Dark circles on the other hand can be a result of actinic changes, allergies, anemia, hyperpigmentation, skin thickness, or even tear trough deformity. Venous pooling in the superficial fat pads in this region can accentuate the periorbital darkening. This becomes prominent especially if the skin is thin.[17,18]

Shadowing over the lower lids can also occur indirectly due to prolapse of orbital fat.[19]

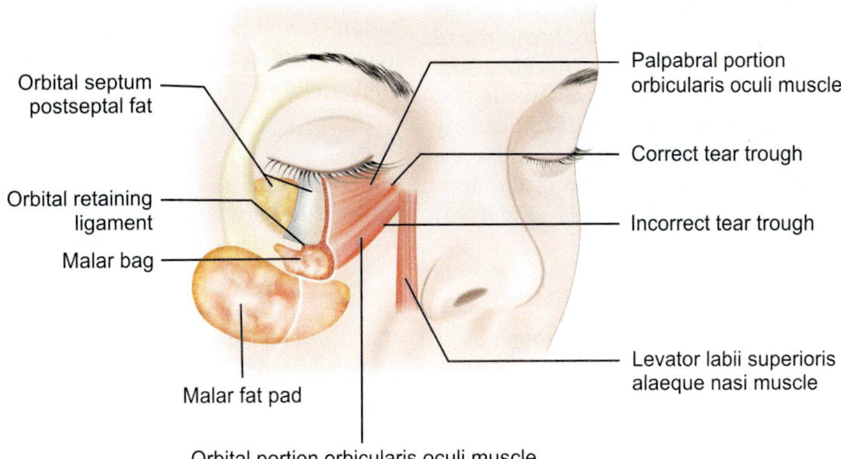

FIG. 12: Anatomy of tear trough deformity.

Causes of Tear Trough Deformity

- Structural: This could be genetic due to bone deficiency or lack of soft tissue overlying the bone in the tear trough area. Hence, it is seen at a young age.
- Changes due to aging: A downward shift of the malar fat pad, atrophy of the deep cheek fat, resorption and recession of inferolateral part of the infraorbital rim and maxilla, tethering of the tear trough ligament, and orbitomalar ligament (OML) as well as thinning of skin under the eyes can all lead to a tear trough deformity.

Anatomy

Haddock et al. described tear trough deformity as the medial periorbital hollow extending obliquely from the medial canthus to the midpupillary line (Fig. 12). It lies lateral to the lacrimal crest and corresponds to the region of the lacrimal sac. Hence, it is called the tear trough. The depression lateral to this is known as the "lid-cheek junction", "palpebromalar groove", or "nasojugal groove".[20]

There are two ligaments described in this region. The tear trough ligament arises from the maxillary periosteum immediately inferior to the orbital rim, and anterior lacrimal crest. It extends up to the midpupillary line, lies and separates the orbital and palpebral parts of the medial orbicularis oculi muscle. It has a single lamina and it terminates at the medial corneoscleral limbus, where it becomes continuous with the orbicularis retaining ligament.[21]

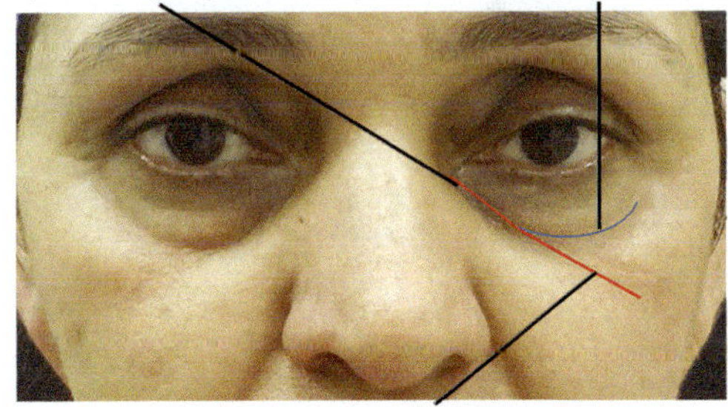

FIG. 13: The tear trough ligament, the orbital retaining ligament, and the zygomaticomalar ligament.

The orbicularis retaining ligament also known as the Orbito-malar ligament (OML) consists of two laminae. The transition from one lamina of tear trough to two laminae of the orbicularis retaining ligament has the aspect of a "Y". The OML penetrates the orbicularis oculi muscle laterally, terminating in multiple cutaneous insertions at the lid-cheek junction and lateral orbital thickening.[22]

The tear trough lies along the tear trough ligament. It is seen as a hollow or depressed line. This line when continuous with the zygomatico-cutaneous ligament is known as the Indian line or the midcheek groove. Between the orbitomalar groove and the Indian line lies the malar mound (Fig. 13).

The entire depression under the eye is best referred to as infraorbital hollow.

The medial part of the infraorbital hollow lies 4-6 mm medial to midpupillary line and corresponds to the course of the facial vein. It consists of two layers: namely (i) the skin, and (ii) orbicularis oculi muscle. The lateral part consists of seven layers: namely (i) skin, (ii) subcutaneous fat, (iii) orbicularis oculi muscle, (iv) SOOF, (v) deep fascia (here it is a continuation of the superficial lamina of the deep temporal fascia), (vi) prezygomatic fat layer, and (vii) periosteum.[13,18,20]

Classification of Volume Loss

Barton's grading system and Hirmand's classification system of the tear trough deformity are described in Tables 3 and 4.[23,24]

Bulges

One also needs to understand that there can be bulges in the infraorbital region which should be kept in mind while filling the infraorbital hollow (Fig. 14).

TABLE 3: Barton's grading system of tear trough based on anatomic analysis[23]

Grade	Description
0	Absence of medial or lateral lines demarcating the arcus marginalis or the orbital rim, and a smooth, youthful contour without a transition zone at the orbit-cheek junction
I	Mild, subtle presence of a medial line or shadow; smooth lateral transition of lid-cheek junction
II	Moderate prominence of a visible demarcation of the lid-cheek junction, extending from medial to lateral
III	Severe demarcation of the orbit-cheek junction, with an obvious step between the orbit and the cheek

TABLE 4: Hirmand's classification system of the tear trough deformity based on clinical evaluation.[24]

Class	Clinical description
I	Patients have loss of volume, limited medially to the tear trough. These patients can also have mild flattening extending to the central cheek
II	Patients exhibit loss of volume in the lateral orbital area in addition to the medial orbit, and they may have moderate deficiency of volume in the medial cheek and flattening of the central upper cheek
III	Patients present with a full depression circumferentially along the orbital rim, medial to lateral

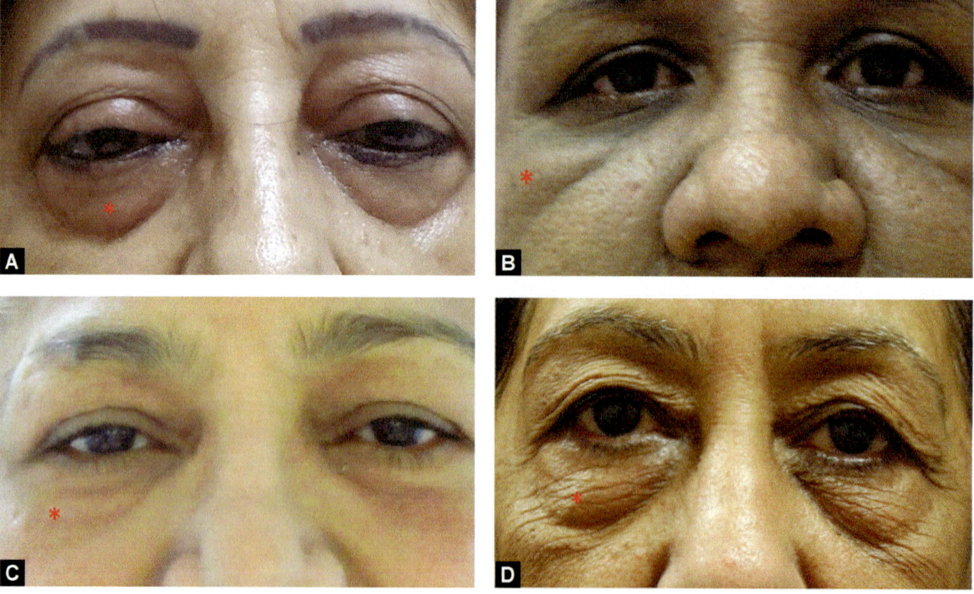

FIG. 14: Bulges: **A,** Orbital fat prolapse; **B,** malar mound; **C,** malar edema; and **D,** festoons and fat prolapse.

Orbicularis Roll

This appears as a pretarsal bulge in the lower eyelid which becomes prominent on closing the eyes or smiling. In younger people, 1–2 units of onabotulinum toxin can be injected into the pretarsal orbicularis in the midpupillary plane to erase this bulge. In older people, the skin is inelastic, hence, a conservative reduction in the muscle would be required surgically.[25]

Orbital Fat Prolapse

Undereye bags are also seen between the eyelid hollow crease and orbital rim hollow as a result of prolapse of the orbital fat from behind the orbital septum. This fat becomes prominent as age advances. Orbital fat can be distinguished from other swellings under the eye by asking the patient to look up. The fat bulge becomes more prominent with upward gaze and reduces on down gaze. The best way to treat this is by blepharoplasty.

Malar Mound

This is seen as a triangular soft tissue bulge between the infraorbital rim and the midcheek junction. This does not change with time of the day or increase or decrease with food, etc. It can be genetic or could also be seen in patients with hypothyroidism. Injection of fillers in the infraorbital hollow should be avoided in patients with malar mound.

Malar Edema

Malar edema is a fluid bag bound by the eyelid crease hollow superiorly but not limited by orbital hollow inferiorly. It appears unaltered on upward and downward gaze. It can worsen during menstrual periods, with allergies, with intake of salt, or alcohol the previous night and is usually more prominent in the mornings. Neither surgery nor fillers will help in these cases. In fact, fillers injected to camouflage the bulge will only worsen the situation.

Festoons

These are seen as hammocks of loose skin and orbicularis muscle hanging between the medial and lateral canthi, between the OML above, and the zygomatic-cutaneous ligament below. They may or may not contain herniated fat. They are seen occurring with advancing age.[26]

ASSESSMENT OF PERIORBITAL REGION BEFORE INJECTION

Skin Elasticity

If the skin under the eye has many folds and has lost its elasticity, it is worth considering a combination of fillers and a resurfacing procedure. Laser resurfacing should be done with proper protection to the eye such as a corneal eye shield. A snap test helps in assessing the elasticity of the skin under the eye.

Snap Test

Pull the skin of the lower eyelid downward and outward gently. Then quickly release it. If the skin returns back to its position immediately without the eye blinking, it indicates that the orbicularis oculi muscle is fully functional. A slow return to its baseline or a sluggish return only on blinking of the eye indicates a positive snap test which means the orbicularis oculi fibers are weak.

Color of Skin

If the skin under the eye is pigmented or acanthotic, you need to assess the cause and treat it. Also, bring it to the patient's notice that a filler will not resolve this issue. In fact, sometimes the dark circles may look more prominent after soft tissue augmentation. However, if there is a tear trough deformity along with hypermelanosis, females prefer to get fillers injected. This reduces the sunken appearance, removes the shadow, and it is easier to conceal the increased pigmentation when the contour is smooth.

Preinjection Preparation

Patients on vitamin E, *Ginkgo biloba*, and nonsteroidal anti-inflammatory drugs (NSAIDs) are asked to discontinue the same for a week before the treatment to prevent bruising.

All the patients are photographed with a standard power shot camera with the same settings and adequate lighting. Written informed consent is taken.

The author prefers to inject with the patient reclined at 45° as the tear trough deformity is better visible in this position than when the patient is lying down. Good lighting is extremely important for better visibility of anatomical landmarks.

Any cosmetic makeup in the area to be treated is completely removed with a cleansing lotion. Cleansing is further done with chlorhexidine and normal saline. The area to be treated is anesthetized with topical anesthesia (usually 2.5% lidocaine/prilocaine or with ice cubes).

Chances of bruising in this area are high due to the rich subdermal vascular plexus.

Stretch the skin under eye to check for any visible blood vessels and avoid injecting through them.

Injection Technique (Video 11)

Use a low-viscosity hyaluronic acid filler to correct the infraorbital hollow or tear trough deformity.

Palpate the orbital rim and mark the injections points along and below the infraorbital rim. Be careful not to deposit filler into the orbit. A three-point injection technique is used most commonly. The first point should be at the center of the orbital hollow. The second point should be 3–5 mm medial to it and the third point 3–5 mm lateral to it.[10,27]

The infraorbital foramen is said to lie 0.7–0.8 mm below the inferior orbital rim 2–3 mm medial to the midpupillary line. This is best palpated and marked as the no go area.

Injections can be given with a 30 G needle using the vertical supraperiosteal depot technique (VSDT) described by Gerhard Sattler.[28] In this technique, vertical injections are given deep on the periosteum. Usually three injection points are used (Fig. 15).[28]

Inject 0.02–0.05 mL of HA filler perpendicularly on the periosteum per injection point. The total volume to be injected depends on the severity of hollowing.

The linear injection technique is preferred if the cheek has been augmented well, using an entry point beneath the lateral canthus.

Use of blunt-tipped cannulas in the tear trough area are said to be less painful. Chances of bruising and edema are also less (Fig. 16).[29]

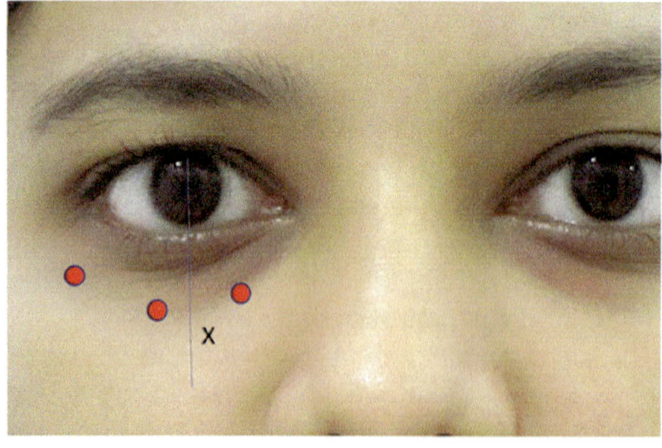

FIG. 15: Injection points for tear trough injection.

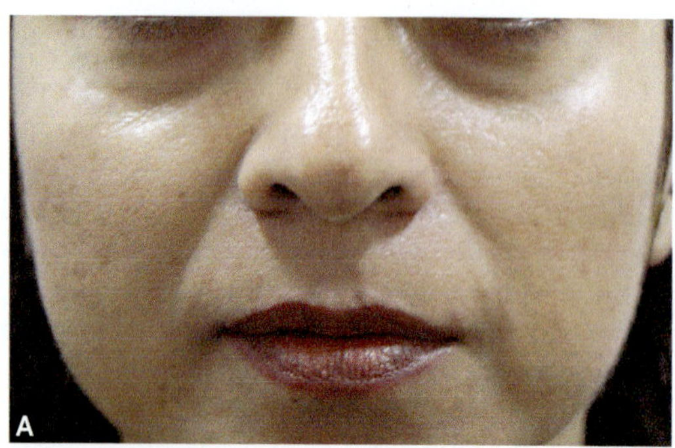

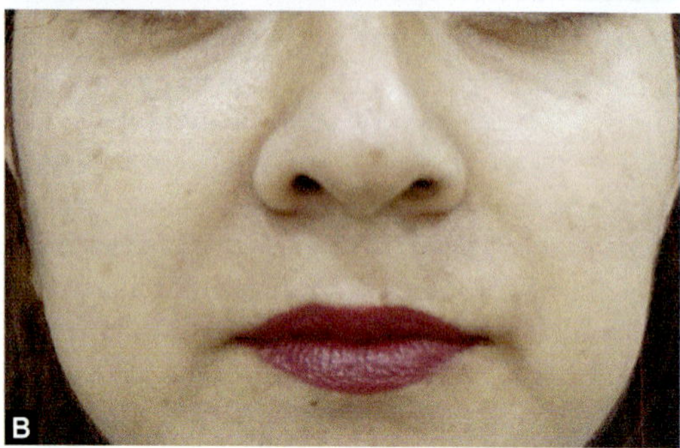

FIG. 16: A, Before injecting tear trough with 1 mL Juvederm Ultra; and **B,** After injecting tear trough with 1 mL Juvederm Ultra.

Immediate Post Injection Management

The injected area is gently massaged to ensure that there are no lumps or irregularities and there is an even distribution of the product. Avoid vigorous massage to prevent bruising or pushing of the product into the globe. Always undercorrect this area if the patient has a history of water retention or facial puffiness. HA can absorb water and increase the swelling.[30] HA can also cause stimulation of de novo production of collagen. Hence, it is best to not to overcorrect the tear trough area to prevent uneven bumps in this area.[31]

A touch-up can be done after 2–4 weeks if required.

Hyaluronic acid in the tear trough area usually lasts for up to 12–15 months.

POST TREATMENT CARE[32]

- Avoid vigorous rubbing or pressing the under eye area or applying too much ice
- Avoid strenuous physical activity, extreme heat, or extreme cold for up to 6 hours after injection
- Avoid cosmetics/makeup for at least 10 hours postinjection
- Ask the patient to preferably keep the head raised during sleep for the first 2 days

- Avoid any kind of facial massages for at least 2 weeks
- Avoid any laser, peel, or radiofrequency treatments for at least a month.

COMPLICATIONS

Immediate Complications

- Erythema
- Pain
- Edema
- Bruising (this can be minimized by applying pressure and ice packs as soon as you see a bleeding point) (Fig. 17)
- Headache
- Asymmetry.

Delayed Complications

The Tyndall Effect

If the HA is injected too superficially, it can lead to a bluish discoloration under the skin due to the Tyndall effect where the blue light spectrum is scattered by the colloid particles more strongly (Fig. 18).[33]

Post Inflammatory Hyperpigmentation

Bruising and hematoma may cause post inflammatory hyperpigmentation (PIH). A vitamin K based cream or treatment with a pulsed dye laser may reduce the bruising if treated on time. PIH may last for 6 weeks or even up to a year.

Orange-brown Staining

Bruising and subsequent deposition of hemosiderin can give an orange brown stain which may take months to resolve on its own. Preinjection ice application, proper depth of injection, discontinuation of anticoagulants at least 7 days before injection, and a smooth, gentle technique may help avoid this complication.[34]

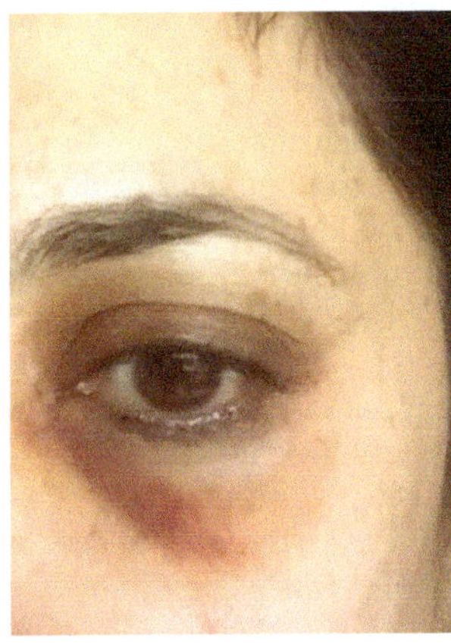

FIG. 17: Bruising.

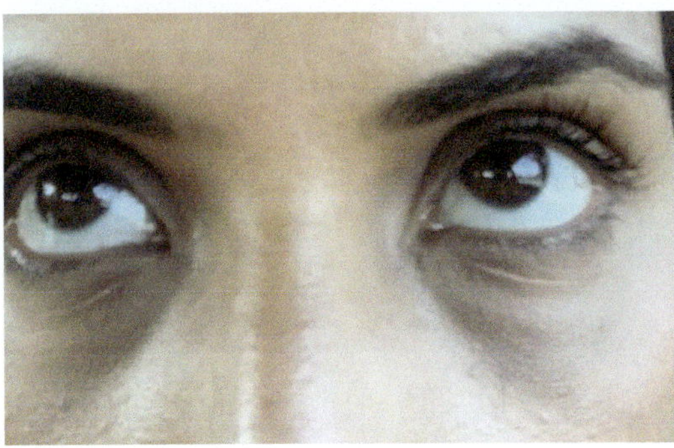

FIG. 18: Tyndall effect.

Puffiness

Patients with prominent inferior orbital fat prolapse, prominent malar fat bulges, and festoons should be injected with caution. Overcorrection will increase bags under the lower eyelid as the HA fillers are hydrophilic in nature.[34]

Infections

Avoid injecting fillers at the site of an infection or even an adjacent site. Though infections are rare, fluctuant nodules may appear and will need antibiotics.

Nodules

Superficial infections can result in nodules. The best way to treat nodules is by injecting hyaluronidase. If the patient has a history of allergic reaction to hyaluronidase, incision and drainage of the product may become necessary (Fig. 19).

Blindness

Blindness may occur due to migration of a filler embolus in a retrograde manner via an arteriole to an antegrade flow through the central retinal artery. Always stay away from the infraorbital foramen and angular artery. Inject small boluses and do not apply too much pressure while pushing the product in order to prevent any such untoward complications.

If the patient complains of inability to see or a lot of pain, the area should be flushed with hyaluronidase. The patient should be sent to an ophthalmologist for retrobulbar injections of hyaluronidase within. Hyperbaric oxygen therapy can be opted too.[35,36]

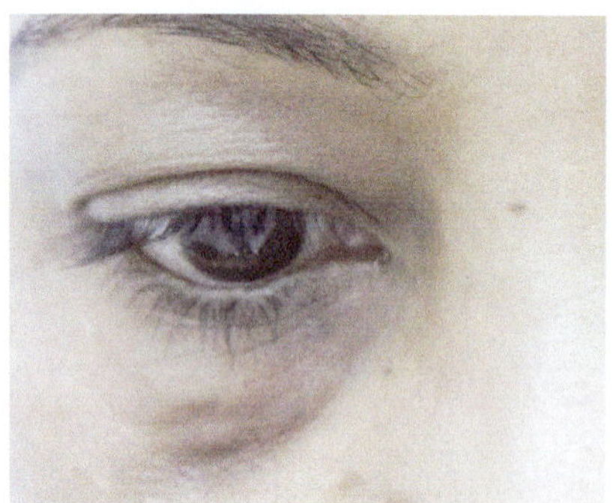

FIG. 19: Nodules.

NASOLABIAL FOLDS

Commonly known as laugh lines, there can be nasolabial creases or NLFs. Nasolabial creases occur over the dermis and epidermis due to repetitive muscle movement. They are common in younger individuals and in people with thin skin. Nasolabial folds are deeper wrinkles seen more as folds in older age groups above 35 years. Nasolabial folds with wrinkle severity scale 2-3 respond well to fillers. However, injecting NLFs with wrinkle severity scale 5 results in a more pronounced ridge at the superior aspect of the NLF.[37]

Anatomic studies have shown that the actual NLF position remains unchanged over time, but the downward migration of the malar cheek pads over the anchored base of the NLF creates the true overhanging defect associated with deep NLFs.[6,13,25,26,38,39,40]

Injection Technique

Topical anesthesia works best while injecting NLFs. Linear threading or fern or vertical depot techniques are used to inject the NLFs (Fig. 20). A sandwich technique has also been described by Rubin where a high viscosity filler is injected deep into the dermis or subcutaneous tissue and a low viscosity filler is placed superficially to take care of the creases.[37]

Treatment Pearls

- It is a good idea to stretch and compress the skin to see the NLF
- Always inject medial to the fold for better results and to prevent a bulge on the lateral surface of the NLF[32]

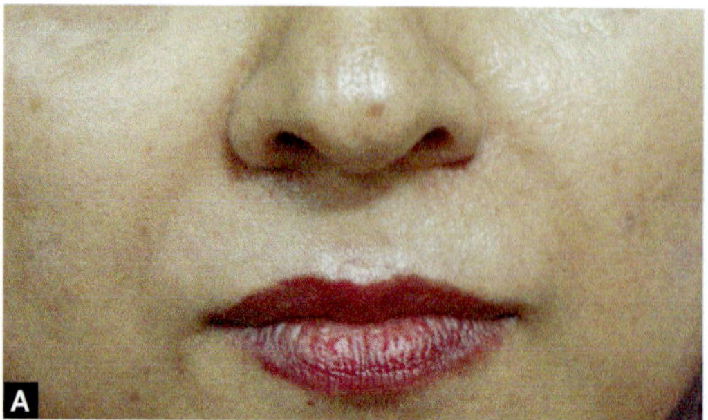

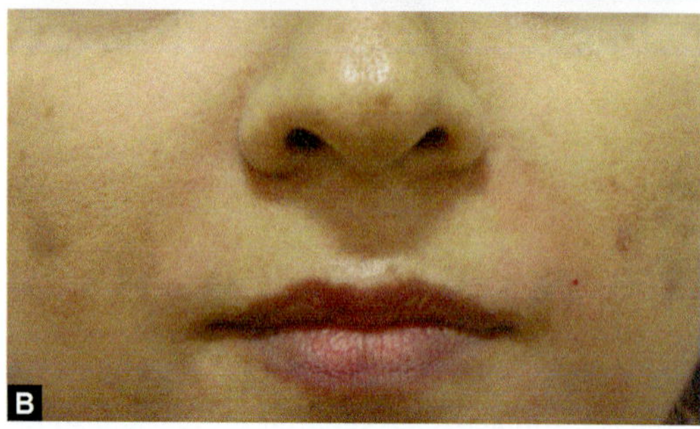

FIG. 20: A, Before injecting nasolabial B, before and after injecting nasolabial fold with 1 mL Restylane.

- Incorrect choice and incorrect placement of the fillers can both result in lumps and bumps
- Keep the angular artery in mind and do not inject anywhere along its said course
- Massage the NLF after placement of the filler for even distribution and avoidance of irregularities in skin
- Avoid injecting if the folds are deep and overhanging. Consider midface volumization instead
- Side effects are as seen in case of any fillers, for example bruising, edema, lumps, or rarely granulomas.

EAR LOBE REJUVENATION

With age, it is seen that ear lobes sag, or become thinner or there are fine lines or deep creases that develop over the lobe. Earrings either droop or the lobes are too thin to bear the weight of heavy earrings.

In such cases, a hyaluronic acid filler can be injected into the lobe to give it volume and support. About 0.3-0.5 mL is usually sufficient for each ear. The effect of the filler is seen to last for up to 18 months. Bruising is the only side effect seen. Too much filler will cause the lobes to become bulky and curl inwards (Fig. 21).[41]

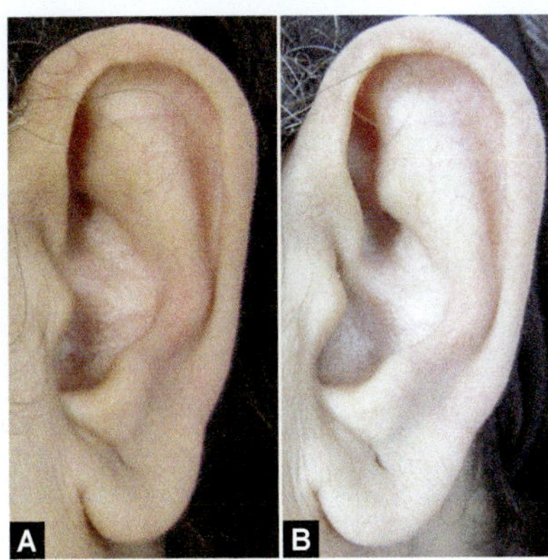

FIG. 21: Before and after injecting ear lobe with 1 mL Perlane.

NOSE

The common concerns that people have when it comes to the nose are a flat nasal bridge, an indistinct dorsal aesthetic line, a broad nasal tip, a wide alar base, and a retracted columella.

Most of these can now be treated with neuromodulators and fillers.

Anatomy

The nose consists of a framework of bone, cartilage, and skin that is supported by ligaments and connective tissue. The skin is thinner and more mobile in the upper two thirds and thicker and adherent in the lower third of the nose.

The superior labial artery forms the columellar branch and the angular artery forms the lateral nasal branch. Both of them supply the tip of the nose. The dorsal nasal and the external nasal arteries are branches of the ophthalmic artery. The lateral nasal vessels are 2–3 mm above the alar groove, and together with the columellar artery arise deep at the nasal base and end at the tip in the subdermal plexus.[42]

The skeleton of the nose consists of cartilage and bone. The bony component consists of a pair of nasal bones placed centrally and the frontal process of the maxilla laterally. The upper lateral cartilages are continuous with the nasal bones. The lower lateral cartilage comprises of lateral, middle, and medial crura. The nasal tip is supported by cartilage, ligaments, and skin.

Points to assess before doing a filler:

- Nasofrontal angle
- Radix breakpoint and dorsum
- Alar base and nostril shape
- Nasal tip, columella, and nasolabial angle
- Look for any deviations along the nasal bridge
- Width of the alar base should be same as the intercanthal distance
- The columella should be only slightly visible on the frontal view.

Indications of Nose Filler

- Augmentation of nose—dorsum, tip, and columella
- Correction of minor deviations and minor humps
- Correction of minor asymmetry of nose
- Correction of postrhinoplasty issues.[13]

Types of Filler

Hyaluronic acid fillers and calcium hydroxyapatite can be used on the nose. The author chooses to do HA fillers with high G prime and cohesivity. Less hydrophilic fillers are preferred to reduce the risk of swelling due to fluid absorption or risk of spread of the filler to the adjacent areas.

Injection Technique

A nerve block is usually preferred and fibers of the ophthalmic and maxillary nerve branch are anesthetized using 2% lignocaine.

Perpendicular supraperiosteal and supracartilaginous injections are given keeping the needle in the midline. A cannula may be used in order to inject along the length of the nose. The cannula is inserted from the columella, a little below the nasal tip. The cannula is kept on the midline and deep in order to avoid any vascular damage. The nondominant hand is used to pinch the nose while injecting the filler so that the filler does not migrate to the sides. To create a support to the columella and a tip projection, the filler can be injected into the columella at an entry point just superficial to the caudal septum and medial crura (Fig. 22).[43]

Pearls

- Observe for skin blanching
- Watch for severe localized or distant pain, both during and after injection. Blanching and pain are signs of a vascular compromise
- Inject slowly, with continuous micromovements of the tip of the needle to reduce risks of intravascular accidents. Give small boluses and preferably retrograde injections. Aspirate before injecting. But remember, negative aspirate is not a sure shot sign of being free from the danger of a vessel damage. Use a 25 G cannula or 30 G needle
- The dorsum of the nose should be straight postinjection.

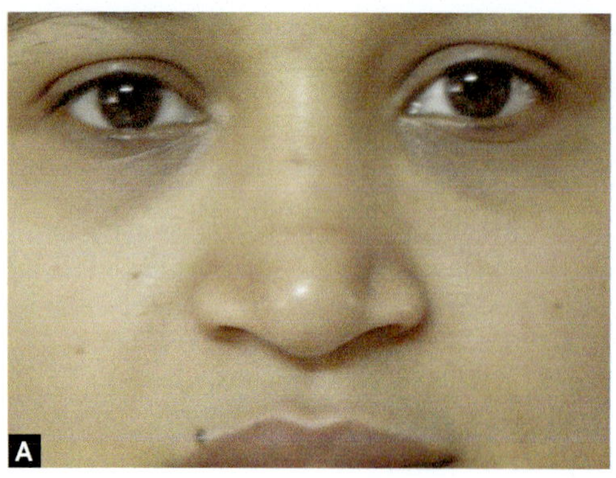

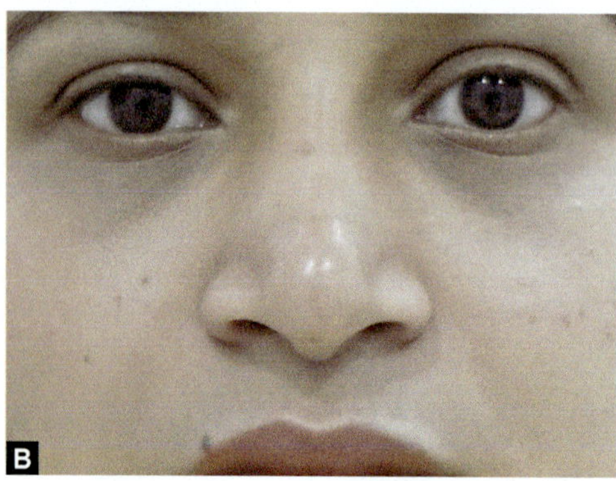

FIG. 22: A, Before reshaping nose with 1 ml Juvederm Ultra plus; and **B,** After reshaping nose with 1 ml Juvederm Ultra plus

Complications

- Blindness[44]
- Necrosis
- Infection (surgical level of asepsis needed while injecting)
- Hematoma
- Excessive filler
- Uneven nose.

CONCLUSION

A three dimensional augmentation of the midface with hyaluronic acid fillers gives a more natural lift to the face, enhancing the appearance. The paradigm shift from injection lines to volumizing the face has been a revolution. The injector should be well versed with the anatomy of the face and should have an eye for beauty in order to be able to create youthful faces. Midface fillers should be combined with fillers for the upper face and lower face in order to create the perfect balance.

REFERENCES

1. Raspaldo H. Volumizing effect of a new hyaluronic acid subdermal facial filler: a retrospective analysis based on 102 cases. J Cosmet Laser Ther. 2008;10:134-42.
2. Ramirez OM, Volpe CR. Double ogee facial rejuvenation. In: Panfilov DE (Ed). Aesthetic Surgery of the Facial Mosaic. Berlin: Springer; 2007. pp. 288-99.
3. Swift A, Remington K. BeautiPHIcation™: a global approach to facial beauty. Clin Plast Surg. 2011;38(3):347-77.
4. Kahn DM, Shaw RB. Aging of the bony orbit: a three-dimensional computed tomographic study. Aesthet Surg J. 2008;28:258-64.
5. Mendelson BC, Hartley W, Scott M, et al. Age-related changes of the orbit and midcheek and the implications for facial rejuvenation. Aesthetic Plast Surg. 2007;31:419-23.
6. Rohrich RJ, Pessa JE. The fat compartments of the face: anatomy and clinical implications for cosmetic surgery. Plast Reconstr Surg. 2007;119(7):2219-27.
7. Rohrich RJ, Arbique GM, Wong C, et al. The anatomy of suborbicularis fat: implications for periorbital rejuvenation. Plast Reconstr Surg. 2009;124:946-51.
8. Moradi A, Watson J. Current Concepts in Filler Injection. Facial Plast Surg Clin North Am. 2015;23(4):489-94.
9. Liew S. Ethnic and Gender Considerations in the Use of Facial injectables: Asian Patients. Plast Reconstr Surg. 2016;137(2):747.
10. Carruthers J, Rzany B, Sattler G, et al. Anatomic guidelines for midface volumetric augmentation. Dermatol Surg. 2012;38:1223-33.
11. Fitzgerald R, Rubin AG. Filler placement and the fat compartments. Dermatol Clin. 2014;32(1):37-50.
12. Rohrich RJ, Pessa JE, Ristow B. The youthful cheek and the deep medial fat compartment. Plast Reconstr Surg. 2008;121(6):2107-12.
13. Cotofana S, Schenck TL, Trevidic P, et al. Midface: Clinical Anatomy and Regional Approaches with Injectable Fillers. Plast Reconstr Surg. 2015;136(5 Suppl):219S-234.
14. Braz AV, Sakuma TH. Midface rejuvenation: an innovative technique to restore cheek volume. Dermatol Surg. 2012;38:118-20.
15. Rho NK, Chang YY, Chao YY, et al. Consensus Recommendations for Optimal Augmentation of the Asian Face with Hyaluronic Acid and Calcium Hydroxylapatite Fillers. Plast Reconstr Surg. 2015;136(5):940-56.
16. de Maio M. Ethnic and Gender Considerations in the Use of Facial Injectables: Male Patients. Plast Reconstr Surg. 2015;136(5 Suppl):40S-43.
17. Lambros V. Observation on periorbital and midface aging. Plast Reconstr Surg. 2007;120:1367-76.
18. Sadick NS, Bosniak SL, Cantisano-Zilkha M, et al. Definition of the tear trough and the tear trough rating scale. J Cosmet Dermatol. 2007;6:218-22.
19. Goldberg RA, McCann JD, Fiaschetti D, et al. What causes eyelid bags? Analysis of 114 consecutive patients. Plast Reconstr Surg. 2005;115:1395-402.
20. Haddock NT, Saadeh PB, Boutros S, et al. The tear trough and lid/cheek junction: anatomy and impli-

cations for surgical correction. Plast Reconstr Surg. 2009;123:1332-40.

21. Wong CH, Hsieh MK, Mendelson B. The tear trough ligament: anatomical basis for the tear trough deformity. Plast Reconstr Surg. 2012;129(6):1392-402.
22. Muzaffar AR, Mendelson BC, Adams WP. Surgical anatomy of the ligamentous attachments of the lower lid and lateral canthus. Plast Reconstr Surg. 2002;110:873-84.
23. Barton FE, Ha R, Awada M. Fat extrusion and septal reset in patients with the tear trough triad: A critical appraisal. Plast Reconstr Surg. 2004;113:2115-21.
24. Hirmand H. Anatomy and nonsurgical correction of the tear trough deformity. Plast Reconstr Surg. 2010;125:699-708.
25. Goldberg RA. Nonsurgical Filling of the Periorbital Hollows. Aesthet Surg J. 2006;26(1):69-71.
26. Kpodzo DS, Nahai F, McCord CD. Malar mounds and festoons: review of current management. Aesthet Surg J. 2014;34(2):235-48.
27. Sharad J. Dermal Fillers for the Treatment of Tear Trough Deformity: A Review of Anatomy, Treatment Techniques, and their Outcomes. J Cutan Aesthet Surg. 2012;5(4):229-38.
28. Sattler G. The tower technique and vertical supra-periosteal depot technique: novel vertical injection techniques for volume-efficient subcutaneous tissue support and volumetric augmentation. J Drugs Dermatol. 2012;11:45-7.
29. Trevidic P. The use of blunt-tipped cannulas for tear trough correction. J Drugs Dermatol. 2012;11:S38-40.
30. Gold MH. Use of hyaluronic acid fillers for the treatment of the aging face. Clin Interv Aging. 2007;2:369-76.
31. Wang F, Garza LA, Kang S, et al. In vivo stimulation of de novo collagen production caused by cross-linked hyaluronic acid dermal filler injections in photodamaged human skin. Arch Dermatol. 2007;143:155-63.
32. Vedamurthy M, IADVL Dematosurgery Task Force. Standard guidelines for the use of dermal fillers. Indian J Dermatol Venereol Leprol. 2008;74 Suppl:S23-7.
33. Kim JE, Sykes JM. Hyaluronic acid fillers: history and overview. Facial Plast Surg. 2011;7:523-8.
34. Sherman RN. Avoiding dermal filler complications. Clin Dermatol. 2009;27:S23-32.
35. Coleman SR. Avoidance of arterial occlusion from injection of soft tissue fillers. Aesthet Surg J. 2002;22:555-7.
36. Loh KT, Chua JJ, Lee HM, et al. Prevention and management of vision loss relating to facial filler injections. Singapore Med J. 2016;57(8):438-43.
37. Rubin MG. Treatment of nasolabial folds with fillers. Aesthet Surg J. 2004;24(5):489-93.
38. Yousif NJ, Gosain A, Sanger JR, et al. The nasolabial fold: a photogrammetric analysis. Plast Reconstr Surg. 1994;93:70-7.
39. Gosain AK, Amarante MT, Hyde JS, et al. A dynamic analysis of changes in the nasolabial fold using magnetic resonance imaging: implications for facial rejuvenation and facial animation surgery. Plast Reconstr Surg. 1996;98:622-35.
40. Hoefflin SM. The ligamentous facial fence: the cause of nasolabial folds and jowling. Plast Reconstr Surg. 1998;101(4):1148.
41. Qian W, Zhang YK, Cao Q, et al. Clinical Application of Earlobe Augmentation with Hyaluronic Acid Filler in the Chinese Population. Aesthet Plast Surg. 2017;41(1):185-90.
42. Rohrich RJ, Gunter JP, Friedman RM. Nasal tip blood supply: an anatomic study validating the safety of the transcolumellar incision in rhinoplasty. Plast Reconstr Surg. 1995;95(5):795-9.
43. Liew S, Scamp T, de Maio M, et al. Efficacy and Safety of a Hyaluronic Acid Filler to Correct Aesthetically Detracting or Deficient Features of the Asian Nose: A Prospective, Open-Label, Long-Term Study. Aesthet Surg J. 2016;36(7):760-72.
44. Carruthers JD, Fagien S, Rohrich RJ, et al. Blindness caused by cosmetic filler injection: a review of cause and therapy. Plast Reconstr Surg. 2014;134(6):1197-201.

25 CHAPTER

Dermal Fillers in Lower Face Rejuvenation

Maya Vedamurthy

INTRODUCTION

Aging of lower face is one of the most common indications of dermal fillers along with neurotoxin. Aging of the lower face occurs as an interplay of skeletal resorption combined with soft tissue descent of midface giving rise to formation of jowls, marionette lines, prejowl sulcus and loss of jawline definition.[1]

Therefore, rejuvenation procedures of the lower face should be addressed as a single unit with the aim of giving an overall lift effect rather than correcting the defects individually.[2]

Volume loss which occurs with aging is combined with descent of midface fat pads leading to downturned oral commissures and occurrence of marionette lines which is accentuated by pull of depressor anguli oris. Therefore, when treating lower face all the components need to be treated as a unit to get the desired result.

CHOICE OF FILLERS FOR LOWER FACE

It is extremely important to remember that lower face is extremely mobile and that fillers need to be placed supraperiosteally or in subdermal plane. It has to be nonpalpable but mobile, and be able to easily integrate with movement of facial muscles in and around this region. The ideal filler should therefore have moderate G′ and medium cohesivity.[3] But to have a lift capacity, a filler with higher G′ and high cohesivity will provide a better correction. So a careful selection of both the products in the lower face will yield better result.

NEEDLE VERSUS CANNULA

Both needles and cannulas are used interchangeably for lower face indications based on the depth and length of the area to be treated.

INJECTION PROTOCOL

The patient is counseled regarding the procedure and an informed consent is obtained. Clinical photographs are taken in all five views which includes one frontal view, two oblique view and two lateral view.[4]

The lower face is supplied by mental nerve and the procedure in this area is painful. Hence, it is advisable to use a product premixed with lidocaine to add comfort to the patient while treating this area. Alternatively, after taking necessary precautions local anesthesia is infiltrated at the site of entry of the cannula which is usually a point lateral to the marionette line.

Also, it should be remembered that the facial artery runs 3 cm in front of the angle of the mandible and its pulsation can easily be felt for confirmation. Therefore, it is advisable to use a cannula to avoid bruising in lower face.

INDICATIONS FOR FILLERS IN LOWER FACE

- Jawline
- Prejowl sulcus
- Chin
- Marionette lines.

Jawline (Video 12)

With aging the jawline becomes ill defined due to atrophy of superior and inferior mandibular fat compartments. The resorption of the underlying mandibular bone along with skin laxity leads to jowl formation. The atrophic ill-defined jawline can be treated by placing the filler material over the periosteum of the inferior mandible.[5]

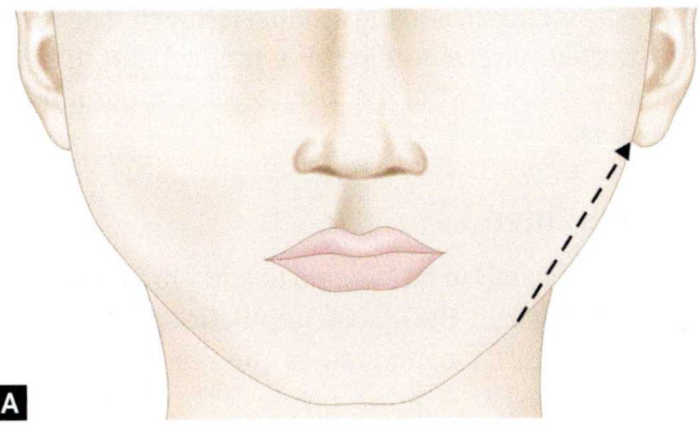

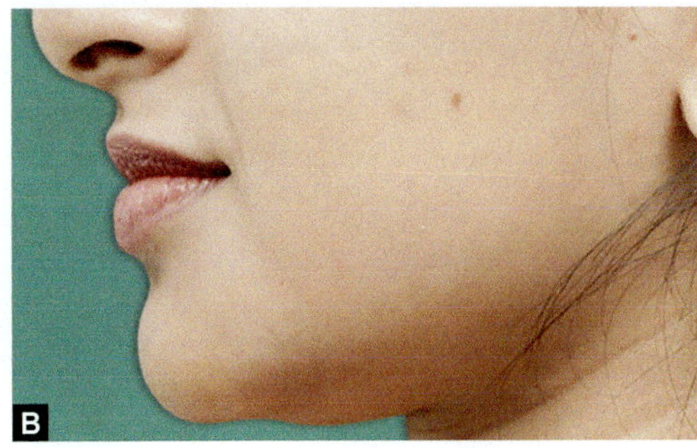

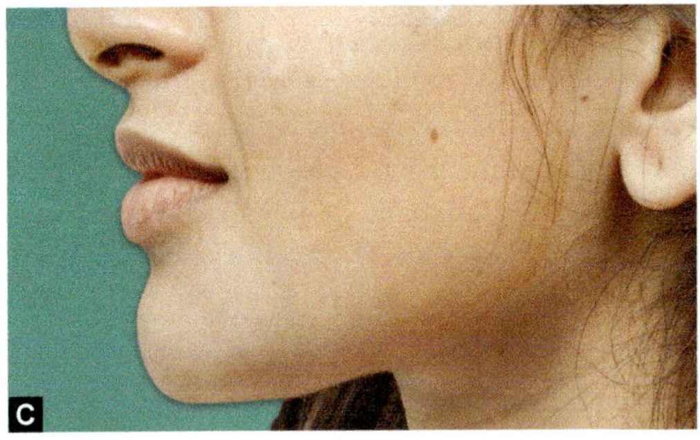

FIG. 1: A, Injection technique for jawline; **B,** before; and **C,** after hyaluronic acid filler.

Most often people have jawlines which are not well defined and this may be due to excessive fat or skin laxity. Patient selection is important because people with prominent double chin or excessive subcutaneous fat are not good candidates. People with thin jawline are ideal candidates. The choice of product will be with a high G′ and high cohesivity which needs to be injected using a cannula. An 18 G cannula is chosen and an entry point is made using a sharp 18 G needle. The entry point is made further away from the facial artery to avoid inadvertent vascular injury. The cannula is introduced along the periosteum of the mandible toward the angle of the mandible and the product is injected as linear threads both antegrade and retrograde to create a well-defined jawline (Fig. 1). A total of 0.5–1 mL may be necessary to inject on either side to give an aesthetic effect.

There is also a consensus recommendation by Dallara et al. for jawline rejuvenation.[6]

A total of six points is chosen (Fig. 2) and a highly viscous product is injected into the surrounding zones (Fig. 3) through this selected point. The volume injected is based on the severity of sagging.

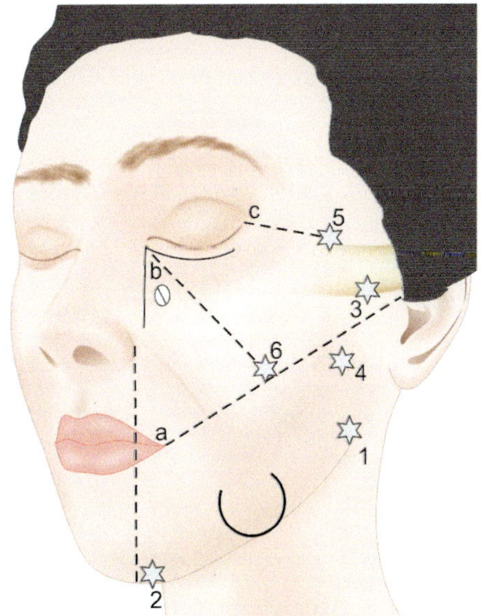

FIG. 2: Points of insertion.

Prejowl Sulcus

The jowl fat begins after the mandibular ligament and extends up to the gonial angle. The jowl fat adheres to the depressor anguli oris and is bound inferiorly by the mandibular retaining ligament. The area between the jowl fat compartment and chin appears atrophic and sunken with aging.

For treating the prejowl sulcus a product with high G′ is chosen to give a volumizing effect. A 23 G

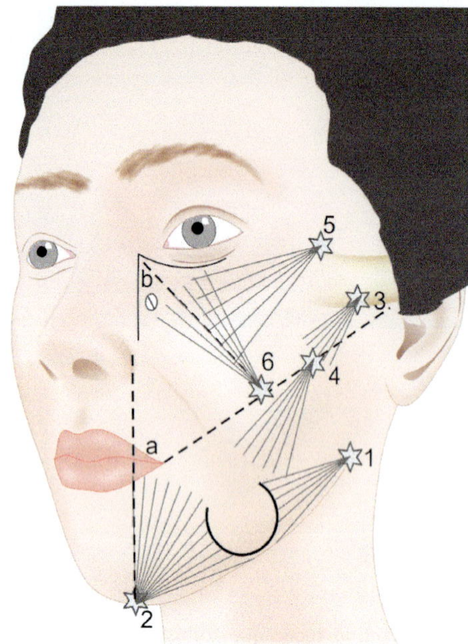

FIG. 3: Zones of injection.

needle is chosen and the product is injected on to the periosteum to camouflage the prejowl and to bring the chin and jowl to the same level without a break (Fig. 4).

Chin (Video 13)

The chin needs to be injected to add Phi proportions to the face. In the Asian population, the chin is usually shorter compared to the rest of the facial proportions. It is advisable to relax the mentalis muscle using neurotoxin before injecting fillers into the chin. The product chosen is a volumizing filler to add volume to the chin or to lengthen the chin. The center is marked and product is injected on either side of the midline using a 23 G needle. The product is injected deep on to the bone and massaged well. Sometimes the middle of the chin is also injected to avoid a cleft chin and to give a smooth rounded contour. Hence, a total 0.5 mL per side may be needed to give a smooth rounded contour.

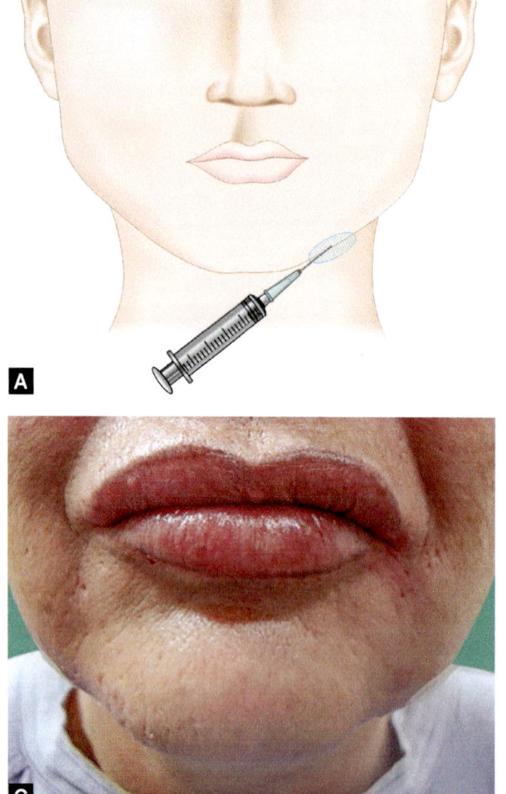

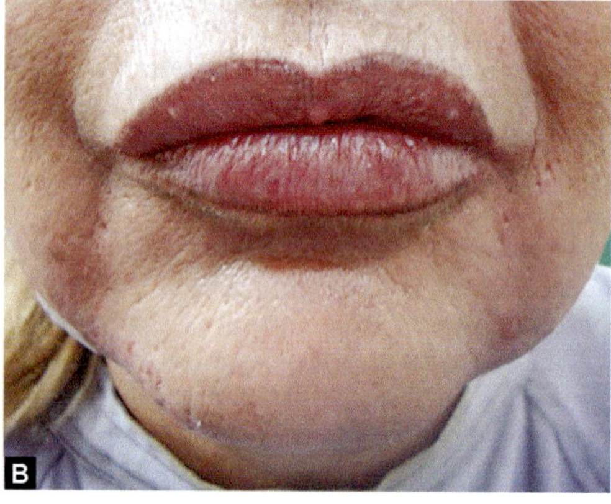

FIG. 4: **A,** Injection technique for prejowl; **B,** before; and **C,** after hyaluronic acid filler.

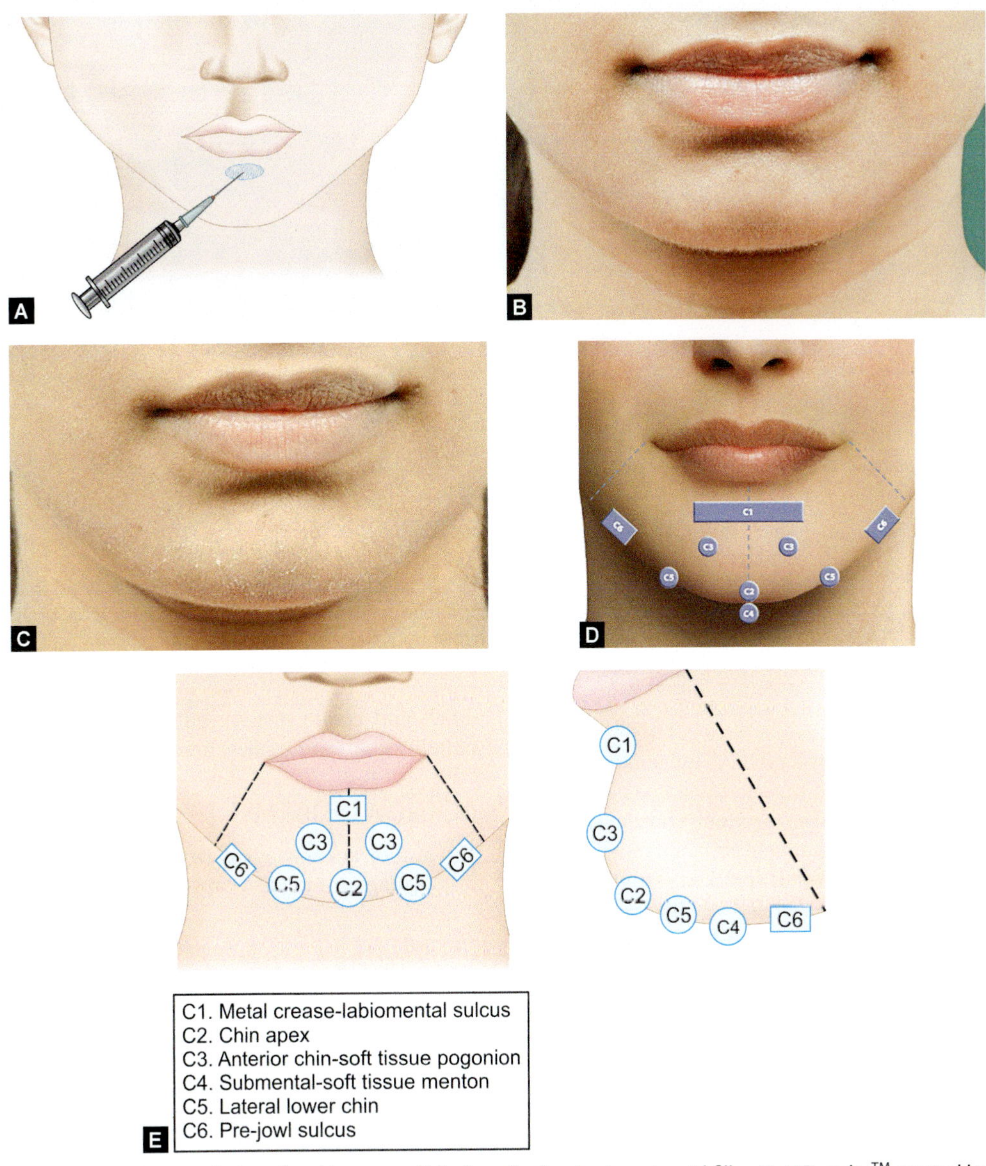

FIG. 5: A, Injection technique for chin crease; **B,** before; **C,** after hyaluronic acid filler; **D,** MD codes^{TM} created by Mauricio de Maio; and **E,** six points for chin.

In patients with prominent mental grooves, the dermal filler is injected subcutaneously using a linear threading technique to efface the crease (Fig. 5).

A micrognathic chin can be volumized by deep supraperiosteal injections using a filler with a high G′. The six point chin reshape as described by Mauricio DeMaio is a good technique in these cases (Table 1).

The areas of injection are the mental crease, chin apex, anterior chin, submental, lateral lower chin and prejowl sulcus (Fig. 5E).

TABLE 1: MD^{TM} codes and injection points for chin

Code	Injection area
C1	Mental crease/labial mental angle
C2 (Jw5)	Chin apex
C3	Anterior chin/soft tissue pogonion
C4	Submental/soft tissue menton
C5	Lateral lower chin
C6 (L6, Jw4)	Prejowl sulcus

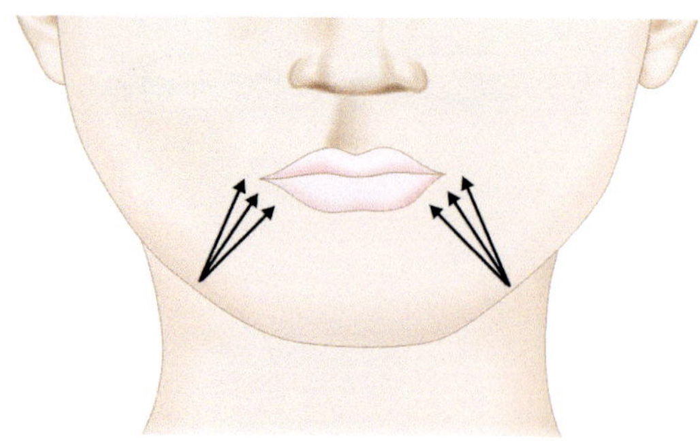

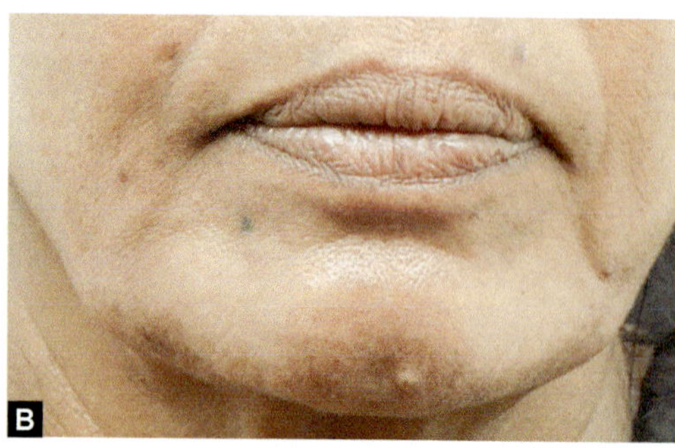

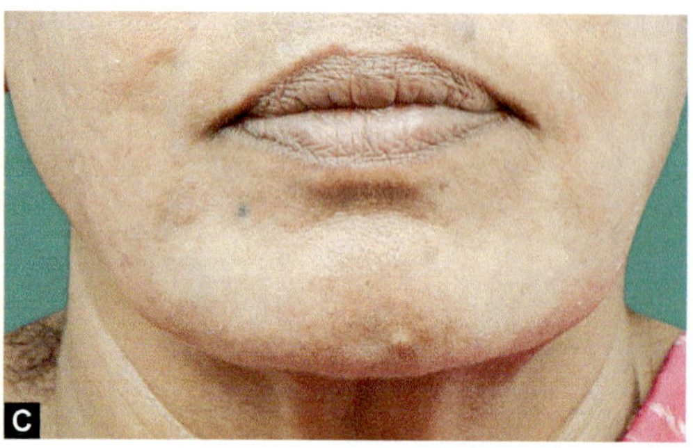

FIG. 6: A, Injection technique for marionette lines; **B,** marionette lines—before; and **C,** marionette lines after hyaluronic acid filler.

Marionette Lines

Marionette line is exacerbated by constant pull of depressor anguli oris muscle causing a downturned oral commissure.[1] The product chosen is with a medium G′ as it is an area of constant movement.

A triangular area is marked extending from the oral commissure down to the jawline. First the product is injected deep on to the bone as a bolus. At a little higher level the product is injected subcutaneously using a fan-shaped technique so as to give support to the oral commissure (Fig. 6). This area can also further be strengthened using a cross hatching technique.[7] So in this area a sandwich technique may be used by using different products at different levels. A total 0.5–1 mL of the product may be required to correct the deficit. The product is massaged well to avoid visible lumps and bumps.[8]

CONCLUSION

Lower face rejuvenation is an important aspect of facial rejuvenation in antiaging therapies. Successful lower face rejuvenation starts with a thorough history, careful assessment, correct choice of filler, and proper technique. It is good to remember that a patient's goal is to achieve a natural age-appropriate look. The best way is to maintain PHI proportions intact and create realistic outcome to achieve the patient's goal within safety limits.

ACKNOWLEDGEMENT

The author acknowledges Dr Divya Sachdev DDVL for the diagrams in this chapter.

REFERENCES

1. Bray D, Hopkins C, Roberts DN. A review of dermal fillers in facial plastic surgery. Curr Opin Otolaryngol Head Neck Surg. 2010;18(4):295-302.
2. Cohen SR, Born TM. Facial Rejuvenation with Fillers. Codner: Elsevier; 2009. pp. 39-52.
3. Pierre S, Liew S, Bernardin A. Basics of dermal filler rheology. Dermatol Surg. 2015;41(Suppl 1):S120-6.
4. Bhatia AC. The clinical image editorial. Arch Dermatol. 2006;142:96-8.
5. Carruthers A, Carruthers J. Calcium hydroxylapatite: microspheres in facial augmentation. In: Jones D (Ed). Injectable Fillers: Principles and Practice. New York: Blackwell Publishing; 2010. pp. 27-42.
6. Dallara JM, Baspeyras M, Bui P, et al. Calcium hydroxylapatite for jawline rejuvenation: consensus recommendations. J Cosmet Dermatol. 2014;13(1):3-14.
7. Braz A, Humphrey S, Weinkle S, et al. Lower Face: Clinical Anatomy and Regional Approaches with Injectable Fillers. Plast Reconstr Surg. 2015;136(5 Suppl):235S-57.
8. Sclafani AP. Soft tissue fillers for management of the aging perioral complex. Facial Plast Surg. 2005;21(1):74-8.

26

CHAPTER

Hyaluronic Acid Fillers for Lip Rejuvenation

Jaishree Sharad

INTRODUCTION

Lips and eyes form the most expressive parts of the face. Full, well-defined lips are considered attractive and are desired by most women and sometimes men too.

Beautification of lips is an ancient culture being practiced for centuries. While African tribes have used lip plates, the ancient Egyptians used henna and carmine to paint their lips, others used crushed rose petals to color their lips. Lip augmentation is one of the most sought after aesthetic procedures in today's time by all age groups starting from late teens to even eighties.

ANATOMICAL LANDMARKS OF LIPS (FIG. 1)

The lips consists of skin and mucosa and is seen as an entire anatomic unit from the base of the nose to the upper part of the chin. The border of the lip is known as the white roll or vermilion border. The body of the lip is called the vermilion. The vermilion consists of a wet lip and a dry lip. The center of the upper vermilion is known as the tubercle. The two paramedian elevations known as philtral columns arise from the base of the nasal septum and end on either side of the tubercle of the upper lip forming an M-shaped cupid's bow. Between the philtral columns lies the philtrum. The lower lip has two tubercles. The upper and lower lip meet at an angle known as the lateral commissures. The crease below the lower lip is known as the labiomental crease. The marionette lines, or labiomandibular folds, as well as the perioral rhytides develop as the face ages.[1]

ANATOMY

From superficial to deep, the layers of the upper and lower lips include the epidermis, superficial fat compartment, orbicularis oris muscle fibers, deep fat compartment, and the mucosa (Fig. 2). The vermilion is composed of nonkeratinized squamous epithelium that covers numerous capillaries, which

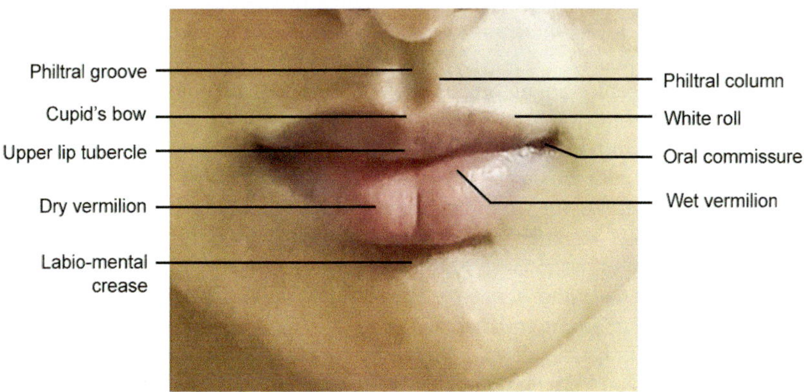

FIG. 1: Anatomical landmarks of lips.

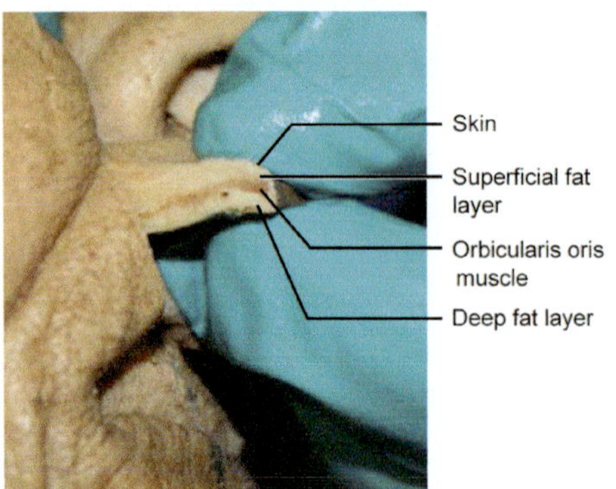

FIG. 2: Layers of the lip
Courtesy: Dr Sebastian Cotofana.

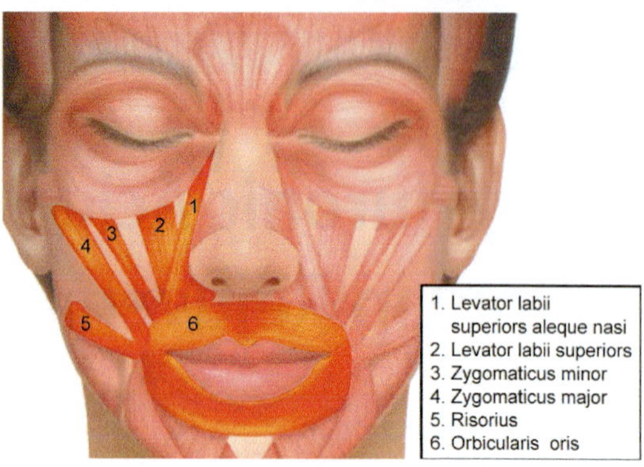

FIG. 3: Perioral and lip muscles.

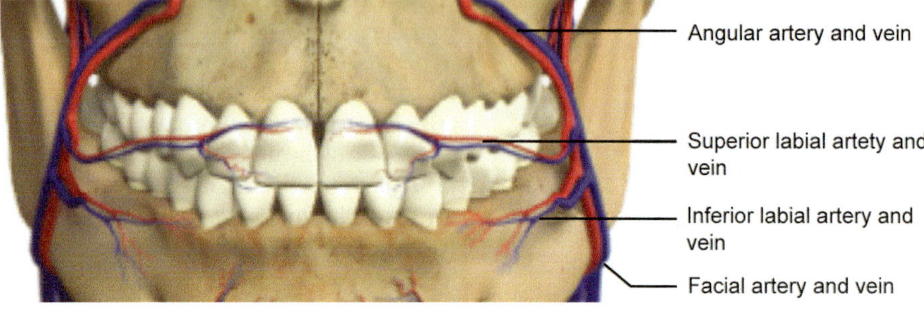

FIG. 4: Arterial supply of lips.

give the vermilion its characteristic pink color. The superficial fat compartment lies below the vermilion or semimucosa and above the orbicularis oris muscle. The deep fat compartment lies below the orbicularis muscle and above the lip mucosa.[2]

The orbicularis oris muscle is a circumferential muscle responsible for the sphincter function of the mouth. It inserts its fibers at the boundary between the vermilion and lip mucosa. Fibers of the levator labii superioris alaeque nasi (LLSAN), levator labii superioris, and zygomaticus minor insert into the upper lip. These are all lip elevators.

The zygomaticus major, levator anguli oris, risorius, buccinators, and depressor anguli oris (DAO) insert at the oral commissure and form the modiolus. The zygomaticus major and levator anguli oris elevate the upper lip. The risorius draws the commissure laterally. The DAO is the most superficial mimetic muscle and it depresses the commissure, responsible partially for the marionette line. The lower lip is inserted by the depressor labii inferioris and mentalis, with mentalis also inserting into chin dermis. Both interlace with platysma fibers and are lip depressors (Fig. 3).[3]

The lips are supplied by the superior and inferior labial arteries [superior labial artery (SLA), inferior labial artery (ILA)] which are branches of the facial artery. Superior labial artery runs between the white and red lips and is covered by the oral mucosa. It anastomoses with the contralateral artery and separates into superficial and deep ascending branches to supply the mucosa and skin. The upper lip has a submuscular arterial arcade at the vermilion mucosa junction. The arteries lie in the submucosa, among the beads of the minor salivary glands, between the lower border of the orbicularis oris and the mucosa of the upper lip. The ILA courses over the alveolar margin of the mandible, far from the vermilion of the lower lip, before giving off ascending branches to the vermilion. Most of the labial branches enter the vermilion perpendicularly, and the marginal artery connecting these terminal branches in the vermilion is very small (Fig. 4).[4]

The upper lip is innervated by the infraorbital nerve. The lower lip is innervated by the mental nerve. The motor innervation of the orbicularis oris is provided by the buccal branches of the facial nerve. The perioral muscles are either innervated by the buccal, or the marginal mandibular branches of the facial nerve.

ARCHITECTURE OF AN IDEAL LIP[5,6]

- An ideal aesthetic lip should lie parallel to a line drawn between the pupils of the eyes with the patient in the postural head position
- The upper lip should be 18–20 mm from the nose and the lower lip should be 36–40 mm from the chin (Fig. 5A)
- In a profile view, a line drawn from the midpoint of the columella of the nose to the chin is known as the Steiner's line. The Steiner's line should barely graze the upper and lower lips (Fig. 5B)
- The nasolabial angle should be 85–105° in a facial profile (Fig. 5C)
- As the upper lip turns from glabrous skin to mucosa, there is a slight elevation or ski jump at the tip of the cupid's bow known as the Glogau-Klein (GK) point (Fig. 5C)
- The philtral ridges, cupid's bow, and the white roll should all be well defined in ideal lips (Fig. 5D)
- The ideal feminine youthful lower lip should be fuller but the upper lip should project more on profile by 1–2 mm (Fig. 5D)
- The upper lip to lower lip ratio in Caucasians is 1:1.6 (phi ratio). However, this golden ratio is not applicable in Asian and African lips. Asian and African lips are usually of equal ratio (Fig. 5E).

CHANGES DUE TO AGING[7,8] (BOX 1)

Maxillary retrusion is evident in both fully dentated patients and those with loss of teeth. Deepening of the maxilla leads to a posterior positioning of the upper lip and the nasolabial fold. The body of the mandible reduces, the ramus becomes oblique, and the angle of the mandible becomes obtuse at an angle of 140° as opposed to a 100–110° angle in a youthful face. The alveolar process is absorbed, reducing the height of the mandible (Fig. 6). This adds to the prominence of the labiomandibular crease and thinning of the lower lips. There is fat loss as well as collagen degradation resulting in the lips to become thin and cave in. Overuse of the orbicularis oris muscle breaks down the soft tissue,

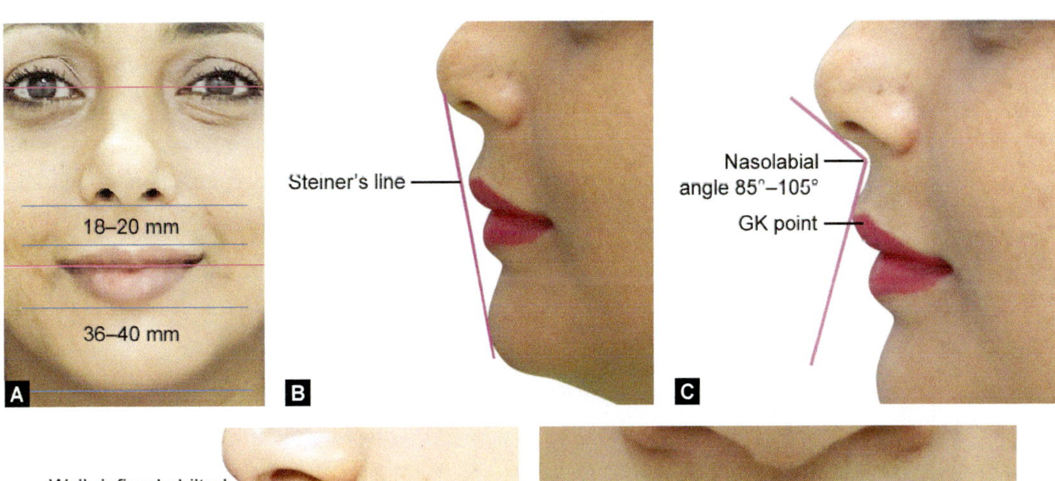

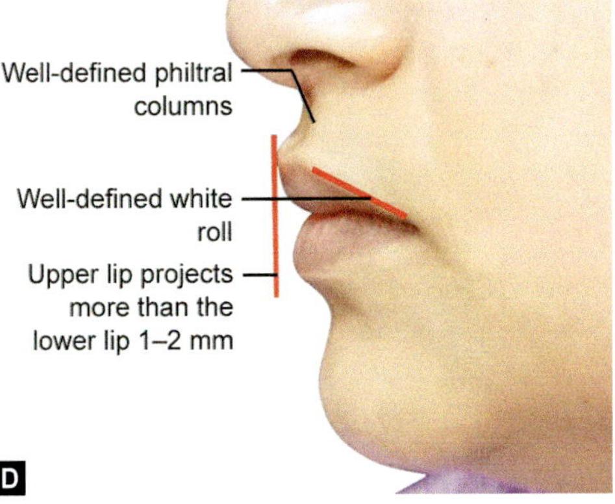

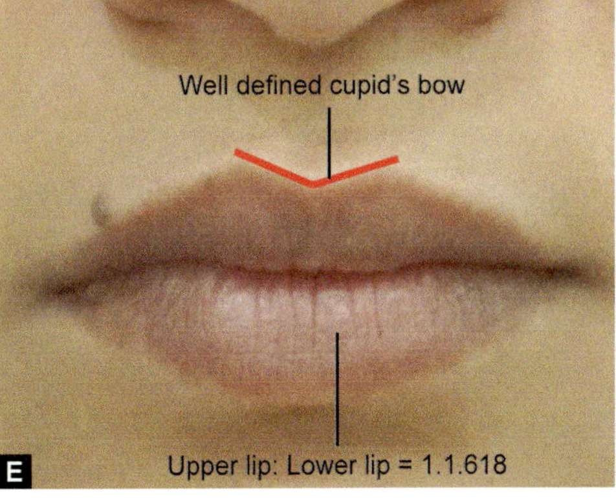

FIG. 5: Architecture of an ideal lip.

BOX 1 Changes in lip due to aging (Fig. 7)

- Flattened philtral columns
- Loss of cupid's bow
- Loss of definition of the lip border
- Lengthening of the vermilion border
- Depleted volume
- Loss of projection of the upper lip
- Downturned oral commissures
- The lips become more vertical and receded

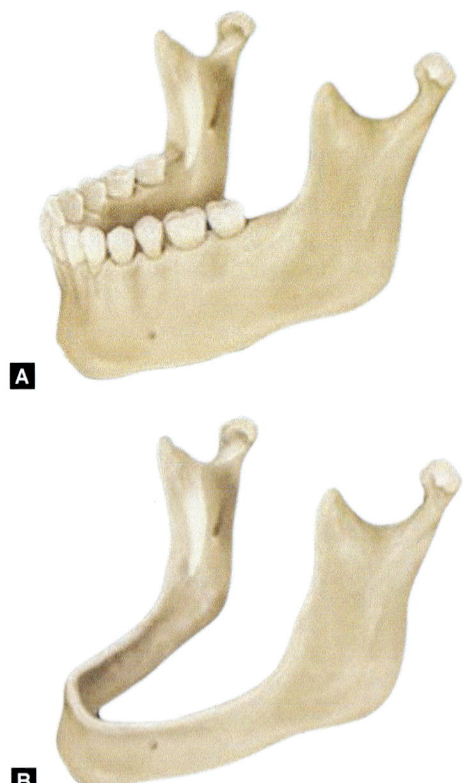

FIG. 6: Changes in the mandible with aging.

creating perioral rhytides or "lipstick lines" and perioral wrinkles.

ASSESSMENT OF LIPS BEFORE INJECTING FILLERS

There are three categories of patients who want lip fillers:

1. Group 1: Patients who have a perfect definition and shape but who wish to augment certain features of their lips. These patients are usually young, in the age group of 20–40 years (Fig. 8)
2. Group 2: Patients who have thin lips and require augmentation. These patients may have genetically thin lips. They could be in the age group of 20–45 years (Fig. 9)
3. Group 3: Patients who have loss of lip definition, volume, and/or perioral rhytides. These are usually old patients who have lost bone, fat, and collagen (Fig. 10).
    - It is important to assess the lips both at rest and in motion
    - Assess the lip architecture: Check if the vermilion border, cupid's bow, and philtral columns are well defined. Assess the vermilion volume. The upper lip and lower lip ratio should be in proportion. Check for the upper lip projection about 2 mm in front of the lower lip
    - Assess the active contraction of muscles. Check for perioral rhytides, marionette lines, and nasolabial folds
    - Assess the dental arcade.

Inclination of Teeth

It is difficult to inject too much filler into the upper lip if there is an anterior inclination of the upper teeth (Fig. 11). With age, there is loss of alveolar bone

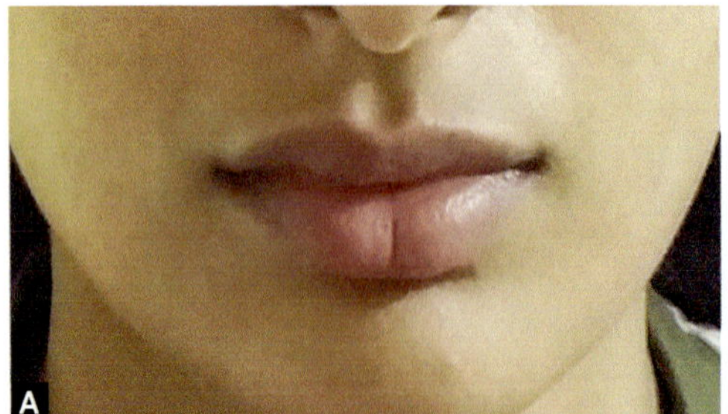

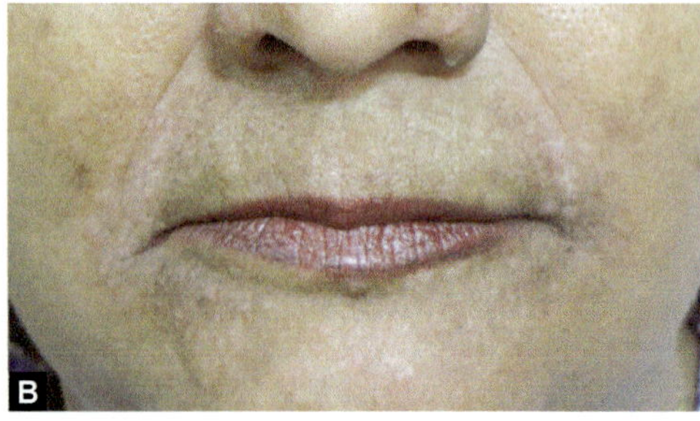

FIG. 7: Changes in lip due to aging. **A,** Youthful lips and **B,** aging lips.

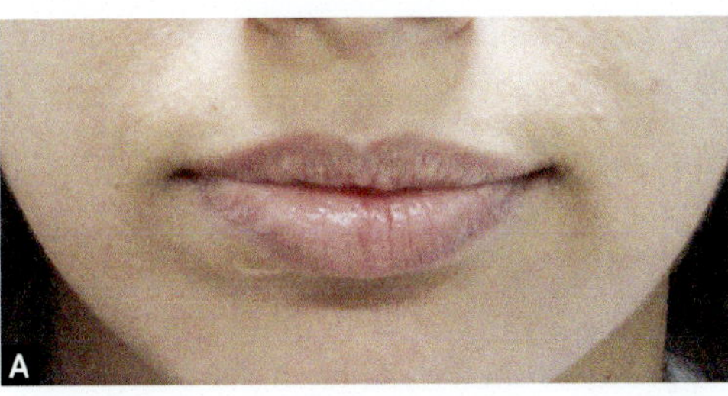

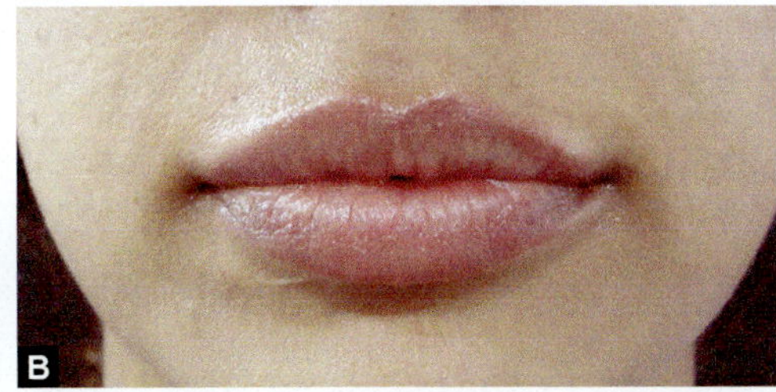

FIG. 8: **A,** Patient with perfect definition, wanted more lip volume and **B,** after 1 mL Juvederm Ultra injection.

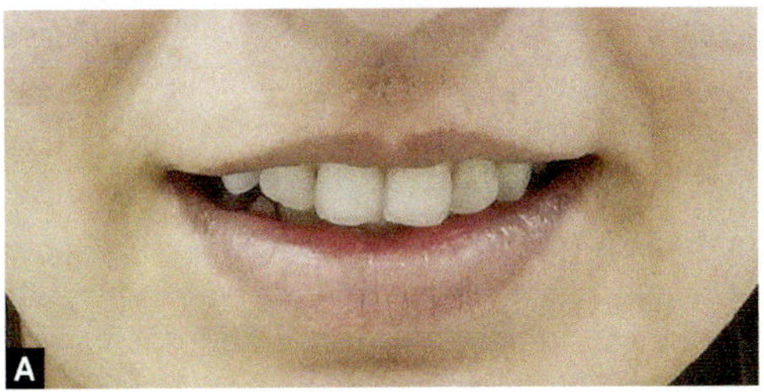

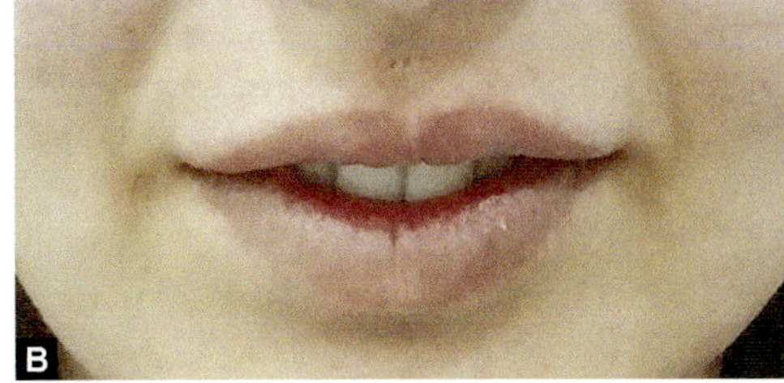

FIG. 9: **A,** Patient with thin upper lips and **B,** after 1 mL of Restylane lip injection.

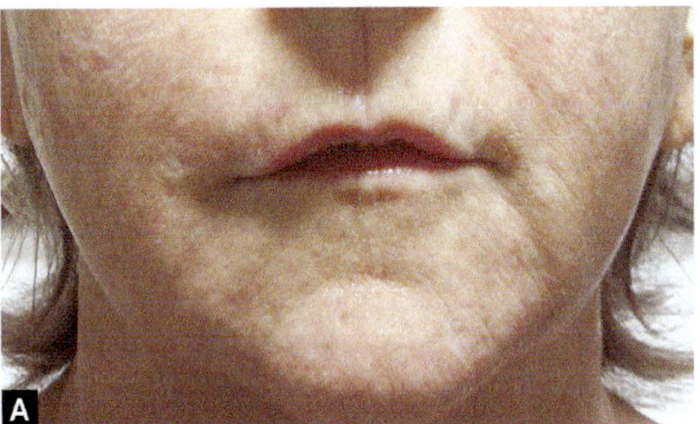

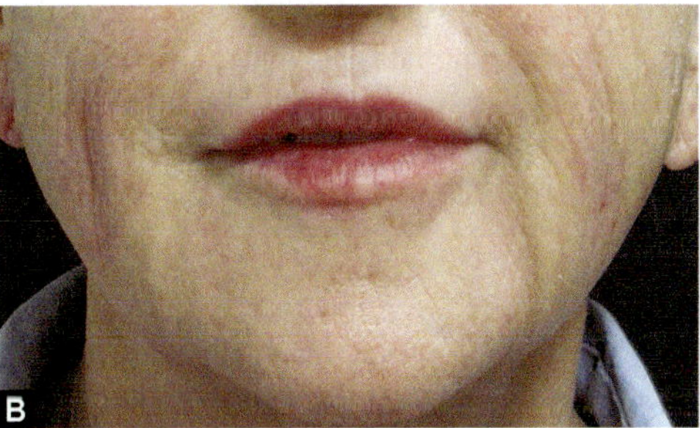

FIG. 10: **A,** A 65-year-old lady before filler injection and **B,** a 65-year-old lady after injection with 1 mL Juvederm Ultra plus into the lip.

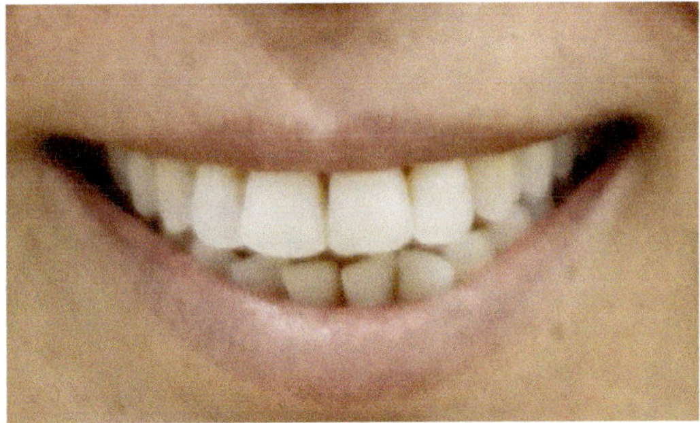

FIG. 11: Anterior inclination of upper teeth.

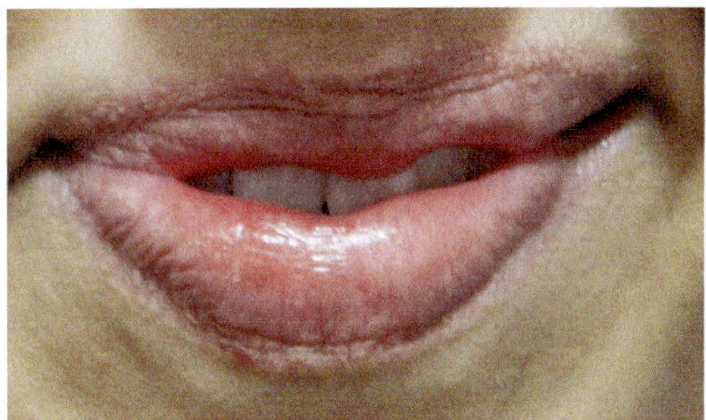

FIG. 12: Asymmetrical smile.

and dental enamel, leading to inversion of lips or reduced vertical dimension resulting in thin lips.

Symmetry

Look for asymmetries upon smiling and at rest (Fig. 12).

TYPES OF SMILE

Assess the type of smile the patient has, in order to be able to maintain the smile even after injecting fillers.[9]

- Mona Lisa smile: Also known as the commissural smile, the oral commissures are pulled upward with or without a show of teeth. The dominant muscle here is the zygomaticus major (Fig. 13A)[10]

- Canine smile: The central upper lip forms the highest point in this type of smile. The dominant muscle is the levator labii superioris (Fig. 13B)
- Full denture or Hollywood smile: The "Hollywood lip" refers to upper and lower lips of equal size, both with exaggerated width, and a flattened cupid's bow.[9] Approximately, 2% of the population have this smile (Fig. 13C)
- Gingival smile: Upon smiling, gingival to lip distance of 4 mm or more is known as gingival or gummy smile and is considered unattractive. In such cases, botulinum toxin injections should be given into the LLSAN muscle to soften the gummy smile (Fig. 13D).

CHOICE OF FILLER

Avoid using a filler with a very high G′. Depending on the part to be injected, a filler with low G′ or mid G′ should be used. Hyaluronic acid (HA) is preferred for lips as it can be molded well and is very forgiving. There are fewer chances of lumps and the filler can be dissolved, if the patient does not like the shape of the lip after injecting fillers.

INJECTION TECHNIQUE (VIDEO 14)

Topical prilocaine may be applied or infraorbital and mental nerve blocks may be given for anesthesia.

Dental topical anesthetic and gingival "miniblocks" (small injections of anesthesia made into the gingival sulcus) can also be given in order to anaesthetise the lips.[11]

The lips are assessed both in frontal profile, and side view, and photographs are taken in all views.

Philtrum

Philtral columns travel from the GK points on the upper lip to the columella of the nose, forming an inverted V. Pinch the skin with the nondominant hand to lift the philtral column and inject superficially into each philtrum column maintaining the inverted V. About 0.1 mL of filler is sufficient for each column.

Cupid's Bow

A full central portion of the upper lip known as the cupid's bow forms the most desirable pout. To create the cupid's bow, inject from the base of the philtral column at the vermilion-cutaneous junction advancing to the vermilion-mucosal junction (wet line). Inject 0.1 cc thin thread of filler in a retrograde fashion to enhance the cupid's bow or create a pout.

The White Roll

This is the vermilion-cutaneous junction of the lip and gives definition to the lip. Inject a light HA into the white roll superficially using the linear threading technique. Some authors prefer to inject just medial to the white roll instead of injecting on the border. Inject from the base of the philtral column toward the oral commissure. Avoid injecting the white roll of upper lip at the oral commissure. Also, avoid injecting

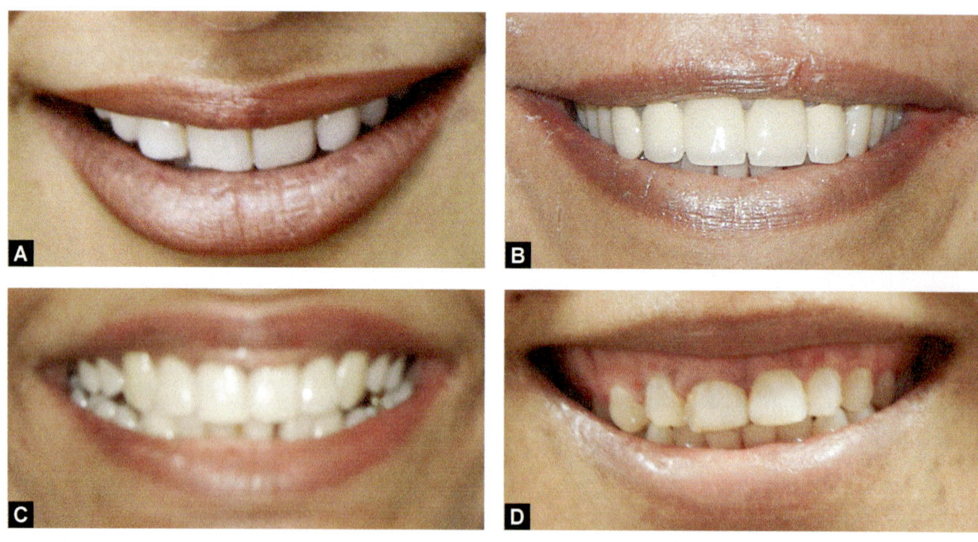

FIG. 13: **A,** Mona Lisa smile; **B,** canine smile; **C,** hollywood smile; and **D,** gingival smile.

the white roll at the cupid's bow. Injecting here will obliterate the cupid's bow creating the undesired lips. The SLA runs along the vermilion border of the upper lip to the facial sagittal midline at a depth of 3 mm (Fig. 14).[12]

Hence, it is important to stay superficial, inject slowly, and in small quantities.

The Vermilion Body

The vermilion body is injected to give volume to the lips (Fig. 15).

Inject in a retrograde linear threading fashion along the wet dry junction of the lip. To fine tune or fill small gaps, a serial puncture technique could be

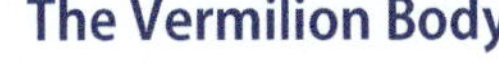

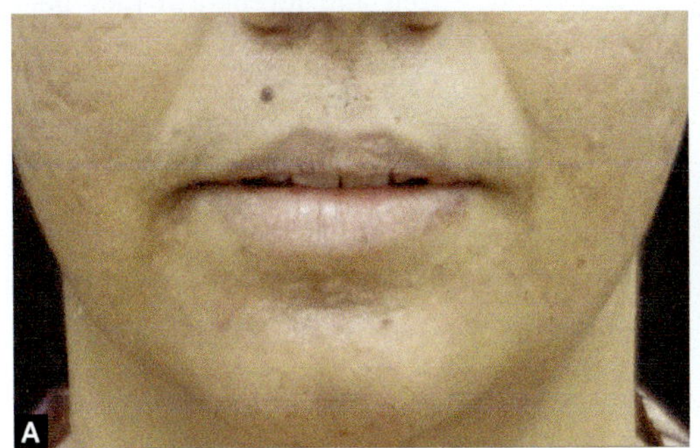

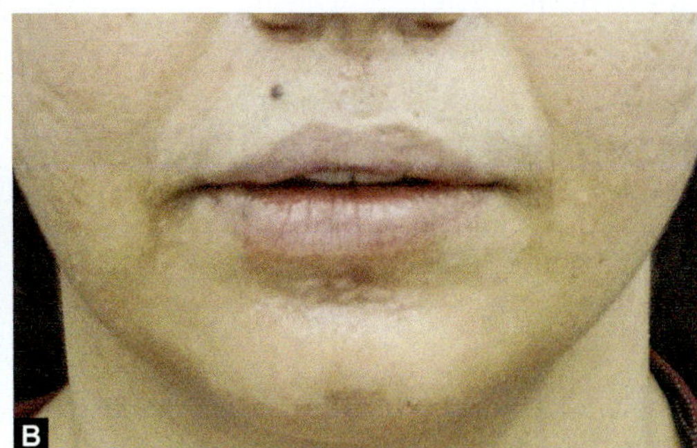

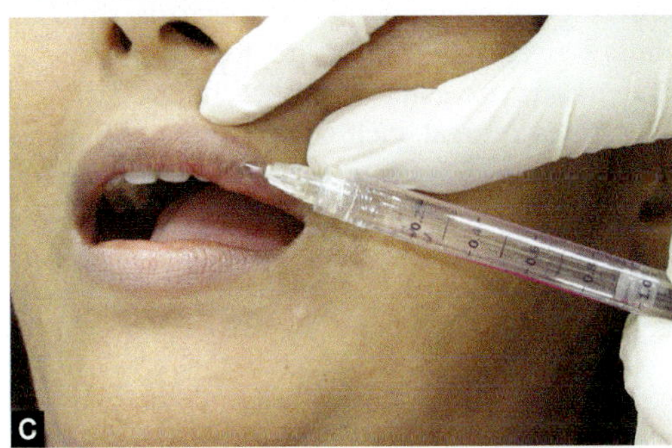

FIG. 14: **A,** Before filler injection into the vermilion body; **B,** after filler injection into the vermilion body; **C,** injecting hyaluronic acid filler into the vermilion body (1 mL Emervel lip used).

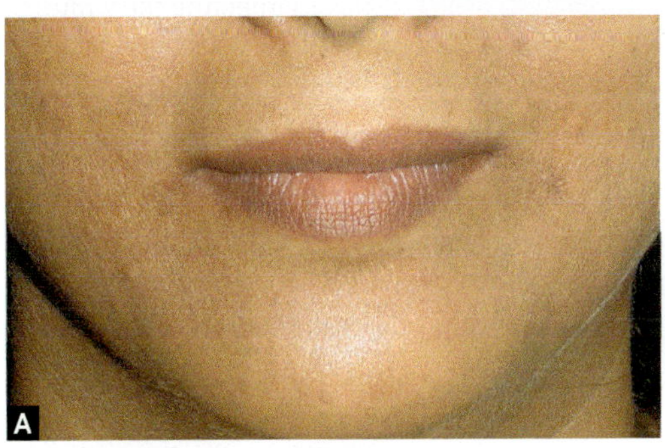

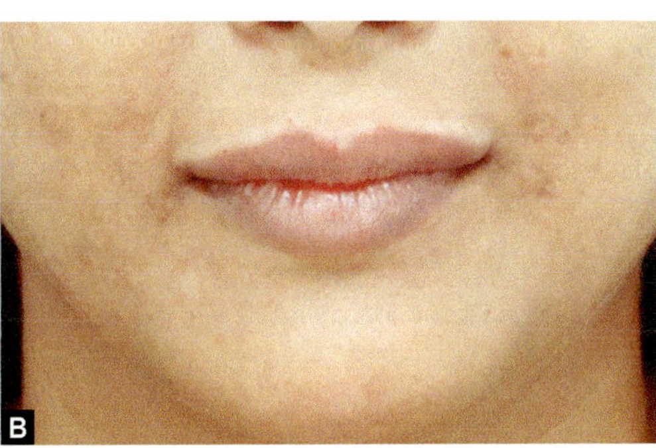

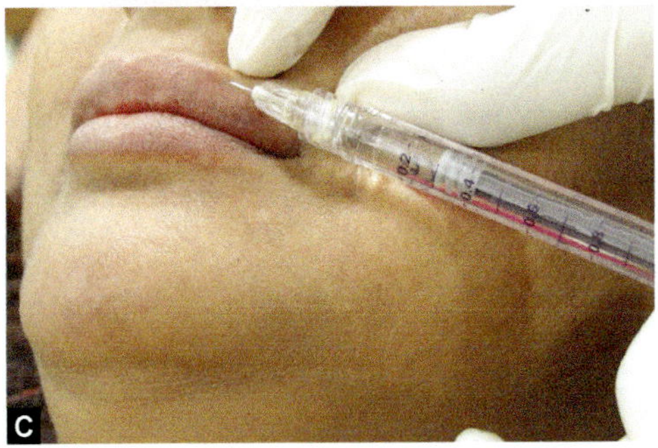

FIG. 15: **A,** Before filler injection into the white roll; **B,** after filler injection into the white roll; **C,** injecting hyaluronic acid filler into the white roll (1 mL Emervel lip used).

used. Usually, 0.4–0.5 mL each is injected into the upper lip and lower lip.

In older patients with thin lips and lip inversion, it is better to inject HA in the deep fat pad behind the orbicularis oris muscle. This plumps up the lip and causes lip eversion.[13]

Oral Commissures

One may inject into the lateral aspect of the cutaneous part of the lower lip to provide support to the oral commissures. Also, inject the marionette line using the tower technique. Adding 2 units of botulinum toxin into the DAO muscle on either side makes the muscle prominent, and helps to turn the oral commissures upward (Fig. 16).

Perioral Lines

A softer filler injected superficially into each line as a bolus effaces the perioral rhytides. Sometimes, just treating the white roll does the trick (Fig. 17).

COMPLICATIONS

- Swelling for 1–3 days. This usually subsides on its own (Fig. 18A)
- Bruising which may persist for up to a week to 10 days (Fig. 18B)
- Temporary redness and tenderness at the site of the injection
- Asymmetrical lip, can be corrected either by doing touch-ups or injecting hyaluronidase
- Lumps and irregularities of lip. These lumps can be massaged and levelled. If they persist, hyaluronidase may be injected to dissolve the lumps
- Infection, a course of antibiotics should be given if there are any signs of infection and inflammation
- Granuloma, more common with permanent fillers like polymethylmethacrylate (PMMA). Non-HA fillers need to be excised.

Vascular Complications

These complications include necrosis and blindness. Hyaluronidase, nitroglycerin paste, and hyperbaric oxygen within 72 hours have been described to treat such complications. However, it is best to avoid the deep plane and stay up to 3 mm deep in the lip, above the muscle. Secondly, watch for blanching.

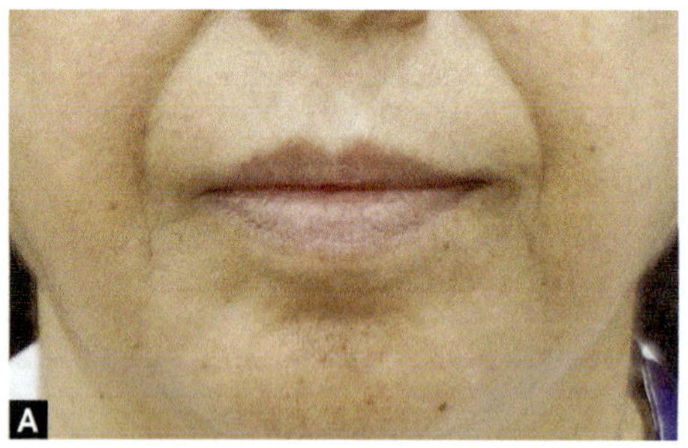

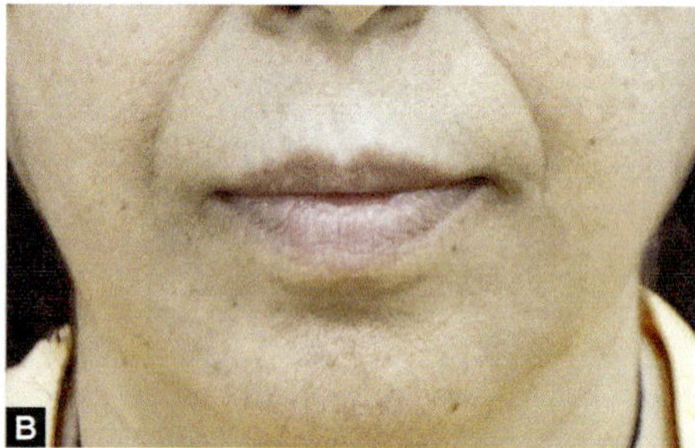

FIG. 16: A, Before filler injection into oral commissure and marionette line (0.1 mL Juvederm Ultra injected into each commissures and 0.5 mL of Voluma injected each marionette line) and **B,** after filler injection into oral commissure and marionette line.

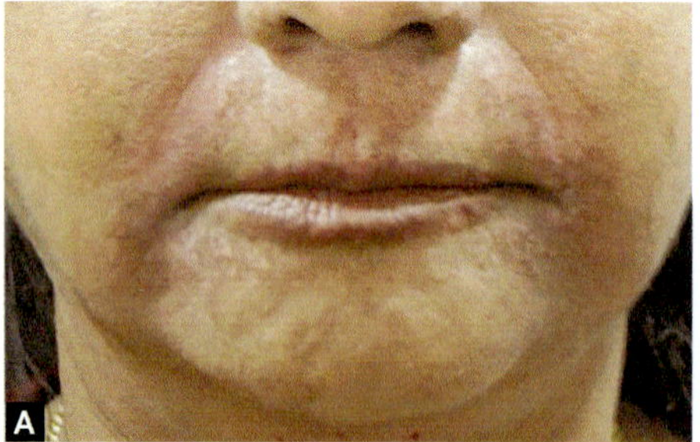

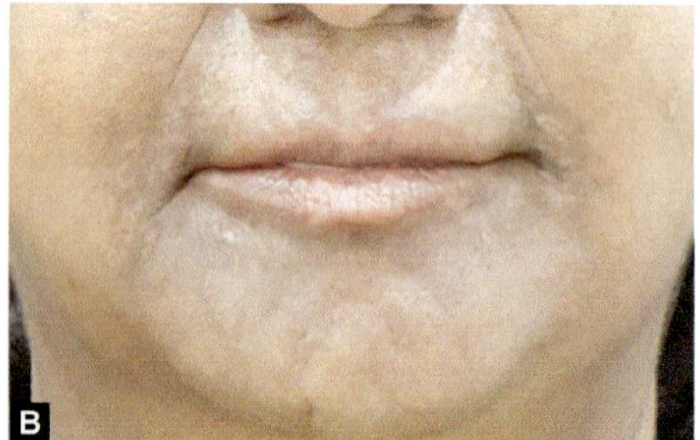

FIG. 17: A, Before filler injection into perioral lines (1 mL Juvederm Ultra used) and **B,** after filler injection into perioral lines.

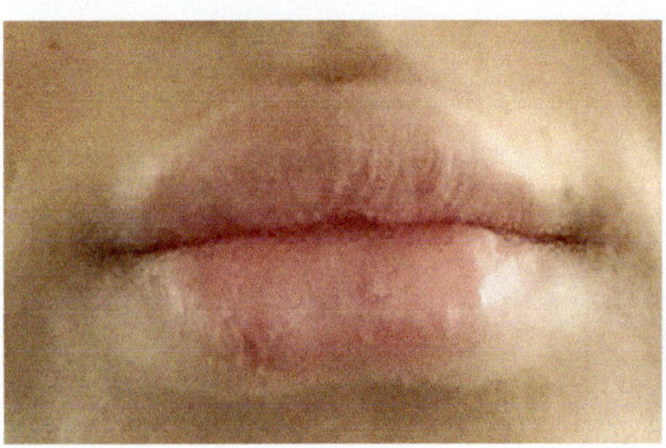
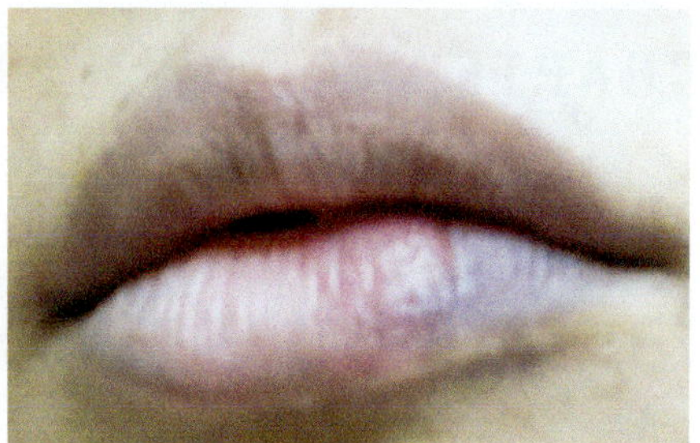

FIG. 18A: A, Temporary swelling and **B,** temporary bruising.

TREATMENT PEARLS

- Always ask for a history of herpes labialis (human papillomavirus) infection. In case of a positive history, give systemic antivirals before injecting fillers
- Stretch the lip with the noninjecting hand, while injecting the lip. This will allow uniform flow of HA and a smooth injection
- Inject slowly to prevent pressure over labial artery and to facilitate uniform placement of product
- Always watch for blanching of the lip. Blanching could indicate direct injection or external compression of the labial artery, either of which can lead to ischemia or necrosis
- After injection, mold the product between two fingers into the philtrum ridge or the white roll to prevent lumps
- To prevent duck lips, avoid overfilling the lip, especially the area of the cupid's bow of the upper lip
- Use 27–30 gauge needles to prevent bruising. To inject along the entire lips behind the muscle as in older and thinner lips, 25 gauge cannulas could be used to prevent arterial complications
- Always underfill the lips, overfilling gives an artificial look, and changes the smile contour
- Consider injecting tiny doses of botulinum toxin into the LLSAN, DAO, mentalis, and orbicularis oris wherever needed in order to treat the perioral complex
- Never inject lips if the patient has any important event or public appearance or party within a week of injection. Always inject a week to 10 days in advance in order to allow the product to settle well and to allow the swelling or tenderness or bruise if any, to subside.

CONCLUSION

Lip augmentation with hyaluronic acid fillers can change the look of the face, making one look youthful and sensuous. The key lies in keeping it natural and not creating the all so famous duck lips. Lip augmentation can also be done with autologous fat. Permanent synthetic fillers into the lip are avoidable to prevent delayed complications.

REFERENCES

1. Mauricio M, Rzany B. Injectable Fillers in Aesthetic Medicine. Berlin-Heidelberg: Springer-Verlag; 2014.
2. Rohrich RJ, Pessa JE. The anatomy and clinical implications of perioral submuscular fat. Plast Reconstr Surg. 2009;124:266-71.
3. Pendergast PM. Anatomy of the face and neck. In: Shiffman MA, Di Guiseppe A (Eds). Cosmetic Surgery. Berlin-Heidelberg: Springer-Verlag; 2012. pp. 29-45.
4. Tansatit T, Apinuntrum P, Phetudom T. A typical pattern of the labial arteries with implication for lip augmentation with injectable fillers. Aesthetic Plast Surg. 2014;38(6):1083-9.
5. Arthur S, Remington K. BeautiPHIcation™: a global approach to facial beauty. Clin Plast Surg. 2011,38(3):347-77.
6. William KA. In search of the perfect lip: 2005. Dermatol Surg. 2005;31(4):1599-603.
7. Wollina U. Perioral rejuvenation: restoration of attractiveness in aging females by minimally invasive procedures. Clin Interv Aging. 2013;8:1149-55.
8. Sarno DS, Gotkin RH. Six steps to the "perfect" lip. J Drugs Dermatol. 2013;11(9):1081-8.
9. Sclafani AP. Soft tissue fillers for management of the aging perioral complex. Facial Plast Surg. 2005;21(1):74-8.
10. Rubin LR. The anatomy of a smile: its importance in the treatment of facial paralysis. Plast Reconstr Surg. 1974;53:384-7.
11. Beer KR. Rejuvenation of the lip with injectables. Skin Ther Lett. 2007;12:5-7.
12. Robertson KM, Dyer WK. The use of fillers in the aging patient. Facial Plast Surg. 1996;12(3):293-301.
13. Braz A, Humphrey S, Weinkle S, et al. Lower Face: Clinical Anatomy and Regional Approaches with Injectable Fillers. Plast Reconstr Surg. 2015;136(5 Suppl):219S-34S.

27 CHAPTER

Hand Rejuvenation

Maya Vedamurthy

INTRODUCTION

Photoaging of hands occurs as a result of combination of intrinsic aging and exposure to ultraviolet rays. Although hand ages at the same rate as the face, hands are the first areas in the body to show visible signs of aging. Dermatoheliosis of the hands manifests coarsening of skin texture, appearance of age spots along with atrophy of the subcutaneous fat and dermis, giving rise to a skeletonized look to the hands.

Rejuvenation of hands becomes an important demand by the patients as the discrepancy between a youthful face and aged appearance of the hand becomes more evident after facial rejuvenation procedures, indicating a person's true age.[1]

HAND AESTHETICS

It is important to understand the various functional and anatomical types of hands which will serve as a guide in rejuvenation procedures.

Hands have been classified by Kretschner and are based on body habitus as follows:[2]

- The leptosome: Asthenic type
- The athletic type: Rough wider hands
- The pyknic type: Short wide dorsum and short conical fingers.

Understanding the Anatomy

The dorsum of the hand has three fatty areolar lamina separated by three thin fascial layers. The dorsal superficial lamina has no apparent structure within it. Below this is the dorsal superficial fascia followed by the dorsal intermediate lamina which has large veins and sensory nerves of the dorsum of the hand. The deepest, which is the dorsal deep lamina, contains the extensor tendons of the hand. Below the dorsal deep lamina are the dorsal interosseous muscles and metacarpal bones. Usually dermal fillers are placed into deep lamina above the metacarpal bones (Fig. 1).

SIGNS OF AGING HANDS

Hand rejuvenation involves various procedures based on the anatomical changes for rejuvenation (Table 1).

Rejuvenation of Skin

Rejuvenation of skin includes the epidermis and dermis. Topical agents—products that are used in

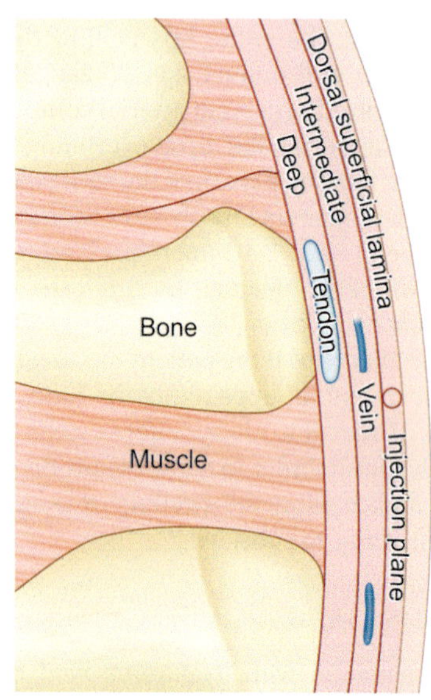

FIG. 1: Cross-sectional anatomy of the dorsal hand.

TABLE 1: Extrinsic and intrinsic signs of aging hands

Extrinsic	Intrinsic
• Dyspigmentation • Solar lentigines • Solar purpura • Actinic keratosis	• Fat loss • Wrinkles • Dermal thinning • Prominent tendons, veins and joints

photoaging such as retinoids, peptides and antioxidants such as vitamin C may be used beneficially in hand rejuvenation.

CHEMICAL PEELS

Chemical peels are commonly performed to treat dyspigmentation, textural changes and age spots. Superficial and medium depth peels are chosen because of the function of the hands, thinness of the skin and fewer adnexal structures. The chemical peels chosen are 50–70% glycolic acid, 30% salicylic acid and 10–20% trichloroacetic acid peels.

PHLEBOLOGY

The prominent veins of the hands can be treated by

- Sclerotherapy
- Endovenous laser ablation.

Sclerotherapy

Sclerotherapy of dorsal veins of the hands is performed using 0.5% sodium tetradecyl sulfate. New foam sclerotherapy using room air or carbon dioxide (CO_2) gas along with sclerosant is carried out for better results.

Endovenous Laser Ablation

Veins are treated using a diode laser leading to ablation of unwanted veins on the dorsum of the hands.

LIGHTS AND LASERS

Intense pulsed light, Q-switched laser, neodymium-doped yttrium aluminum garnet (Nd:YAG), fractionated CO_2, erbium YAG are some of the lasers useful in skin resurfacing of the hands. The age spots and lentigines are treated using lasers for selective photothermolysis of melanin.

This chapter will focus on hand rejuvenation using dermal fillers.

HAND REJUVENATION WITH DERMAL FILLERS

Treatment with dermal fillers helps to restore volume loss and improve the effects of aging hands. Plumping of the hands with dermal fillers helps to improve skin laxity and decreases the prominence of joints, tendons and veins.

The product commonly used in revolumization of hands includes:

- Autologous fat
- Hyaluronic acid
- Calcium hydroxylapatite
- Poly-L-lactic acid
- Polycaprolactone.

Autologous Fat

Autologous fat was one of the first substances to be used in volumization of the hand. The procedure involved aspiration and harvesting of fat from a donor area usually the inner thigh and injecting into the dorsa of hand using a cannula.[3]

Hyaluronic Acid

Hyaluronic acid (HA) is known to bind and retain water and thereby increase turgor and volume of tissue. Since plumping of dorsa of hand is required in hand rejuvenation, hyaluronic acid is a suitable agent in hand volumization. The injection of cross-linked HA is also thought to stimulate collagen production.[4] Cross linked hyaluronic acid degrades slowly thereby stays in the tissue longer and acts as a volume filler. The longevity of HA filler depends on the degree of cross linking, gel particle size and varies usually from 3 months to 18 months. Hyaluronic acid may be used on the hand for increasing the hydration or as a volume filler. Hydrating HA fillers used for rehydrating the skin is injected into the superficial dermis and dermoepidermal junction. These fillers rehydrate the skin and restore the quality and texture of the skin.

Revolumizing HA fillers are placed within mid-deep dermis and subcutaneous planes and intended to restore volume and give the skin a smooth surface.[5]

Poly-L-Lactic Acid

Poly-L-lactic acid (PLLA) is a biodegradable synthetic filler known to stimulate the production of collagen in areas of volume loss.[6] Poly-L-lactic acid was first used by Redaclli for hand rejuvenation in 2006.[7] Poly-L-lactic acid is available as lyophilized powder to be mixed the day before treatment with 1 mL of 1% lidocaine with or without epinephrine and 5 mL of sterile water. Larger dilutions and longer reconstitution time are recommended for safety reasons. Usually the product is placed in the subcutaneous layer and massaged diligently.

Calcium Hydroxylapatite

Calcium hydroxylapatite (CaHA) is the first Food and Drug Administration approved injectable filler for hand rejuvenation. Calcium hydroxylapatite is a biodegradable substance that follows the same metabolic pathway as bone debris that results from common bone fractures. After 2–3 months the carboxymethyl cellulose is replaced by collagen leading to permanent results.[8] The product is injected subdermally using 25 gauge 1 inch long, several sessions may be needed to achieve final results.

Preprocedure Evaluations

- Assessment of volume loss
- History of current medications especially blood thinners
- History of bleeding abnormalities
- History of type of work/hobbies that may require lots of hand utilization.

Procedure

After proper counseling, an informed consent is obtained. Photographs of both hands lying prone on a flat surface with fingers extended are taken. It is necessary to remove all ornaments such as finger rings and wash the hands thoroughly with antiseptic solution. A topical anesthetic agent may be used for 30–40 minutes prior to the procedure. Putting the patient in Trendelenburg position can reduce vein pressure to potentially reduce bleeding.[9] The area to be treated should diligently be cleaned with appropriate antiseptic solutions.

Techniques

Several techniques are available and may be used depending on the indication and comfort of the injector. The dermal filler for hands may be injected using a needle or a cannula based on product choice and technique. A cannula is used to inject the product distally and radially with withdrawing the needle.[10] This is also known as tunneling as linear threads are placed along tendons.

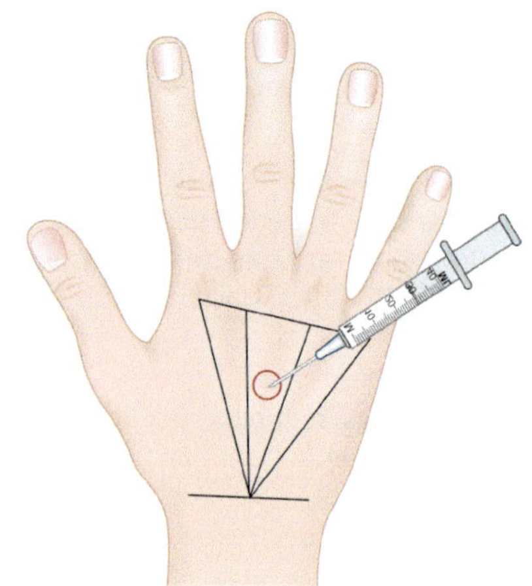

FIG. 2: Bolus technique.

Bolus-tenting Technique

This technique is quite useful when using CaHA or volumizing HA filler. Here, the entire product is injected as a single bolus at a point midway between the dorsal crease of the wrist and the metacarpophalangeal joints. The product is then evenly massaged to cover the entire dorsum of the hand. This panic bolus technique minimizes the entry points and thereby bruising (Fig. 2).

Postprocedure Instructions

Performing a gentle hand massage after injection is recommended using ultrasound gel, vitamin K cream, or arnica cream.

The technique for hand rejuvenation may be a combination of the following:

- Microdroplets
- Linear threading
- Fanning
- Bolus technique.

Microdroplet Technique

Microdroplet injections involves injecting minute amounts of the filler randomly avoiding the vessels. The product is placed into the superficial dermis using a 27 gauge needle. This technique is used for hydrating the skin (Fig. 3).

Linear Threading

Linear threading may be antegrade to push aside the vessels as the material is being injected or may be retrograde. Here, a cannula is used to inject the material along the tendons (Fig. 4).

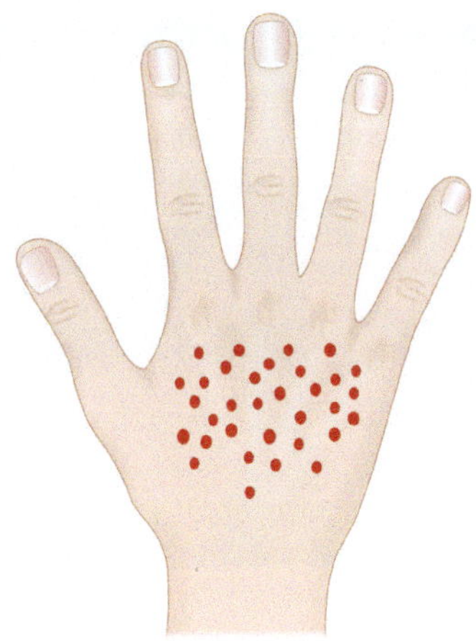

FIG. 3: Microdroplets technique.

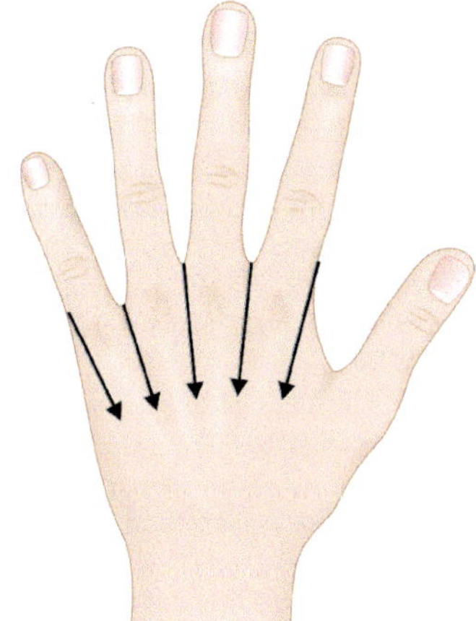

FIG. 4: Linear threading technique.

Fanning

This is used to inject the material radially across the dorsa of the hand through a single entry point usually below the wrist (Fig. 5).

Patients are requested to ice the area for 10 minutes. Some physicians recommend bandaging the hand with compression, arthritis gloves, or wrap. Patients should avoid carrying heavy objects or workouts for 2 days and keep their upper limb elevated above the level of their heart several times that day for a period of 15–20 minutes, to minimize swelling. Patients may resume normal activities after 2 days or as soon as they are comfortable. A follow up is needed after 14 days to assess the results.

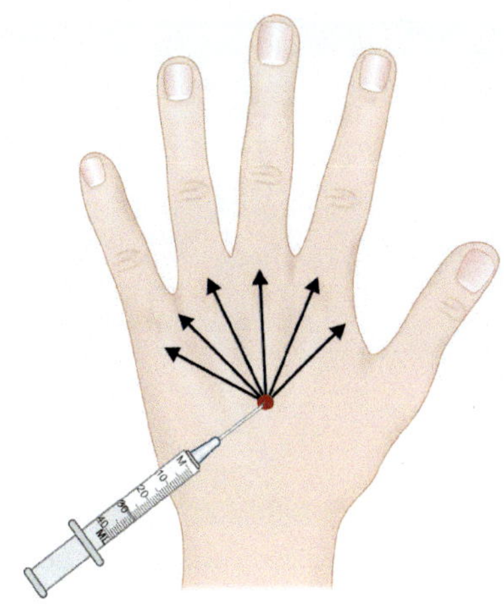

FIG. 5: Fanning technique.

COMPLICATIONS

Complications after hand rejuvenation with filler are uncommon, if performed judiciously.

However, complications that may arise may be classified as:

Minor

- Bruising
- Temporary swelling
- Tenderness
- Temporary numbness
- Tyndall effect (hyaluronic acid).

Major Adverse Reactions

- Difficulty performing activities with hands (e.g., keyboard, piano, etc.,)
- Infections
- Nodule formation
- Granuloma
- Management algorithm[10,11]

TIPS

- A good pretreatment assessment
- Good counseling
- Choose temporary fillers for the first time
- Avoid overcorrection
- Avoid inadvertent vessel injury
- Combination approach gives better results
- Identify and manage complications early.

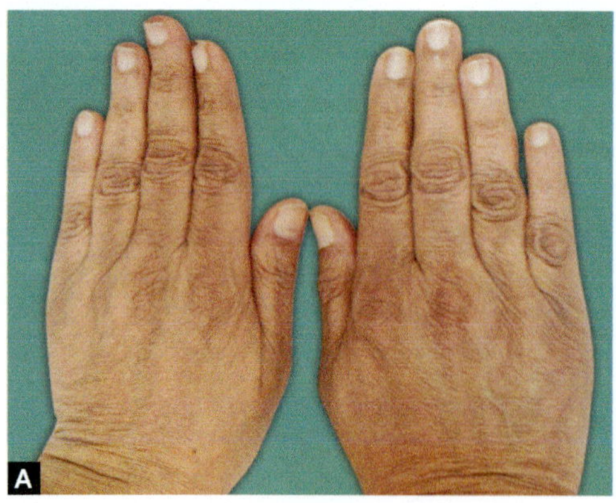
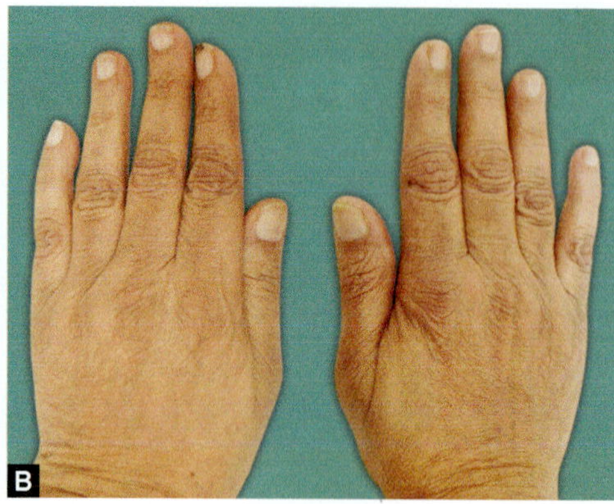

FIG. 6: Hand rejuvenation with **A,** fillers before and **B,** fillers after.

CONCLUSION

Hand rejuvenation with dermal fillers complements rejuvenation procedures in antiaging protocol (Fig. 6). A thorough knowledge of the anatomy, products, and techniques gives the best and safe results. Combination approach with other procedures aimed at improving the overall appearance of the aged hand gives cosmetically pleasing results.

REFERENCES

1. Fabi SG, Goldman MP. Hand rejuvenation. A review and our experience. Dermatol Surg. 2012;38(7 Pt 2):1112-27.
2. Jakubietz RG, Jakubiet MG, Kloss D, et al. Defining the basic aesthetics of the hand. Aesthet Plast Surg. 2005;29(6):546-51.
3. Villanueva NL, Hill SM, Small KH, et al. Technical refinements in autologous hand rejuvenation. Plast Reconstr Surg. 2015;136(6):1175-9.
4. Wang F, Garza LA, Kang S, et al. In vivo stimulation of de novo collagen production caused by cross-linked hyaluronic acid dermal filler injections in photodamaged human skin. Arch Dermatol. 2007;143(2):155-63.
5. Dallara JM. A prospective, noninterventional study of the treatment of the aging hand with Juvederm Ultra® 3 and Juvederm Hydrate. Aesthet Plast Surg. 2012;36(4): 949-54.
6. Sadick NS, Anderson D, Werschler WP. Addressing volume loss in hand rejuvenation, a report of clinical experience. J Cosmet Laser Surg. 2008;10(4):237-41.
7. Redaclli A. Cosmetic use of polylactic acid for hand rejuvenation: report on 27 patients. J Cosmet Dermatol. 2006;5(3):233-8.
8. Jacovella PF. Calcium hydroxylapatite facial filler. Clin Plast Surg. 2006;33(4):511-23.
9. Fathi R, Cohen JL. Challenges, considerations and strategies in hand rejuvenation. J Drug Dermatol. 2006;15(7):809-15.
10. Kühne U, Imhof M. Treatment of the ageing hand with dermal fillers. J Cutan Aesthet Surg. 2012;5(3):163-9.
11. Park TH, Yeo KK, Seo SW, et al. Clinical experience with complications of hand rejuvenation. J Plast Reconstr Aesthet Surg. 2012;65(12):1627-31.

28

CHAPTER

Complications of Fillers

Maya Vedamurthy

INTRODUCTION

With the increasing demand of soft tissue augmentation, there is an increase in the number of procedures performed leading to an increased incidence of complications. Documentation and reporting of all complications including new and rare ones have created awareness among injectors. Complications with hyaluronic acid fillers can occur with technique, site of filler placement, property of the filler substance, and lastly the tissue response to the filler substance. The complications may range from early to late reactions, and may be classified as temporary or permanent. Therefore, it is necessary for the physician to have a sound knowledge of the products available, the complications that may arise, and also the knowledge of avoiding and treating dermal filler complications.

PATIENT EVALUATION

A patient undergoing a filler treatment needs to be evaluated for a safe and expected outcome with the procedure.

HISTORY

A thorough history with regard to allergies, bleeding tendencies and a proper drug history is essential. History of previous fillers in the treatment area and the response to treatment is essential, to choose the right product.

EXAMINATION

Aging of the face varies from individual to individual based on extrinsic and intrinsic factors. So examination is necessary to determine the area and platform on which the filler should be placed. Fat compartments of the face need to be evaluated with respect to volume loss and descent which occurs with aging, and the volume that would be required to correct the defect should be calculated to avoid overcorrection.

CHOICE OF FILLER

Hyaluronic acid fillers are classified based on the gel hardness and gel cohesivity. Fillers premixed with the anesthetic agent should be chosen for patients who are not allergic to xylocaine. The thickness of the skin should be taken into consideration while choosing a filler. Similarly, a hyaluronic acid filler with lift capabilities need to be selected while repositioning fat pads which have descended with aging.

DISCUSSION

Complications with hyaluronic acid fillers may be classified as early and late complications (Table 1).

TABLE 1: Complications of fillers[1]

Early	Late
Hypersensitivity	Granuloma
Infections	Infection and biofilm
Embolism	Nodules
Reactivation of herpes simplex	Migration
Overcorrection	Hypertrophic scarring
	Telangiectasia
	Lipoatrophy

Early Complications

Early complications with hyaluronic acid fillers may be injection related or substance related.

Injection-related Complications

The procedure-related events are erythema, bruising and tenderness which may be due to improper technique. These reactions usually subside spontaneously within a week. However, erythema can be reduced by using topical corticosteroids and avoiding sun exposure. Bruising can be treated by rubbing in arnica cream for 5 minutes and five times a day for 5 days. Pulsed dye laser and intense pulse pulsed dye laser are useful in treating bruising more effectively. Tenderness can be managed by administering systemic nonsteroidal anti-inflammatory agents for a few days.

Filler Substance-related Complications

Hypersensitivity Reactions

Hypersensitivity reaction to hyaluronic acid per se is rare but reported. With the advent of filler mixed with local anesthetics one has to be more vigilant and determine the eliciting compound for hypersensitivity reactions. Localized hypersensitivity reactions are more common than generalized systemic reactions. The localized reactions may range from erythema to late abscess like reactions.[2]

Infections[3]

Infections can be prevented by a good history, instituting prophylactic antivirals or antibiotics as per need and by following strict asepsis throughout the procedure. In patients requiring antivirals, administration of acyclovir 200 mg qid for 5 days starting 2 days prior to procedure or valacyclovir 500 mg bid or famciclovir 250 mg tid is recommended. For patients requiring antibacterials, oral antibiotics (ofloxacin 200 mg bid, azithromycin 500 mg od or amoxyclavulic acid 500 mg tid) are administered 2 days prior to the procedure and continued for 3 days post procedure.

For abscesses, a culture sensitivity followed by appropriate antibiotics and incision and drainage is advised.

Embolism

The complications arising due to embolism may range from tissue necrosis to blindness. It occurs due to accidental blockage of subdermal artery when filler is injected through a resting needle, due to decreased tissue perfusion by vascular compromise by undesirable amount of filler material, surrounding edema and inflammation due to filler per se, or because of direct entry of filler into the vessel.[4]

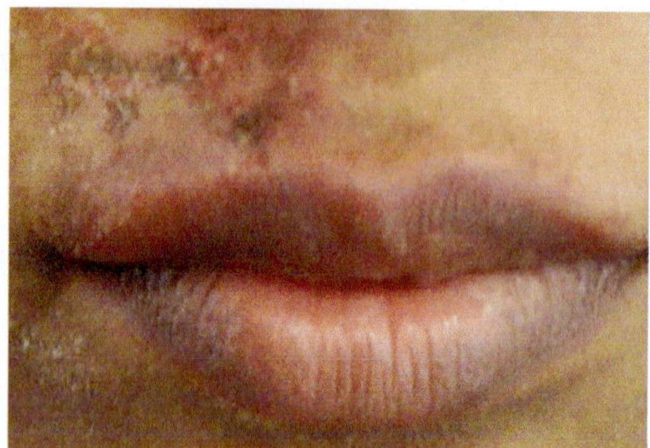

FIG. 1: Skin necrosis due to vascular occlusion.

In case of arterial occlusion, there will be immediate blanching with severe pain whereas in case of venous occlusion there will be delayed dull pain with bluish discoloration of the injected area[5] (Fig. 1).

Methods to avoid or minimize vascular embolism would be to aspirate before injecting, utilize a smaller needle or a blunt cannula and inject using minimal pressure. Once intralesional injection is suspected it is wise to stop the procedure and inject hyaluronidase along with topical warm compresses, 2% nitroglycerine paste or topical oxygen infusion cream. In case of blindness referral to an ophthalmologist for emergency measures is advised.[6]

Overcorrection

Injection of too much material can lead to undesired results such as lumpiness, bumpiness or nodule formation. Inappropriate placement of dermal filler especially in areas of thin soft tissue coverage can give rise to Tyndall effect. Excess amount of filler or improper placement can be corrected by injecting hyaluronidase (Fig. 2).

Late Complications

Granulomas[7]

Granulomas are delayed hypersensitivity reactions to a foreign body. The dermal filler incites a foreign body reaction based on the physiochemical properties of the substance, the amount of filler injected and biofilm formation. Although permanent fillers carry a higher risk of granuloma formation, nonanimal stabilized hyaluronic acid have been reported to induce granuloma. Clinically they appear as papules, nodules, or plaques which may lead to ulceration and fibrosis. A histopathology of the suspected lesion

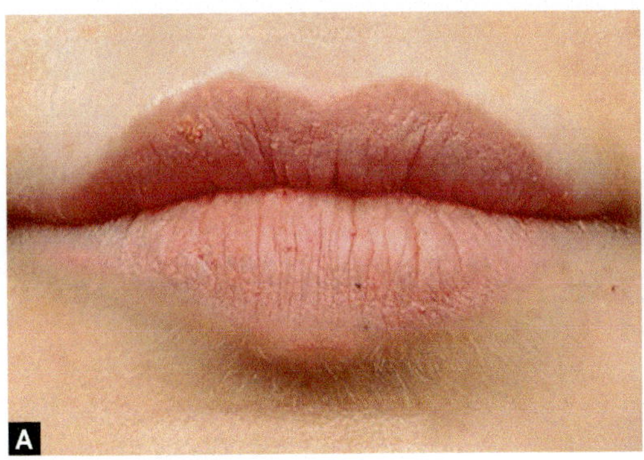

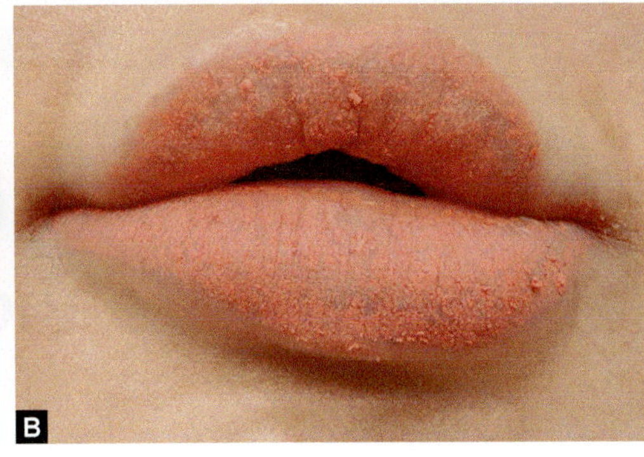

FIG. 2: A, Before filler and **B,** overcorrection of lips after filler.

will help to confirm the diagnosis and the probable nature of the filler material used.

Management includes ruling out biofilm formation, use of appropriate antibiotic as needed before proceeding to treat the granuloma. If sterile, the granuloma may be injected with corticosteroids and 5-fluorouracil and or hyaluronidase in case of hyaluronic acid filler. Oral minocycline 100 mg bid is said to have anti-inflammatory and antigranulomatous properties. An alternative approach is to remove the material by microliposuction cannulas or surgical excision.

Migration

Migration is generally more common with permanent fillers but in the author's experience migration is seen with hyaluronic acid fillers when used where the skin is thin as in the periocular region or where there is not enough structural support as in the chin area especially when highly dense material are used in such places. Migration occurs early and can be prevented by using adhesive tapes for a few days in these areas till the filler settles in place. In case of excessive migration, the product is removed using hyaluronidase.

Telangiectasia

Telangiectasia is quite visible in areas where the skin is thin and more in light colored individuals. This can happen at the injection site and this can be treated with pulsed dye laser or intense pulsed light.[8]

Lipoatrophy[9]

Lipoatrophy occurring with fillers is a paradox as dermal fillers are indicated in the treatment of human immunodeficiency virus lipoatrophy.[10] However, facial lipoatrophy has been reported with hyaluronic acid fillers.

CONCLUSION

Complications with dermal fillers can be avoided if product selection and patient selection is stringent. However as described by Carruthers, the aesthetic benefit the patient achieves with temporary fillers is 90% technique and 10% substance.[11] Therefore, the experience of the injector along with safety measures is the best way to avoid complications and have a happy patient.

REFERENCES

1. Hexsel DM, Hexsel CL, Iyenger V. Liquid injectable silicone: history, mechanism of action, indications, technique and complications. Semin Cutan Med Surg. 2003;22(2):107-14.
2. Shafir R, Amir A, Gur E. Long-term complications of facial injections with Restylane (injectable hyaluronic acid). Plast Reconstr Surg. 2000;106(5):1215-6.
3. De Boulle K. Management of complications after implantation of fillers. J Cosmet Dermatol. 2004;3(1):2-15.
4. Weinberg MJ, Solish N. Complications of hyaluronic acid fillers. Facial Plast Surg. 2009;25(5):324-8.
5. Sclafani AP, Fagien S. Treatment of injectable soft tissue filler complications. Dermatol Surg. 2009;35(Suppl 2): 1672-80.
6. Ozturk CN, Li Y, Tung R, et al. Complications following injection of soft-tissue fillers. Aesthet Surg J. 2013;33(6): 862-77.
7. Kohli M, Davda R. Complications of fillers. In: Pai GS (Ed). Complications in Cosmetic Dermatology Crafting Cures, 1st Edition. New Delhi: Jaypee Brothers Medical Publishers; 2016. pp. 90-108.
8. Lemperle G, Duffy DM. Treatment options for dermal filler complications. Aesthet Surg J. 2006;26(3):356-64.
9. Lemperle G, Rullan RP, Gauthier-Hazan N. Dermal filler complications. Plast Reconstr Surg. 2006;112(33):93-107.
10. Andre P, Wechsler J, Revuz J. Facial lipoatrophy: report of five cases after injection of synthetic fillers into nasolabial folds. J Cosmet Dermatol. 2002;1(3):120-3.
11. Carruthers J. Review of Long-Lasting Dermal Fillers. Aliso Viejo, CA: Medical Insight, Inc.; 2006. pp 6-23.

29

CHAPTER

Nonhyaluronic Acid Fillers: Science and Techniques

Jason J Emer, Heidi Waldorf

INTRODUCTION

Noninvasive facial rejuvenation procedures such as soft tissue filling are popular alternatives for patients who are adverse to traditional surgery and demand antiaging treatments with minimal recovery time and limited complication risk. Soft tissue fillers can smooth, reshape, and/or recontour skin by filling and lifting depleted areas directly, as well as by improving the overall appearance of skin by hydration and neocollagenesis. With proper training and techniques, and appropriate filler selection based on the patient's individual aesthetic goals, soft tissue filling procedures have few limitations.[1,2]

Synthetic filling agents such as poly-L-lactic acid (PLLA), calcium hydroxylapatite (CaHA), polymethylmethacrylate (PMMA), and silicone oil offer alternative options for patients in desire of long-lasting results (ranging from a year to permanence) or in situations where volumization or recontouring requires additional substances with higher viscosity and/or the ability to promote collagenesis. Nonhyaluronic acid (HA) fillers such as those that are biostimulators (PLLA, CaHA), semipermanent (PMMA), and permanent (silicone oil) differ in respect to the chemical composition, dynamics, and interaction with the surrounding host tissue.

CLASSIFICATION

The non-HA fillers can be classified as:

- Biodegradable fillers:
    - Calcium hydroxylapatite gel (Radiesse)
    - Polylactic acid (Sculptra, New-Fill)
- Nonbiodegradable fillers:
    - Polyacrylamide gel [polyacrylamide hydrogel (PAAG), Aquamid and Amazingel]
    - Polymethylmethacrylate (Artecoll and Artefill)

They can also be classified as:

- Semipermanent: Longevity between 1 year and 2 years
- Permanent: Longevity more than 2 years.

CALCIUM HYDROXYLAPATITE (RADIESSE)

Calcium hydroxylapatite, also known as CaHA, is represented by the formula $Ca_5(PO_4)_3(OH)$ and is the principle component of human teeth and bone. The pure powder is white and can be modified to form a gel or a paste. Calcium hydroxylapatite is a synthetic soft tissue filler composed of suspending CaHA (30%) in a gel carrier (70%) consisting primarily of water, glycerin, and carboxymethylcellulose. Because it is biocompatible, no skin testing is necessary.[3] It has a large particle size range of 25–45 μm, which impedes phagocytosis and provide longevity. Calcium hydroxylapatite has Food and Drug Administration (FDA) approval for radiographic tissue marking, treatment of vocal cord insufficiency, dental defects, for the improvement of moderate to severe facial wrinkles and folds, and facial lipoatrophy (Fig. 1).[4,5] Despite rumors, to the contrary, when injected in this formulation, CaHA does not turn into bone or interfere with evaluation of diagnostic radiographic imaging in regions of soft tissue augmentation.[6]

Indications

Calcium hydroxylapatite has been approved by the US FDA for injecting the dorsum of hands (Fig. 2). Off-label use of CaHA has included volume restoration of mid-face, jawline, buttocks, neck, post rhinoplasty contour correction, acne scar correction, ear lobule augmentation, and wrinkling of the décolletage (Figs 2–4). The FDA approved use is to

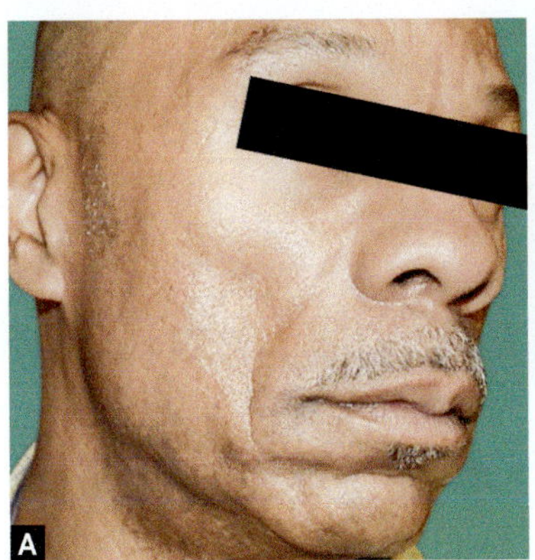
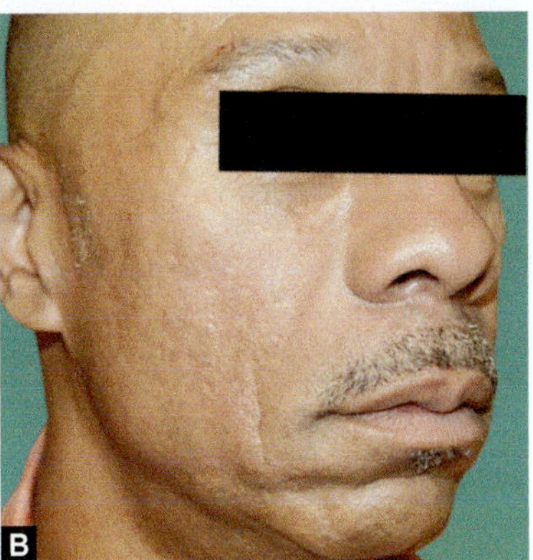

FIG. 1: Calcium hydroxylapatite (CaHA) for facial lipoatrophy. **A,** Before and **B,** after CaHA [2, 1.5 cc syringes each mixed with 0.5 cc of lidocaine hydrochloric acid 1% and 1:100,000 epinephrine] injected using a cross-hatching technique on the midface. Significant improvement in volume and contour is seen immediately after injection.

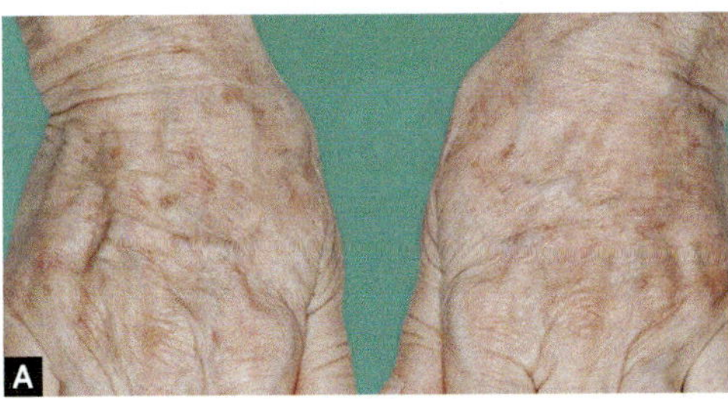
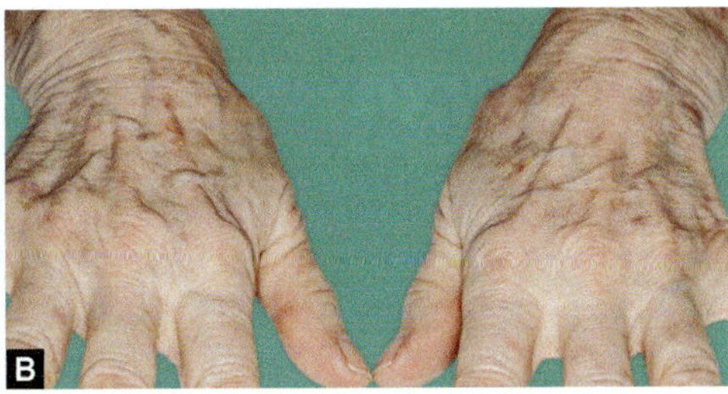

FIG. 2: Calcium hydroxylapatite (CaHA) for hand rejuvenation. **A,** Before and **B,** after CaHA (a single 1.5 cc syringe mixed 1:1 with lidocaine hydrochloric acid 1% and 1:100,000 epinephrine) injected into each dorsal hand using a flexible microcannula (25 gauge, 2 inch) to avoid any complications. Immediate improvement in tendon and vessel show, as well as superficial wrinkling is noted with no evidence of bruising or swelling.

mix the prepared 1.5 mL syringe of CaHA with 0.3 mL of 2% lidocaine without epinephrine and to inject with a 27 gauge needle with Luer lock fittings.[7] Many practitioners, including both contributing authors dilute the material further to help reduce pain and injection force, with little reported change in efficacy or longevity.[8]

A benefit of CaHA over other filling agents is its high viscosity and elasticity (G prime or G') allowing for large areas of augmentation and lift with little product, correlating with sustained clinical results reported lasting between 12 months and 3 years.[9-11] So called "touch up" injections 3 months after the initial injection may prolong the duration of effect.[12] Injection volumes are considerably less with CaHA as compared to other fillers for a similar clinical effect due to these intrinsic product properties.

As compared to HA fillers, CaHA is considered to have high viscosity and high elasticity, which gives it the ability to lift, sculpt, and support more readily and in a predicable manner.[13] Mixing lidocaine into the filler will reduce both elasticity and viscosity and should be taken into account. These properties give CaHA the advantages of longevity with the subsequent ability for facial shaping and large volume enhancements as compared to HA fillers.[14,15]

Indications

Nasolabial folds (NLFs), cheeks, acne scars, and prejowl sulcus, buttocks, decolletage, dorsum of hands, and mid-face.[16]

Advantages

High safety profile, high patient satisfaction, and durability in a period of 4 years of CaHA injected into various facial areas of aesthetic concern such as the NLFs, marionette lines/oral commissures, lips, glabella, and cheeks.[17]

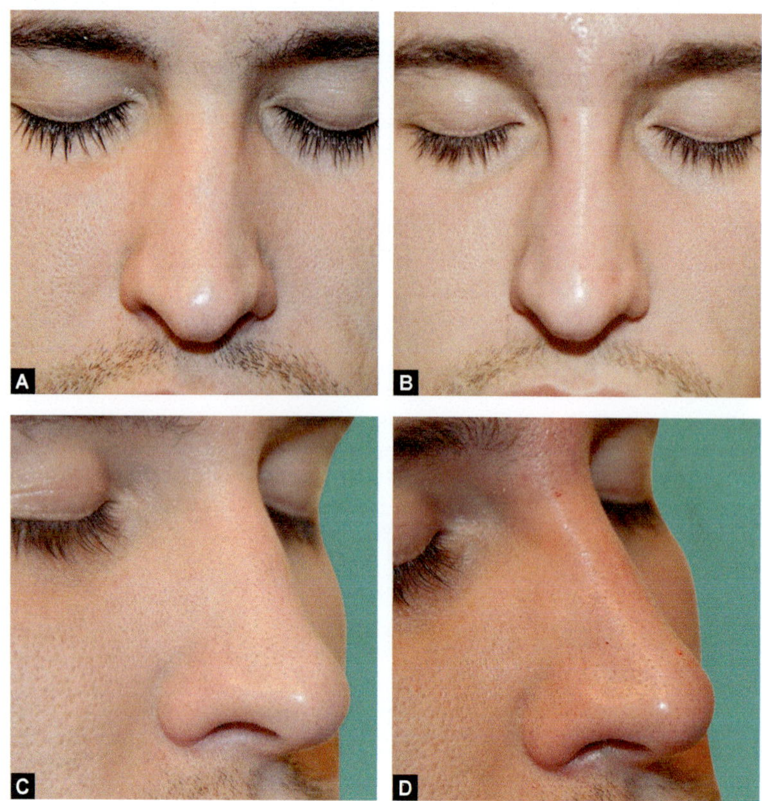

FIG. 3: Calcium hydroxylapatite (CaHA) for nasal recontouring. Before **(A,C)** and after **(B,D)** 0.6 cc of CaHA (a 0.8 cc syringe mixed with 0.1 cc lidocaine hydrochloric acid 1% and epinephrine 1:100,000) injected supraperiosteally into the nasal dorsum and nasal midline to improve contour (mild saddle deformity/bone irregularity).

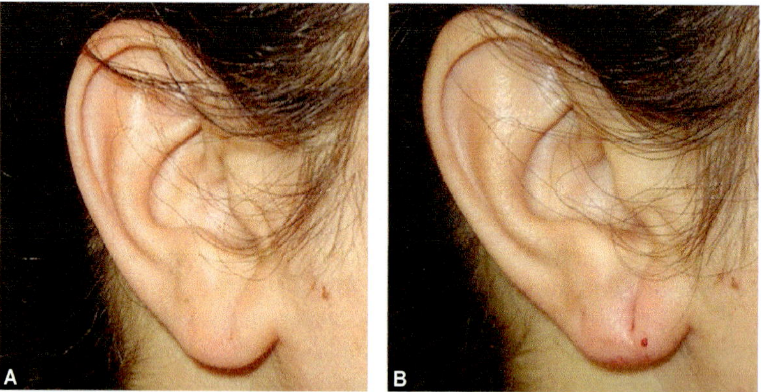

FIG. 4: Calcium hydroxylapatite (CaHA) ear lobule augmentation. **A,** Before and **B,** after 0.2 cc of CaHA (a 0.8 cc syringe mixed 1:1 with lidocaine hydrochloric acid 1% and epinephrine 1:100,000) injected into the ear lobule using serial puncture and linear threading techniques in a three-dimensional approach to revolumize and give support.

One further advantage of CaHA is its ability for neocollagenesis. The initial volume replacement is substituted with natural collagen from attracted histiocytes and fibroblasts that forms a scaffold around CaHA microspheres after the gel carrier dissolves.[18,19] Preauricular biopsies 6 months after

CaHA injection demonstrated deposition of collagen around, and infiltration into, the filler microspheres with a fibroblastic and mild histiocytic tissue response.[20] Both type I and III collagen were seen on polarized, picrosirius red (PSR) staining, and immunohistochemical (IHC) analysis.

Injection Techniques (Figs 5 and 6)

Calcium hydroxylapatite is indicated for placement into the subcutaneous space or on the periosteum and are safe and effective. Given the high viscosity and particulate nature, it is recommended to use a 25–27-gauge needle. Alternatively, blunt-tipped microcannulas (22–27 gauge) can be used instead of sharp hypodermic needles as they may be less painful, atraumatic, and allow for a single entry point to be used to deposit large amounts of material in a wide treatment area.[21-23] Sharp needle or blunt-tipped cannula length can vary and it is common to use a 1.25 inch needle and/or 1.5–2.0 inch cannula in the subcutaneous plane when treating large/wide areas such as the midface, prejowl, lateral zygoma, or preauricular areas. For periosteal placement, smaller needle lengths such as a 0.5–1 inch are recommended over use of the blunt-tipped cannula.

Superficial placement, such as into the periocular or perioral or forehead lines, is contraindicated with CaHA because of the risk of visible and/or palpable white nodules. It is generally suggested that CaHA be avoided for injections within the orbital rims. As discussed previously, nodule formation—due to product accumulation/"clumping"—may occur if injected in areas that are frequently mobile such as the lips due to the "pumping action" of orbicularis oris muscle and should be avoided.[24,25]

The tear troughs, malar eminence, lateral zygoma, and the mental crease are particularly vulnerable to filler visibility. Treatment of these areas requires periosteal placement or deeper subcutaneous placement. Increasing the volume of lidocaine that is mixed before treatment may also reduce the risk of nodule formation by reducing viscosity and elasticity. The decreased viscosity and elasticity translates into

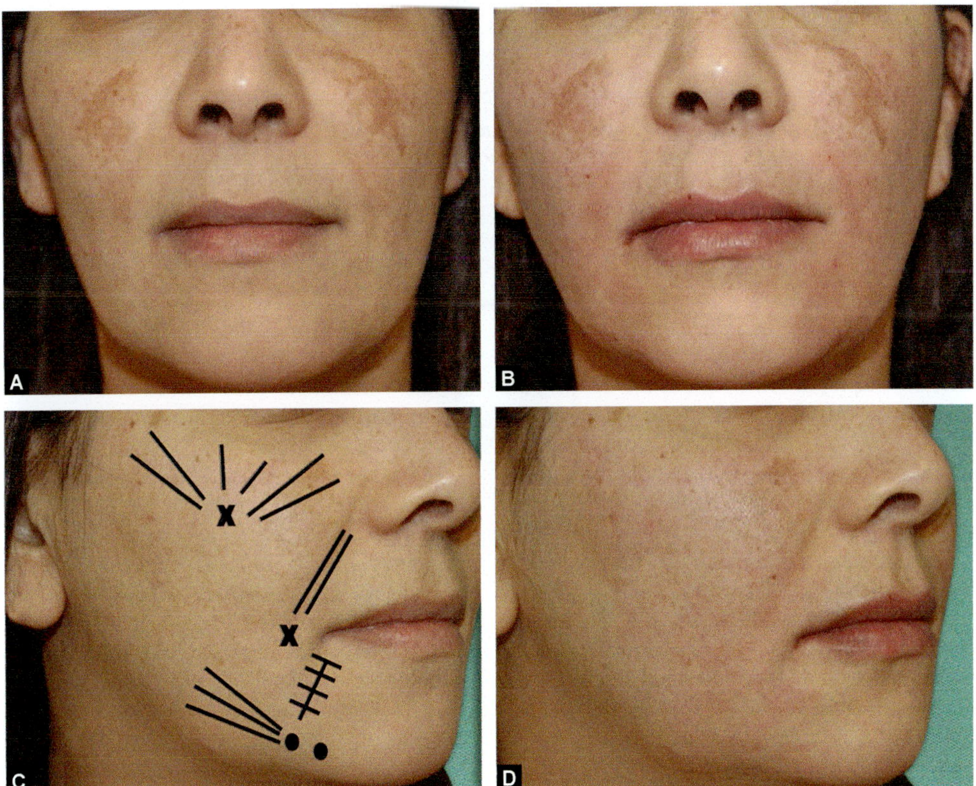

FIG. 5: Calcium hydroxylapatite (CaHA). **A**, Before CaHA injection; **B**, after CaHA injection; **C**, markings for injection; and **D**, after injection, side view.

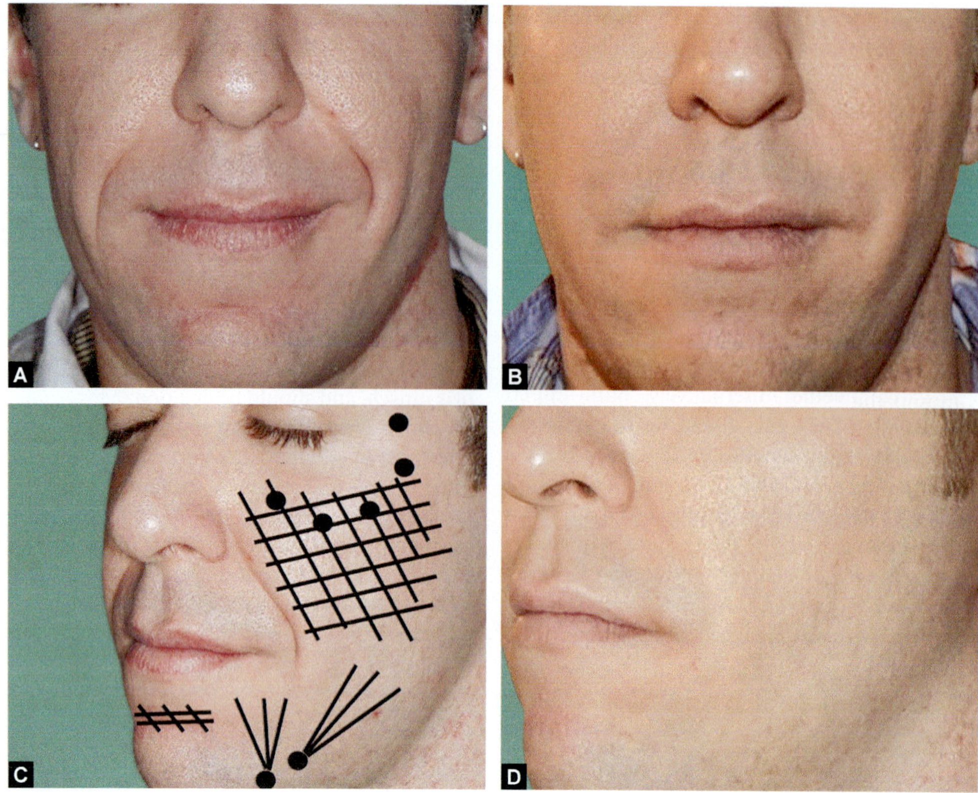

FIG. 6: Calcium hydroxylapatite (CaHA) for pan-facial rejuvenation. **A,** Before and **B,** 3 months after CaHA injected in a cross-hatching pattern using **C,** retrograde linear threads (lines) in the midface, chin/lower cutaneous lip, and prejowl, as well as supraperiosteally (dots) on the jawline, tear trough, and periocularly. **D,** Sustained improvements in volume and lifting are noted. The nasolabial folds were not directly injected, but are improved due to recontouring of the midface fat compartments (suborbicularis oculi fat and deep medial cheek fat).

reduced extrusion force and more malleable product for massage as well as less product opacity.[26] This is particularly helpful in areas such as the hands, perioral region, or in the mental crease where nodule formation is more common due to a propensity for localized product accumulation. In both the authors' opinion, CaHA has the added benefit of providing an opaque background to the hands where an HA filler could leave the area looking bruised.

For periosteal injections, the needle is inserted and passed through tissue till the periosteum is "tapped" and small aliquots of material are deposited until the desired corrected result is seen. Some authors like a "tower technique"—a variation on the depot and layering techniques—where via a perpendicular injection into the periosteal plane, a depot injection is made with a gradual tapering of product deposition as the needle is withdrawn.[27,28] A series of towers or filler "struts" are created in a vertical fashion providing both lifting and support to bony architecture as well as the surrounding soft tissue. Anatomical areas most amenable to this technique include the lateral brow, NLFs, marionette lines, prejowl sulcus, lateral tear trough, lateral zygoma, and mental area.

After injection, aggressive immediate massage may help in ensuring adequate dispersion and prevent clumping of product. When they occur, nodules may be punctured with a 16 to 18-gauge needle or #11 blade to facilitate extrusion of the material or can be removed later with a 2 or 3 mm punch. Unfortunately—unlike hyaluronidase for HA-type fillers—there is no "antidote" available to dissolve unwanted CaHA. The use of intralesional saline injection followed by massage in order to mechanically break up the product has been described. Subcision of nodules may facilitate their breakdown as well. Intralesional corticosteroids [with or without 5-fluorouracil (5-FU)] have also been used, however, they carry a risk of atrophy peripheral to the retained filler, making it more, rather than less visible. Fractional carbon dioxide laser has been recently reported to aid in nodule resolution.[29] Radiofrequency treatment atop the nodule may create enough dermal heating and edema to disperse the nodule.[30,31] One author (JE) had success in using fractional nonablative laser (Fraxel; Solta Medical) and fractional radiofrequency (Sublative; Syneron Candela) with and without microneedling (Eclipse Micropen) to treat superficial irregularities. Finally, injecting additional filler, for example a HA-type filler around the nodule to blend the surface with the surrounding skin contours—can reduce the appearance of the nodule until it resolves over time. Because there is no immediate antidote to CaHA placement, it is contraindicated for use in glabellar lines and the piriform aperture where compromise of vital vessels is a high risk (Fig. 7).

Side Effects

Side effects such as ecchymosis and edema may occur. Some of the rare complications reported are submucosal nodules of lip, cellulitis, nodule formation, biofilm formation and skin necrosis (Fig. 7).[16,32-37]

POLY-L-LACTIC ACID (SCULPTRA)

Poly-L-lactic acid was initially approved for the use of pan-facial volumization of lipoatrophy secondary to human immunodeficiency virus (HIV) or acquired immunodeficiency syndrome (AIDS) therapy as New Fill in 1999, with subsequent approvals for the correction of shallow to deep NLF contour deficiencies and other facial wrinkles as Sculptra Aesthetic in 2009. Unlike static filling agents, PLLA does not augment the skin directly, but instead indirectly improves contour by tissue stimulation with neocollagenesis. Instead of an immediate effect, volume is restored gradually over several weeks.[38,39] PLLA is a synthetic polymer related to α-hydroxy acids, similar to absorbable suture material. It is manufactured as a lyophilized preparation containing microparticles of PLLA, carboxymethylcellulose, and mannitol.[40] It is stored at room temperature, and is reconstituted with sterile or bacteriostatic water and/or lidocaine at least 2 hours prior to use. In the author's opinion, longer reconstitution time (>24–72 h up to 6 weeks) and higher dilution (>9 mL total volume) limits adverse events such as nodule formation and asymmetries.

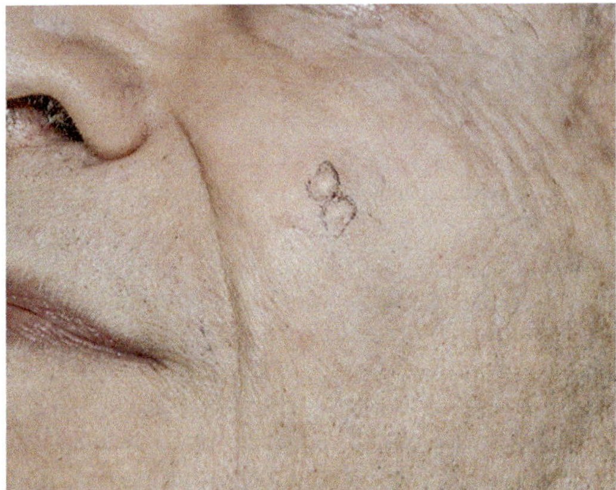

FIG. 7: Calcium hydroxylapatite nodule of the cheek. Two yellow-white nodules are seen superficially on the left cheek 2 weeks after midfacial revolumization in a patient with human immunodeficiency virus lipoatrophy

Once injected, the PLLA microparticles induce an inflammatory response with subsequent collagen deposition by local fibroblasts.[41] PLLA particles are 40–60 μm and impede phagocytosis and diffusion. Volume restoration is a result of a granulomatous inflammation that stimulates collagen production in the deep dermis or subcutaneous tissue. Initial clinical changes are evident immediately after injection, but are short lived as the carrier solution is absorbed in the following hours to days. Patients desiring immediate results or with social constraints requiring little downtime may be unhappy if expectations are not discussed.

Histologically, a capsule of macrophages, mast cells, foreign-body giant cells, lymphocytes, and vascular structures are seen surrounding the PLLA particles a month after implantation.[42] The particles are degraded into naturally occurring lactic acid, carbon dioxide, and water, with subsequent deposition of type I collagen.[43] By 18 months, there is no evidence of granulomatous inflammation, but evidence of new collagen deposition is sustained.

In a study of 20 patients injected with two to six PLLA treatment sessions, three-dimensional (3D) digital surface imaging demonstrated a gradual but sustained statistical improvement in midfacial (maximum, 1.82 mL) and nasolabial (maximum, 1.11 mL) volume.[44]

A recent review suggested that three treatment sessions with a minimum of 3 to 4 weeks intervals between treatment sessions to allow for the cellular cascade, responsible for collagen repair and restoration to occur is an optimal regimen for the majority of patients.[45]

At least greater than two injection sessions are required to achieve visible and sustainable results.

The most recent long-term studies have documented safety and sustained efficacy from up to 2 years and continuing up to 5 years posttreatment.[46-49] One study reported longer-term maintenance with the use of one to two touch-up sessions between years 2 and 4.[46] All in all, excellent and safe improvements in appearance are seen in all populations if a conservative, systematic approach is taken in non-HIV patients.

Additionally, many studies have also highlighted the ability of PLLA to provide not only physical, but also psychological improvements up to 25 months.[50,51]

Delayed nodule formation is the primary concern after PLLA injection. The reported incidence of nodule formation varies from less than 5% to greater than 40%; higher rates may be dependent on variables such as study design, patient reporting, product preparation, and injection techniques.[40,52] Most PLLA-induced nodules develop several months to a year after treatment and can frustratingly persist.[49]

As touched upon earlier, new treatment protocols have markedly reduced the incidence of nodule formation and improved cosmetic results. Utilizing higher dilution volumes (8–12 mL total; 5–10 mL of sterile water plus 1–2 mL of 1% lidocaine with or without epinephrine) and earlier reconstitution (a minimum of 24–72 hours before injection) improves product hydration and reduces clumping of dried product within the tissue. Further, the addition of lidocaine in the injection mixture limits pain after a small amount has been delivered to the treatment area. Topical anesthetic, "stress balls", and "talkesthesia", or ice packs, are useful to defer pain during primary needle entry when using PLLA as with other injectables. A maximum of 10 mL can be contained within the glass vial provided.[53] Thus, in areas such as a décolletage or arm or knees, larger dilution volumes (15–16 mL) must take place outside of the supplied sterile vial in either the injection syringes or an additional larger sterile vial.[54,55] It is important to maintain sterility during this process to avoid infectious complications.

Deep product placement in the subcutaneous and periosteal planes and vigilant avoidance of intramuscular injections (i.e., lip, perioral, and periocular) has reduced the development of visible papules and nodules as well. Other helpful techniques include limiting volume injected per session, aggressive massage by the patient after treatment (the *5/5/5* rule: 5 minutes, 5 times a day, for 5 days) and waiting 4 to 8 weeks between injection sessions.[56-58] Like CaHA, another particulate agent, PLLA should not be injected into the lips. The periorbital area is particularly vulnerable to the formation of nodules and foreign body granulomas so treatment with PLLA above the orbital rim is generally not suggested.[59] Although, PLLA may be injected in the hands in a "depot" method below the muscle at a significantly diluted volume, the authors do not inject PLLA in that area because of the high incidence of visible persistent nodules.[60-62] The temples, midface, preauricular area, piriform aperture, prejowel sulcus, and jawline are ideal locations for periosteal placement and can rejuvenate through structural volume restoration of these areas.[63,64] Patients should be warned that even if not visible, palpable nodules may occur, which are asymptomatic and not dangerous and will resolve over time.

Injection Techniques

Poly-L-lactic acid should be injected into the deep dermis or subcutaneous layer using a 25–26 gauge sharp-needle or blunt-tipped, larger-gauge (22 or 25) microcannula. The authors prefer using 3 mL syringes for product delivery as this allows less interruption during injections, however, for novice injectors a 1 mL syringe can be used to allow for a smaller precise product placement as is done with autologous fat injections by one author (JE). Injections are typically made using a linear threading, cross-hatching, or fanning technique but depot injections on periosteum can also be used. Superficial injections may be associated with increased local adverse events such as nodules and papules, especially with low dilution volumes so it is recommended that pressure on the syringe plunger be stopped well before reaching the skin surface.

In additional to decreased skin elasticity and loss of facial fat volume with aging, there is a profound loss of the craniofacial skeletal support that contributes to facial contour changes.[65] The authors spend a significant time during the cosmetic consultation discussing the process of facial aging and the cumulative effects of how changing skin, muscles, bone, and soft tissue affect facial appearance. Periosteal depot injections of PLLA to address age-related structural deficiencies in the bony architecture of the face and add structural support have been well described.[66] Along with volume restoration, this globally translates to a more youthful appearance and helps persistence of the product and is a therapeutic technique that can be extrapolated to the use of other volumizing fillers.

The authors typically use two main techniques for injection: (i) supraperiosteal placement (temples, piriform aperture, zygoma, and mandible), and (ii) retrograde fanning/linear threading (midface/cheek, preauricular, NLFs, marionette lines, and mental crease). Injections should be performed with a 25–26-gauge sharp-needle (1–1.5 inch) or 25-gauge, blunt-tipped cannula (1.5–2 inch) on a 3 mL syringe (Figs 8 and 9). Adequate hydration/mixing of

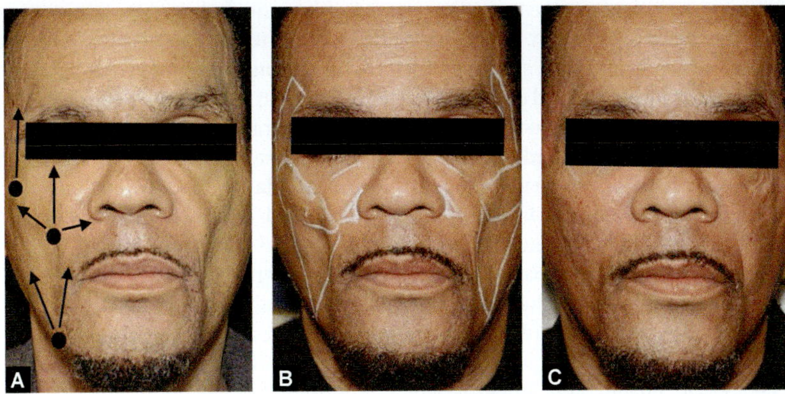

FIG. 8: Poly-L-lactic acid (PLLA) for facial lipoatrophy. **A,** Before; **B,** planning/marking; and **C,** after microcannula injections of PLLA. With only a few entry points (dots), pan-facial contouring and volumization (midface, zygoma, temple, and pyriform aperture) can be obtained with multiple vectors (arrows) of retrograde injections in the subcutaneous plane.

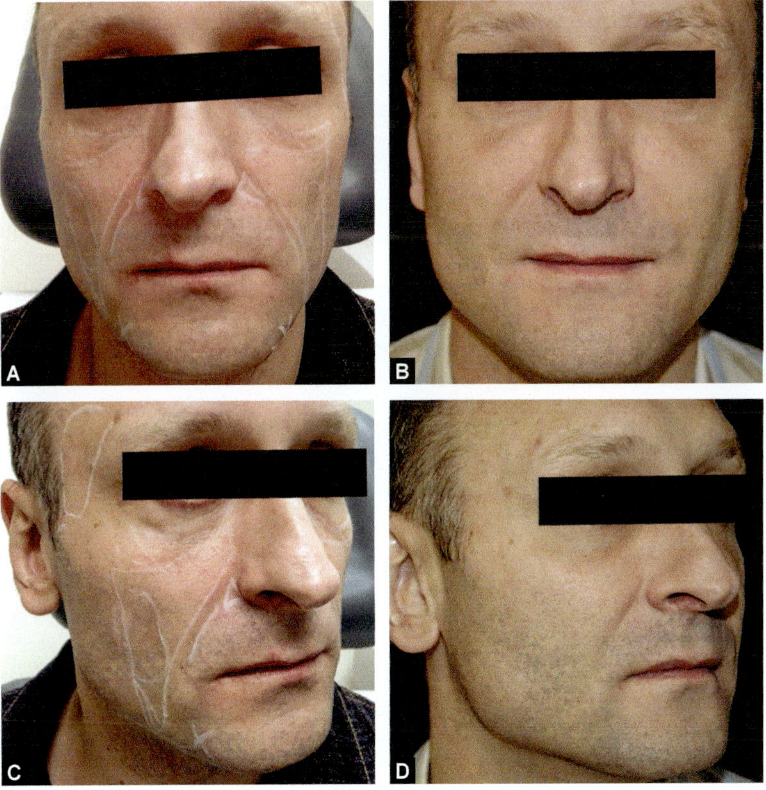

FIG. 9: Poly-L-lactic acid: **A and C,** Before; **B and D,** after.

product should be performed 24 to 72 hours prior to usage, and once drawn into syringes, it should be consistently rocked by nursing staff or well mixed using a vortex mixer (common in laboratories to mix liquid vials) to ensure homogenous dispersion of product and limit potential clogging. Leaving 0.5 cc of air in each syringe will allow mixing while being held.[67] Clogging is most often due to settling of product in the syringe prior to injection, and is more common if the material is drawn into syringes and left to sit on the Mayo stand for a period of time prior to the procedure. It is best to avoid product settling as it can lead to uneven application and contributes to nodule formation, so some advocate warming the solution or drawing from the vial and injecting one syringe at a time. If particulate separation is seen, pull the plunger back and rock the syringe back and forth to allow easier mixing and then force the material to back out through the needle or cannula to ensure it is clear before injecting. Smaller-gauge needles or cannulas (i.e., 27–30 guage) and longer-length needles (i.e., 1.25–1.5 inch) become more easily clogged. Keeping the injecting thumb (or hypothenar eminence) off the plunger until in the plane of injection will help limit clogging of the needle. Of note, supraperiosteal placement may be more prone to needle clogging than in the subcutaneous planes.

Each thread should be equally dispersed and limited to small aliquots (0.1–0.5 mL), especially in areas with less subcutaneous fat such as the periocular or perioral areas, tear trough, lateral zygoma, prejowl/mandible, or preauricular areas. Areas requiring more volumization may need more product placement, but it is better to use more threads with less volume to avoid overcorrection or an unpredictable result. For depot injections in a serial puncture technique along the periosteum such as on the chin, prejowl/mandibular, lateral zygoma, pyriform aperture, and/or temples/forehead, a sharp needle should be used with only small aliquots of material deposited. It is better to have multiple sessions with lower injection volumes than higher volumes in fewer sessions. No more than two vials are used per visit every 4–8 weeks until a desired effect is seen.

Temporal augmentation is the best example of using the bolus, depot injection technique to describe the semipermanent biostimulatory effects on facial contouring and volumization. One of several (usually 4–8 per temple) deep depot injections below the temporalis muscle and above the periosteum—with aspiration before each injection to avoid intravascular product placement—are started along the frontal hairline and moved anteriorly toward the medial aspect of the eyebrow but superior to the lateral zygoma.[63,67] The needle is inserted perpendicular to the skin surface and pressed deeply through facial planes till the periosteum is reached.[68] The patient will experience a "cracking" or "snapping" sound along with pressure, but little pain, as the needle reaches its placement point. Overtime, there is a gradual increase in volumization of the temporal/forehead region and a lifting effect of the tail of the eyebrow.

Injection of the lateral eyebrow (tail) and suprabrow can also help to give a lifting effect and improve temporal contouring (Fig. 10). Depot injection along the supralateral orbit can give lift and fullness, while linear threading with sharp needle or microcannula with the injection point beginning at the tail of the brow, can provide contouring. Small aliquot depot injections along the zygoma can help balance midface volumization as well as supply recontouring manifested by a lifting effect on the NLFs/lateral cheek or oral commissures. Fanning in the deep dermal or subcutaneous planes atop the area of depot injections can provide even more contouring, if desired.

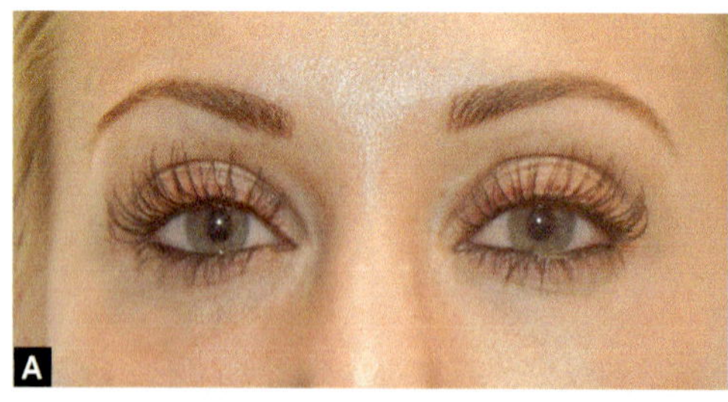

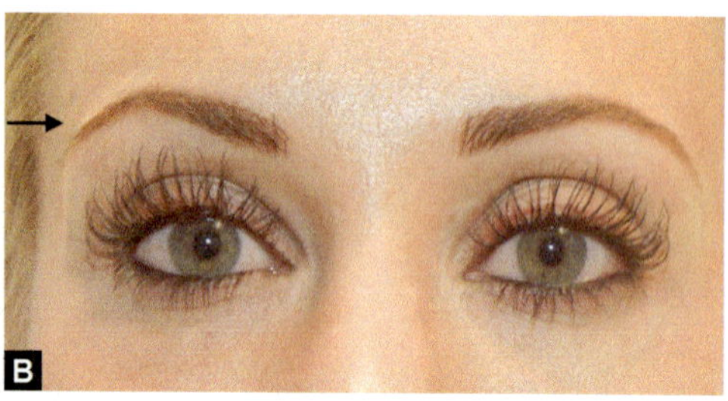

FIG. 10: Poly-L-lactic acid (PLLA) for eyebrow and temple contouring. Before **A,** and after **B,** right eyebrow and temple rejuvenation with supraperiosteal depot injections of PLLA (total 9 cc dilution) along the orbital rim and temporal fossa. Notice immediate lift of the right lateral eyebrow (arrow) without direct injection into this area, but rather more superior and lateral injections into the temporal fossa.

The pyriform aperture/canine fossa supports the superior NLF and nasal tip. With aging, bony resorption of this area can cause nasal tip depression and lack of support of the NLFs.[69] Supraperiosteal depot injection with sharp needle or access with long (1.5–2 inch) blunt-tipped microcannula from an entry point at the lateral oral commissure can help alleviate this loss of structural support. A similar, supraperiosteal injection technique can be used to improve the mandibular grove/mandibular angle with depot injection.

Until the availability of Voluma, PLLA was the most studied agent in the United States for midface volumization in the deep dermal or subcutaneous plane. Filling of the majority of the midface can be accomplished with a few injection points if using the fanning or bolus technique, but requires multiple injection points and passes of the needle if using cross-hatching. Fanning/linear threading can also be useful in the preauricular, marionette, and mental crease from single injection points in those areas. When injecting the periocular (orbicularis oculi) or perioral (orbicularis oris, modiolus, and depressor anguli oris) areas it is important to avoid muscular injection to limit PLLA particle clumping. The treating physician can then mold and massage the treated area to confirm dispersion of the diluted product. Firm massaging throughout treatment and in the subsequent days to weeks after treatment will help adequate spread and positioning of product and aid in symmetrical results with avoidance of papules and nodules. Ice packs help to limit immediate posttreatment edema, bruising/hematoma, and erythema commonly seen with soft tissue filler augmentation and reduce the discomfort common with patient massage. Some suggest the use of oral or topical *Arnica montana*, bromelain (derivative of pineapple), topical vitamin K, and/or oral vitamin C to reduce posttreatment ecchymosis and swelling starting 2 days before and continuing up to 5 days after treatment, particularly in those with busy social schedules or on anticoagulants. However, any patient with significant cardiac disease should check with a primary physician prior to starting any homeopathic supplement.

Although, not studied in clinical trials, it has become standard of care to inject a given patient with more than one filler in a given treatment session. Combining a "palette" of agents allows the physician to take advantage of their different rheologic and biologic characteristics to improve both deep and superficial defects in multiple anatomic regions. For example, CaHA can be injected in the periosteal plane under PLLA injected in the subcutaneous plane in the same visit to provide the patient with both immediate and sustained results. Products can also be layered in the same plane with one filler injected into the deep subcutaneous and the other into the deep dermal or superficial subcutaneous planes. This is particularly helpful in addressing superficial lines with HA-type fillers, diluted CaHA, or liquid silicone after the volume deficiency (i.e., lifting/recontouring) has been addressed (Figs 11 and 12).[70]

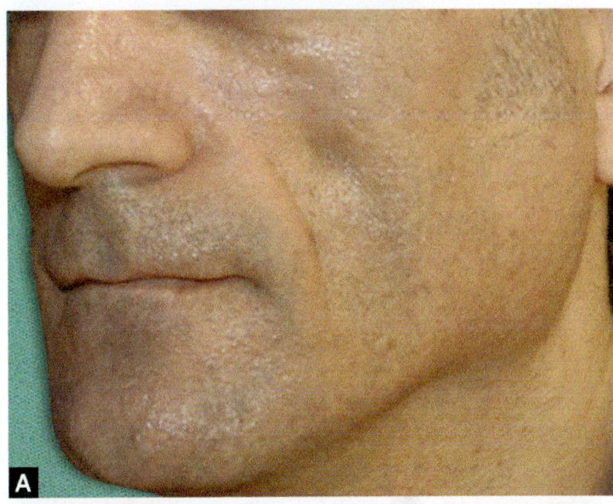

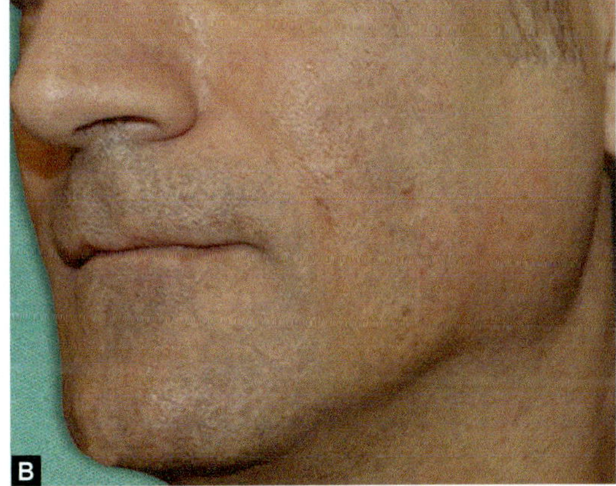

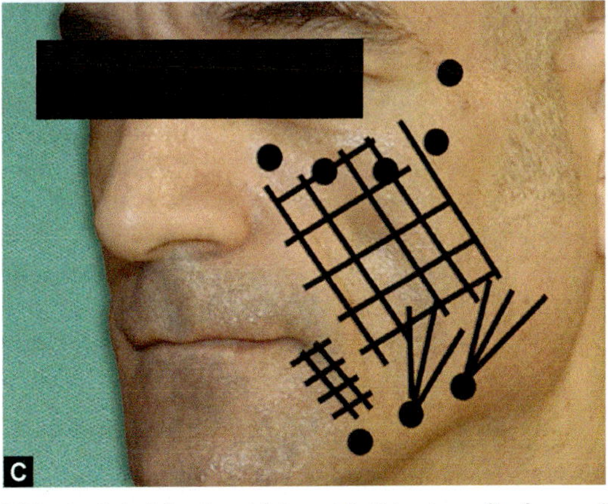

FIG. 11: Poly-L-lactic acid. **A** and **B,** Side view of before and after; **C** Injection markings.

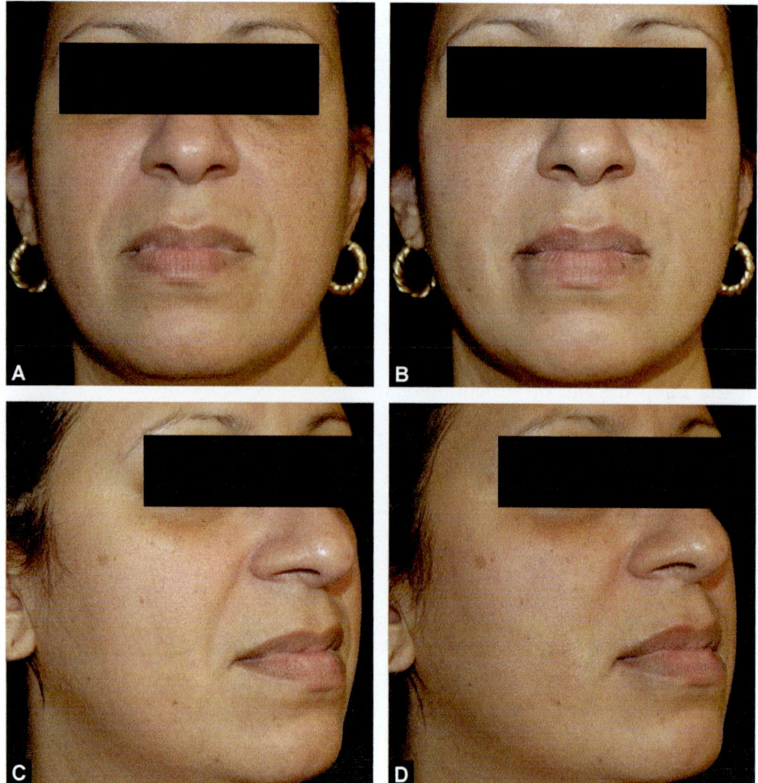

FIG. 12: Poly-L-lactic acid combined with hyaluronic acid filler for mid-face and nasolabilal fold improvement. **A** and **B**, Front view of before and after; **C** and **D**, Side view of before and after.

POLYMETHYLMETHACRYLATE (BELLAFILL) (ARTEFILL HAS BEEN RENAMED)

Polymethylmethacrylate (Bellafill, previously known as Artefill) is the only FDA approved permanent filling agent and the only one that contains bovine collagen. The exact composition is 20% implant volume of nonbiodegradable PMMA microspheres, 80% implant volume of purified bovine collagen gel (3.5%), lidocaine hydrochloride (0.3%), and water for injection (92.6%). Because it contains bovine collagen, the approval in the United States (but not in Canada) requires skin testing prior to use.[71] The PMMA available in the USA differs from that originally available in Europe (Artecoll) as it is derived from a closed USA bovine herd, it has a more consistent (uniform and smooth) particle size and shape, and has a larger particle size (30–50 μm). The larger particle size helps carry a lower risk of immunogenicity and digestion by macrophages, as early nanoparticles (<20 μm) were thought to be associated with increased granulomatous reactions. The resultant foreign body/granulomatous reaction provides delayed augmentation through long-lasting collagenesis.[72] The collagen carrier of this product is of bovine origin and thus, carries the same potential allergenicity of 1–5% reported in the literature for bovine collagen.[73,74] The collagen carrier prevents clumping of the product and migration to adjacent areas, as well as an immediate short-lived volumization.[75,76] Within 1 month after treatment, the bovine collagen carrier is replaced with increased connective tissue growth. No acute sensitivity reactions have been documented to date.[77-79]

A recent study listed delayed onset complications of PMMA injection such as persistent redness, telangiectasia, hypertrophic scarring, nodules, and delayed granulomatous reactions, as having a 3% complication rate in the literature.[80]

Granulomas generally occur 6–24 months post-treatment and frequently after multiple procedures or when multiple types of fillers are injected.[77,81,82] However, a recent report presented a patient who developed granulomatous/inflammatory lip, chin, and cheek nodules 15 years after being treated with an injectable collagen and another "unknown" substance, later found to be PMMA microspheres.[83] Granulomas can be caused by incorrect positioning of filler material or filler migration, muscle-induced displacement, capsular contraction from the surrounding inflammatory and fibrotic response, and/or as a result of a foreign-body reaction to the filler depot. Some believe all granulomatous reactions are delayed-type hypersensitivity reactions, where others hypothesize they are a result of subclinical low-grade infections (biofilm). It is still unknown what mechanisms are responsible for provoking these complications, but it is likely a combination of patient-dependent and filler-specific effects.

Clinical persistence of PMMA is secondary to the nonbiodegradable nature of the product. If nodules develop, treatment includes repeated intralesional corticosteroid injections (2.5–5 mg/mL) with or without 5-fluorouracil (5-FU, 50 mg/mL) at increasing concentrations every 3 to 4 weeks till improvement is seen. Other reported therapies such as oral anti-inflammatory antibiotics, subcision with 16 to 18 gauge Nokor needles, and/or surgical extraction can be immediately beneficial. In one case, the use of allopurinol showed resolution and in another a high-frequency 100 watt probe using a modified endocoagulation method directly into the nodules showed improvement.[84-86] It is important to distinguish this type of nodule formation versus superficial beading and ridging representing a impending hypertrophic scar due to superficial placement of PMMA, as the latter may require more aggressive therapies such as laser or excision.[87]

Injection Techniques

Polymethylmethacrylate is supplied as 0.8 mL syringes with 26-gauge, 5/8 inch needles and indicated for the treatment of NLFs, preferentially injected into the deep dermis or subcutis (dermal/subdermal junction) since, superficial placement is associated with long-lasting pruritus, redness, and hypertrophic scarring in association with delayed-onset inflammatory nodules or hypersensitivity reactions (Fig. 13). Fortunately, localized pruritus and redness can be treated with topical or injectable corticosteroids and/or topical calcineurin inhibitors. Hypertrophic scarring can sometimes be softened by topical or injectable corticosteroids, topical silicone, topical or injectable 5-FU, topical imiquimod, cryotherapy, or various laser technologies such as pulsed dye, potassium titanyl phosphate (KTP), and/or fractional ablative or nonablative laser, or fractional radiofrequency; however, results can be permanent and emotionally devastating to both the physician and patient.[88-91]

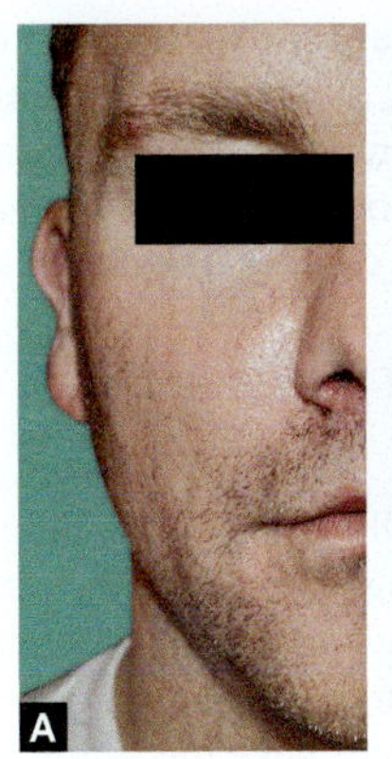

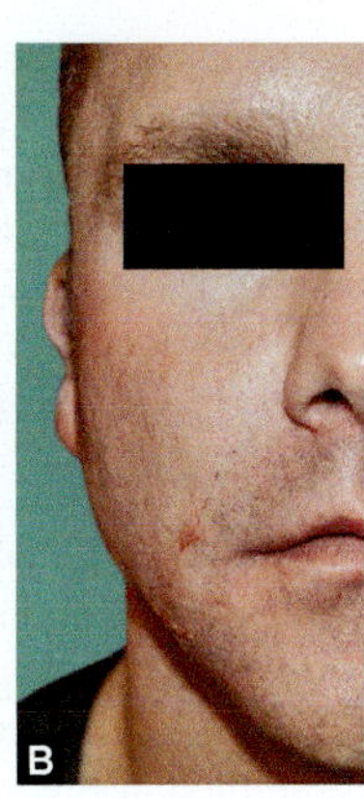

FIG. 13: Polymethylmethacrylate for jawline contouring. **A,** Before, **B,** After; A series of three treatments with periosteal depot injections and small subcutaneous linear threads were used to widen the jawline and give a more masculine apperance.

To avoid these complications, it important to avoid a large, localized accumulation of product during injection. Although, the package inserting recommends a tunneling/linear threading injection technique, the microdroplet technique as described with the use of silicone oil is likely the best method to minimize complications. Multiple treatment sessions with small aliquots (0.1–0.5 mL per site) of material injected with a 26 or 27 gauge needle into the desired treatment areas will help to optimize volume. Caution to overcorrect should be taken with any long-lasting particulate/permanent filler. As described earlier, it is best to avoid areas which are highly mobile such as the lips/perioral or ocular areas, as product clumping can lead to irregularities and nodule formation. Complications have also been seen in the use of PMMA in the hands, similar to PLLA, and it is best to avoid the use of these products in this location.[92] Off-label improvement in the treatment of acne scars was recently published and treatment for HIV lipoatrophy was presented at a national conference poster session.[93,94]

Skin testing is required prior to use and consists of the patient receiving a 0.1 mL intradermal injection of collagen into the volar forearm 4 weeks prior to treatment. A positive response consists of erythema to any degree, induration, tenderness, and swelling, with or without pruritus. An equivocal response is where no localized skin reaction occurs but the patient develops a systemic reaction such as a rash, arthralgia, or myalgia any time during the 4-weeks observation period. Patients demonstrating a positive skin test or two equivocal skin tests should not receive treatment.

CONCLUSION

The demand for minimally invasive aesthetic treatments providing safe long-lasting results continues to increase. Most commonly used for facial reshaping and wrinkle treatment are HA type fillers as they are the best studied agents and have the safety benefit of reversibility. However, practitioners and patients are sometimes frustrated with shorter lived results and limited versatility. The use of biostimulatory, semipermanent, and permanent fillers provides an enhanced option for patients requiring facial contouring, shaping, or increased volumization. Permanent filling is a particular need for patients with static defects like acne or surgical scars that tend to be more resistant to other fillers and to alternate modalities like laser resurfacing. Knowledge regarding product availability and proper use is of the utmost importance to limit complications and deliver superior clinical results.

REFERENCES

1. André P. Evaluation of the safety of a non-animal stabilized hyaluronic acid (NASHA—Q-Medical, Sweden) in European countries: A retrospective study from 1997 to 2001. J Eur Acad Dermatol Venereol. 2004;18(4):422-5.
2. Bray D, Hopkins C, Roberts DN. A review of dermal fillers in facial plastic surgery. Curr Opin Otolaryngol Head Neck Surg. 2010;18(4):295-302.
3. Radiesse Injectable Implant. (2014). Instructions for use. [online] Available from: www.fda.gov/ohrms/dockets/ac/06/briefing/2006-4233b1_04.pdf. [Accessed November 16, 2017].
4. Radiesse® Injectable Implant. (2014). Instructions For Use. [online] Available from: www.radiesse.com/wp-content/uploads/RADIESSE_Wrinkle_Filler_Instructions_for_Use.pdf. [Accessed December 24, 2014].
5. Radiesse Voice Gel. Injectable Implant: Instructions for use. [online] Available from: www.radiesse-voice.com/docs/RADIESSE_Voice_Gel_Instructions_for_Use.pdf. [Accessed December 16, 2014].
6. Carruthers A, Liebeskind M, Carruthers J, et al. Radiographic and computed tomographic studies of calcium hydroxylapatite for treatment of HIV-associated facial lipoatrophy and correction of nasolabial folds. Dermatol Surg. 2008;34(Suppl 1):S78-84.
7. Marmur E, Green L, Busso M. Controlled, randomized study of pain levels in subjects treated with calcium hydroxylapatite premixed with lidocaine for correction of nasolabial folds. Dermatol Surg. 2010;36(3):309-15.
8. Lupo MP, Swetman G, Waller W. The effect of lidocaine when mixed with large gel particle hyaluronic acid filler tolerability and longevity: A six-month trial. J Drugs Dermatol. 2010;9(9):1097-100.
9. Silvers SL, Eviatar JA, Echavez MI, et al. Prospective, open-label, 18-month trial of calcium hydroxylapatite (Radiesse) for facial soft-tissue augmentation in patients with human immunodeficiency virus-associated lipoatrophy: One-year durability. Plast Reconstr Surg. 2006; 118(3 Suppl):34S-45.
10. Jansen DA, Graivier MH. Evaluation of a calcium hydroxylapatite-based implant (Radiesse) for facial soft-tissue augmentation. Plast Reconstr Surg. 2006;118(3 Suppl):22S-30.
11. Carruthers A, Carruthers J. Evaluation of injectable calcium hydroxylapatite for the treatment of facial lipoatrophy associated with human immunodeficiency virus. Dermatol Surg. 2008;34(11):1486-99.
12. Redbord KP, Busso M, Hanke CW. Soft-tissue augmentation with hyaluronic acid and calcium hydroxylapatite fillers. Dermatol Ther. 2011;24(1):71-81.
13. Sundaram H, Voigts B, Beer K, et al. Comparison of the rheological properties of viscosity and elasticity in two categories of soft tissue fillers: calcium hydroxylapatite and hyaluronic acid. Dermatol Surg. 2010;36(Suppl 3):1859-65.
14. Moers-Carpi M, Vogt S, Santos BM, et al. A multicenter, randomized trial comparing calcium hydroxylapatite to two hyaluronic acids for treatment of nasolabial folds. Dermatol Surg. 2007;33(Suppl 2):S144-51.
15. Bass LS, Smith S, Busso M, et al. Calcium hydroxylapatite (Radiesse) for treatment of nasolabial folds: Long-term safety and efficacy results. Aesthet Surg J. 2010;30(2):235-8.
16. Sadick NS, Katz BE, Roy D. A multicenter, 47-month study of safety and efficacy of calcium hydroxylapatite for soft tissue augmentation of nasolabial folds and other areas of the face. Dermatol Surg. 2007;33(Suppl 2):S122-6.
17. Tzikas TL. A 52-month summary of results using calcium hydroxylapatite for facial soft tissue augmentation. Dermatol Surg. 2008;34 Suppl 1:S9-15.
18. Marmur ES, Phelps R, Goldberg DJ. Clinical, histologic and electron microscopic findings after injection of a calcium hydroxylapatite filler. J Cosmet Laser Ther. 2004;6(4):223-6.
19. Laeschke K. Biocompatibility of microparticles into soft tissue fillers. Semin Cutan Med Surg. 2004;23(4):214-7.
20. Berlin AL, Hussain M, Goldberg DJ. Calcium hydroxylapatite filler for facial rejuvenation: A histologic and immunohistochemical analysis. Dermatol Surg. 2008;34(Suppl 1):S64-7.
21. Fulton J, Caperton C, Weinkle S, et al. Filler injections with the blunt-tip microcannula. J Drugs Dermatol. 2012;11(9):1098-103.

22. Zeichner JA, Cohen JL. Use of blunt tipped cannulas for soft tissue fillers. J Drugs Dermatol. 2012;11(1):70-2.
23. Emer J, Sundaram H. Aesthetic applications of calcium hydroxylapatite volumizing filler: An evidence-based review and discussion of current concepts: (part 1 of 2). J Drugs Dermatol. 2013;12(12):1345-54.
24. Beer KR. Radiesse nodule of the lips from a distant injection site: Report of a case and consideration of etiology and management. J Drugs Dermatol. 2007;6(8):846-7.
25. Ridenour B, Kontis TC. Injectable calcium hydroxylapatite microspheres (Radiesse). Facial Plast Surg. 2009;25(2):100-5.
26. Busso M, Voigts R. An investigation of changes in physical properties of injectable calcium hydroxylapatite in a carrier gel when mixed with lidocaine and with lidocaine/epinephrine. Dermatol Surg. 2008;34(Suppl 1):S16-23.
27. Bartus CL, Sattler G, Hanke CW. The tower technique: a novel technique for the injection of hyaluronic acid fillers. J Drugs Dermatol. 2011;10(11):1277-80.
28. Sattler G. The tower technique and vertical supraperiosteal depot technique: novel vertical injection techniques for volume-efficient subcutaneous tissue support and volumetric augmentation. J Drugs Dermatol. 2012;11(8):545-7.
29. Reddy KK, Brauer JA, Anolik R, et al. Calcium hydroxylapatite nodule resolution after fractional carbon dioxide laser therapy. Arch Dermatol. 2012;148(5):634-6.
30. Cassuto D, Marangoni O, De Santis G, et al. Advanced laser techniques for filler-induced complications. Dermatol Surg. 2009;35(Suppl 2):1689-95.
31. Cassuto D, Sundaram H. A problem-oriented approach to nodular complications from hyaluronic acid and calcium hydroxylapatite fillers: Classification and recommendations for treatment. Plast Reconstr Surg. 2013;132(4 Suppl 2):48S-58S.
32. Graivier MH, Bass LS, Busso M, et al. Calcium hydroxylapatite (Radiesse) for correction of the mid- and lower face: consensus recommendations. Plast Reconstr Surg. 2007;120(6 Suppl):55S-66.
33. Daley T, Damm DD, Haden JA, et al. Oral lesions associated with injected hydroxylapatite cosmetic filler. Oral Surg Oral Med Oral Pathol Oral Radiol. 2012;114(1):107-11.
34. Daines SM, Williams EF. Complications associated with injectable soft-tissue fillers: A 5-year retrospective review. JAMA Facial Plast Surg. 2013;15(3):226-31.
35. Goulart JM, High WA, Goldenberg G. Evidence of calcium hydroxylapatite migration: Distant nodule formation in the setting of concurrent injection with nonanimal stabilized hyaluronic acid. J Am Acad Dermatol. 2011;65(2):e65-6.
36. Lemperle G, Gauthier-Hazan N. Foreign body granulomas after all injectable dermal fillers: part 2. Treatment options. Plast Reconstr Surg. 2009;123(6):1864-73.
37. Lemperle G, Gauthier-Hazan N, Wolters M, et al. Foreign body granulomas after all injectable dermal fillers: part 1. Possible causes. Plast Reconstr Surg. 2009;123(6):1842-63.
38. Gogolewski S, Jovanovic M, Perren SM, et al. Tissue response and in vivo degradation of selected polyhydroxyacids: Polylactides (PLA), poly(3-hydroxybutyrate) (PHB), and poly(3-hydroxybutyrate-co-3-hydroxyvalerate) (PHB/VA). J Biomed Mater Res. 1993;27(9):1135-48.
39. Lacombe V. Sculptra: a stimulatory filler. Facial Plast Surg. 2009;25(2):95-9.
40. Sculptra Aesthetic. (2016). Doctor Discussion Guide. [online] Available from http://sculptraaesthetic.com/sculptra_aesthetic.pdf [Accessed December 16, 2017].
41. Schierle CF, Casas LA. Nonsurgical rejuvenation of the aging face with injectable poly-L-lactic acid for restoration of soft tissue volume. Aesthet Surg J. 2011;31(1):95-109.
42. Humble G, Mest D. Soft tissue augmentation using sculptra. Facial Plast Surg. 2004;20(2):157-63.
43. Vleggaar D. Soft-tissue augmentation and the role of poly-L-lactic acid. Plast Reconstr Surg. 2006;118(3 Suppl):46S-54.
44. Lowe P, Lowe NJ, Patnaik R. Three-dimensional digital surface imaging measurement of the volumizing effect of injectable poly-L-lactic acid for nasolabial folds. J Cosmet Laser Ther. 2011;13(2):87-94.
45. Bauer U, Graivier MH. Optimizing injectable poly-L-lactic acid administration for soft tissue augmentation: The rationale for three treatment sessions. Can J Plast Surg. 2011;19(3):e22-7.
46. Rendon MI. Long-term aesthetic outcomes with injectable poly-L-lactic acid: observations and practical recommendations based on clinical experience over 5 years. J Cosmet Dermatol. 2012;11(2):93-100.
47. Butterwick K, Lowe NJ. Injectable poly-L-lactic acid for cosmetic enhancement: Learning from the European experience. J Am Acad Dermatol. 2009;61(2):281-93.
48. Bassichis B, Blick G, Conant M, et al. Injectable poly-L-lactic acid for human immunodeficiency virus-associated facial lipoatrophy: cumulative year 2 interim analysis of an open-label study (FACES). Dermatol Surg. 2012;38(7 Pt 2):1193-205.
49. Levy RM, Redbord KP, Hanke CW. Treatment of HIV lipoatrophy and lipoatrophy of aging with poly-L-lactic acid: a prospective 3-year follow-up study. J Am Acad Dermatol. 2008;59(6):923-33.
50. Nelson L, Stewart KJ. Psychological morbidity and facial volume in HIV lipodystrophy: Quantification of treatment outcome. J Plast Reconstr Aesthet Surg. 2012;65(4):439-47.
51. Ong J, Clarke A, White P, et al. Objective evidence for the use of polylactic acid implants in HIV-associated facial lipoatrophy using three-dimensional surface laser scanning and psychological assessment. J Plast Reconstr Aesthet Surg. 2009;62(12):1627-35.
52. Burgess CM, Quiroga RM. Assessment of the safety and efficacy of poly-L-lactic acid for the treatment of HIV-associated facial lipoatrophy. J Am Acad Dermatol. 2005;52(2):233-9.

53. Palm M, Chayavichitsilp P. The "skinny" on sculptra: a practical primer to volumization with poly-L-lactic acid. J Drugs Dermatol. 2012;11(9):1046-52.
54. Fabi S, Bolton J, Goldman MP, et al. The Fabi-Bolton chest wrinkle scale: A pilot validation study. J Cosmet Dermatol. 2012;11(3):229-34.
55. Peterson JD, Goldman MP. Rejuvenation of the aging chest: A review and our experience. Dermatol Surg. 2011;37(5):555-71.
56. Lam SM, Azizzadeh B, Graivier M. Injectable poly-L-lactic acid (Sculptra): Technical considerations in soft-tissue contouring. Plast Reconstr Surg. 2006;118(3 Suppl):55S-63.
57. Woerle B, Hanke CW, Sattler G. Poly-L-lactic acid: A temporary filler for soft tissue augmentation. J Drugs Dermatol. 2004;3(4):385-9.
58. Narins RS. Minimizing adverse events associated with poly-L-lactic acid injection. Dermatol Surg. 2008; 34(Suppl 1):S100-4.
59. Beer K. Clinicopathologic correlation of delayed-onset periorbital poly-L-lactic acid nodules. Dermatol Surg. 2009;35(Suppl 1):399-402.
60. Apikian M, Roberts S, Goodman GJ. Adverse reactions to polylactic acid injections in the periorbital area. J Cosmet Dermatol. 2007;6(2):95-101.
61. Stewart DB, Morganroth GS, Mooney MA, et al. Management of visible granulomas following periorbital injection of poly-L-lactic acid. Ophthal Plast Reconstr Surg. 2007;23(4):298-301.
62. Redaelli A. Cosmetic use of polylactic acid for hand rejuvenation: report on 27 patients. J Cosmet Dermatol. 2006;5(3):233-8.
63. Rose AE, Day D. Esthetic rejuvenation of the temple. Clin Plast Surg. 2013;40(1):77-89.
64. Sadick NS, Manhas-Bhutani S, Krueger N. A novel approach to structural facial volume replacement. Aesthetic Plast Surg. 2013;37(2):266-76.
65. Vleggaar D, Fitzgerald R. Dermatological implications of skeletal aging: a focus on supraperiosteal volumization for perioral rejuvenation. J Drugs Dermatol. 2008;7(3):209-20.
66. Fitzgerald R, Vleggaar D. Using poly-L-lactic acid (PLLA) to mimic volume in multiple tissue layers. J Drugs Dermatol. 2009;8(10 Suppl):s5-14.
67. Goldman MP. Cosmetic use of poly-L-lactic acid: My technique for success and minimizing complications. Dermatol Surg. 2011;37(5):688-93.
68. Sykes JM. Applied anatomy of the temporal region and forehead for injectable fillers. J Drugs Dermatol. 2009;8(10 Suppl):s24-7.
69. Fitzgerald R, Vleggaar D. Facial volume restoration of the aging face with poly-L-lactic acid. Dermatol Ther. 2011;24(1):2-27.
70. Beer K. Dermal fillers and combinations of fillers for facial rejuvenation. Dermatol Clin. 2009;27(4):427-32.
71. Bellafill. (2017). Introduction. [online]. Available from www.bellafill.com/sites/default/files/Bellafill_IFU.pdf. [Accessed December 16, 2017].
72. Piacquadio D, Smith S, Anderson R. A comparison of commercially available polymethylmethacrylate-based soft tissue fillers. Dermatol Surg. 2008;34(Suppl 1):S48-52.
73. Krauss MC. Recent advances in soft tissue augmentation. Semin Cutan Med Surg. 1999;18(2):119-28.
74. Kamer FM, Churukian MM. Clinical use of injectable collagen: a three-year retrospective review. Arch Otolaryngol. 1984;110(2):93-8.
75. Lemperle G, Morhenn VB, Pestonjamasp V, et al. Migration studies and histology of injectable microspheres of different sizes in mice. Plast Reconstr Surg. 2004;113(5):1380-90.
76. Lemperle G, Morhenn V, Charrier U. Human histology and persistence of various injectable filler substances for soft tissue augmentation. Aesthetic Plast Surg. 2003; 27(5):354-66.
77. Cohen SR, Berner CF, Busso M, et al. ArteFill: A long-lasting injectable wrinkle filler material—summary of the U.S. Food and Drug Administration trials and a progress report on 4- to 5-year outcomes. Plast Reconstr Surg. 2006;118(3 Suppl):64S-76.
78. Cohen SR, Berner CF, Busso M, et al. Five-year safety and efficacy of a novel polymethylmethacrylate aesthetic soft tissue filler for the correction of nasolabial folds. Dermatol Surg. 2007;33(Suppl 2):S222-30.
79. Cohen SR, Holmes RE. Artecoll: a long-lasting injectable wrinkle filler material: Report of a controlled, randomized, multicenter clinical trial of 251 subjects. Plast Reconstr Surg. 2004;114(4):964-76.
80. Kadouch JA, Kadouch DJ, Fortuin S, et al. Delayed-onset complications of facial soft tissue augmentation with permanent fillers in 85 patients. Dermatol Surg. 2013;39(10):1474-85.
81. Alcalay J, Alkalay R, Gat A, et al. Late-onset granulomatous reaction to Artecoll. Dermatol Surg. 2003;29(8): 859-62.
82. Kim KJ, Lee HW, Lee MW, et al. Artecoll granuloma: a rare adverse reaction induced by microimplant in the treatment of neck wrinkles. Dermatol Surg. 2004;30(4 Pt 1):545-7.
83. Wu W, Chayavichitsilp P, Hata T. Extremely delayed granulomatous reaction to soft-tissue injectables (polymethyl methacrylate). J Am Acad Dermatol. 2012; 67(5):e206-7.
84. de Barros Silveira LK, de Oliveira FL, Alves Tde B, et al. The therapeutic benefit of allopurinol in the treatment of foreign body granulomas caused by polymethylmethacrylate microspheres. Case Rep Dermatol Med. 2012;2012:945205.
85. Yagima Odo ME, Mayumi Odo L, Fujimoto Nemoto NC, et al. Treatment of nodules caused by polymethylmethacrylate. A pilot study. Dermatol Surg. 2008;34(12):1746-8.
86. Park TH, Seo SW, Kim JK, et al. Clinical experience with polymethylmethacrylate microsphere filler complications. Aesthetic Plast Surg. 2012;36(2):421-6.

87. Carruthers JD, Carruthers A. Facial sculpting and tissue augmentation. Dermatol Surg. 2005;31(11 Pt 2):1604-12.
88. Eke U, Diaz C, Abdullah A. Keloid scars in type VI skin successfully treated with combined surgery and pulsed dye laser therapy. Br J Dermatol. 2013;168(6):1360-2.
89. Levy LL, Zeichner JA. Management of acne scarring, part II: A comparative review of non-laser-based, minimally invasive approaches. Am J Clin Dermatol. 2012;13(5):331-40.
90. Gupta S, Sharma VK. Standard guidelines of care: Keloids and hypertrophic scars. Indian J Dermatol Venereol Leprol. 2011;77(1):94-100.
91. Juckett G, Hartman-Adams H. Management of keloids and hypertrophic scars. Am Fam Physician. 2009;80(3):253-60.
92. Al-Qattan MM. Complications related to Artecoll injections for soft tissue augmentation of the hand: 3 case reports. J Hand Surg Am. 2011;36(6):994-7.
93. Epstein RE, Spencer JM. Correction of atrophic scars with artefill: an open-label pilot study. J Drugs Dermatol. 2010;9(9):1062-4.
94. Eviatar J, Barbarino S. Artefill: A long lasting filler used to treat HIV lipoatrophy. Presented at: 26th Annual Scientific Meeting of the American Academy of Cosmetic Surgery. Orlando, FL; 2010.

30 CHAPTER

Noncosmetic Indications for Fillers

Rasya Dixit

INTRODUCTION

In this day of instant gratification, often times, it becomes necessary to provide moderate to excellent solutions for various skin conditions in short periods of time. Noting the effects of fillers which deliver predictable and seemingly instant results with minimal downtime, they have been adapted to suit noncosmetic skin indications as well. The following chapter deals with these indications. By no means are these the complete list, however, they offer a glimpse of what can be achieved in various conditions, and how to use the fillers in these indications. The reader is free to use these guidelines as a framework and identify potential new indications in their patients.

ADVANTAGES OF FILLERS OVER OTHER TREATMENT OPTIONS

Fillers are noninflammatory or cause minimal inflammatory changes. This makes them very desirable in patients who have usually developed significant adverse effects with inflammatory procedures that breach the skin like laser or dermal surgical techniques. Especially the skin types prone to side effects of dyspigmentation or keloid formation (which are triggered by inflammation) are good candidates for these procedures.

Fillers also offer the advantage of instant results, making this procedure great for patients who need quick results often to meet social deadlines.

Fillers come with minimal downtime, which is often not the case with most light or laser-based technologies. Again, it is a treatment option for those patients who desire the results with no downtime as well as faster result time.

BOX 1 Contraindication to filler treatments for noncosmetic treatments

- Pregnancy
- Lactation
- Autoimmune diseases
- Infection at the site
- Unrealistic expectations
- Severe scarring and postsurgery (proceed with caution as there may be vascular compromise)

Many times, a filler treatment may be the one treatment available after all other treatments are done and patient desires further enhancement of results. Sometimes, it may offer the last bit of results and at other times, it may remain a ray of hope for patients.

The disadvantage remains as the need for a repeat treatments as the filler undergoes its metabolism. However, the results and request for repeat treatments make this a definite therapeutic option.

Contraindications to filler treatments are given in box 1.

INDICATIONS

Acne Scars

There are currently many dermatosurgical, laser, and microneedle-based treatments available to treat acne scars.[1,2] However, the search for the perfect treatment for the scars goes on. Lasers and dermatosurgical techniques have a limitation of needing multiple sessions, needing months to complete the schedule. Many of these treatments also have downtime, which make it troublesome for some patients.[3]

Role of Fillers in Acne Scars (Box 2)

Multiple clinical trials using various filler materials have been described. A medical-grade silicone microdroplet treatment has been described as a permanent filler for scars with good results.[4] Polymethylmethacrylate, poly-L-lactic acid, and calcium hydroxyapatite have all been used with good results.[5-7] Hyaluronic acid (HA) fillers with good lifting properties show significant improvement and have been reported in multiple studies.[8] These products earlier gave good as well as long-lasting results. However, as any irregularity or in case of undesired result, it may also persist for a longer time as these molecules cannot be readily dissolved. Therefore, HA fillers remain the filler of choice for the author as these are more forgiving and can be moulded with gentle pressure in case of an overfill. Also, the availability of hyaluronidase which can be used to correct any lumps or overfilling that makes this product ideal for beginners.[9]

When should dermal fillers be considered in acne scar management? Dermal fillers, just like many of the laser techniques used for acne scar treatment, work best in soft atrophic scars of the rolling type. The HA fillers offer the additional advantage of improvement of hydration of the overlying skin, thus improving the results as well. These fillers can be used to easily combined with traditional methods of scar treatment. However, it is advised to use the filler as the last treatment after all the other treatment modalities have been completed. This is to prevent any inflammation from the other techniques which may enhance the resorption of the filler.

The data of use of fillers as a method of treatment of acne scars comes mostly from case reports and uncontrolled studies. The outcome and longevity of the tissue augmentation depend not only on the filler type and injection technique but also on the scar type. As observed with traditional acne scar treatments, rolling scars and depressed box scars respond best to fillers, with minimal or no improvement seen in ice pick scars. As expected, fillers are not indicated in the management of hypertrophic or keloidal acne scars.[10]

In clinical practice, often a combination of multiple techniques is used to achieve patient satisfaction. The newer developments in fillers include techniques to combine them with stem cells and stimulate extracellular matrix (ECM) and target the activation of white adipose tissue stem cells to enhance and sustain tissue augmentation. Animal studies to provide medical evidence are in process.[11,12]

Different injecting techniques have been described to target the acne scars. Goodman and Van Den Broek described the modified tower vertical filler technique using high lift HA.[13] The filler was injected perpendicular to the base of the scar, and a depot was created and product was deposited as the needle was withdrawn, giving a support like a tent pole. In this case series, patients found a three time reduction in the mean scar count by the second session.

Hussain et al. described a two-plane technique using two different fillers of different consistency in a deep and superficial plane.[14] Though the technique was used to correct a traumatic scar, the same method can be used to correct acne scars associated with lipodystrophy. Here the HA filler with a better lifting profile is injected in a deeper plane, and the one with the lighter lifting profile in a superficial plane.

Subcision is recommended before either of the earlier techniques are used. This allows the fibrous bands which hold the base of the scar to be broken. The filler can be introduced at a session after a week. If the filler is done in the same session, there may be under or overfilling as the subcision itself causes edema. If the subcision step is skipped, the presence of the fibrous bands causes the filler to migrate around the scar making the scar more prominent. Figure 1 shows a patient of about 40 years of age who had undergone multiple treatments including laser resurfacing with mild to minimum improvements. A subcision was performed, and 1 week later an HA of medium lifting capacity was injected with a cannula using a grid technique. Quantity of 1 mL was used for each cheek. Note the improvement in the texture of the skin. The cannula also provides additional subcision as well as induces neocollagenogenesis. A second session with a filler can be used to address the individual scars if needed.

Though fillers are not thought to be useful in ice pick scars, using a thin HA filler to hydrate the

BOX 2 Role of fillers in acne scars

- Immediate results
- Can be used in those who had poor response to other treatments for acne scars
- Can be used in patients where postinflammatory hyperpigmentation is a concern
- Improves the lipodystrophy in patients with severe scarring
- Hyaluronic acid fillers also improve skin quality of the overlying skin

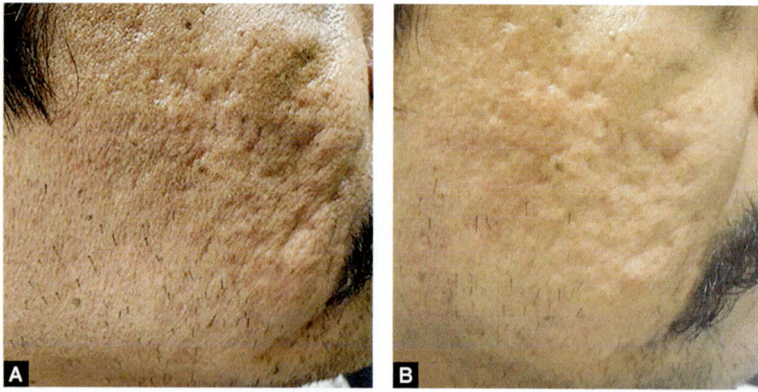

FIG. 1: Acne scars in 40 year old man given two sessions: **A,** Before and **B,** after subcision and filler.

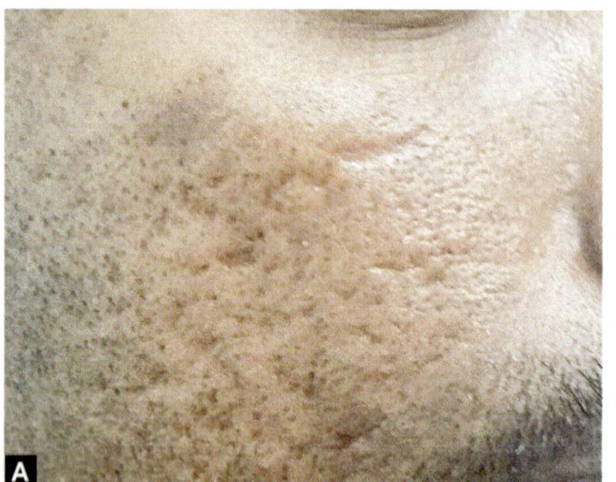

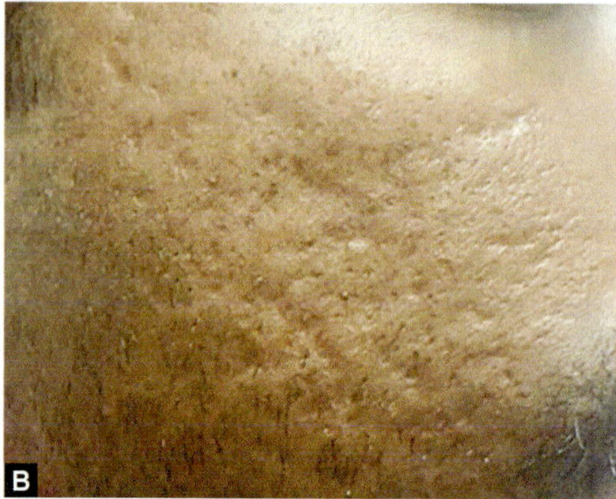

FIG. 2: Acne scars after subcision and filler.

skin will help to reduce the appearance of the scars in the author's experience. The patient in figure 2 was a 25-year-old young man who needed to get his scars treated for a social occasion which was a month away. He had one treatment of subcision and 1 mL of medium lifting capacity. Hyaluronic acid filler was used in the linear threading technique under all the linear scars. Some fillers were also deposited at mid-dermis depth as microdroplets in regular interval in the area of open pores. Note the significant improvement in the improvement in the pores posttreatment.

En Coup De Sabre/Morphea

Morphea and localized scleroderma often leave residual deformities. The patients who have active disease need to be assured that the skin does soften and the process is self limiting, however, the active disease needs to be addressed with a combination of oral medications with or without phototherapy.[15,16] If the atrophic scars are disfiguring and cause distress to the patients, then a search for treatment option includes soft tissue augmentation with fat or fillers.[17,18]

Fat grafting as well as fillers have been described to manage the residual atrophy. The advantage of the HA fillers in the bone overlay technique has been hypothesized to deliver a semipermanent volumization by Mashiko et al.[19] They followed up 12 patients with localized scleroderma, who had been injected with high lifting HA over a mean of 21 months. An interesting observation of the magnetic resonance imaging (MRI) images showed that the area which was injected was actually persistently volumized by the formation of new capsule fibrosis and calcification/ossification. This made them speculate that using the technique of bone overlay was contributing to these changes, possibly due to the activation of periosteal stem cells.

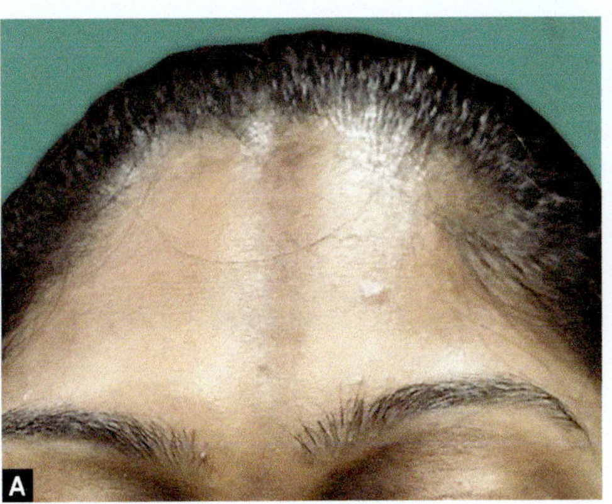

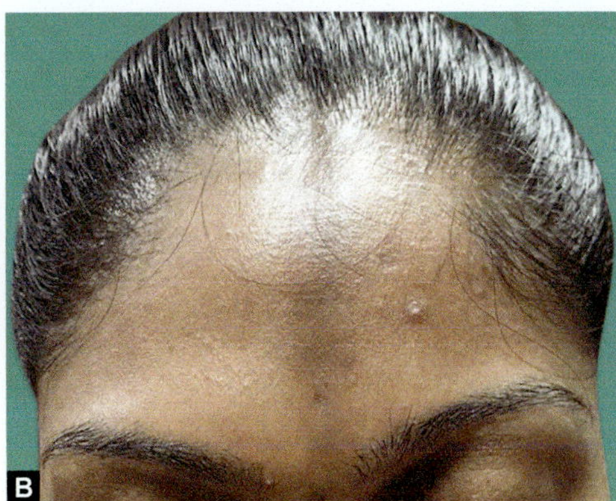

FIG. 3: Fillers for en coup de sabre, **A,** before and **B,** after.
Courtesy: Dr Aarthi L, Chennai.

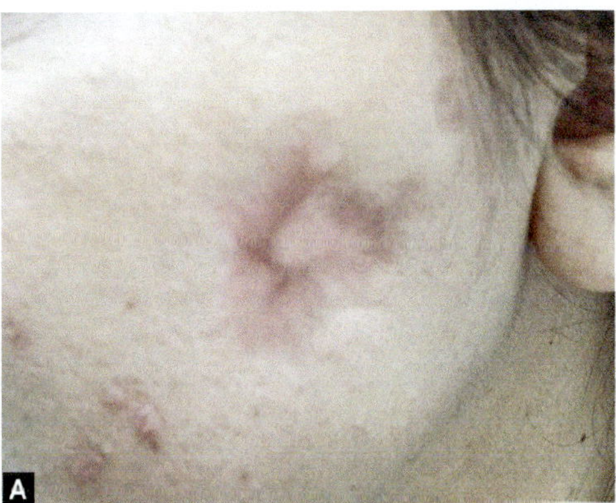

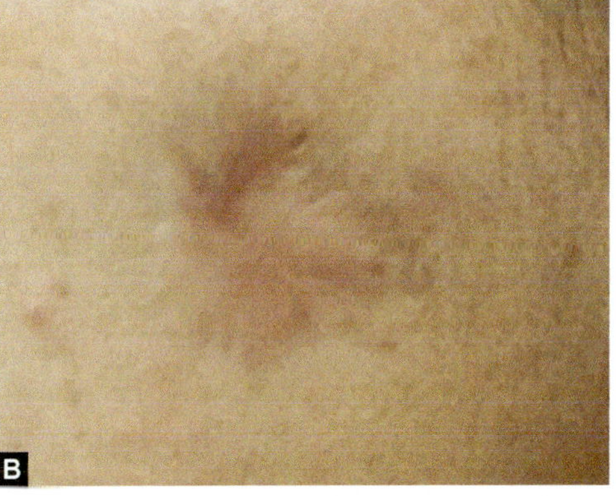

FIG. 4: Depressed traumatic scar **A,** before and **B,** after HA filler.

The filler can be introduced once the disease process has died down. The overlying pigment can be managed by a Q-switched yttrium aluminum garnet (YAG) laser (Fig. 3). This patient with en coup de sabre was treated with 2 mL of high lifting capacity HA filler. The treatment was done using a bone overlay technique using a needle. Caution is recommended in this site as the supratrochlear vessels are present in the treatment zone. Q-switched YAG laser treatment is deferred for 2 weeks postprocedure.

Postsurgical Defect/Posttraumatic Scar

Fillers have been documented in the management of acne scars quite frequently, however, the same techniques can be used for any atrophic scars which cannot be managed otherwise. Also, fillers form an alternative to surgery in such patients.

In the management of a patient with a traumatic atrophic scar over the zygoma, where the alternative was surgery, the patient requested for a trial of HA filler. An HA filler of medium lifting quality was used with a cannula and deposited as a mesh under the base of the scar. Both the improvement of the depth of scar as well as the color and texture of the skin was noted after the treatment, with patient reporting good satisfaction posttreatment (Fig. 4). This patient with a depressed scar over the zygoma was treated with 1 mL of high lifting capacity HA injected as tower technique under the scar to lift the scar. A cross hatching with cannula was also done to hydrate the scar. The improvement was seen both in the depth as well as in the color of the scar. Note thick scars are likely to have poor vascular supply, inject with caution, and do not inject too much volume at one sitting.

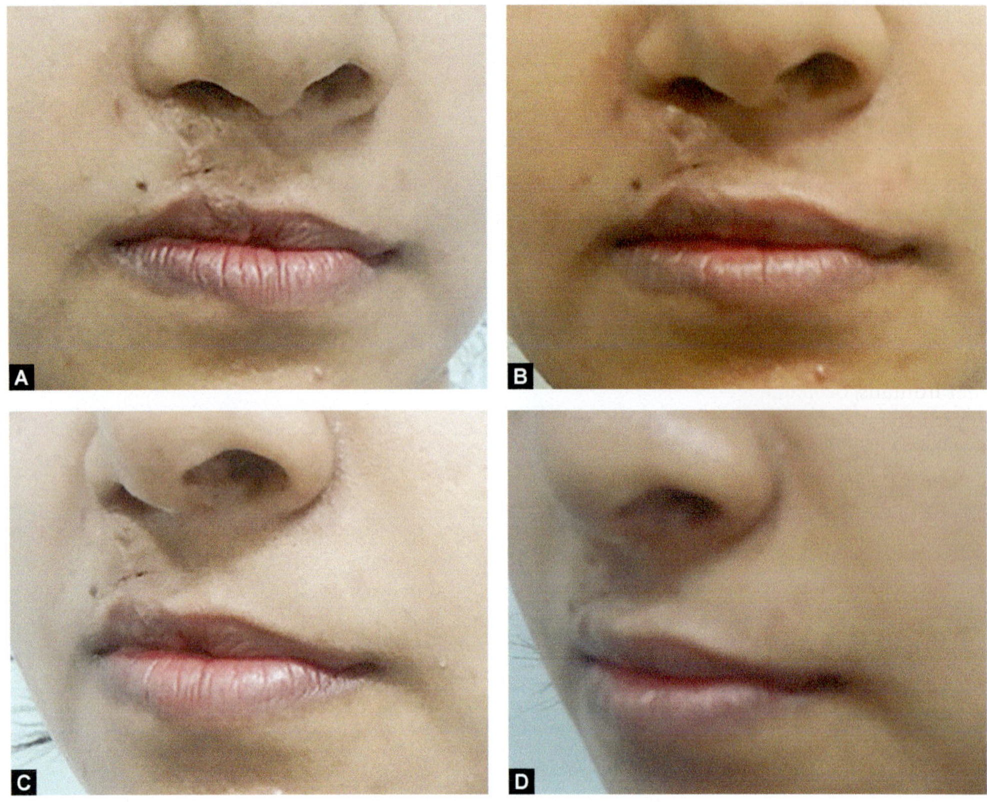

FIG. 5: Filler for postsurgical scar lip: **A,** before , **B,** after , **C,** before, **D,** after.

Postlip Surgery/Posttrauma/Cleft Lip Repair/Postcancer Treatment Lip Repair

The lips form one of the focal points of the face with any involvement of the lip causing imbalance in the harmony of the face. Surgery forms the first stage of the improvement and a HA implant follows to restore the balance to the face.[20]

A medium lift HA product is placed to recreate symmetry as much as possible. Multiple surgeries of innate cleft palate is usually followed by corrective intervention of plastic surgeons requires hospitalization of patients, causes postoperative swelling, and takes longer time to recover. Patients desire a painless, comfortable treatment to correct the aesthetic defect. The combination of treatments with fillers and surgical procedures may help process and provide more natural results than are possible with any of these techniques alone. Figure 5 shows a young girl with a surgical scar after trauma to the face. The scar was treated with fractional carbon dioxide laser and lip was balanced with a HA filler with medium lifting properties. The improvement was perceived especially on animation, where the scar did not pull at the lip as it did previously.

Lipodystrophy

Both fat as well as fillers have been documented to be very successful in the management of lipodystrophy of various etiology. When the volume to be replaced is substantial, fat as a filler is more appropriate as the economics work in its favor. However, HA fillers are a safe and effective treatment option.[21]

In lipodystrophy, HA product of high lifting capacity with a cannula in a mesh or cross-hatching technique in the deep dermis using a cannula. The use of the cannula offers a dual advantage of subcision during the procedure and prevents inadvertent intravascular deposition of filler product.

RESTORATION OF FACIAL SYMMETRY BY MYOMODULATION

Facial paralysis of various etiologies causes functional as well as aesthetic problems to the patient. Various surgical techniques are described to treat chronic facial paralysis, however, when the problem is acute, a combination of neuromodulators along with fillers can be used to balance the face so that the symmetry is restored.

Ali et al. described a patient with facial nerve paralysis postmiddle ear surgery, who was treated with a combination of neuromodulators injected into her frontalis, orbicularis oculi, and levator labii superioris. Hyaluronic acid was used to enhance the left medial and middle cheek fat for reconstruction of the left zygomatic arch, to contour the left nasolabial fold, and HA was injected to raise the left eyebrow.[22]

The author also notes the modification of muscle action after the injection of filler in certain areas, especially the nasolabial folds and marionette lines where the improvement is not only due to the improvement of volume, but also by the reduction or modification of muscle movement. In the hyperkinetic lower face, where some muscles cannot be targeted using neuromodulator, because of the overlapping muscular actions, a filler can provide a resistance and prevent full contraction of the muscle.

CONCLUSION

Our understanding of the fillers has expanded the universe of indications for their use. When we can provide a nonsurgical and immediate aesthetic improvement, fillers score over surgical techniques. Often the use of these products changes our view of how the skin and underlying tissues like bone, fat, and fibrous tissues respond to these treatments, producing better understanding of the physiology of these structures. This makes for infinite learning and interesting observations on our journey to the discovery of newer indication and better techniques to perfect and supplement or replace surgical techniques of yore.

REFERENCES

1. Davis EC, Callender VD. A review of acne in ethnic skin: pathogenesis, clinical manifestations, and management strategies. J Clin Aesthet Dermatol. 2010;3(4):24-38.
2. Fabbrocini G, Annunziata MC, D'Arco V, et al. Acne scars: pathogenesis, classification and treatment. Dermatol Res Pract. 2010;2010:893080.
3. Jansen T, Podda M. Therapy of acne scars. J Dtsch Dermatol Ges. 2010;8 Suppl 1:S81-8.
4. Barnett JG, Barnett CR. Treatment of acne scars with liquid silicone injections: 30-year perspective. Dermatol Surg. 2005;31(11 Pt 2):1542-9.
5. Epstein RE, Spencer JM. Correction of atrophic scars with artefill: an open-label pilot study. J Drugs Dermatol. 2010;9(9):1062-4.
6. Beer K. A single-center, open-label study on the use of injectable poly-L-lactic acid for the treatment of moderate to severe scarring from acne or varicella. Dermatol Surg. 2007;33(Suppl 2):S159-S67.
7. Goldberg DJ, Amin S, Hussain M. Acne scar correction using calcium hydroxylapatite in a carrier-based gel. J Cosmet Laser Ther. 2006;8(3):134-6.
8. Wollina U, Goldman A. Hyaluronic acid dermal fillers: safety and efficacy for the treatment of wrinkles, aging skin, body sculpturing and medical conditions. Clin Med Rev Ther. 2011;3:107-21.
9. Rzany B, Becker-Wegerich P, Bachmann F, et al. Hyaluronidase in the correction of hyaluronic acid-based fillers: A review and a recommendation for use. J Cosmet Dermatol. 2009;8(4):317-23.
10. Halachmi S, Ben Amitai D, Lapidoth M. Treatment of acne scars with hyaluronic acid: an improved approach. J Drugs Dermatol. 2013;12(7):e121-3.
11. Wollina U. Midfacial rejuvenation by hyaluronic acid fillers and subcutaneous adipose tissue—a new concept. Med Hypotheses. 2015;84(4):327-30.
12. Nowacki M, Pietkun K, Pokrywczyńska M, et al. Filling effects, persistence, and safety of dermal fillers formulated with stem cells in an animal model. Aesthet Surg J. 2014;34(8):1261-9.
13. Goodman GJ, Van Den Broek A. The modified tower vertical filler technique for the treatment of post-acne scarring. Australas J Dermatol. 2016;57(1):19-23.
14. Hussain SN, Goodman GJ, Rahman E. Treatment of a traumatic atrophic depressed scar with hyaluronic acid fillers: A case report. Clin Cosmet Investig Dermatol. 2017;10:285-7.
15. Marzano AV, Menni S, Parodi A, et al. Localized scleroderma in adults and children. Clinical and laboratory investigations on 239 cases. Eur J Dermatol. 2003;13(2):171-6.
16. Kroft EB, Berkhof NJ, van de Kerkhof PC, et al. Ultraviolet A phototherapy for sclerotic skin diseases: A systematic review. J Am Acad Dermatol. 2008;59(6):1017-30.
17. Onesti MG, Troccola A, Scuderi N. Volumetric correction using poly-L-lactic acid in facial asymmetry: Parry Romberg syndrome and scleroderma. Dermatol Surg. 2009;35(9):1368-75.
18. Narins RS, Dayan SH, Brandt FS, et al. Persistence and improvement of nasolabial fold correction with nonanimal-stabilized hyaluronic acid 100,000 gel particles/mL filler on two retreatment schedules: Results up to 18 months on two retreatment schedules. Dermatol Surg. 2008;34 Suppl 1:S2-S8.
19. Mashiko T, Mori H, Kato H, et al. Semipermanent volumization by an absorbable filler: onlay injection

technique to the bone. Plast Reconstr Surg Glob Open. 2013;1(1):e4-14.
20. Stolic D, Jankovic M, Draskovic M, et al. The Surgical Lips Deformity Corrected with Hyaluronic Fillers: A Case Report. Open Access Maced J Med Sci. 2015;3(3):423-5.
21. Teplica D. Discussion: Autologous fat grafting and injectable dermal fillers for human immunodeficiency virus-associated facial lipodystrophy: a comparison of safety, efficacy, and long-term treatment outcomes. Plast Reconstr Surg. 2013;131(3):507-9.
22. Sahan A, Tamer F. Restoring facial symmetry through non-surgical cosmetic procedures after permanent facial paralysis: a case report. Acta Dermatovenerol Alp Pannonica Adriat. 2017;26(2):41-2.

4

SECTION

ADJUNCTIVE TREATMENTS

31 CHAPTER

Basic Peels

Shehnaz Z Arsiwala

INTRODUCTION

Prevalent since time immemorial, chemical peels have now become a valuable asset in the therapeutic armamentarium of a cosmetic dermatologist.

Chemical peeling is a simple office procedure, easy to learn and practice, safe and effective in learned hands, affordable to most, and with minimal to none side effects as they have advantages like ease of performance, cost effectiveness, and optimum results when chosen for appropriate indications. Chemical peels are used for enhancing and improving the skin texture, pigmentation, and rejuvenation. Basic peels and techniques, however, form the crux of understanding and performing peels.

CONCEPT OF PEELING

Chemical peels create epidermal destruction, its subsequent elimination is followed by tissue replacement through regeneration and remodeling through a controlled stage of inflammation. The mechanism by which epidermal destruction occurs varies from one peeling agent to another.[1] The different molecular composition of epidermis and dermis, different pH, and the variable interactions with various peeling agents defines the clinical endpoint and the outcome of a peel. The tissue targets and their characteristics for peels are highlighted in table 1. The initial chemical peels concept was that a peeling agent is largely pH dependant and works by acidity. As proposed by Rubin the new concept is that peels work by different mechanisms (Table 2).[1] These include:

- Caustic action: Acidity dependent-trichloroacetic acid (TCA).
- Metabolic action: pH dependent-alpha hydroxy acids (AHAs), retinoic acid, and azelaic acid.
- Toxic action: Phenol-salicylic acid (SA), resorcinol.

TABLE 1: Tissues which are targets in peels[1]

Epidermis	Dermis
• Keratinocytes	• Glycosaminoglycans, collagen, and elastin
• Protein rich (keratin)	• Sugars rich
• Water (lesser than dermis)	• Lipids (more than epidermis)
• More acidic: pH 5.5	• Water (more than epidermis)
• Skin barrier: Lipid, sebum, and sweat	• Less acidic: pH 6.5.

GROUND RULE FOR PEELS

Peels should be conducted on well informed, sun protected, and compliant patients with realistic expectations. Broad-spectrum sunscreen with sun protection factor of 15 or above and ultraviolet A (UVA) coverage should be started well in advance. A newer photostable sunscreen with a physical block should be chosen.

PRIMING AND ITS IMPORTANCE FOR SKIN OF COLOR

Priming involves home care regimen with sun protection and lightening creams to make the skin conducive for peeling. It involves usage of the products 4–7 weeks before executing peels and is essential as it allows uniform penetration of the peeling agent and reduces wound healing time.[2-4]

TABLE 2: Mechanism of action of peels[1]

Mechanism	Characteristic feature	Peeling agent	Target action
Caustic (destruction of cells locally)	Acidity dependent	Trichloroacetic acid	Coagulation and destruction of epidermis, elimination, regeneration, and remodeling. No systemic action
Metabolic (modifies cell structure and synthesis)	pH dependent	• Alpha hydroxy acids • Retinol • Azelaic acid	• Keratinocytes dyscohesion, exfoliation, regeneration, and remodeling • Retinoid receptors, keratinocyte regulation and regeneration, and remodeling • Reactive oxygen species, antibacterial
Toxic (localized and systemic actions if absorbed)	Non-pH dependent	• Salicylic acid • Phenol • Resorcinol	• Noncaustic, keratolytic, anti-inflammatory, lipophilic, and sebolytic but • Systemic absorption • Keratolysis by protein denaturation. Toxic effects on cells. Systemic action

Priming Tips[5-9]

Broad-spectrum sunscreen with UVA coverage is mandatory and should be applied as an adequate film every 5 hourly and reapplied on washing or wiping. Glycolic acid (GA) is used for priming when textural improvements with peels are sought. Tretinoin is used for priming when treating acne and acne scars with chemical peels. Kojic acid and hydroquinone (HQ) are used as priming agents when treating pigmentation and melasma with peels. Combination of earlier priming agents acts by synergism and are often used for priming in dark skin types to improve the peel outcome. In author's experience while priming patient's mature skin, a hydrating agent of nonocclusive variety is also introduced as a part of priming regimen.

BASIC PEELS

Classification of Peeling Agents

The peels are classified according to the depth of injury they create (Box 1). The depth of peel is dependent upon the agent used for peeling, its modality of action: Caustic, metabolic, or toxic, strength and concentration of the peeling used, and the pH of the peeling agent. Also, patient factors like skin type, indication, prepeel preparation, and priming influence peel penetration. These variables need to be considered while executing a successful peel procedure and enhancing outcome.

BOX 1 Depth of peels

- Superficial wounding: Light peel—stratum granulosum, papillary dermis
- Medium depth wounding: Medium peel—upper reticular dermis
- Deep depth wounding: Deep peel—midreticular dermis

Peeling Agents

Peeling agents are alcohol acids which have a carboxyl group and a hydroxyl base. Depending on the position of hydroxyl group they can be AHA or beta hydroxy acids (BHAs). Phenol, TCA, and retinoic acids are not alcohols but acids.[5,10]

Types of Basic Peeling Agents

- Alpha hydroxy acids
- Beta hydroxy acids
- Trichloroacetic acid
- Retinol
- Phenol.

Alpha hydroxy acids[1,11,12] also known as fruit acids are the most commonly used peels. These have acid carboxyl group in the first carbon and hydroxyl group in alpha position. Alpha hydroxy acids are metabolic peels and are pH dependent for their actions. The AHA peels are listed in boxes 2 and 3. Low strength acids achieve a superficial peel at acidic pH and aqueous base compared to large molecular weight acids. With high pH these have moisturizing properties. The irritation associated with AHAs is more due to formulation rather than the acid itself. The AHA peels have a metabolic action and are pH dependent and require termination by neutralizing

BOX 2 Subgroups of alpha hydroxy acid

Three subgroups of AHA

- Monocarboxylic acids: Glycolic, lactic
- Dicarboxylic: Malic
- Tricarboxylic: Citric

BOX 3 Alpha hydroxy acids

- Glycolic acid (sugarcane)
- Lactic acid (milk)
- Malic acid (apples)
- Citric acid (citrus fruits)
- Mandelic acid (bitter almonds)
- Glycolic acid + ammonium glycolate
- Alpha hydroxyethanoic acid + ammonium alpha hydroxyethanoate

BOX 4 Endpoint in alpha hydroxy acid peels

Sheer vigilance in AHA peels

- First sign of erythema: Means early dyscohesion of stratum corneum
- Blanching (frosting): Means epidermolysis (medium depth)
- Desquamation: Epidermal detachment—more than medium depth

AHA, alpha hydroxy acid.

TABLE 3: Degree of epidermolysis with alpha hydroxy acid

Peeling	pH	pKa	Molecular size	Features
Pyruvic acid	0.6	2.39	Smallest	Potent peeling agent
Glycolic acid (free)	0.6–1.7	3.83	Small	Good peeling agent
Lactic acid	2.5	2.23	Largest AHA	Moisture holding
Mandelic acid	1.0	3.41	Larger	Less irritant

AHA, alpha hydroxy acid.

with water or 5% sodium bicarbonate solution (Box 4). Table 3 highlights the pH, pKa, and degree of epidermolysis caused by various AHAs.

Actions of Glycolic Acid

The GA are weak acids, pKa is 3.8. Glycolic acid is diluted with alcohol or propylene glycol, acetone, or tap water to achieve 20, 25, 30, and up to 70%. Glycolic acid has long shelf life and formulated as either:

- Free acid (nonneutralized, aqueous pH 0.6–1.7)
- Partially neutralized (less irritant)
- Buffered (resists pH change)
- Esterified (glycol citrate).

The small molecular size of GA enables rapid penetration through the horny layer and reaches the dermis. At low concentration GA decreases coenocytes adhesion by enzyme interference at the surface of corneocytes, thus, increasing desquamation and thinning of stratum corneum. At high concentration it causes corneocytes detachment (epidermolysis). Chemically stimulated epidermopoiesis is seen as thicker epidermis with thinner stratum corneum. By increasing the epidermal thickness, GA regulates keratinization, reduces intercorneocyte cohesion, enhances hydration, improves quality of elastin, and decreases density of collagen. Glycolic acid also reduces pigmentation. The endpoint of the peel is time dependant and appropriate endpoint should be achieved before termination. Patient discomfort is a rough gauge and a verbal communication of discomfort on 1–10 range is sought. In absence of endpoint, the peel must be neutralized at the score above 7. Time of application is decided according to the indication and patient tolerance. Depending on concentration and time of contact they can be repeated weekly, bimonthly or monthly (Fig. 1).[1,11]

Alpha Keto Acids[13-15]

Pyruvic acid (PA) has a keto group in alpha position. PA is physiologically converted to lactic acid (LA) in the skin and forms natural moisturizing factor. It has a small molecular size and a low pKa and thus a potent peeling agent. It is soluble in water and alcohol. It is a keratolytic, antimicrobial, sebostatic, and has collagen remodeling actions. PA is available as 40–60% solution or gel base. 100% PA produces epidermal necrosis in 30–60 seconds, dermal effects occur in 2 minutes (60%). The PA peel when applied causes frosting seen in 2–15 minutes of application and needs to be neutralized. Postpeel erythema may persist for 2 weeks to 2 months. Pyruvic acid has no systemic toxicity like phenol. It is used for photoaging, postacne pigmentation as well as melasma; it is used for acne and improves mild scars. It is also beneficial in verruca plana.[16]

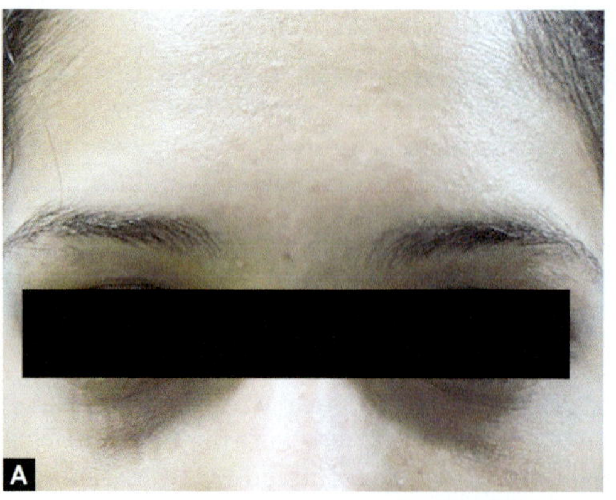

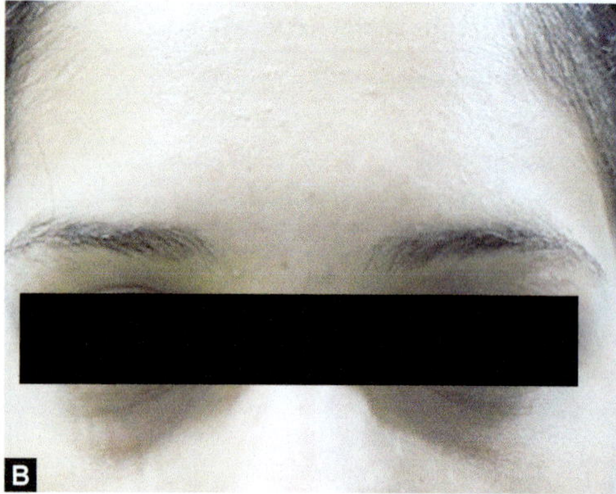

FIG. 1: A, Before and B, after 35% glycolic acid peels.

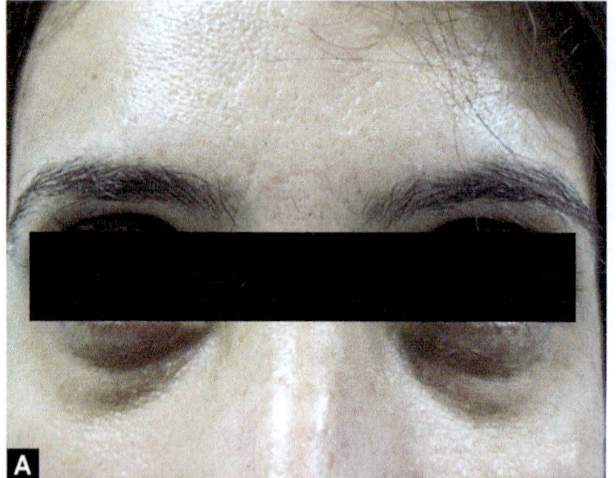

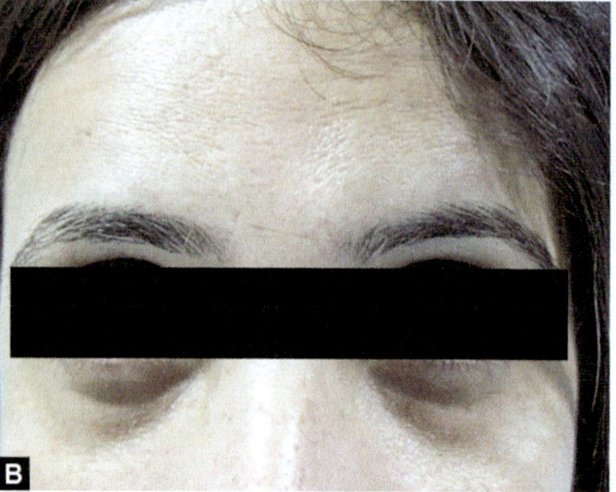

FIG. 2: A, Periorbital pigmentation—before and B, after five sessions of lactic acid + arginine peels.

Lactic Acid

Derived from milk, they are superficial peels with little to no downtime. Lactic acid is largely used for rejuvenation, photodamage, and textural improvements especially in periorbital area. It is used safely in skin of color. Ranging from 40–70% in strength, 70% gel peels are less irritating and suitable for sensitive skin. Lactic acid has ability to moisturize the skin and used for patients with dry skin (Fig. 2).[11,17]

Mandelic Acid[18]

Derived from almond extracts known as phenoxy-glycolic acid/amygdalic acid. It is a low-molecular weight agent obtained from bitter almonds. Mandelic acid (MA) has antibacterial and anti-inflammatory properties and helpful adjuvant in active acne. Mandelic acid used from 20–50% is also known to improve hyperpigmentation and so helpful in acne with pigmented scars in Asian skins, it is a less irritant peel compared to GA (Fig. 3).

Beta Hydroxy Acids

Beta hydroxy acid is simple organic acids derivatives of aspirin and is a hydroxyl derivative of benzoic acid. Salicylic acid naturally found in sweet birch, willow bark, and wintergreen leaves and highly water soluble. This includes SA and alpha lipohydroxy acids. Salicylic acid powder dissolved in 95% ethanol. Crystallizes on skin to form pseudofrost. Available as 20–30% peeling solution. It has a pKa of 3. Salicylic acid peels were first described by Unna and is used for many years by clinicians for chemical peeling.

Actions of Salicylic Acid[19-23]

Salicylic acid has a toxic mode of action (Table 2). It is a keratolytic and dissolves desmosomes between corneocytes thus causing exfoliation and accelerates cell turnover. Salicylic acid specially decreases surface roughness, reduces fine lines, and improves texture of the skin. The lipophilic nature makes it sebolytic and is considered far superior to AHA in

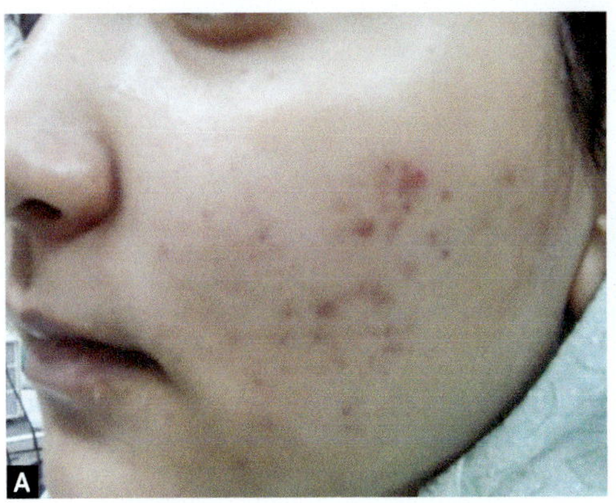

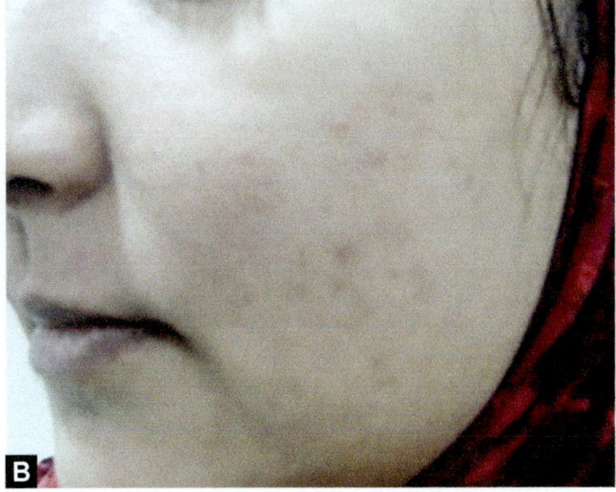

FIG. 3: A, Postacne macules before mandelic acid (MA) peels and **B,** improvement after MA peels.

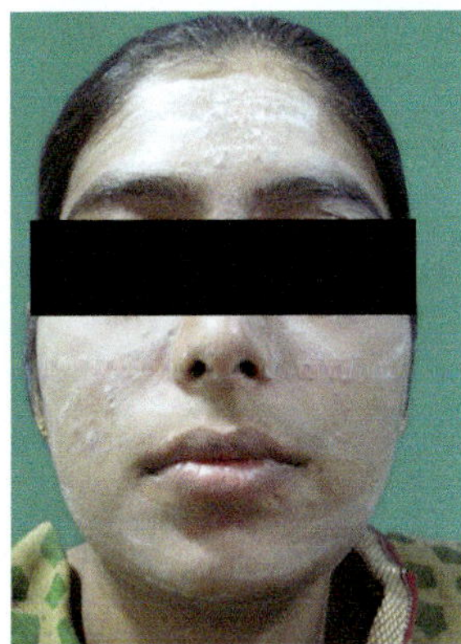

FIG. 4: Pseudofrost of salicylic acid.

acne and seborrhea as it can exfoliate even within oil rich pores thus reducing comedones. Salicylic acid has additional anti-inflammatory effects and inhibits prostaglandins, through arachidonic cascade, a factor useful in inflammatory acne. Salicylic acid fades pigment spots, exfoliating pigmented keratinocytes, and accelerates cell cycle preventing new pigment transfer thus very useful in postacne pigmented macular phase (Fig. 4).

Salient features of SA peels are:

- Salicylic acid peels are relatively safer for dark skin types
- Best outcome in early erythematous acne scars along with comedogenic or papular inflammatory acne
- Used for truncal and upper arm acne and postacne pigmented macules
- Reduces associated seborrhea
- Used as adjunctive to medical therapy in melasma, postinflammatory hyperpigmentation (PIH), photodamage, and textural improvement (Fig. 5)
- As a prepeel before TCA peels and best combined with MA/retinol peel
- Contraindicated in pregnancy, lactation, and sensitivity to aspirin
- Adequate hydration while performing large areas
- Look out for manifestations of salicylism. Complains of tinnitus, giddiness while executing peels on large surface areas
- Excellent as a priming peel before fractional lasers.

JESSNER'S PEEL[2,24]

Introduced by Max Jessner, this is a popular peel which is a combination of AHA and BHA and resorcinol. The combination works by synergism to improve outcome for acne, acne scars, photodamaged skin, and wrinkles. The peel contains SA, LA and resorcinol, and the modified one has resorcinol replaced by citric acid. Safety and tolerance is better with citric acid as resorcinol is a toxic agent with potential for strong irritation. Storage is in amber colored bottles due to its light sensitive property. This peel is to be avoided in pregnancy and in patients with known allergy to SA or resorcinol. The peel can be applied in 2–3 coats with a slight rubbing technique. Increasing coats increases the depth of penetration. Sufficient interval between coats is essential to prevent inadvertent deeper penetration and patchy coating. The peel does not require neutralization. Jessner's peel can be combined with TCA for deeper penetration.

TRICHLOROACETIC ACID[25-29]

Trichloroacetic acid is a self neutralizing caustic peel with pKa of 0.26. Trichloroacetic acid is a stronger acid than GA and are not pH dependent. It is nontoxic when applied to the skin as it is not transported to capillary dermal vessels. Tissue destruction occurs by protein

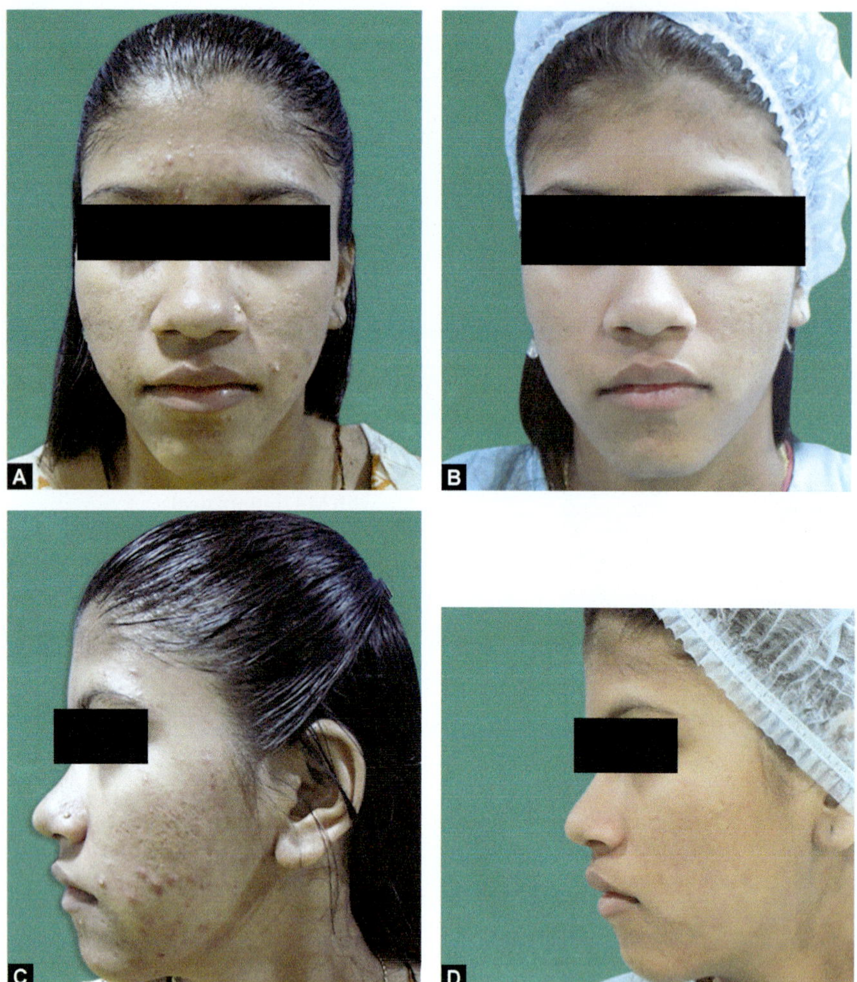

FIG. 5: A, Papular acne and postacne macules—before; **B,** papular acne and postacne macules—before; **C,** after five sessions of salicylic acid (SA) peels; and **D,** after five sessions of SA peels.

precipitation. Once protein precipitation occurs they are neutralized automatically. Endpoint is frosting. Action of TCA is proportional to concentration applied, greater the amount applied more the destruction.

Mechanism of Action of Trichloroacetic Acid

- Precipitation of epidermal proteins
- Epidermal necrosis
- Sloughing and dermal inflammation
- Collagen remodeling.

Injury induced depends on concentration of the peel, so repeat coats cautiously. Single coat of TCA peel creates a superficial peel, increasing number of coats can make it medium depth. Frosting here acts as a guide to depth control. High strength associated with pigmentary side effects.[25] Usage of 15-25% optimum for skin types 4-6. Low strength TCA can reach desired depth by multiple coats, vigorous application, or by combining with other agents.

Trichloroacetic acid level of frosting and peel depth are gauged by time required for frost to appear, time required for frost to fade, and evident epidermolysis (Box 5).

Trichloroacetic Acid Peel Technique

- Surface anesthesia may be needed for medium depth peels

BOX 5 Clinical indicator for depth of trichloroacetic acid peel[26]

- Degree of frosting = Depth of penetration
- Grade 1—Erythema with streaky frost = Superficial peel
- Grade 2—White frosting with visible erythema = Medium depth peel
- Grade 3—White enamel frosting, no erythema = Deep peel

- Prepeel cleansing and degreasing
- Patient should be in a comfortable semirecline position
- Trichloroacetic acid is applied through cotton soaked in acid but squeezed dried to prevent pooling or dripping
- Sequence of application is forehead, temple cheeks, perioral, and chin
- Single coat applied at a time
- A slight pressure can be applied but overcoating by vigorous to and fro movements repeated in same area to prevent inadvertent deeper penetration should be avoided
- The first coat left on for 2-5 minutes and skip areas covered
- Second coat applied if required only after sufficient interval and frosting from first coat is seen
- Frosting is endpoint.

Level of frosting gauged according to endpoint seen (Box 5).

Post-TCA peel erythema appears which paves way for dryness or crusting. The TCA treated skin appears dark brown and undergoes exfoliation over 2–7 days.

Trichloroacetic acid peels are used for melasma, postacne scars, actinic keratosis, wrinkles, etc. Deeper depth peels give more long-lasting results but associated with pigmentary complications in darker skin.

The TCA peels are very crucial in improving most types of scars. Depth of the peel can be controlled and generally 15-25% strength peels in four sessions with adequate priming are very helpful in shallow and rolling boxcar type of scars.

Cross Technique

A technique consisting of the focal application of higher TCA concentrations by pressing hard on the entire depressed area of atrophic acne scars. This technique is called chemical reconstruction of skin scars (CROSS). Performed for fibrotic and superficial as well as deep ice pick scars deep rolling and boxcar scars and shows an excellent improvement in 3-5 sittings conducted at monthly intervals. Repeated CROSS application destroys the atrophic pit with restructuring and thickening of dermal collagen. Best results are seen for fibrotic, ice pick, boxcar scars, and dilated pores.

Though the alpha, BHAs, and TCA form the basic peels, we know interplay between these agents is possible and this concept has laid base for development of sound, rational, and evidence-based revolutionary techniques in peels. The segmental, sequential, rotational, and switch peels are the newer techniques used.

RETINOL PEELS[30,31]

Retinol is a natural form of vitamin A. Retinol peels work by keratolytic, sebolytic, comedogenic, and anti-inflammatory actions. Reduce photodamage, fine wrinkles, and improve pigmentation and texture. They are more powerful than SA peels and are very popular for usage in acne, acne scars, melasma, and photodamage. It accelerates cell turnover and useful for rejuvenation. They are available as slow release or liquid peels and have synergistic actions when used along with ascorbyl glucoside. A series of 4–6 sessions is conducted at 3 weekly intervals. Retinol peels are to be used cautiously in dry skin conditions (Fig. 6).

PHENOL PEELS[32-35]

Phenol peels are deep depth peels and were discovered in 1834. Phenol or carbolic acid is a toxic peel derived from coal tar. Liquefied phenol is 88% solution in water. Croton oil, water, septisol, and glycerin are added to improve the penetration by reducing the skin surface tension and improve the peel outcome.

Phenol peels are most inflammatory and are systemically absorbed and are applied on various cosmetic units of the face gradually overtime while observing the endpoint which is white gray frosting. Phenol peels are largely used for wrinkles, dyschromias, and acne scars as well as periorbital rejuvenation. Patients are investigated before phenol peels for heart diseases and an electrocardiogram (ECG) and complete blood count is recommended before phenol peeling.

INFLAMMATORY PROFILE OF BASIC PEELING AGENTS

Amidst the peeling agent's SA is the least inflammatory followed by TCA and GA, the resorcinol, Jessner's, and phenol being the most inflammatory

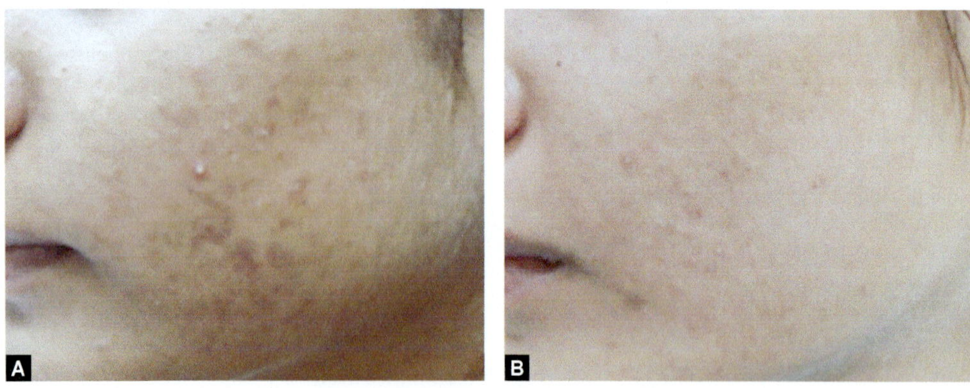

FIG. 6: A, Before four sessions of retinol peels and B, after four sessions of retinol peels.

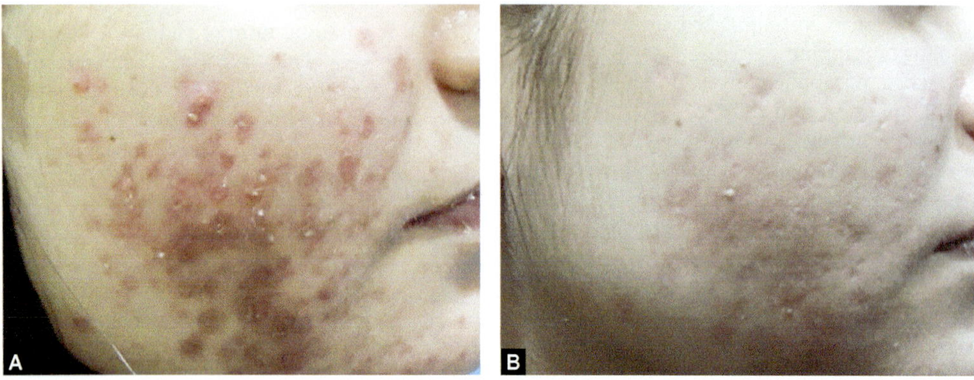

FIG. 7: A, Before postacne erythematous and pigmented scars and B, after six sessions of salicylic acid + mandelic acid peels.

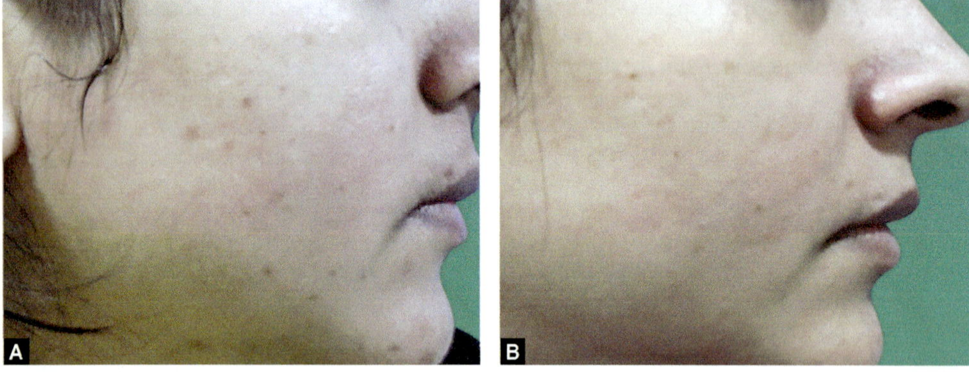

FIG. 8: A, Postacne hyperpigmented macules and B, after six sessions of glycolic acid peels.

peels (Figs 7 and 8). The more inflammation in a dark skin patient the more potential for pigmentary adverse effects hence, right choice of peeling agent, knowledge of its mechanism of action on the target tissues, and inflammatory profile is crucial.

Peels are avoided in:

- Active bacterial/viral infections/fungal infections
- Within 6 months of oral isotretinoin therapy (deep peels)
- Keloidal tendency
- Unrealistic expectations
- Coexisting inflammatory dermatoses

- Poor priming
- Any photosensitive skin conditions or photosensitizing drugs
- Unrealistic expectations.

CLINICAL INDICATIONS FOR BASIC PEELS FOR INDIAN SKIN TYPES (BOX 6)

Indications

Proper case selection and indication for chemical peels is essential, choice of peeling agent varies from person to person, and is different for different indications. See box 6 for common peel indications.[36]

PEELS USED FOR ACNE AND ATROPHIC ACNE SCARS

While treating acne and acne scars peels improve coexisting comedonal and papular acne, alleviate postacne erythema, and improve pigmentation at base of healed lesions. In addition they improve the depth, contour, and cause softening of associated scars. Treating early with chemical peels in postacne phase will help in preventing the progressive scarring of the healing lesions in inflammatory acne and also added improvement in texture glow as well as impart a more youthful appearance of the skin (Box 7).

Commonly used agents are SA for comedonal, papular, and inflammatory acne, and postacne macules, AHA peels for acne, early scars, and textural improvements, TCA for boxcar scars, rolling scars, and CROSS TCA for ice pick scars.

BOX 6 Common indications for chemical peeling

Acne:
- Papular, comedonal, and inflammatory
- Acne scars: Early and atrophic—Grade 1–2
- Postacne pigmented macules.

Pigmentation:
- Postinflammatory hyperpigmentation
- Melasma
- Photodamage
- Freckles.

Wrinkles:
- Fine lines
- Photoaging
- Texture

BOX 7 Favorable features for peels response in melasma

- Melasma <1 year of duration
- Epidermal component more favorable than dermal component
- Heterogeneous pigment pattern more favorable than homogenous pigment pattern

PEELS FOR PIGMENTATION

Chemical Peels and Melasma

While evaluating a case for peels in melasma, one must consider all the possible peel as well as nonpeel options available to improve the melasma. Interventions in melasma are always adjuvant to topical therapies. Peels are introduced for unresponsive or recalcitrant cases. Never as first line or monotherapy. Chemical peels work by removal of melanin. Peels are adjuvant to medical management and useful only for epidermal component in melasma. Helpful in elimination of melanin from the keratinocytes as well as melanosomes transfer to keratinocytes. Peels are useful in epidermal component (Box 8). Peels should not be used before 3 months of basic topical therapy, after adequate suppression of melanogenesis and sun protection. Hyperpigmentation reported to be the most common side effect of high strength peels especially GA and TCA. Low strength combination peels or rotational peels are more commonly used for Indian skin. Clearance of whatever degree requires maintenance with topical therapy like GA, TCA, Jessner's solution, SA, tretinoin, and kojic acid peels are used. Glycolic acid 20–50% are useful in dark skin types.

BOX 8 Chemical peel complications

- Edema
- Erythema
- Irritation
- Dryness
- Hyperpigmentation
- Contact dermatitis
- Bacterial infections
- Photosensitivity
- Reactivation of herpes
- Flare of acne vulgaris
- Acneiform eruptions
- Hypopigmentation
- Scarring and atrophy
- Hypertrophy/keloids

Dermal Melasma does not Respond Well to Chemical Peeling Treatment

Postpeel Care

- Ice compresses
- Restrict emollients for 2 days
- Once peeling occurs start emollients
- Sunscreens are a must
- Moisturizers may be required
- Advise mild gentle neutral pH facial cleansers.

Algorithms for peels in acne, acne scars, and pigmentation are highlighted in flowcharts 1 to 3.

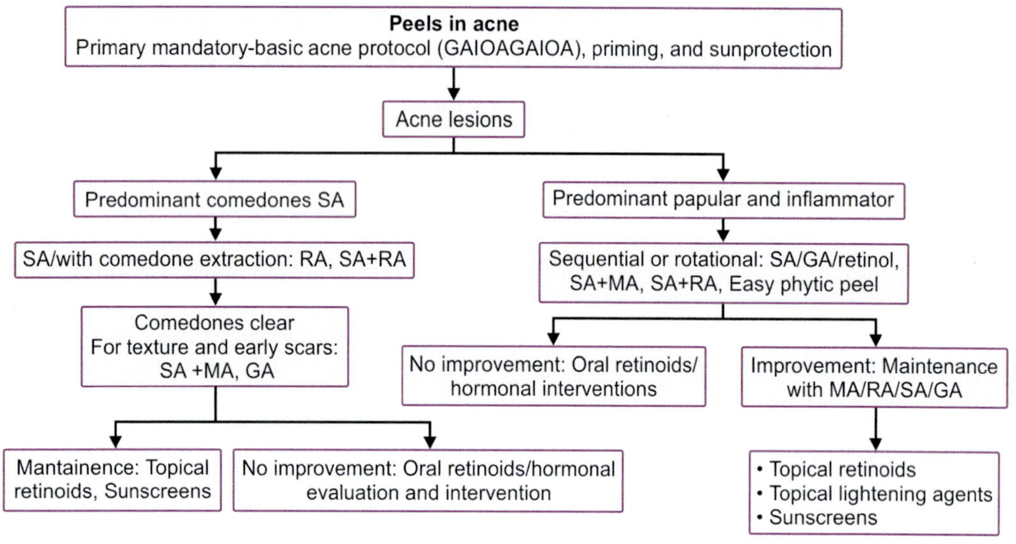

GA, glycolic acid; MA, mandelic acid; SA, salicylic acid.

FLOWCHART 1: Peels in acne.

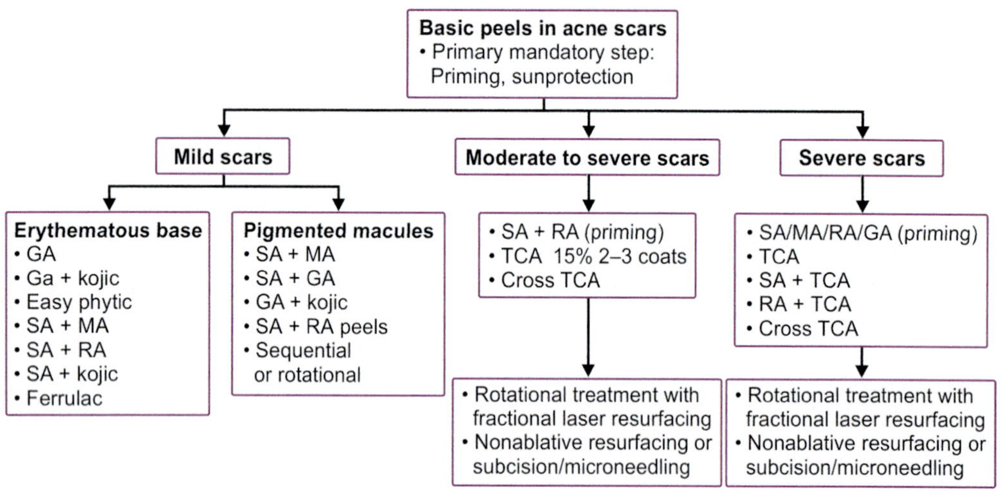

GA, glycolic acid; MA, mandelic acid; SA, salicylic acid; TCA, trichloroacetic acid.

FLOWCHART 2: Basic peels in acne scars.

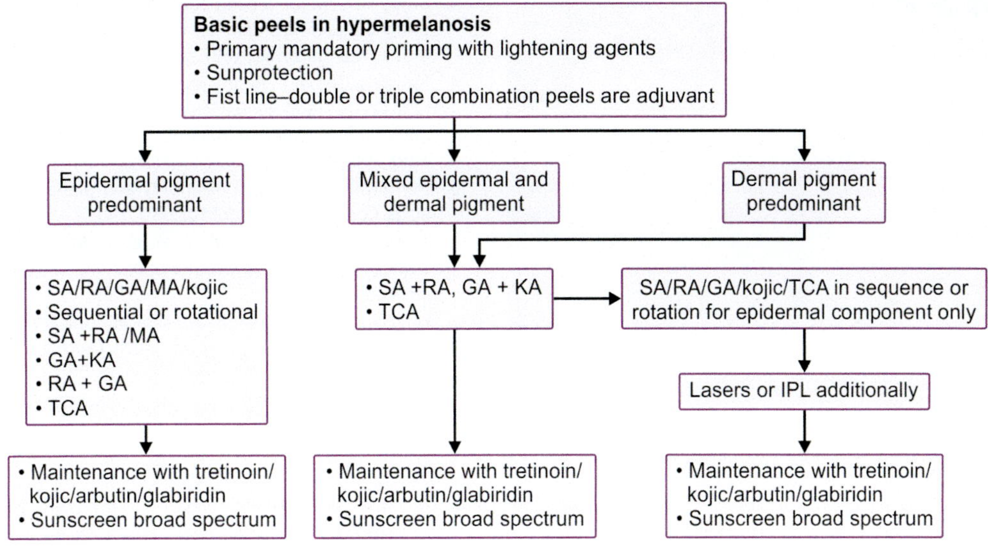

GA, glycolic acid; KA, kojic acid; MA, mandelic acid; SA, salicylic acid; TCA, trichloroacetic acid.

FLOWCHART 3: Basic peels in hypermelanosis.

COMPLICATIONS OF PEELS[29,35,37-40]

Chemical peels are associated with certain unwanted side effects (Box 8). Poor priming, noncompliance, wrong peeling agent, and high concentration peels are associated with more frequent side effects, etc. Treating skin of color demands additional consideration as one has to focus on preventing pigmentary altercations, so adequate priming and achieving right depth of peel is essential. This is simply achieved by getting the right choice of peel agent, right priming, adequate sun protection, interpeel vigilance, and optimum postpeel care (Figs 9 to 11).

The peeling process can result in certain mild transient effects and sometimes moderate or permanent complications especially while dealing with dark skin patients.

For Indian skin the recommendation is to use a low strength peel for an agent like TCA and repeat coats. SA peels are considered safest and high strength GA are associated with risk of epidermolysis, irritation, and PIH. Postinflammatory hyperpigmentation is often transient and lasts for 4–6 weeks and fades in most cases with high percentage of HQ and aggressive sun protection. In some cases it may persist for longer periods. Hyperpigmentation

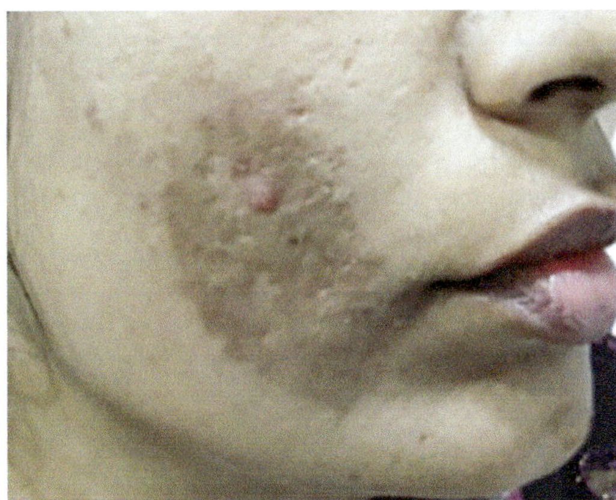

FIG. 9: Postinflammatory hyperpigmentation caused by high strength glycolic acid peels in unprimed patient by unqualified person.

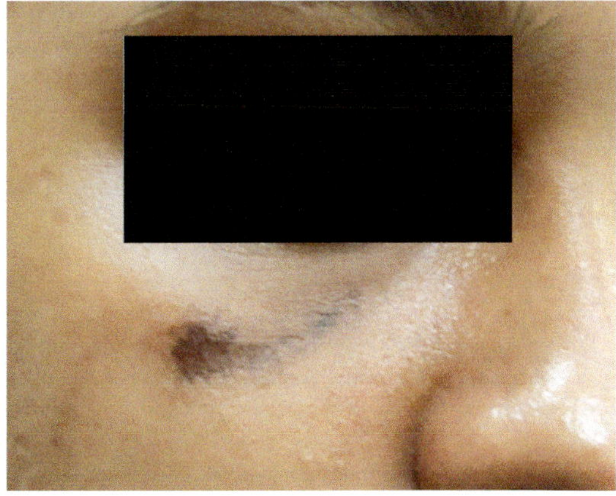

FIG. 10: Post-trichloroacetic acid peel postinflammatory hyperpigmentation—demarcatory line. Peel done by unqualified person.

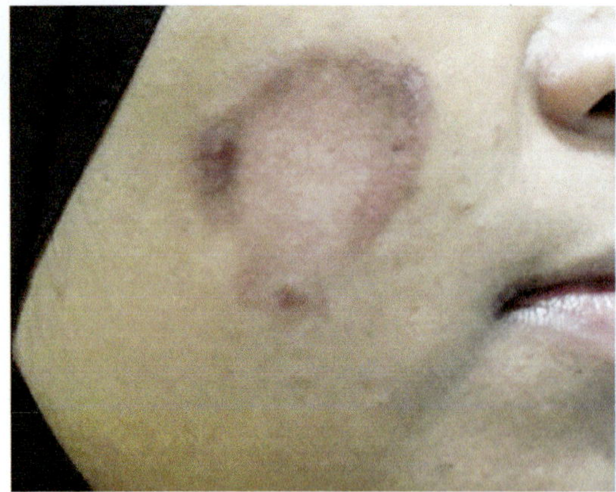

FIG. 11: Post-trichloroacetic acid peel postinflammatory hyperpigmentation—done by unqualified person.

may be focal or seen as demarcatory lines or blotchy and pan facial. Erythema which lasts for more than 2–3 weeks in postpeel phase is likely to result in hyperpigmentation. Hypopigmentation with deep peels like TCA and phenol are difficult to treat complications. Delayed hypopigmentation is a potential risk of phenol peels in skin of color. Contact dermatitis can occur with GA, resorcinol, and even LA peels and should be avoided in patients with dry and sensitive skin types.

CONCLUSION

Chemical peeling is the most popular and economic in office procedure to improve acne, acne scars, pigmentary conditions, and texture. Perfect peels can be executed when one has knowledge of formulations, actions, and techniques for appropriate indications in a well primed, compliant, and sun protected patient. While treating dark skin additional caution while choosing peel strength, optimum priming, and absolute sun protection are mandatory. Understanding peel formulations, their mechanism of action, right choice of peel, and right indication enables one to execute the correct peel response in a conducive patient.

REFERENCES

1. Dewandre L. The chemistry of peels and a hypothesis of action mechanisms. In: Rubin MG, Editor. Chemical Peels, 1st edition. New Delhi: Elsevier Inc.; 2006. pp. 1-12.
2. Savant SS. Superficial and medium depth chemical peeling. In: Savant SS, Editor. Textbook of Dermatosurgery and Cosmetology, 2nd edition. Mumbai: ASCAD; 2005. pp. 177-95.
3. Brody H. General peeling concepts. In: Brody H, Editor. Chemical peeling and resurfacing, 2nd edition. St Louis: Mosby Year book Inc.; 1997. pp. 39-72.
4. Nanda S, Grover C, Reddy BS. Efficacy of hydroquinone (2%) versus tretinoin (0.025%) as adjunct topical agents for chemical peeling in patients of melasma. Dermatol Surg. 2004;30(3):385-9.
5. Hermitte R. Aged skin, retinoids and alpha hydroxyl acids. Cosmet Toilet. 1992;107:63-7.
6. Jimbow K, Obata H, Pathek M, et al. Mechanism of depigmentation by hydroquinone. J Invest Dermatol. 1974;62(4):436-49.
7. Hung VC, Yu-Yun Lee, Zitelli JA, et al. Topical tretinoin and epithelial wound healing. Arch Dermatol. 1989; 125(1):65-9.
8. Hevia O, Nemeth AJ, Taylor JR. Tretinoin accelerates healing after TCA chemical peels. Arch Dermatol. 1991;127(5):678-82.
9. Resnik BI. The role of priming the skin for peels. In: Rubin MG (Ed). Chemical Peels: Procedures in Cosmetic Dermatology, 1st edition. New Delhi: Elsevier Inc.; 2006. pp. 21-6.
10. Allinger NL, Cava MP, de Jongh DC, et al. Chimie Organique (Organic Chemistry). Montreal: McGraw-Hill; 1990.
11. Van Scott EJ, Yu RJ. Control of keratinization with alpha hydroxy acids and related compounds. Arch Dermatol. 1974;110(4):586-90.
12. Van Scott EJ, Yu RJ. Alpha-hydroxy-acids: procedures for use in clinical practice. Cutis. 1989;43(3):222-8.
13. Fabbrocini G, De Padova MP, Tosti A. Chemical peels: what's new and what isn't new but still works well. Facial Plast Surg. 2009;25(5):329-36.
14. Ghersetich I, Brazzini B, Peris K, et al. Pyruvic acid peels for treatment of photoaging. Dermatol Surg. 2004;30(1):32-6.
15. Griffin TD, Van Scott EJ, Maddin S. The use of pyruvic acid as a chemical peeling agent. J Dermatol Surg Oncol. 1989:15:1316.
16. Halasz CL. Treatment of warts with topical pyruvic acid: with and without 5 Fluorouracil. Cutis. 1998;62(6):283-5.
17. Sharique KE, Al-Tikreety MM, Al-Mashhadani SA. Lactic acid chemical peels as a new therapeutic modality in melasma in comparision to Jessner's solution chemical peels. Dermatol Surg. 2006;32(12):1429-36.
18. Taylor MB. Summary of mandelic acid for improvement of skin conditions. Cosmet Dermatol. 1999;12:28.
19. Vedamurthy M. Salicylic acid peels. Indian J Dermatol Venereol Leprol. 2004;70(2):136-8.
20. Lazo ND, Meine JG, Downing DT. Lipids are covalently attached to rigid corneocytes protein envelop eisting predominantly as beta-sheets: a solid state nuclear magnetic resonance study. J Invest Dermatol. 1995;105(2):296-300.
21. KiligmanD, Kligman AM. Salicylic acid peels for treatment of photoaging. Dermatol Surg. 1998;24(3):325-28.
22. Joshi SS, Boone SI, Alam M, et al. Effectiveness, safety, and effect on quality of life of topical salicylic acid peels for treatment of post inflammatory hyperpigmentation in dark skin. Dermatol Surg. 2009;32(4):372-5.

23. Lee HS, Kim IH. Salicylic acid peels for treatment of acne vulgaris in Asian patients. Dermatol Surg. 2003; 29(12):1196-9.
24. Fulton JE. Jessner's peel. In: Rubin M (Ed). Chemical peels: Procedures in Cosmetic Dermatology. New Delhi: Elsevier Inc.; 2006. pp. 57-71.
25. Halaas YP: Medium depth peels. Facial Plast Surg Clin North Am. 2004;12(3):297-303.
26. Monheit GD. Skin preparation: an essential step before chemical peeling or laser resurfacing. Cosmet Dermatol. 1996;9:9-14.
27. Monheit GD, Kayal JD. Chemical peeling. In: Nouri K, Khouri L (Eds). Techniques of Dermatologic Surgery. New Delhi: Elsevier Inc.; 2003. pp. 233-44.
28. Rubin MG. Manual of Chemical Peel: Superficial and Medium Depth, 1st edition. Philadelphia: Lippincott Co; 1995. pp. 110-29.
29. Brody HJ. Complications of chemical resurfacing. Dermatol Clin. 2001;19(3):427-37.
30. Kligman DE. Tretinoin peels versus glycolic acid peels. Dermatol Surg. 2004;30(12 Pt 2):1609.
31. Khunger N, Sarkar R, Jain RK. Tretinoin peels versus glycolic acid peels in treatment of melasma in dark skinned patients. Dermatol Surg. 2004:30(5):756-60.
32. Larson DL, Karmo F, Hetter GP. Phenol-croton oil peel: establishing a scientific model for animal investigation. Aesthet Surg J. 2009;29(1):47-53.
33. Baker TJ, Gordon HL, Seckinger DL. A second look at chemical face peeling. Plast Reconstr Surg. 1966; 37(6):487.
34. Park JH, Choi YD, Kim SW, et al. Effectiveness of modified phenol peel (Exoderm) on facial wrinkles, acne scars and other skin problems of Asian patients. J Dermatol. 2007;34(1):17-24.
35. Landau M. Cardiac complications in deep chemical peels. Dermatol Surg. 2007;33(2):190-3.
36. Garg VK, Sinha S, Sarkar R. Glycolic acid peels versus salicylic-mandelic acid peels in active acne vulgaris and post-acne scarring and hyperpigmentation: a comparative study. Dermatol Surg. 2009;35(1):59-65.
37. Truppman F, Ellenbery J. The major electrocardiographic changes during chemical face peeling. Plast Reconstr Surg. 1979;63(1):44.
38. Lee JB, Chung WG, Kwahck H, et al. Focal treatment of acne scars with trichloroacetic acid: chemical reconstruction of skin scars method. Dermatol Surg. 2002;28:1017-21.
39. Khunger N, Arsiwala S. Step by step chemical peels. In: Khunger N, Editor. Combination and Sequential Peels. New Delhi: Jaypee Brothers Medical Publishers (P) Ltd; 2008. pp. 201-18.
40. IAA Consensus Document. Acne scars. Indian J Dermatol Venerol Leprol. 2009;75.52-3.

32 CHAPTER

Platelet-rich Plasma in Aesthetic Dermatology

Salim Thurakkal

INTRODUCTION

Autologous blood concentrates in the form of platelet-rich plasma (PRP), aimed at the delivery of biologically active substances such as growth factors (GFs), cytokines, fibrin, etc., have recently been involved in a large number of new clinical applications in different medical fields.[1] Basic science and research findings have pointed out the role of platelet-derived growth factors (PDGFs) to be biologically active in many key regenerative steps, such as the development of angiogenesis, the formation of the protein matrix, and the enhancement of cell proliferation.

Platelet-rich plasma has been investigated in several disciplines in medicine for its role in wound healing, especially in orthopedics and dentistry.[2] It has also been shown to promote hair survival and growth, both *in vitro* and *in vivo*.[3] In recent years, there has been a proliferation of reports relating to the usage of PRP for dermatological indications like patterned hair loss, alopecia areata, acne scarring, facial rejuvenation, wound healing, and fat transplantation.[4] Few recent studies have suggested its utility and relevance in aesthetic dermatology and the combination of PRP with other therapies is particularly interesting.

This chapter will focus on the biology of PRP, methodology, and current indications and applications in aesthetic dermatologic practice.

DEFINITION

Platelet-rich plasma: synonyms—autologous platelet gel, plasma rich growth factors, and platelet concentrated plasma.

Platelet-rich plasma means abundant platelets that are concentrated into a small volume of plasma. There is no consensus on the definition of PRP. Some investigators have suggested that PRP should refer to the fraction with a platelet concentration 3–5 times greater than normal levels. However, the most accepted definition at present characterizes PRP as a volume of autologous plasma that contains a platelet concentration above basal concentration (150,000–350,000/μL).[5] Although the optimal PRP platelet concentration is unclear, the current methods by which PRP is prepared is reported to involve 300–700% enrichment.

It is an effective concentration of multiple fundamental GFs by virtue of platelets alone (stored as α-granules in platelets) and plasma proteins, namely fibrin, fibronectin, and vitronectin.[6]

HISTORIC PERSPECTIVES

Since 1970s, PRP has received significant attention as an application for tissue repair and hemostasis during the healing process of ulcers and undermined wound surfaces.[7] After the discovery in the 1980s of the release of bioactive molecules with action in damaged tissue, PRP started to be used in regenerative medicine.[8] Ten years later, PRP started to be used in maxillofacial surgery, taking advantage of the potential of fibrin for adherence and its hemostatic properties.[9] Clinical observation revealed PRP could stimulate cell proliferation and have anti-inflammatory characteristics.

An outpatient method for obtaining PRP for application in implantology was reported by Anitua in the year 1999.[9] Further different techniques have been developed and the range of applications has been extended. Now, PRP is an indispensible therapeutic option in many of the aesthetic dermatologic indications. Figure 1 shows

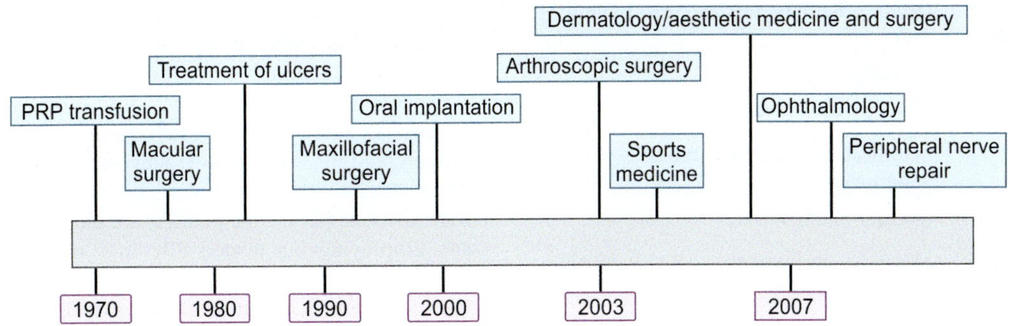

PRP, platelet-rich plasma.

FIG. 1: Timeline for the introduction of platelet-rich plasma in different medical indications.

TABLE 1: Classification and functions of bioactive molecules present in platelet-rich plasma

Category	Proteins	Function
Adhesive proteins	Von Willebrand factor, fibrinogen, fibronectin, vitronectin, lamminin-8	Cell interaction, hemostasis, composition of extracellular matrix
Coagulation factor and associated proteins	Factor V/Va, multimerin, protein S, high-molecular weight kininogen, antithrombin III, tissue factor pathway inhibitor	Thrombin production and regulation
Fibrinolytic factors and associated proteins	Plasminogen, -2 antiplasmin, histidine-rich glycoprotein, -2 macroglobulin	Plasmin production and vascular remodeling
Proteases and antiproteases	Tissue inhibitors of metalloproteases 1-4 (TIMP 1-4), metalloproteases 1, 2, 4, 9, α1 antitrypsin	Angiogenesis, vascular modeling, coagulation regulation
Growth factors	PDGF, TGF- 1 and 2, EGF, IGF-1, VEGF, bFGF, HGF, BMP-2, 4, 6, CTGF	Chemotaxis, cell proliferation and differentiation, angiogenesis
Chemokines, cytokines, and others	IL8, FasL, endostatins, osteonectin, bone sialoprotein	Regulation of angiogenesis, vascular modeling, cell interactions, bone formation
Antimicrobial proteins	Thrombocidins	Bactericidal and fungicidal properties
Membrane glycoproteins	Most of the components of the plasma membrane	Platelet aggregation and adhesion, protein endocytosis, inflammation, thrombin generation, platelet-leukocyte interactions
Others	Chondroitin 4 sulfate, albumin, immunoglobulins, semaphoring	Promote angiogenesis, cartilage regeneration, fibrin production, and platelet adhesion

PDGF, platelet-derived growth factor; TGF-1, transforming growth factor 1; EGF, epidermal growth factor; IGF-1, insulin-like growth factor-1; VGEF, vascular endothelial growth factor; bFGF, basic fibroblast growth factor; HGF, hepatocyte growth factor; CTGF, connective tissue growth factor.

the timeline for the introduction of PRP in different medical indications.[10]

BIOLOGY OF PLATELET-RICH PLASMA

Platelet-rich plasma represents a complex mixture of GFs, cytokines, and chemokines. Classification and functions of bioactive molecules present in PRP is listed in table 1.[9]

Various GFs including PDGF, transforming growth factor (TGF), vascular endothelial growth factor (VEGF), and insulin-like growth factor (IGF), are secreted from the α-granules of concentrated platelets activated by aggregation inducers. These factors are known to regulate processes including cell migration, attachment, proliferation and differentiation, and promote extracellular matrix (ECM) accumulation by binding to specific cell surface

TABLE 2: Various growth factors and their biological role

PDGF	Biological role
αα	Chemotactic for fibroblasts and macrophages
αβ, ββ	Mitogenic for fibroblasts, muscles, endothelial
TGF-β1	Mediate, angiogenesis
TGF-β2	Mitogenic for fibroblasts, smooth muscles Regulate matrix protiens
VGEF	Chemotactic and mitogenic for endothelial cells. Mediates angeogenesis
EGF	Mediates angeogenesis. Mitotic for fibroblasts, keratinocyte, endothel
HGF	Mediates regeneration
FGF2	Mediates tissue organization and regeneration
FGF-9	Mediates follicular generation

PDGF, platelet-derived growth factor; VGEF, vascular endothelial growth factor; EGF, epidermal growth factor; HGF, hepatocyte growth factor; FGF-2, fibroblast growth factor 2; FGF-9, fibroblast growth factor 9; TGF-β1, transforming growth factor beta 1.

receptors.[5] Various GFs present in PRP and their biological role are enumerated in table 2.

The proteins that act to promote cell adhesion (fibrin, fibronectin, and vitronectin) are another essential component of PRP. These provide the structural support necessary for cell migration and for proliferation and 3-dimensional growth of tissues over these structures. Therefore, PRP has effects not only directly related to the target cells for the various GFs but also has a broader effect as an ECM for the stimulation and repair and/or regeneration of the tissue.[8,9,11]

Degranulation of the prepackaged GFs in platelets occurs upon *activation*, i.e., on coming in contact with coagulation triggers. The active proteins are then secreted, binding to transmembrane receptors of target cells, which include mesenchymal stem cells, osteoblasts, fibroblasts, endothelial cells, and epidermal cells.[11] These agonists bound transmembrane receptors then activate an intracellular signal protein that causes the expression of a gene sequence that directs cellular proliferation, matrix formation, osteoid production, collagen synthesis etc. thus provoking tissue repair and tissue regeneration.[12]

The platelet-rich plasma can be activated with different agents like 10% calcium chloride and thrombin. The active secretion of these GFs by platelets begins within 10 minutes after activation, with more than 95% of the presynthesized GFs secreted within 1 hour.[13]

Recent works prove that activation with an external agent is not really necessary. Most commercial PRP kits do not activate PRP. Some replace calcium that was bound by anticoagulant citrate dextrose (ACD) to create a more physiological state. Employing inactivated PRP may result in a more normal physiologic activation by the injected tissue. Collagen is a natural activator of PRP, thus when PRP is used in soft tissue, it does not need to be exogenously activated.

CLASSIFICATION OF PLATELET-RICH PLASMA

The development of a wide range of preparation protocols, devices, and centrifuges for varying indications have led to a number of different platelet concentrates, unfortunately all under the same name as PRP. Dohan Ehrenfest et al. have proposed a classification of platelet concentrates into four categories depending upon their leucocyte and fibrin content as follows. This classification system was largely cited, advocated, and validated by a multidisciplinary consensus conference published in 2012.[14]

Pure platelet-rich plasma (PPRP) or leucocyte poor PRP products are preparations without leucocytes and with a low density fibrin network after activation.

Leucocyte and platelet-rich plasma (LPRP) products are preparations with leucocytes and with a low density fibrin network after activation. It is in this family that the largest number of commercial or experimental systems exists. Particularly, many automated protocols have been developed in the last years, requiring the use of specific kits that allow minimum handling of the blood samples and maximum standardization of the preparations; e.g., Plateltex (Bratislava) and RegenACRR kit (Regen Laboratory). These protocols employ gelifying agents or a separator gel within the centrifugation kit to enhance the complete collection of the buffy coat layer.

Pure platelet-rich fibrin (PPRF) or leucocyte poor platelet-rich fibrin preparations are without leucocytes and with a high density fibrin network. These products only exist in a strongly activated gel form, and cannot be injected or used like traditional fibrin glues; e.g., Fibrinet PRFM kit (Cascade).

Leucocyte and platelet-rich fibrin (LPRF) or second generation PRP products are preparations with leucocytes and with a high density fibrin network. Venous blood is collected in glass tube and centrifuged without anticoagulant. Fibrin polymerized clot that is rich in platelets and leukocytes finally obtained; e.g., Choukroun's PRF.

METHODOLOGY

Manual Double Spin Method

Platelet-rich plasma is separated from whole blood by "light-spin" centrifugation and subsequently the platelets are concentrated by "heavy-spin" centrifugation with removal of the supernatant plasma. Figure 2 shows different fractions obtained after centrifugation of anticoagulated blood.

The first spin step is performed at constant acceleration to separate RBCs from the remaining whole blood volume. After the first spin step, the whole blood separates into three layers: an upper layer that contains mostly platelets and WBC, an intermediate thin layer that is known as the buffy coat and that is rich in WBCs, and a bottom layer that consists mostly of RBCs (Fig. 2). For the production of pure PRP (PPRP), upper layer and superficial buffy coat are transferred to an empty sterile tube. The second spin step is then performed. "g" for second spin should be just adequate to aid in formation of soft pellets (erythrocyte-platelet) at the bottom of the tube. The upper portion of the volume that is composed mostly of platelet poor plasma (PPP) is removed.

The final platelet concentration depends on the volume reduction of PPP. Approximately 3/4 of the supernatant is discarded and the platelet-rich pellet is resuspended in remaining amount of plasma. Figure 3 explains the step by step procedure of double spin method.

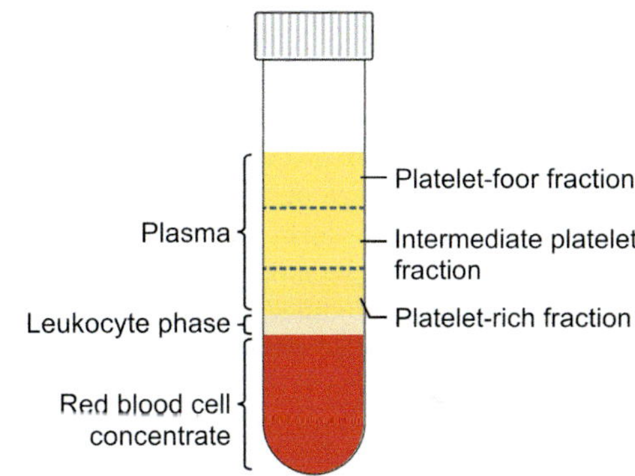

FIG. 2: Different fractions obtained after centrifugation of anticoagulated blood.

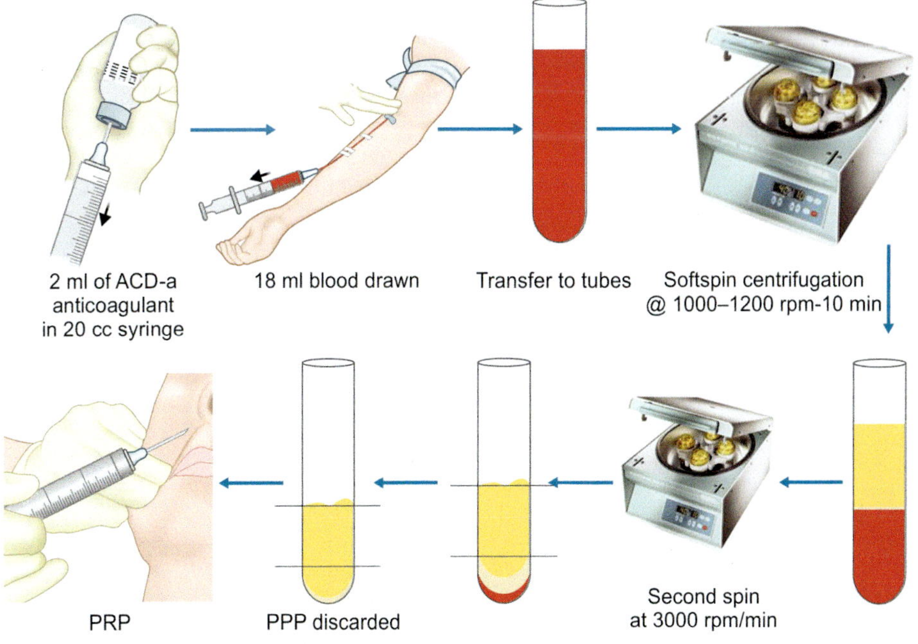

PRP, platelet-rich plasma; PPP, platelet poor plasma; ACD, anticoagulant citrate dextrose.

FIG. 3: Step-by-step procedure of double spin method.

The platelet yield depends mainly on conditional parameters like size and shape of the container used, rate and time of spin, and anticoagulant used. There has been a gross lack of comparative studies to standardize the PRP procedural parameters. The viability of the platelets is assured by carrying out the process in a refrigerated centrifuge at 20°C. Box 1 enumerates the prerequisites for obtaining optimal PRP.

Modified Syringe Method

Excellent yield of PRP can be achieved by using a new unique, cost effective double syringe method (Fig. 4). Author finds this method as one of the most effective "closed system" method and chance of contamination is very minimal. The method consists in a simple modification of a disposable 5 mL syringe that allows insertion into a common centrifuge and positioning of the syringe on the centrifuge so the PRP separates next to the tip of the syringe. Fukaya et al. proposed a double spin method using disposable syringes.[15] We have modified the technique to a single spin method to yield similar quality PRP.

BOX 1 Prerequisites for obtaining optimal platelet-rich plasma

- Informed consent
- Free of antiplatelet drugs like aspirin or other NSAIDs for at least two weeks prior to the procedure
- Avoid heavy fatty meal immediately before procedure
- The process must be carried out under strict aseptic conditions. Use sterile tubes, pipettes, syringes, reagents, vacutainers
- Optimum temperature regulations, i.e., 20–24°C. - Cold centrifugation

NSAIDs, nonsteroidal anti-inflammatory drugs.

The quality and yield of PRP is comparable with automated gel based systems. Figure 3 shows the platelet counts in whole blood and the modified syringe method prepared PRP. The platelet count has increased from 2.66 to 13.13 lakhs/µL.

Procedure

Eighteen milliliter of whole blood was collected from the patient. Four disposable 5 mL twice a day syringes were taken. The finger holders of the syringes were cut using scissors so as to insert the syringe into the centrifuge. Each tube had 0.5 mL of acid citrate dextrose anticoagulant to which 4.5 mL of blood was added. The syringes were closed using sterile stoppers and centrifuged at 3,100 rpm for 15 minutes.

Each syringe was then connected to a 3-way cock and PPP was aspirated and discarded. The plasma along with buffy coat was transferred in the similar way using the same 3-way cock to 1 mL syringes. This was mixed well and then injected (Figs 5–8). The advantages of modified syringe method are listed in box 2. The absolute and relative contraindications for PRP treatment are listed in box 3.

AUTOMATED DEVICES

There are many PRP systems commercially marketed, which facilitate the preparation of ready to apply platelet-rich suspensions in a reproducible manner. These systems differ widely in their ability to collect and concentrate platelets depending on the method and time of its centrifugation. Although time saving, these adapted kits can be quite expensive compared to the manual process. Most of the devices are based on gel separation technique (Fig. 9).

Platelet-rich plasma devices can be usually divided into lower and higher concentration

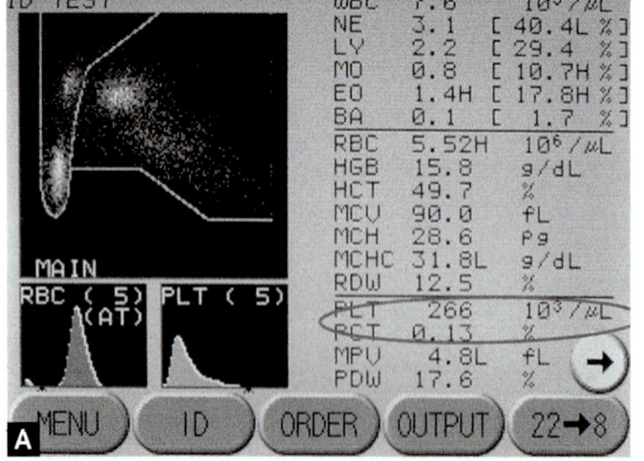

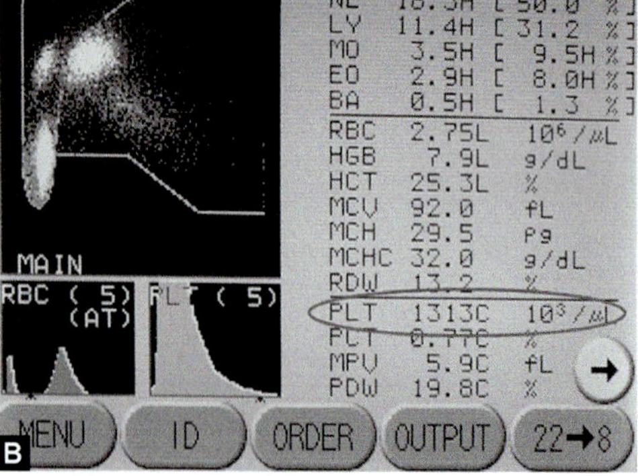

FIG. 4: Platelet counts in **A**, whole blood and **B**, the modified syringe method prepared platelet-rich plasma.

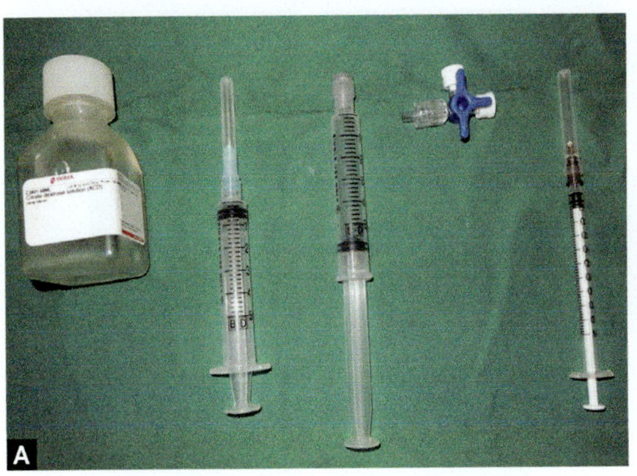

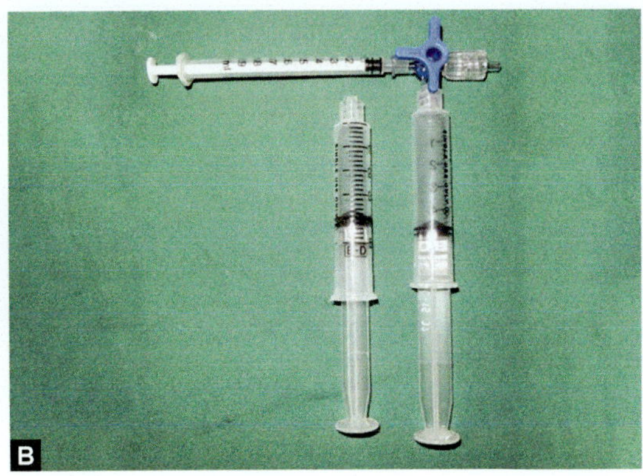

FIG. 5: A, Syringes, three-way cock, sterile stoppers, anticoagulant anticoagulant citrate dextrose used in modified syringe technique. **B,** Syringes connected using three ways.

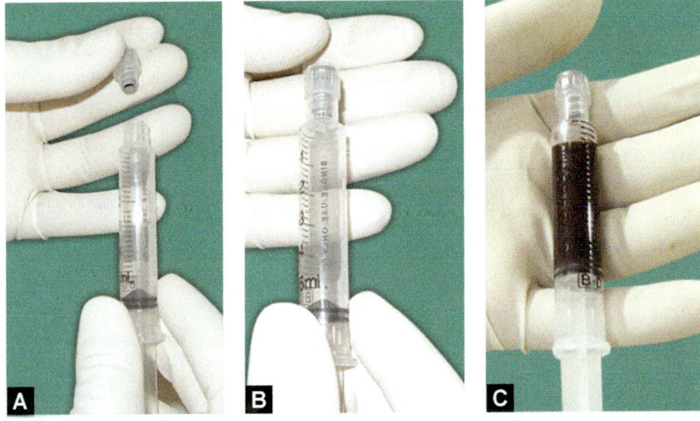

FIG. 6: 5 cc syringe with stopper ready for centrifugation.

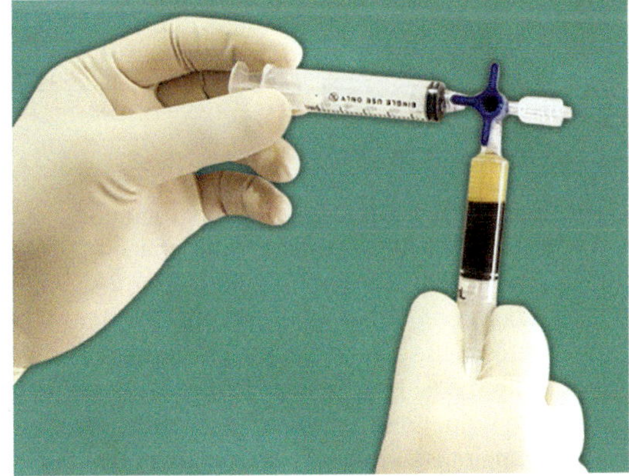

FIG. 7: Empty syringe connected via three ways to transfer the plasma.

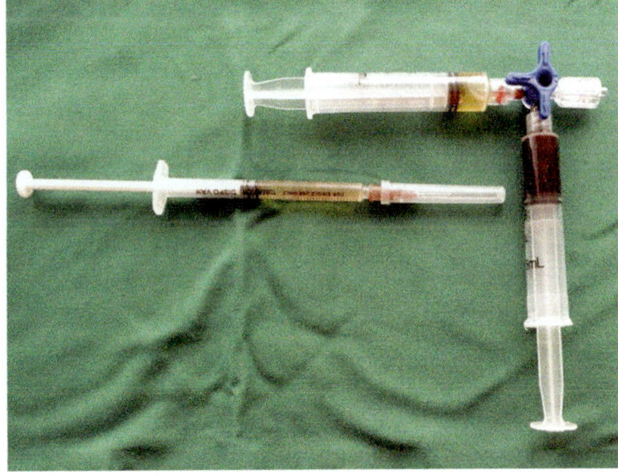

FIG. 8: Platelet-rich plasma collected. Please note that red blood cells are still in the first syringe and not contaminating the plasma.

systems. The approved high yielding devices include Biomet GPS II and III (platelet count 38×); Harvest SmartPReP 2 APC + (46×); and ArterioCyteMedtronic Magellan (37×). The lower concentration systems

BOX 2 Platelet-rich plasma—contraindications

Absolute contraindications:
- Platelet dysfunction syndrome
- Critical thrombocytopenia
- Hemodynamic instability
- Septicemia
- Local infection at the site of the procedure
- Patient unwilling to accept risks

Relative contraindications:
- Consistent use of NSAIDs within 48 hours of procedure
- Corticosteroid injection at treatment site within 1 month
- Systemic use of coriticosteroids within 2 weeks
- Tobacco use
- Recent fever or illness
- Cancer- especially hematopoetic or of bone
- Hemoglobin <10 g/dL
- Platelet count <105/μL

BOX 3 Advantages of modified syringe method
- Closed method.
- Chances of contamination – minimal
- Pure PRP with out RBC's.
- Yield of Platelets high.
- Easy to perform.

PRP, platelet-rich plasma; RBCs, red blood cells.

include Arthrex ACP, Cascade PPR therapy, and PRGF (Biotech Institute Vitoria) and Regen PRP (Regen Laboratory).[13]

MODIFICATIONS OF PLATELET-RICH PLASMA

Takikawa et al.[16] investigated a low-molecular weight heparin as a carrier for PRP. Dalteparin/protamine (DP), in water soluble microparticles, acts as a biomaterial to adsorb, stabilize, and gradually release the GFs in PRP, as almost all of them are known to be heparin binding. Results showed that DP in PRP could further improve the hair thickness compared to PRP alone without any side effects, although effect of DP alone was not assessed as control.

Automated PRP kits containing hyaluronic acid are used in skin rejuvenation and volume loss. Regen Cellular Matrix (Regen Laboratory) is one of the available devices (Fig. 10).

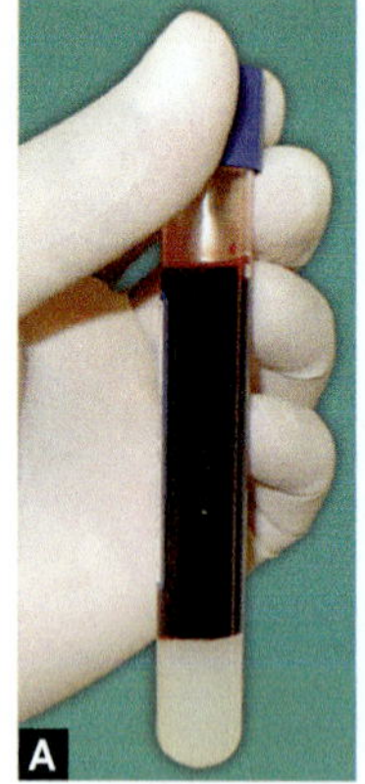

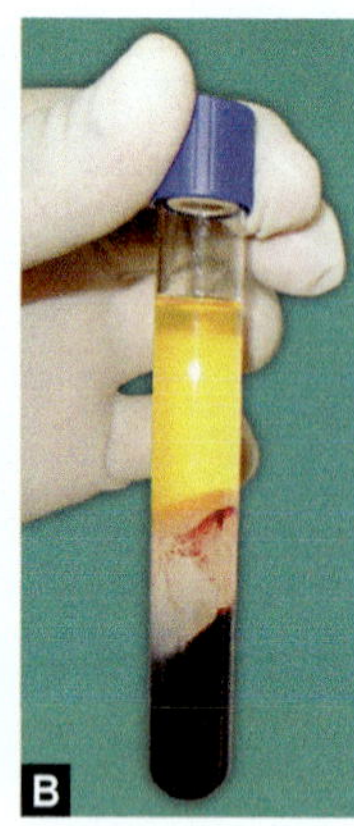

FIG. 9: Automated kit with gel separation before and after centrifugation.

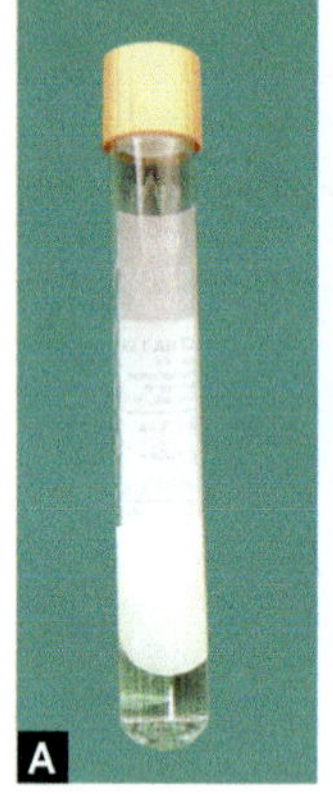

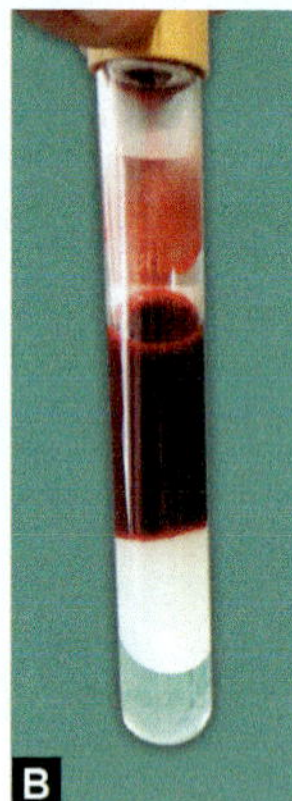

FIG. 10: Platelet-rich plasma kits containing hyaluronic acid.

AESTHETIC DERMATOLOGIC INDICATIONS

Hair Thinning and Androgenetic Alopecia

The hair follicle cycle is responsible for regulating hair growth. Hair follicles transition from anagen (active phase) to catagen (involution due to apoptosis) and subsequently enter in telogen (rest phase). Many GFs participate in the regulation of the follicular cycle, controlling the active phase and promoting catagen or telogen induction.[17]

The angiogenic role of PRP has recently caught the attention of dermatologists and plastic surgeons, to explore its usefulness as a hair growth modality. The role of PRP in promoting hair survival and growth has been demonstrated both *in vitro* and *in vivo*. Published data on PRP in androgenetic alopecia is given in table 3.

TABLE 3: Published data on platelet-rich plasma in androgenetic alopecia

Reference No.	Mode of platelet-rich plasma used	Control group	Split side study	Outcome	Subjects
16	Injections of PRP or PRP/ dalteparin and protamine microparticles	Yes: Saline	Yes	Both treatments increased mean number of hairs and thickened epithelium	26
18	PRP injections onto half of scalp	Yes: Saline	Yes	Increased mean growth rate of hair	1
19	PRP containing CD34+ cells	Yes: Placental extract	No	Improved clinical presentation, hair thickness, and number of hairs	26
20	PRP injections	No	No	Improved pull test results and improved hair volume and quality	42

PRP, platelet-rich plasma.

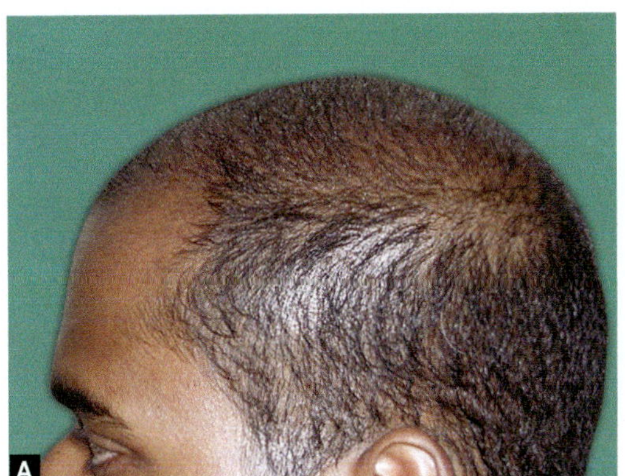

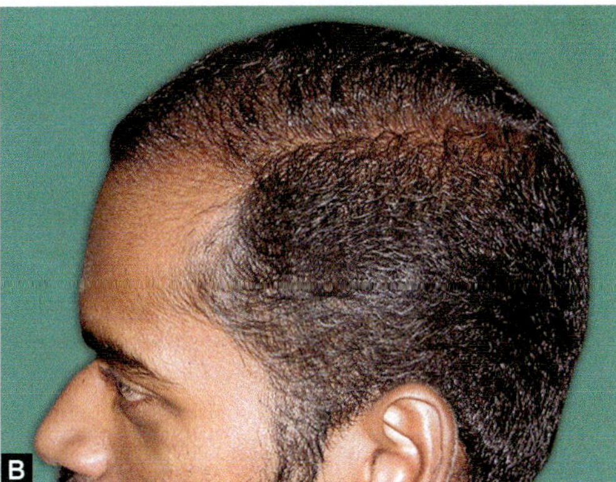

FIG. 11: Three sessions of platelet-rich plasma at monthly interval. **A**, Before and **B**, after in androgenetic alopecia.

Although the specific mechanism of action of PRP on the hair follicle is still unknown, Li et al.[3] found increased secretion of follicular GF 7 and β-catenin, with the subsequent proliferation of cells of the hair papilla and activation of the extracellular kinase- and Akt-dependent signaling pathways.

One study showed how it is possible to stimulate growth and increase hair density if the follicles are embedded in PRP prior to grafting.[18-21] In a pilot study, Kang et al. suggested that the potential benefits of interfollicular injection of a PRP preparation with CD34+ cells in the treatment of female- and male-pattern alopecia were due to their angiogenic action.[19]

Hence, PRP has a significant role in the management of patterned hair loss. Figure 11 shows the result of PRP in androgenetic hair loss.

Alopecia Areata

Platelet-rich plasma is found to be beneficial in the management of alopecia areata. Greco et al.[22] tried it in a single patient of alopecia areata as mesotherapy, with good subjective results at 10 months follow-up.

Another randomized, double-blind clinical trial has been conducted in which the benefit of PRP application was assessed in 45 patients with alopecia areata. On comparing triamcinolone acetonide with placebo, a significant increase in repopulation was found along with a decrease in hair dystrophy and less pruritus and itching.[23] In addition to stimulating cell proliferation, with an increase in Ki-67 in treated areas, the known anti-inflammatory action of PRP could help explain the good outcomes obtained in alopecia areata.

SKIN REJUVENATION AND DERMAL AUGMENTATION

Skin aging leads to decreased vascularization, limited replenishment of cells, and the intercellular matrix, skin appendage disorders, fat atrophy, and loss of

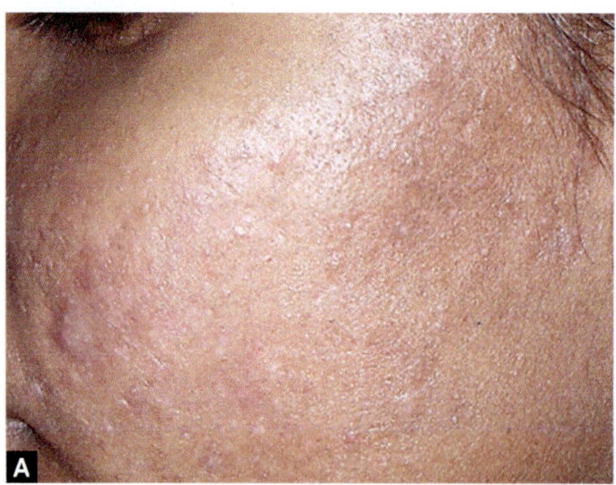

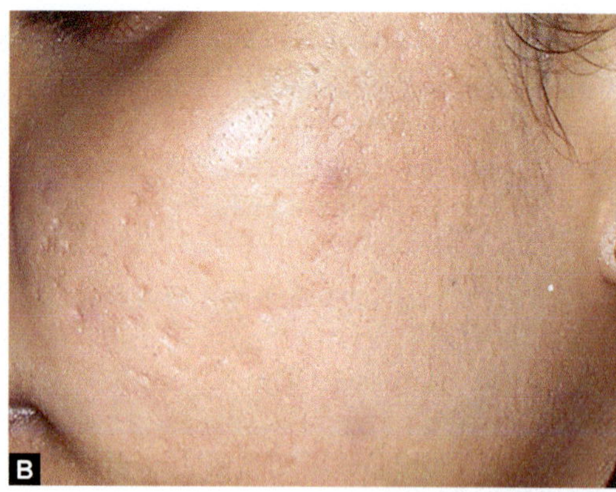

FIG. 12: Platelet-rich plasma with hyaluronic acid (Cellular Matrix); **A,** before and **B,** after 2 months

muscle tone. The few studies that have assessed the clinical benefit of PRP in skin aging used largely subjective outcome measures.[24]

In vivo studies have shown PRP exercises a bioregenerating action through stimulation of fibroblast proliferation, with an increase in anti-inflammatory factors (HGF), angiogenic factors vascular endothelial growth factor (VEGF), and proteins related to ECM remodeling such as procollagen I, hyaluronic acid, and tissue inhibitor of metallopeptidase 1.[25,26]

A uncontrolled study of 23 patients receiving three consecutive monthly facial intradermal PRP injections[24] reported a qualitative improvement in appearance. Another study employed PRP injections in the context of microneedling, reporting a difference in skin firmness as rated by dermatologists; however, it is not possible to distinguish this from the effect of the dermaroller used in isolation.

A split-faced study on the effects of three PRP injections over the course of 12 weeks improved infraorbital wrinkles and skin tone in Asian subjects. Platelet-rich plasma treatment significantly improved both wrinkles and skin tone in infraorbital skin.[27]

We have found PRP along with hyaluronic acid providing excellent results in skin rejuvenation (Fig. 12).

SCARS

Scar tissue represents the replacement of the normal dermal architecture with dense collagen bundles; this may lead to significant cosmetic or functional impairment. Some studies suggest a beneficial role for PRP as an adjuvant for scar treatment techniques. Its use is becoming more commonplace after chemical or physical exfoliation or after laser resurfacing.

In a randomized, nonblinded study, 60 patients with unsightly scars were divided into three groups which were treated with either laser resurfacing, PRP and autologous fat grafting or all three modalities in combination. Results were evaluated by an independent physician at 6 months after treatment according to the Manchester Scar Scale. An improvement was reported in 18% of patients treated with fat grafting and PRP, in 30% treated with 1,540 nm nonablative laser alone and in 45% when all three modalities were employed in combination.[28]

Another noncontrolled study of 64 patients evaluated PRP in combination with fat grafting and fractionated carbon dioxide laser.[29] Patient satisfaction was reported at 6 months; however, there was no independent evaluation of scar appearance.

One study showed how the technique was able to reduce erythema and accelerate healing in patients treated with ablative fractional carbon dioxide laser.[30]

Our personal experience in combining PRP with fractional laser resurfacing and microneedling radiofrequency treatment in acne scars and aging skin is highly encouraging results in a short time (Figs. 13 and 14). Platelet-rich plasma also reduces the downtime of the primary procedure as the healing is accelerated.

LIPOSCULPTING

Another application of PRP is liposculpting, where it is used for optimizing free fatty acid grafts for subsequent infiltration. *In vitro* studies have shown a significant increase in the number of adipocytes. Clinical studies have shown that PRP can prolong the duration of the restorative environment compared to fatty infiltrations by themselves.[31]

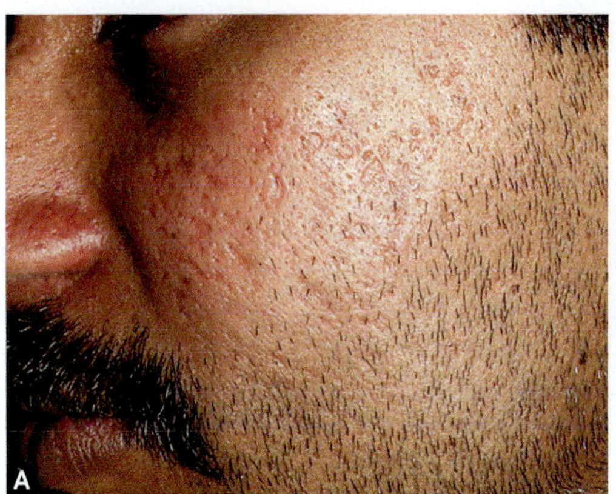
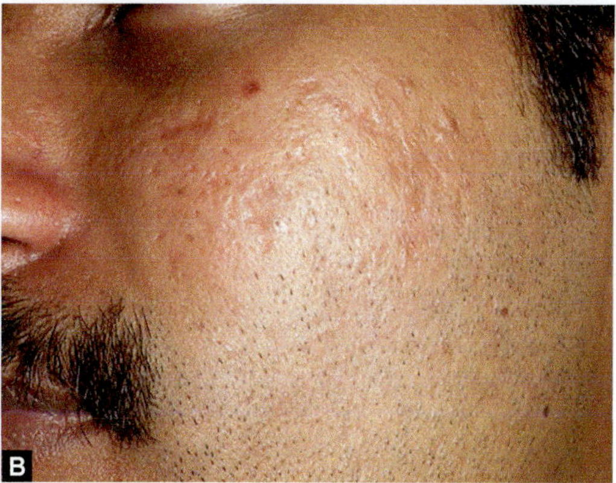

FIG. 13: Platelet-rich plasma and microneedling radiofrequency treatment: **A,** before and **B,** after 6 months

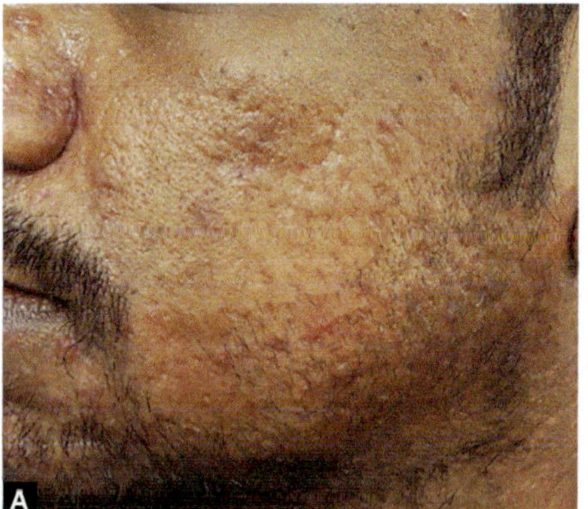
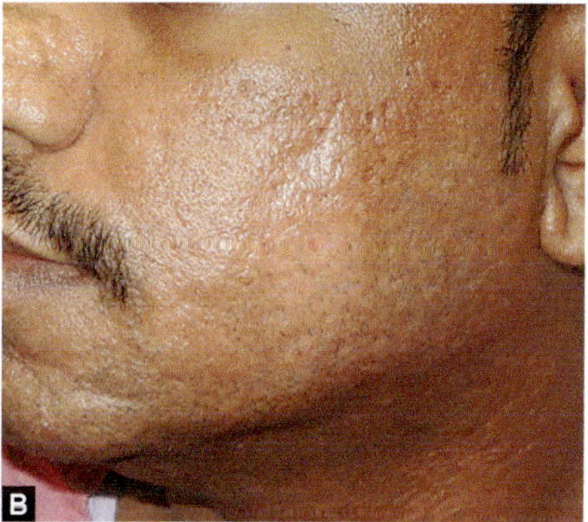

FIG. 14: Platelet-rich plasma and fractional carbon dioxide laser treatment: **A,** Before and **B,** after 3 months. Note the significant dilution of pigmentation and roughness

Fat grafts when mixed with PRP resulted in greater vascularity, fewer cysts and vacuoles, less fibrosis, and overall improved survival and quality of fat grafts compared to saline.[32] This was found to maintain fat graft survival in a patient with facial contour defect for up to 2 years.

STRIAE DISTENSAE

Striae distensae are dermal scars with epidermal atrophy found in skin subjected to continuous stretching. This is a very common presentation in cosmetic dermatologic clinics. There are few promising studies on PRP in the management of striae distensae.

A combination therapy of intradermal radiofrequency and PRP was administered to patients with striae distensae once every 4 weeks. After 12 weeks of treatment, 100% of the 19 patients showed at least mild improvement (0–25% improvement). Overall, 5.3% achieved excellent improvement, 36.8% achieved marked improvement, 31.6% achieved moderate improvement, and 26.3% achieved mild improvement.[33]

In another study on ultrasound-assisted topical PRP therapy has been used to treat striae distensae after plasma fractional radiofrequency therapy.[34] Platelet-rich plasma was applied with ultrasound assistance to enhance transepidermal drug delivery every 2 weeks for 8 weeks. The average width of the widest striae reduced in size from 0.75 to 0.27 mm. In total, 71.9% of the patients reported good or very good improvements in their striae distensae as well.[36] Furthermore, post-treatment abdominal biopsies showed increased collagen density and elastic fibers in the dermis.[35]

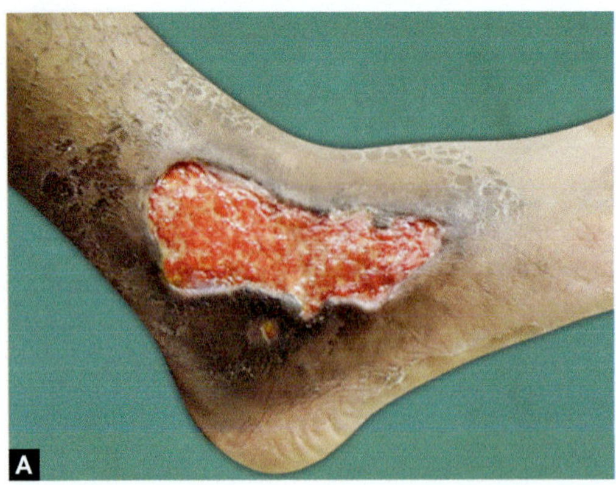

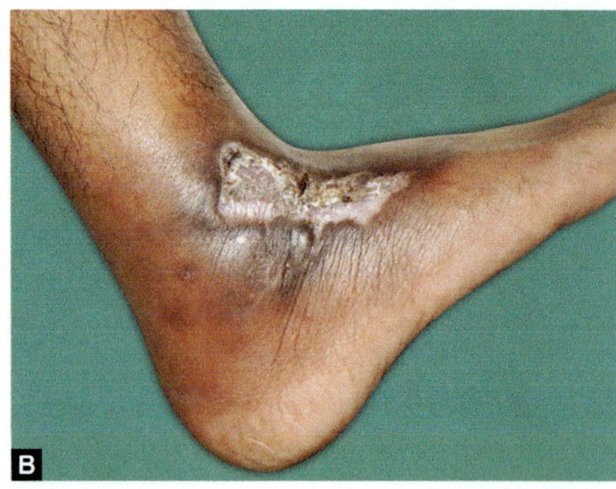

FIG. 15: Platelet-rich plasma in ulcer: ulcer: **A,** before and **B,** after three injections.

LIPODERMATOSCLEROSIS

Lipodermatosclerosis, also known as sclerosing panniculitis, is a chronic, painful process affecting the lower legs and believed to be caused by venous insufficiency. It is characterized by skin induration, erythema, edema, and hyperpigmentation giving an inverted champagne bottle appearance.

In an isolated case report, refractory lipodermatosclerosis was treated with intralesional subcutaneous injections of PRP in five sessions at 2 weeks interval that led to complete reepithelialization of venous ulcer and marked improvement in hyperpigmentation and induration at the treated site (Fig. 15).[36]

PLATELET-RICH PLASMA IN OTHER APPLICATIONS

With the proven activity of PRP in promoting tissue regeneration, various other applications have been proposed.

The activity of PRP as a biological glue is the rationale for using it to improve the viability of skin flaps in recipient tissue beds. It is used in plastic surgery and dermatological surgery in processes that require the use of flaps to accelerate healing, improve sealing by eliminating dead space, decrease bleeding and the need for drainage and compression dressing, and reduce edema and postoperative pain.[37]

It also helps in faster healing and reduction of downtime associated with various ablative laser procedures.

Platelet-rich plasma has shown promising results in chronic ulcers. It is used as topical spray or as perilesional injections. Kim et al.[38] treated 16 patients affected by various acute and chronic ulcers including stasis ulcers, diabetic ulcers, livedoid vasculitis, claw foot and traumatic ulcers with PRP. Topical application of PRP significantly accelerated the re-epithelialization process, shown to be through the upregulation of cell cycle regulatory proteins like cyclin A and CDK4.

Nicoli et al.[39] reported a case of hidradenitis suppurativa resistant to multiple treatments with good response to the combination of surgery, PRP, and Hyalomatrix, a system that releases hyaluronic acid.

Multilayer PRP injections used along with autologous fat transfer have found to improve lichen sclerosus of vulva.[40]

Practical tips while preparing PRP are listed in boxes 3 and 4.

COMPLICATIONS OF PLATELET-RICH PLASMA

Being an autologous preparation, PRP is devoid of any serious adverse effects, apart from local injection

BOX 4 Practical tips

- To avoid unintentional activation of platelets, most protocols use large bore needles (>22) to draw the blood and re-inject PRP.
- Cold centrifugation prevents unintentional degranulation.
- There are different centrifuge protocols with different spin speeds and times. The optimal regimen to prevent unintentional activation is unclear.
- Collagen is a natural activator of PRP, thus when PRP is used in soft tissue, it does not need to be exogenously activated.

PRP, platelet-rich plasma.

site reactions like pain or secondary infection, which can be avoided with proper precautions.

Platelet-rich plasma does not induce any mitogenic activities. It is limited to augmentation of the normal healing process and is theoretically not mutagenic, as the GFs released do not enter the cell or its nucleus, but only bind to the membrane receptors and induce signal transduction mechanisms.

CONCLUSION

Platelet-rich plasma has been shown to be potentially beneficial as a bioregenerator in many applications in different fields of medicine, including aesthetic dermatology. It has found to be effective and acts synergistic to other treatment modalities when combined. Most studies have evaluated the potential utility of PRP in combination therapies with other modalities such as lasers, radiofrequency, and autologous fat grafting.

In summary, platelet-rich plasma therapies are in general well tolerated with few complications and further evaluation is justified in the context of organized trials. The potential role of PRP in dermatology and aesthetic medicine is an exciting frontier that may eventually lead to superior therapies in the near future. More clinical studies are needed to support the efficacy of this safe and simple technique with multiple potential benefits and help establish it as a routine treatment with well-defined indications in cosmetic dermatology.

REFERENCES

1. Schiavone G, Raskovic D, Greco J, et al. Platelet-rich plasma for androgenetic alopecia: A pilot study. Dermatol Surg. 2014;40:1010-9.
2. Rogers N. Commentary on autologous platelet-rich plasma: A potential therapeutic tool for promoting hair growth. Dermatol Surg. 2012;38:1047-8.
3. Li ZJ, Choi HI, Choi DK, et al. Autologous platelet-rich plasma: A potential therapeutic tool for promoting hair growth. Dermatol Surg. 2012;38:1040-6.
4. Lynch MD, Bashir S. Applications of platelet-rich plasma in dermatology: a critical appraisal of the literature. J Dermatol Treat. 2016;27(3):285-9.
5. Wroblewski AP, Melia HJ, Wright VJ. Application of platelet-rich plasma to enhance tissue repair. Oper Tech Orthop. 2010;20:98-105.
6. Arshdeep, Kumaran M S. Platelet-rich plasma in dermatology: boon or a bane? Indian J Dermatol Venereol Leprol. 2014;80:5-14.
7. Pierce GF, Mustoe TA, Altrock BW, et al. Role of platelet-derived growth factor in wound healing. J Cell Biochem. 1991;45:319-26.
8. Knighton DR, Ciresi KF, Fiegel VD, et al. Successful treatment with autologous platelet-derived wound healing factors (PDWHF). Ann Surg. 1986;204:322-30.
9. Anitua E. Plasma rich in growth factors: preliminary results of use in the preparation of future sites for implants. Int J Oral Maxillofac Implants. 1999;14:529-35.
10. Sánchez M, Andia I, Anitua E, et al. Platelet-rich plasma (PRP). Biotechnology: concepts and therapeutic applications in orthopedics and sports medicine. In: Agbo EC (Ed). Innovations in Biotechnology. Rijeka, Croatia: In Tech; 2012. pp. 113-38.
11. Marx RE. Platelet-rich plasma (PRP): what is PRP and what is not PRP? Implant Dent. 2001;10:225-8.
12. Marx RE, Carlson ER, Eichstaedt RM, et al. Platelet-rich plasma: growth factor enhancement for bone grafts. Oral Surg Oral Med Oral Pathol Oral Radiol Endod. 1998;85:63846.
13. Dhurat R, Sukesh M. Principles and methods of preparation of platelet-rich plasma: A review and author's perspective. J Cutan Aesthet Surg. 2014;7:189.
14. Dohan Ehrenfest DM, Rasmusson L, Albrektsson T. Classification of platelet concentrates: from pure platelet-rich plasma (P-PRP) to leucocyte- and platelet-rich fibrin (L-PRF). Trends Biotechnol. 2009;27:158-67.
15. Fukaya M, Ito A. A new economic method for preparing platelet-rich plasma. Plast Reconstr Surg Glob Open. 2014;2(6):e162.
16. Takikawa M, Nakamura S, Nakamura S, et al. Enhanced effect of platelet-rich plasma containing a new carrier on hair growth. Dermatol Surg. 2011;37:1721-9.
17. Price VH. Treatment of hair loss. N Engl J Med. 1999;341:964-73.
18. Park KY, Kim HK, Kim BJ, et al. Letter: platelet-rich plasma for treating male pattern baldness. Dermatol Surg. 2012;38:2042-4.
19. Kang JS, Zheng Z, Choi MJ, et al. The effect of CD34+ cell containing autologous platelet-rich plasma injection on pattern hair loss: a preliminary study. J Eur Acad Dermatol Venereol. 2014;28:72-9.
20. Betsi EE, Germain E, Kalbermatten DF, et al. Platelet-rich plasma injection is effective and safe for the treatment of alopecia. Eur J Plast Surg. 2013;36:407-12.
21. Uebel CO, da Silva JB, Cantarelli D, et al. The role of platelet plasma growth factors in male pattern baldness surgery. Plast Reconstr Surg. 2006;118:1458-66.
22. Greco J, Brandt R. The effects of autologous platelet -rich plasma and various growth factors on non-transplanted miniaturized hair. Hair Transplant Forum Int. 2009;19:49-50.
23. Trink A, Sorbellini E, Bezzola P, et al. A randomized, double-blind, placebo and active controlled, half-head study to evaluate the effects of platelet-rich plasma on alopecia areata. Br J Dermatol. 2013;169:690-4.
24. Redaelli A, Romano D, Marcianó A. Face and neck revitalization with platelet-rich plasma (PRP): clinical outcome in a series of 23 consecutively treated patients. J Drugs Dermatol. 2010;9:466-72.
25. Kim DH, Je YJ, Kim CD, et al. Can platelet-rich plasma be used for skin rejuvenation? Evaluation of effects of

platelet-rich plasma on human dermal fibroblast. Ann Dermatol. 2011;23:424-31.

26. Park HB, Yang JH, Chung KH. Characterization of the cytokine profile of platelet-rich plasma (PRP) and PRP induced cell proliferation and migration: upregulation of matrix metalloproteinase-1 and-9 in HaCaT cells. Korean J Hematol. 2011;46:265-73.
27. Kang BK, Shin MK, Lee JH, et al. Effects of platelet-rich plasma on wrinkles and skin tone in Asian lower eyelid skin: preliminary results from a prospective, randomized, split-face trial. Eur J Dermatol. 2014;24:100-1.
28. Cervelli V, Nicoli F, Spallone D, et al. Treatment of traumatic scars using fat grafts mixed with platelet-rich plasma, and resurfacing of skin with the 1540 nm non-ablative laser. Clin Exp Dermatol. 2012;37:55-61.
29. Nita AC, Orzan OA, Filipescu M, et al. Fat graft, laser CO(2) and platelet-rich-plasma synergy in scars treatment. J Med Life. 2013;6:430-3.
30. Na JI, Choi JW, Choi HR, et al. Rapid healing and reduced erythema after ablative fractional carbon dioxide laser resurfacing combined with the application of autologous platelet-rich plasma. Dermatol Surg. 2011; 37:463-8.
31. Cervelli V, Gentile P, Scioli MG, et al. Application of platelet-rich plasma to fat grafting during plastic surgical procedures: Clinical and in vitro evaluation. Tissue Eng Part C Methods. 2009;15:625-34.
32. Oh DS, Cheon YW, Jeon YR, et al. Activated platelet-rich plasma improves fat graft survival in nude mice: A pilot study. Dermatol Surg. 2011;37:619-25.
33. Kim IS, Park KY, Kim BJ, et al. Efficacy of intradermal radiofrequency combined with autologous platelet-rich plasma in striae distensae: a pilot study. Int J Dermatol. 2012;51:1253-8.
34. Suh DH, Lee SJ, Lee JH, et al. Treatment of striae distensae combined enhanced penetration platelet-rich plasma and ultrasound after plasma fractional radiofrequency. J Cosmet Laser Ther. 2012;14(6):272-6.
34. Suh DH, Lee SJ, Lee JH, et al. Treatment of striae distensae combined enhanced penetration platelet-rich plasma and ultrasound after plasma fractional radiofrequency. J Cosmet Laser Ther. 2012;14:272-6.
35. Jeong KH, Shin MK, Kim NI. Refractory lipodermato-sclerosis treated with intralesional platelet-rich plasma. J Am Acad Dermatol. 2011;65:e157-8.
36. Findikcioglu F, Findikcioglu K, Yavuzer R, et al. Effect of preoperative subcutaneous platelet-rich plasma and fibrin glue application on skin flap survival. Aesthetic Plast Surg. 2012;36:1246-53.
37. Kim SA, Ryu HW, Lee KS, et al. Application of platelet-rich plasma accelerates the wound healing process in acute and chronic ulcers through rapid migration and up regulation of cyclin A and CDK4 in HaCaT cells. Mol Med Rep. 2013;7:476-80.
38. Nicoli F, Balzani A, Lazzeri D, et al. Severe hidradenitis suppurativa treatment using plateletrich plasma gel and Hyalomatrix. Int Wound J. 2013;12(3):338-43.
39. Casabona F, Priano V, Vallerino V, et al. New surgical approach to lichen sclerosus of the vulva: the role of adipose-derived mesenchymal cells and platelet-rich plasma in tissue regeneration. Plast Reconstr Surg. 2010;126:e210-1.

33 CHAPTER

Thread Lift

Madhuri Agarwal

INTRODUCTION

In the last decade, there is an explosive increase in the demand by patients for anti-aging treatments that are nonsurgical, high on safety, and results but have less downtime. Currently, physicians have a vast choice of technologies for treating skin concerns of aging and ill-defined contours such as botulinum toxin, soft tissue fillers, radiofrequency, and high-intensity focused ultrasound.

Thread lift is a procedure that is in demand with the advent of newer options of nonsurgical threads.

Thread lift provides an actual "lift," and is a semi-invasive procedure. It has a long-lasting effect and in a milder form matches the effect of brow lift or a lower face and neck lift.

HISTORY OF THREADS

In the late 1990, barbed suture thread was used by Russian surgeon Marlen Sulamanidze to lift and improve the sagging of face.[1] Since then many adaptations of this native suture, Aptos, have been tried by physicians. In these alternatives, the threads are placed along a planned course, then the threads are pulled, anchored appropriately, and the extra ends are snipped off at the entry point.[2]

Some aesthetic physicians view the procedure of thread lift with certain degree of suspicion. The Contour Threadlift system (Surgical Specialties Corporation) was approved by the Food and Drug Administration (FDA) in 2005. However, due to the high occurrence of postprocedure complications, it lost its FDA approval,[3] even though new cogged suture alternatives are currently available.[4] While reviewing the literature for threads, it is crucial to consider that even though initial data displayed inconsistent results and early relapse, with the development of new devices and the refinement of indications for each technique, the occurrence of complications has reduced subsequently in later studies.[5] Thread lifting performed correctly has minor complications and adverse effects.

TYPES OF THREADS

There are various options of threads available for thread lift procedure. The common material currently used in nonsurgical threads are polydioxanone (PDO), poly-L-lactic acid (PLLA), and polycaprolactone (PCA). The types of thread can be divided into four main categories as follows.[6]

Mode of Absorption

- Absorbable threads that are absorbed with time depending on the material used in threads, e.g., PDO thread,[6-9] silhouette soft thread (PLLA or sculptra in solid form)[6,10]
- Nonabsorbable thread including Aptos thread, contour thread, silhouette lift thread, Woffles thread (polypropylene), and gold thread.

Method of Thread Insertion

- Free-floating method refers to insertion of the thread into the skin without fixation
- Fixed method requires fixation of the thread to the tissue under the skin.

Barbed and Nonbarbed Thread (Smooth Threads)

- Barbed thread: There are three types of barbed thread:[6,11-13]
    - Bidirectional thread (long suture) are inserted into a hollow needle and then placed in

the treated area. Examples include the Aptos thread, Aptos 2 G (double needle), silhouette soft, and Woffles thread
    - Unidirectional barbed threads (long sutures) are designed to be anchored to a fixed structure, such as the deep temporal fascia. Examples include contour thread and silhouette lift thread
    - Cogged threads (short sutures): Examples include PDO unidirectional cogged thread, PDO bidirectional cogged thread, and PDO multidirectional cogged thread[6,14]
- Nonbarbed threads (smooth thread): There are two types of nonbarbed thread:
    - Monofilament plain: Examples include Miracu plain thread and TR lift thread[6,14]
    - Monofilament screw or spiral: Examples include K2 screw lifting and T screw lifting thread.

The value of bidirectional thread over unidirectional thread and nonbarbed thread is that bidirectional thread cannot move in either direction because of the two-way fixation provided by the barbs. However, if there is asymmetry of the face from the thread insertion, unidirectional threads or nonbarbed threads allow easier postoperative correction.[6,15,16]

Length of Threads

The threads are also classified based on its length, because different lengths are used for different lift techniques such as the short suture technique and long suture technique.[6]

- Short suture is defined by any thread shorter than 90 mm in length
- Long suture is defined by any thread longer than 90 mm in length.

MECHANISM OF ACTION

The procedure is also known as biorevitalization with threads. In thread lift procedure, a fine sterile biodegradable thread in inserted into the dermal layer of the skin to induce the formation of collagen (Flowchart 1).

Implantation of loose tissues caused by physical lifting and fixing by the thread

↓

First phase is inflammatory phase of platelet and neutrophil aggregation

↓

Then the second phase of proliferation and scaffolding for the tissue regeneration is triggered Fibroblast activity is stimulated on the surrounding parts of the thread leading to neocollagenesis

↓

This newly formed collagen will help by providing a lifting effect and reduce appearance of sag, double chin, nasolabial folds

FLOWCHART 1: Mechanism of action.

HISTOPATHOLOGICAL ANALYSIS

There are studies performed that have demonstrated histologically the actual changes in dermal structures after thread lift. In a study conducted by Savoia et al, the histological analysis was performed 2 and 6 months after the thread lift.[17] Two months after the procedure, observation with an optical microscope enabled the detection of a fragment of thread in the subcutaneous tissue to which a connective structure adhered. The latter was structured around a roughly ovoid-shaped cavity with a maximum diameter of around 0.3 mm (Fig. 1). The internal section of this structure, looking into the cavity, was made up of larger and rounder "fibroblastic" cells surrounding a "free floating" thread that appears dark following the histological preparations, but when fresh, was white.[17]

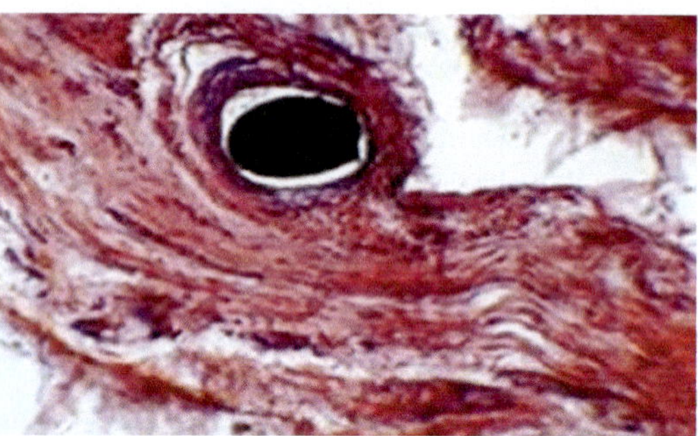

FIG. 1: Fragment of skin removed 2 months after the procedure from the right cheek containing a white microscopic filament (Happy Lift™ Revitalizing). (H&E, original magnification ×920).

Source: Savoia A, Accardo C, Vannini F, et al. Outcomes in thread lift for facial rejuvenation: A study performed with happy lift revitalizing. Dermatol Ther (Heidelb). 2014;4:103-14.

Indications

- Cheek enhancement
- Jawline lift
- Brow lift

- Nose augmentation
- Crow's feet and periorbital zone
- Forehead
- Cheeks
- Skin rejuvenation
- Neck lift
- Double chin reduction
- Hair rejuvenation
- Upper arm and chest tightening
- Abdominal tightening and reduction
- Cellulite
- Knee lift.

Patient Selection for Thread Lift

Ideal Candidates for Thread Lift

- People with initial signs of aging who need definition and contouring of face
- Women and men from mid-30–40s
- Patients with mild to moderate looseness of the jaw, start of sagging in mid-face, or slight bags under the eyes or on the neck.

Poor Candidates for Thread Lift

- Patients with excessive laxity of skin and are at an advanced age will show a very negligible improvement
- Patients who have very coarse, rugged skin, and are obese will not show any improvement.

Contraindications

Absolute Contraindications

- Pregnancy/lactation
- Oral steroids/immunosuppresants/anticoagulant therapy
- Autoimmune disorders, uncontrolled diabetes, active infection
- Keloidal tendencies
- Unrealistic expectations.

Relative Contraindications

- Herpes simplex or fever blisters
- Skin infection (bacterial/fungal/viral) on the face
- Multiple acne lesions
- Alpha-hydroxy acids/retinoids in last 2 weeks.

RESULT ORIENTATION FOR THREAD LIFT

- Benefit of the threads will be seen in the form of smoothening of the skin, decrease in the sagging of the skin
- Results can be appreciated after the first session immediately and improve over the next few months
- Threads can be combined with other treatments like botulinum toxin, dermal fillers, chemical peels, lasers, and other rejuvenation services
- Maintenance can be done once in 3 month or as and when required.

PREPROCEDURE PREPARATION

- Anesthesia: The anesthesia used is in cream form applied over the selected area. At times, a local tumescent anesthesia is delivered along the expected track of thread lift to ensure complete comfort of the patient
- A surgical asepsis is vital for thread lift to prevent any secondary infections. Clean the area thoroughly with alcohol and betadine after the requisite anesthesia is done
- The trolley for thread lift procedure must be prepared as shown in figure 2.

POSTPROCEDURE CARE

After treatment, slight edema or bruising may occur. There may also be some depression or some puckering of the skin. These transient effects will usually resolve few days after treatment. At times the thread end may pop out of the entrance to the skin. Trimming the protruding end can rectify this procedural issue.

An antibiotic cream is applied to the entry and exit points. Ice may be applied to reduce any bruising and anti-inflammatory tablets may be taken in case of pain for 2–3 days if necessary.

Postprocedure recommendations include the following:

- Keep the head elevated and sleep face up for the first 3–5 nights
- Avoid excessive facial movements while chewing, talking, and yawning for a week
- Wash and dry the face and apply make-up gently for 5 days
- Avoid sports, in particular contact sports, for 2–3 weeks
- Avoid facial massage and facial aesthetic treatments for 3 weeks
- Avoid dental surgery for 3 weeks.

Side Effects

- Bruises
- Edema

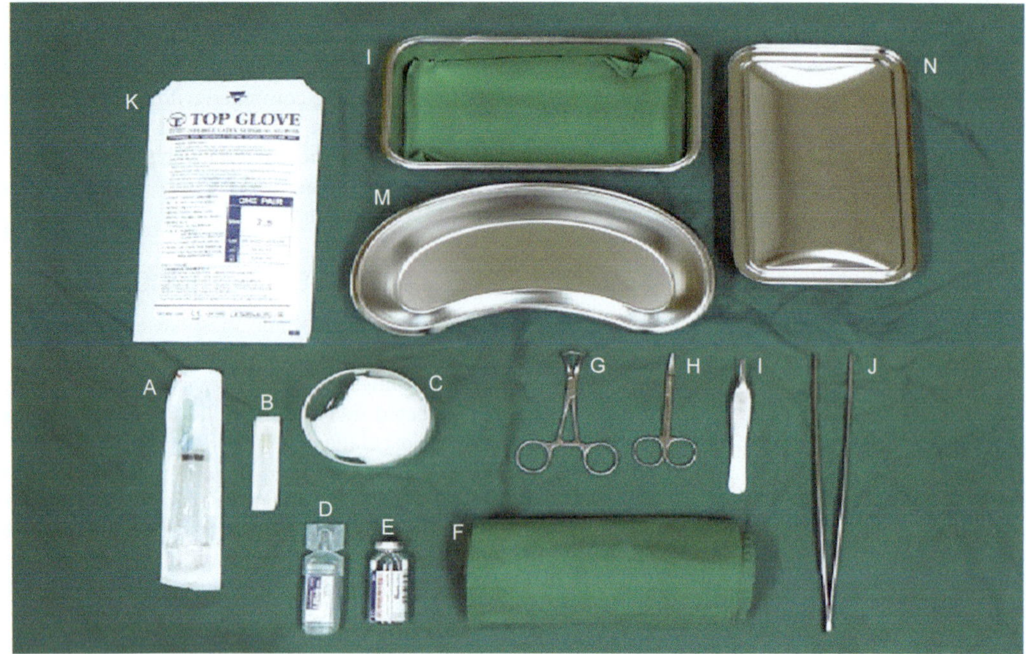

FIG. 2: An array of surgical instruments for thread lifting. **A,** 10 cc syringe; **B,** 25 G long needle (38 mm); **C,** alcohol swab; **D,** sodium chloride injection 20 mL; **E,** epineprin, lidocaine HCL hydrate 2% (20 mL); **F,** operation drape (60 cm × 60 cm); **G,** tower clip; **H,** Iris operating scissors; **I,** Iris forceps; **J,** dressing forceps; **K,** sterile latex surgical glove 6 half; **L,** dressing package tray; **M,** emesis basin; **N,** tray cover. Additional needs: Puncture needle 18 G, 27 G.

- Pain
- Sense of muscle contraction/skin pulling.

Adverse Effects from Improper Procedure

- No change
- Asymmetry
- Aggravation of problem (complication)
- Visible threads
- Dimpling result.

Thread lift procedural technique depends on the type of thread used. The procedure is described in detail below with respect to the popular threads currently in use.

Polydioxanone Threads

Polydioxanone threads are threads in use for some time with appreciable results. They take about 6 months to be absorbed, longer than both Vicryl and Dexon. Ruff proposed that PDO, a very gradually absorbed polymer, is adequate to lift intact tissue sufficiently with nominal concern about long-term side effects.[18]

The various parts of PDO thread is shown in figure 3. Polydioxanone threads used for facial rejuvenation can be classified into three different types:[19]

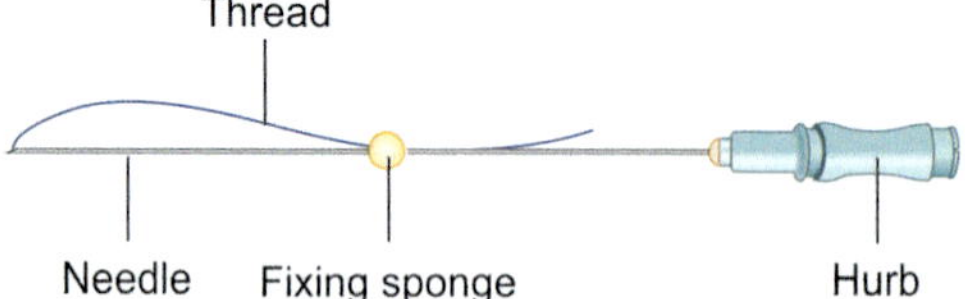

FIG. 3: The different parts of polydioxanone thread.

1. Mono PDO thread: Nonbarbed, monofilament, and thin (0.07–0.15 mm)
2. Spring or twin thread: It is made from a twined single monofilament or 2 braided monofilaments and is more tensile compared to mono-PDO thread
3. Cog PDO thread: It has barbs that, on insertion, adhere to tissues for the lifting effects. Cog PDO thread, depending on the direction of the spikes, is classified as unidirectional, bidirectional, or multidirectional (Fig. 4).

When inserted to a needle, the thread forms a V-shape with an inner half inserted in the caliber of the needle and the other half on the outside. Removal of the needle or cannula by itself results in the thread

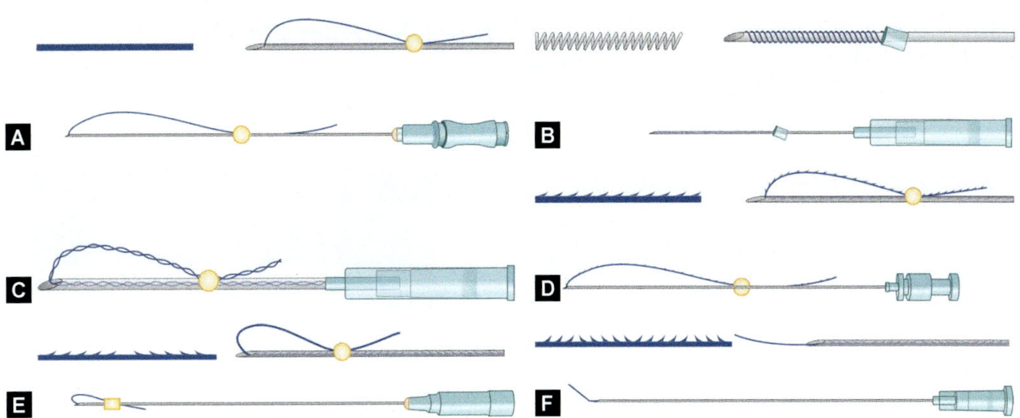

FIG. 4: Types of polydioxanone thread. **A,** Mono thread; **B,** spring thread; **C,** twin thread; **D,** unidirection cogged thread; **E,** bidirection cogged thread; and **F,** multidirection cogged thread.

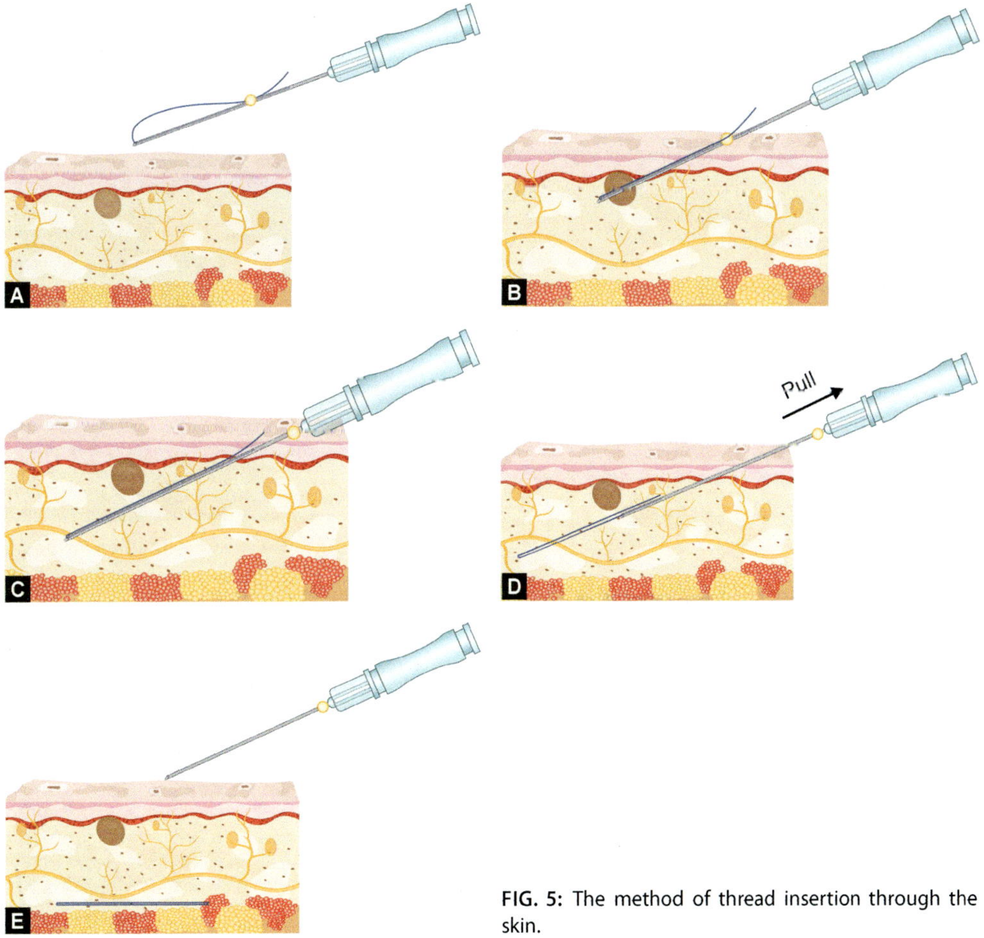

FIG. 5: The method of thread insertion through the skin.

remaining intact in the tissue, after insertion of the needle or cannula (Fig. 5). Variable length and thickness are available of needle thicknesses of 18–31 gauge and threads. Depending on the length of skin length in the insertion area, appropriate thread length is selected. For lifting and rejuvenating purposes, combination of cog and twin threads can be used, in all patients.[14]

Polydioxanone Insertion Techniques

The various methods of PDO thread insertion is elaborated in detail with illustrations. The AquaLift mono and Cogs threads are commonly used in PDO category.

Chin (Fig. 6)

- Insert the thread along the mandible margin for 1 cm below the chin
- Insert the thread up to the neck area
- Insert into the subcutaneous layer and rotate more than 10 times.

Double Chin (Fig. 7)

- 0.5 cm distance, sewing technique
- Performing the procedure in a sewing fashion that extends across the subcutaneous layer and the dermis
- Using a 9 mm 5-0 PDO is advised
- A meshed shape insertion.

Cheek Sag (Fig. 8)

- Inserting the thread parallel to the nasolabial wrinkle in 0.5 mm distances up to the front of the ear
- Inserting in 0.5 mm distances in a diamond-shaped mesh pattern
- If the skin sags easily, shorten the distances or insert in double or triple structures.

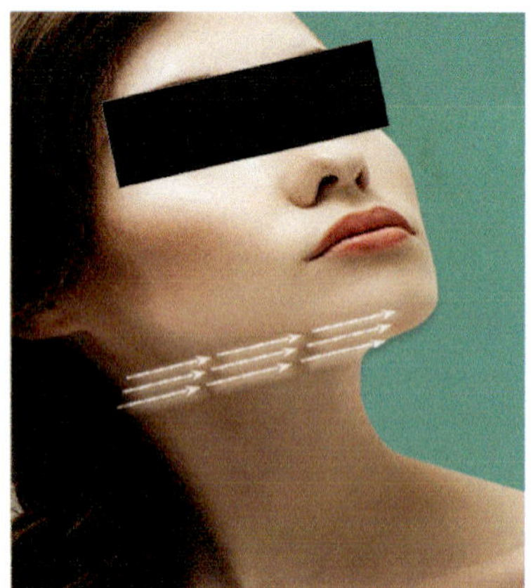

FIG. 6: Chin polydioxanone insertion method.

Nasolabial Folds (Fig. 9)

- Using 29 G, 50 mm, 6-0 PDO or 27 G, 70 mm, 5-0 PDO for good effect

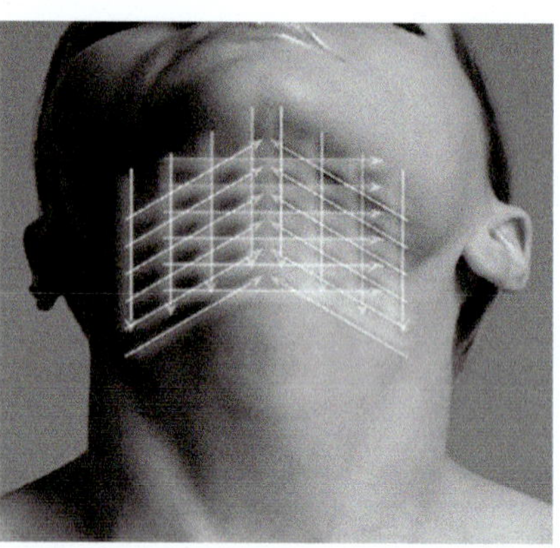

FIG. 7: Double chin polydioxanone insertion method.

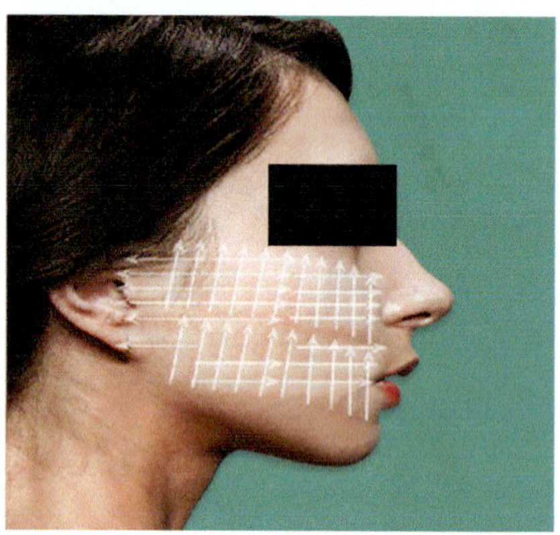

FIG. 8: Cheek sag polydioxanone insertion method.

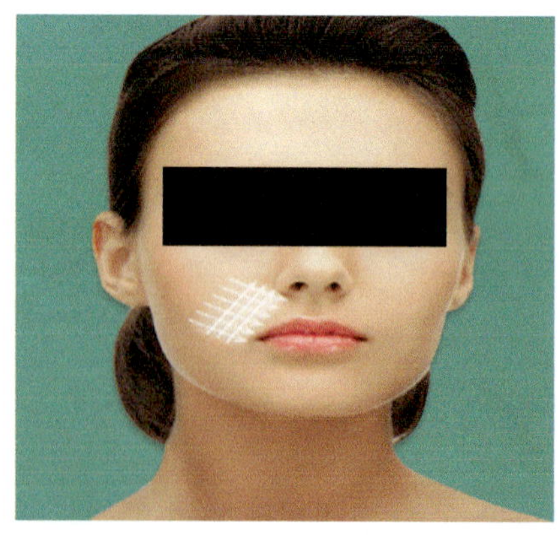

FIG. 9: Nasolabial folds polydioxanone insertion method.

- In order to minimize the discomfort, 29 G, 50 mm, 6-0 PDO insertion is advised
- Inserting the thread into the dermal layer in 0.5 mm distances from the nose ends where the nasolabial wrinkles begin to the mouth ends
- Deep wrinkle: Inserted parallel to the line directly below the wrinkle, 0.3 cm distance, deep dermal layer.

Marionette Lines (Fig. 10)

- Inserting into the dermal layer in a direction perpendicular to the wrinkle as with the marionette lines
- The deeper the wrinkle: Use more number of threads.

Crow's Feet (Fig. 11)

- Using a 30 G, 30 mm, 7-0 PDO
- Inserting the thread into the dermal layer parallel to the wrinkles and perpendicular to the threads insert at 0.5 cm distances so that a diamond-shaped mesh pattern.

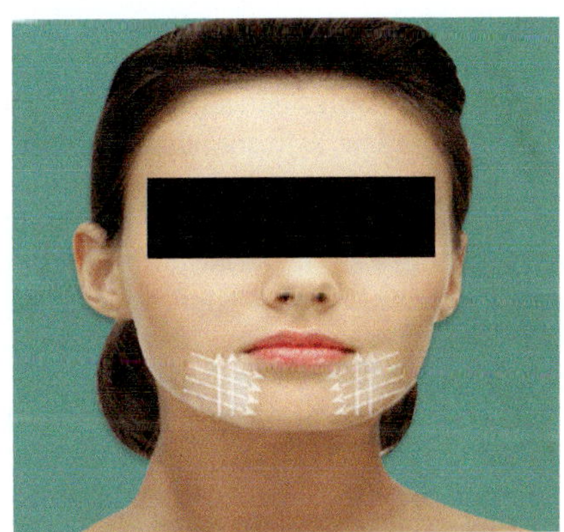

FIG. 10: Marionette lines polydioxanone insertion method.

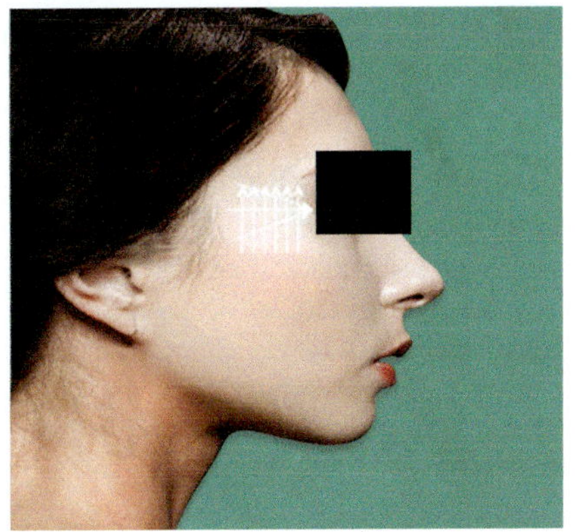

FIG. 11: Crows feet polydioxanone insertion method.

Forehead Lines (Fig. 12)

- Inserted in the dermis under the wrinkles along the wrinkle lines
- 0.5 cm distance, deep dermal layer.

The PDO thread results are subtle immediately after the procedure and gradually appreciable results are seen over 2–3 months as seen in figure 13.

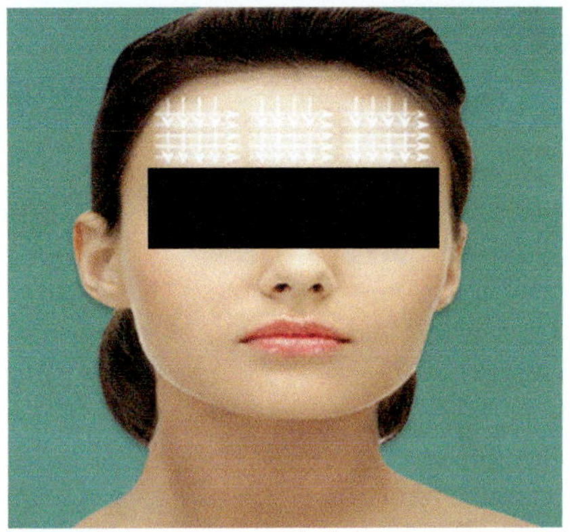

FIG. 12: Forehead lines polydioxanone insertion method.

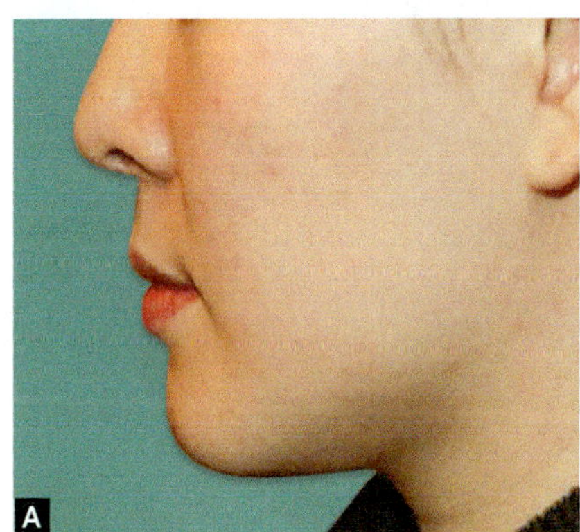

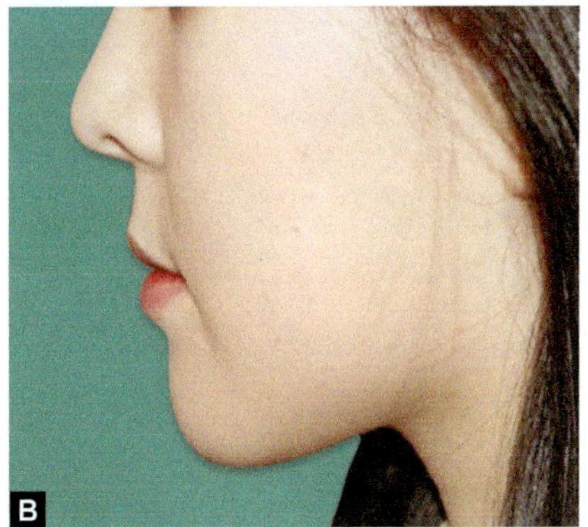

FIG. 13: Before and after (2 months) polydioxanone threads
Source: Alfa AquaLift.

Cogs Thread Insertion Method

Jowl Line (Fig. 14)

- By inserting 14 cm 3-0 bidirectional barbed threads from the front of ear and the upper part of zygomatic arch boundary
- Make the ends of thread locate in the lateral portion of face.

Nasolabial Folds (Fig. 15)

- By inserting 14 cm 3-0 bidirectional barbed threads from the front of ear and the upper part of zygomatic arch boundary
- Make the ends of thread locate to 1 cm before the nasolabial fold boundary.

Latero Mental Lift (Fig. 16)

- By inserting 14 cm 3-0 bidirectional barbed threads from the front of earlobe
- Make the ends of thread locate to the place 1 cm past the labiomental fold boundary.

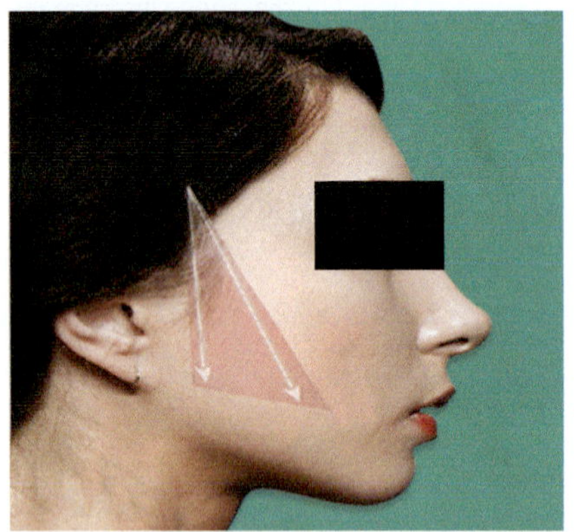

FIG. 14: Jowl line Cogs insertion method.

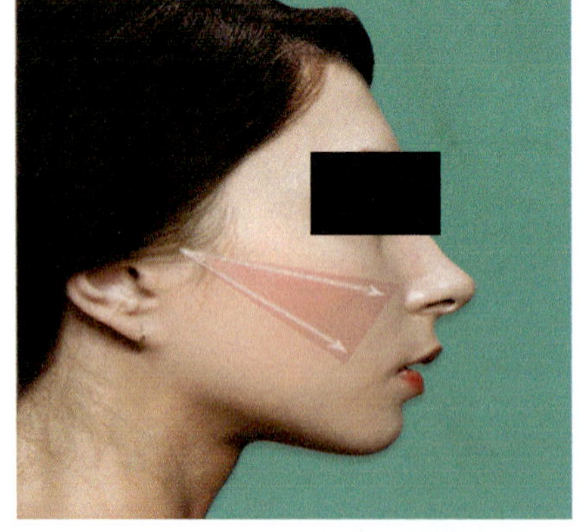

FIG. 15: Nasolabial folds Cogs insertion method.

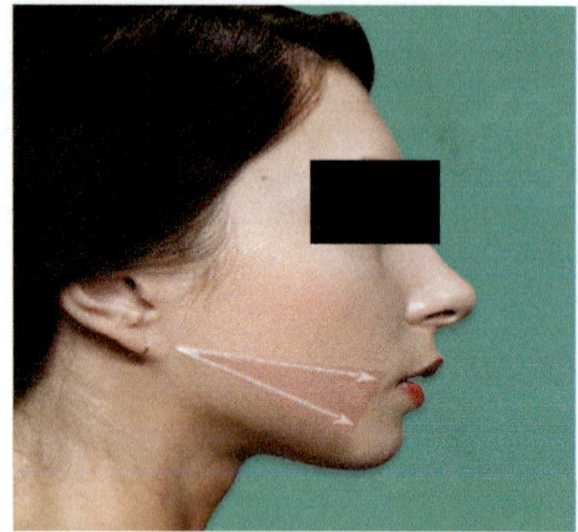

FIG. 16: Latero mental lift Cogs insertion method.

Polydioxanone thread lift shows results after 4 weeks of the procedure and the best results take about 2–3 months after one session as seen in figure 17.

Poly-L-lactic Acid

Polylactic acid (PLA) is a well-known polymer that has been used for many years in a number of biomedical and pharmaceutical applications. It has a long history of use as resorbable suture, a drug delivery system and in surgery—in particular in orthopedic fixation devices such as pins, rods, and screws.[19] It is also a key material in the development of tissue engineering.[20] These applications have been approved for human use by the FDA. Polylactic acid is generally classified as a safe material.[21]

Silhouette Soft is the patented PLLA thread approved for use. The physical and chemical configuration of the Silhouette sutures supports facial tissue repositioning by applying immediate traction and repositioning of the soft tissue of the face. It also leads to building up of new collagen fiber formation around its structure, augmenting tissue support against the gravitational pull.

The presence of the slow-absorbing cones creates initial traction and this is reinforced by the buildup of new collagen formation. The tissue traction is maintained by the collagen around and inside a series of knots intercalated between the cones after the cones are reabsorbed.

These sutures can be repositioned or readjusted in the future (1.5–2 years later). This can be done by pulling them from the temporal area, where all of them converge. Additionally, sutures can be added then to reinforce the previous ones or to treat other areas. The sutures can be also inserted at different

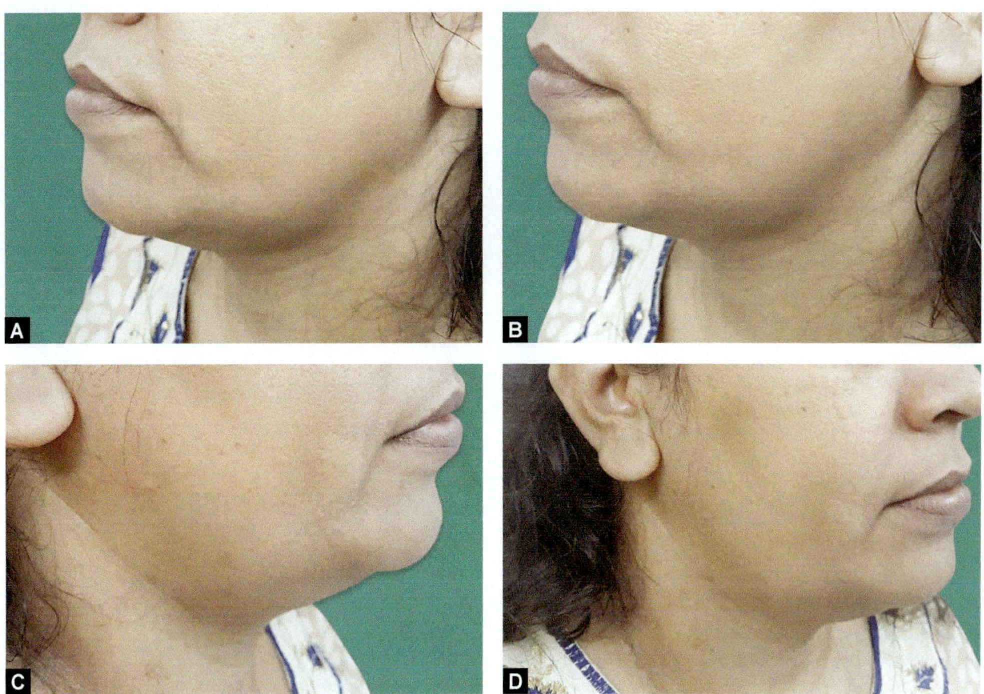

FIG. 17: Before and after Cogs thread lift for lower face and mono threads for Jawline.
Courtesy: Dr Madhuri Agarwal.

TABLE 1: Silhouette Soft threads family

Products	Soft 8 cones	Soft 12 cones	Soft 16 cones
USP designation	3.0	3.0	3.0
Length	30 cm	27.5 cm	26.8 cm
Number of cones	8	12	16
Direction of cones	Bidirectional	Bidirectional	Bidirectional
Space between cones	5 mm	8 mm	8 mm
Material	Polylactic acid	Polylactic acid	Polylactic acid
Needle	2 needles (23 G) of 12 cm each	2 needles (23 G) of 12 cm each	2 needles (23 G) of 12 cm each

USP, United States Pharmacopeia.

planes of the facial soft tissues such as superficial, intermedium, or deep.

Description of Thread

Silhouette Soft® suture is made of poly-L-lactic acid, while its cones are made of lactide/glycolide (82% lactide and 18% glycolide). These components are totally resorbable, biocompatible, and biodegradable.[22]

On each suture, there are two series of cones. Each series has the same number of cones, which face in opposite directions towards the extremity of each suture, hence the term "bidirectional." The cones are separated by tied knots, placed at 0.5 cm (8 cones) or 0.8 cm (12 cones) and (16 cones) intervals from each other, free floating between the knots (Table 1).

The central section of the suture is 2 cm long. This section is delimited by two knots and is free of cones. These two knots are at an equal distance from the middle of the suture.

It is important to assess each case in order to decide where and in which direction the skin needs to be lifted. This will determine the length of suture required and the type of pattern used.

The suture lengths are 10 cm with eight cones, 16 cm with 12 cones, and 20 cm with 16 cones. The cones are bidirectional with half the cones facing in one direction and the other half in the opposite direction. They can be inserted in a straight pattern, an obtuse angle or U-shaped pattern.

The straight-line suture is most suitable if, in addition to skin traction, an increase in the volume of the treated area is sought, thanks to the compression of adipose tissue. The angled sutures create lift in the direction placed.

Prepare the Patient

Determine the areas to be treated and vectors. Draw patterns with a ruler, respecting the 6, 9, and 11 cm rules. Choose the size of the sutures accordingly. Clean and disinfect the area to treat for the first time. Lay down the patient and cover the chest with a sterile field. Cover hair with bouffant cap. Additionally, place a sterile field over the bouffant cap. The area to be treated must be clear of hair, make-up, and piercings. Carry out a second, high-level disinfection of the area.

Remove Material from Pouches

The aluminum pouch is not sterile (Fig. 18). The external part of the transparent pouch is not sterile (Fig. 19). The white plastic pouch is sterile (Fig. 20).

Twist the plastic clip to remove Silhouette Soft® from the pouch. Prepare the thread with slight traction to tighten the knots. Do not overtighten with excessive pulling.

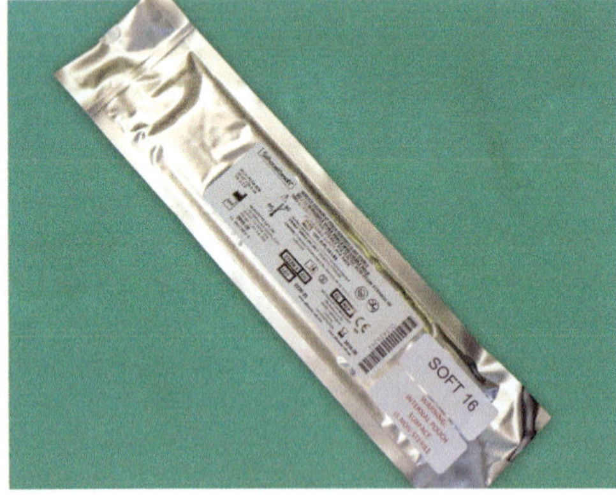

FIG. 18: Outside not sterile.

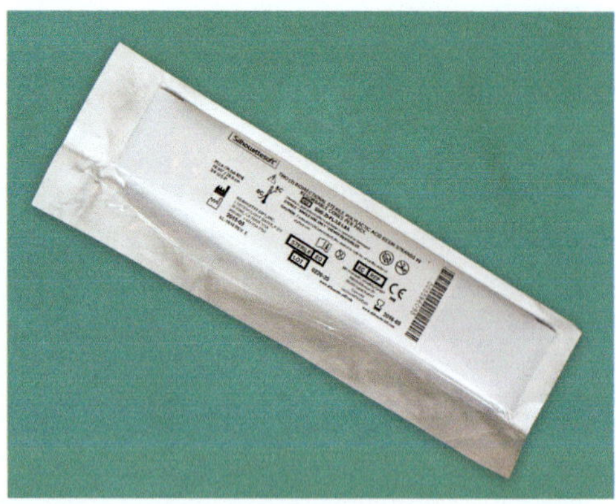

FIG. 19: Outside not sterile, inside sterile.

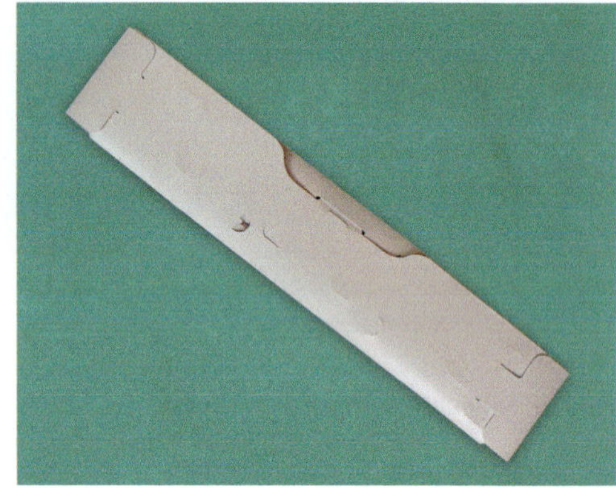

FIG. 20: Inside sterile.

Local Anesthesia

Disinfect the area to be treated for the third time. Local anesthesia procedures are always the same, regardless of the pattern applied—0.5 cc of lidocaine 1% with adrenaline 1:200,000 injection in each entry and exit point of any pattern. Administer local anesthesia to the entry and exit points.

- Lidocaine 1% with adrenaline 1:200,000
- 0.5 cc each point.

Silhouette Soft Premarking Techniques

- Entry points
- Exit points.

Preoperative marking aims to determine the position and the direction of the sutures on the areas to be treated.

Mid Face and Jaw Line (Fig. 21)

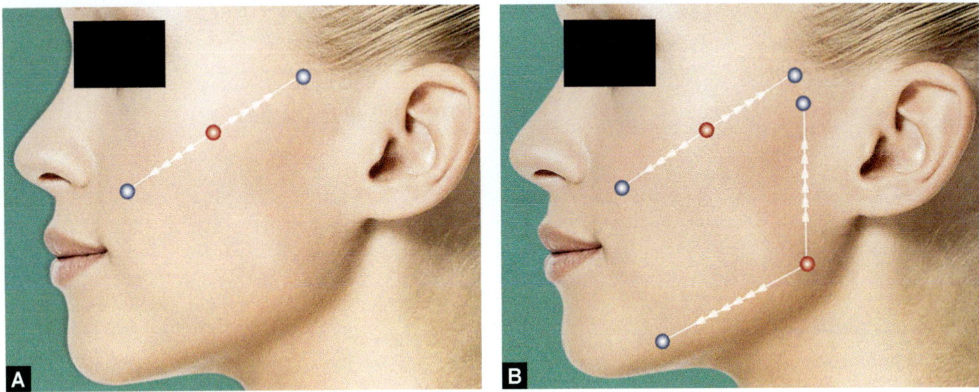

FIG. 21: **A,** Straight patterns and **B,** combined patterns: Straight and angle.

Neck (Fig. 22)

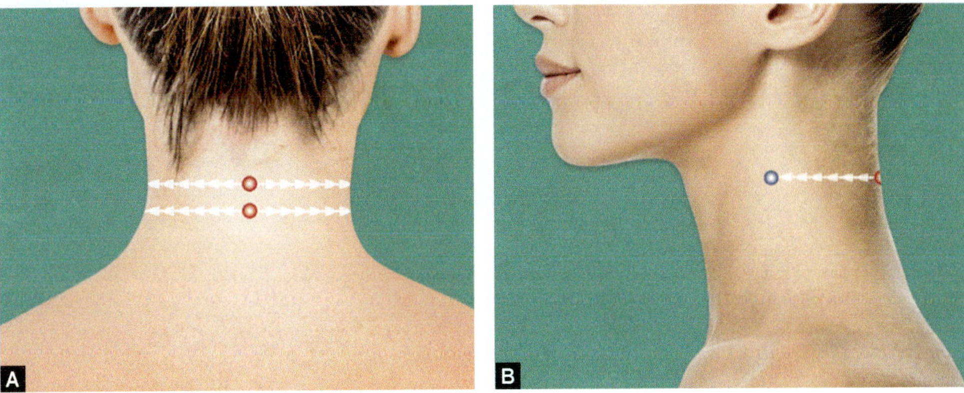

FIG. 22: Rein technique for the neck. **A,** Back view rein technique for the neck and **B,** side view.

Eyebrow (Fig. 23)

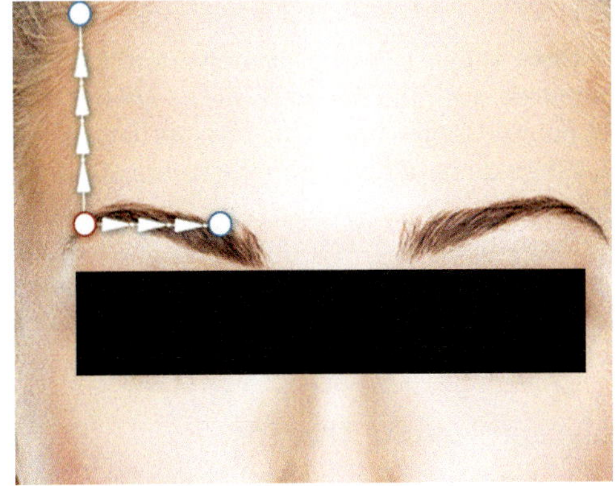

FIG. 23: L technique for eyebrow.

Creating the Entry Point (Fig. 24)

Create the entry hole with an 18 G needle.

Insertion of the Suture

Silhouette Soft® sutures are inserted at a depth of 5 mm beneath the skin in the subcutaneous tissue. The black line at the end of the needle tip indicates the limit of 5 mm.

Insert the point of the first suture needle perpendicularly to the skin through the entry point to a depth of 5 mm into the subcutaneous tissue (Fig. 25) until the black line disappears. Then turn the needle horizontally and guide it through the subcutaneous tissue. Depth may be adapted according to patient indications.

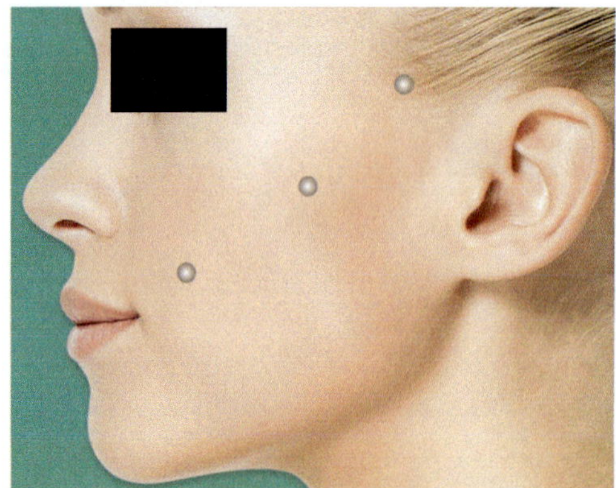

FIG. 24: Entry point site.

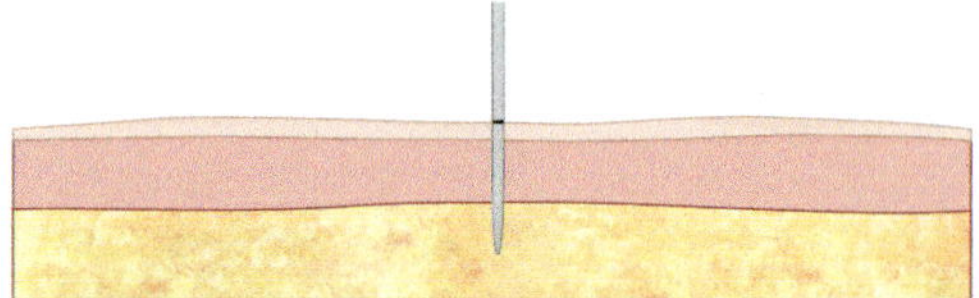

FIG. 25: Needle tip 5 mm (black mark) in the tissue in a vertical position.

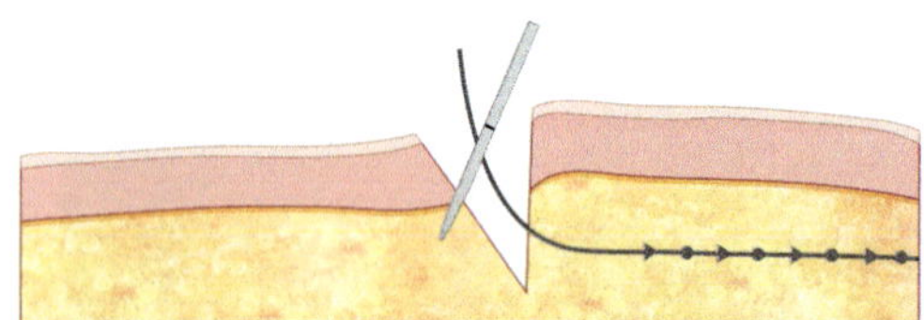

FIG. 26: Needle insertion in the first half of the suture.

Extract the needle through the first exit point. Gently pull it and by way of traction, the first series of cones will enter in the adipose tissue. When the last cone is inserted (Fig. 26), stop the traction and start with the insertion of the second half of the suture.

Introduce the needle located at the second end of the suture, perpendicularly to the skin in the same entry hole, respecting the depth of 5 mm into the adipose tissue. Proceed in the direction of the second exit point (Fig. 27).

Prick the skin at the pre-established exit point (Fig. 28). Extract the needle, with a gentle pull so the second series of cones are inserted in the tissue (Fig. 29).

The entire suture has now been implanted (Fig. 30). Cut thread leaving the free ends long. Repeat these actions with each suture, then on the other side.

This is the modeling phase applied to the treated area. With all the fingers of one hand, pinch the tissue, while applying gentle pressure (Fig. 31).

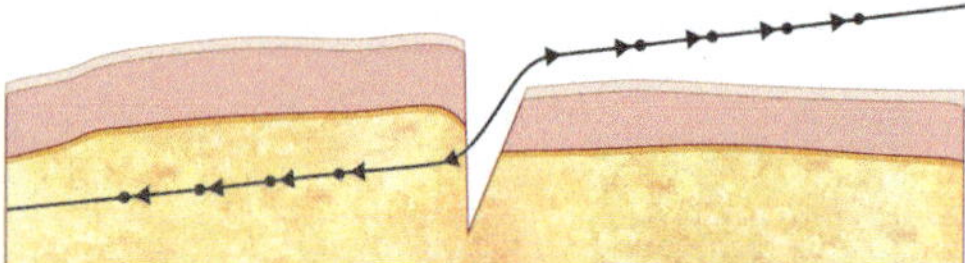

FIG. 27: Suture insertion

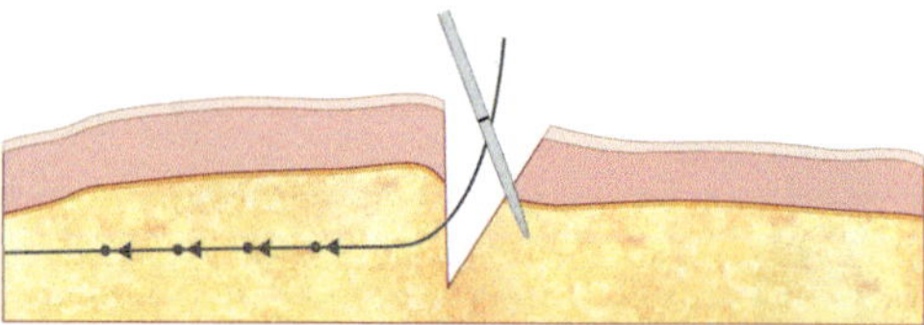

FIG. 28: Needle insertion in the second half of the suture pattern.

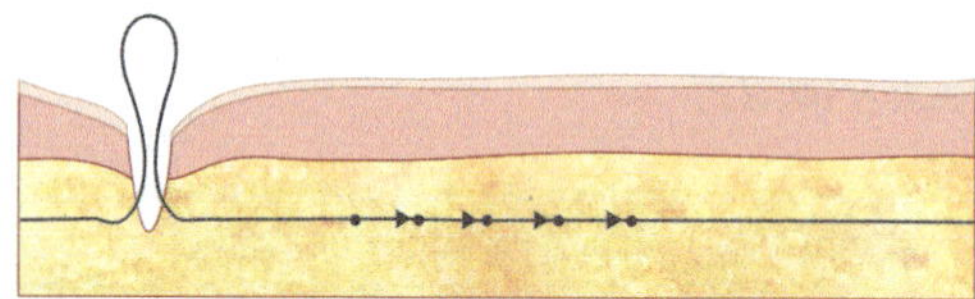

FIG. 29: Suture insertion second half.

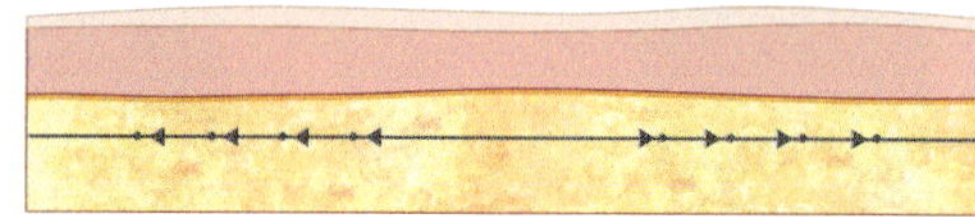

FIG. 30: Complete suture insertion.

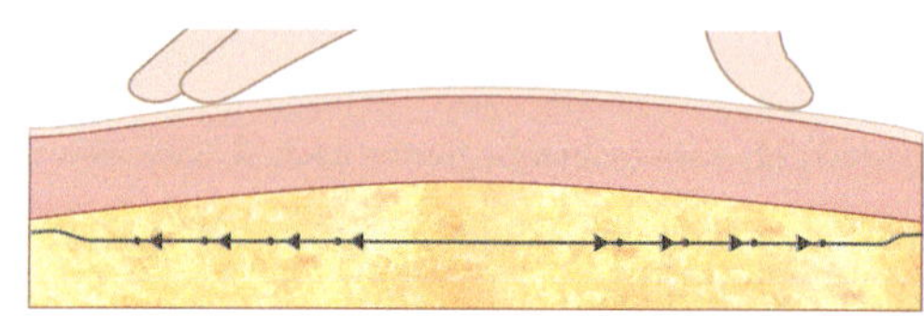

FIG. 31: Modeling phase of suture.

Once adipose tissue compression has been completed, trim the free ends of the sutures at the exit points. Use the tips of the scissors to gently pull back the skin in order to trim the suture at a deeper level.

Clean the treated area, apply antiseptic ointment.

Poly-L-lactic acid threads such as Silhouette Soft threads are known to show long-lasting, global facelift results seen in figures 32 and 33.

Polycaprolactone Threads

Polycaprolactone is another known polymer employed in various forms in multiple fields of medicine.

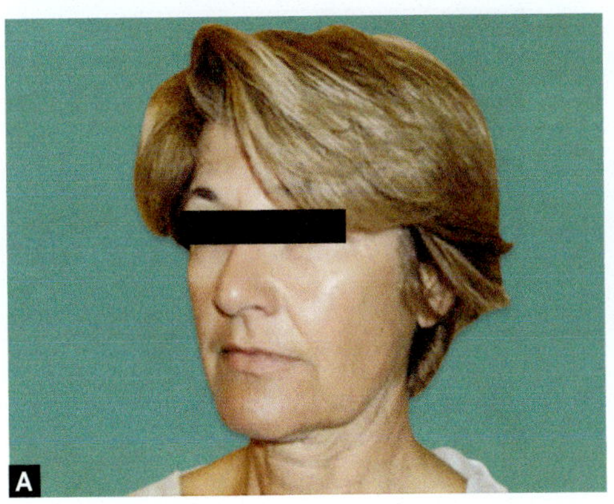

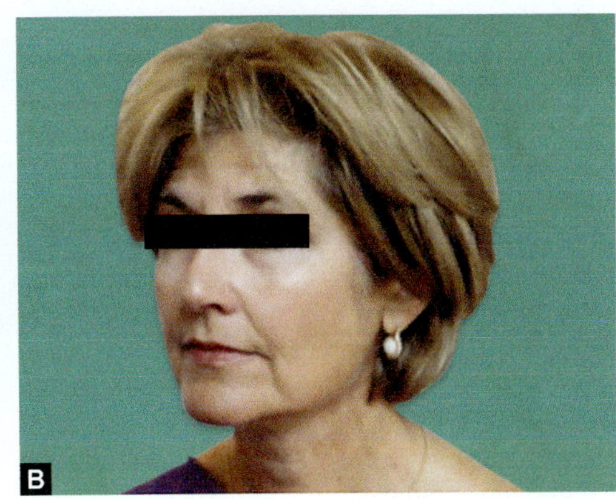

FIG. 32: Pre- and post-Silhouette Soft results.
Source: Silhouette Product presentation.

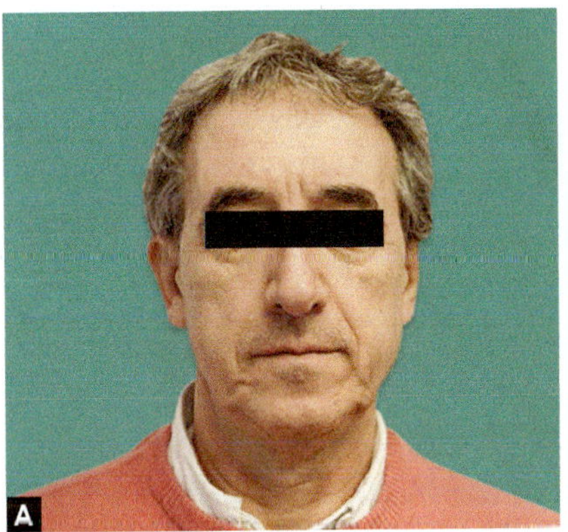

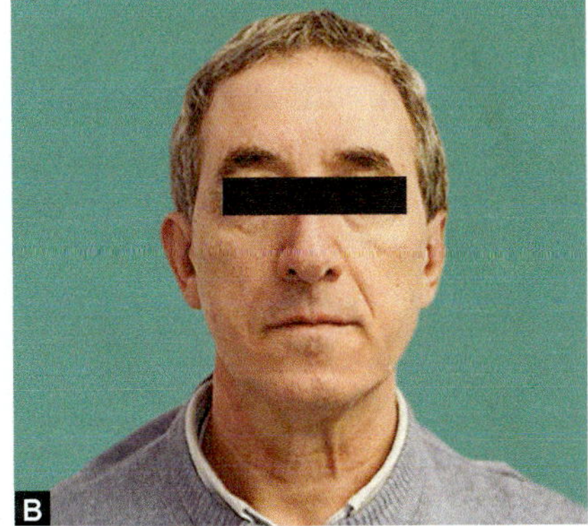

FIG. 33: Pre- and post-30 days Silhouette Soft results.
Source: Silhouette product presentation.

It has been in use for some time as a soft tissue filler for skin hydration and volumization, PCA threads is known to have long lasting results in skin rejuvenation. These threads induce both collagen type I and III, thus delivering a more comprehensive result.

Happy Lift range of PCA threads are popularly used by physicians. The Happy Lift™ Revitalizing range is an absorbable, monofilament, suspension thread of synthetic origin (caprolactone) manufactured by Assut Europe Spa for Promoitalia International Spa. This product belongs to the category 07 of inactive implanted devices, in the reabsorbable thread group, and in class III of medical devices.[17,22] Moreover, the device has the CE mark 0373 released by the Istituto Superiore della Sanita` dell'Italia (Italian Board of Health, Rome, Italy).

In this range, the types of threads are:

- Double needle threads are convergent bidirectional threads (length 12–23 cm, 2.0 USP caliber) with straight needle (lengths 9 or 15 cm, 24 G caliber) at the ends
- Free floating threads are convergent bidirectional threads (length 12–23 cm, 2.0 USP caliber), which are introduced into the hypoderm with the assistance of cannula (length 9/15 cm, 21 G caliber)
- Anchorage are unidirectional, barbed threads (length 12.5 cm, 2.0 USP caliber).

The immediate effect is the lifting of the tissue, due to the mechanical action produced by the thread, which contrasts the falling of the area treated. This is possible due to the arrangement of the threads' barbs, disposed in two directions (divergent and opposite), compared to the middle point of the thread. The reaction strength produced on both its sides, in fact, allows the connection of the tissue on each barb that functions as a hook and at the same time, prevents the sliding, and movement of the thread in the two opposite directions. Thanks to this specific geometry of the Happy Lift™ Revitalizing, anchorage points are not required on the superior and inferior part of the facial anatomic region to lift. Once positioned in the subcutaneous tissue, they will continue to practice their sustaining action on the tissues. It is an advantage compared to the unidirectional barbed threads as these barbs are positioned in one direction. Therefore, even if widespread, they lift the tissue in only one direction.[12,15,17,23] The histological valuations have highlighted that the subdermal suspension thread used in the study by Savoia et al. connects itself to the high and lateral dermis retinacula cutis system, to the superficial muscular aponeurotic system and to the downward muscular bands to exercise an effective anchoring and lifting action.[17]

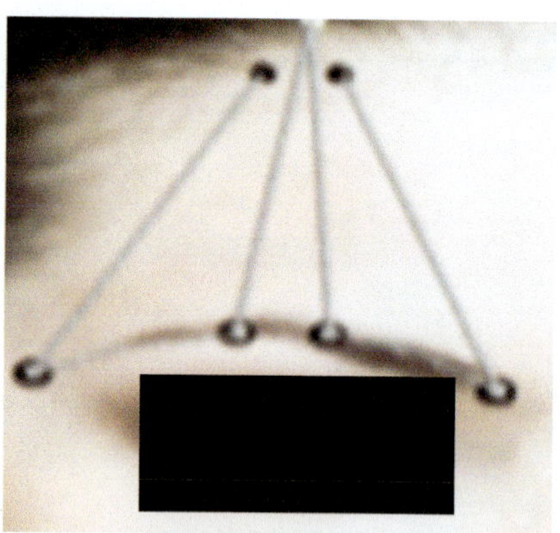

FIG. 34: Double needle for the treatment of the eyebrow.
Source: Savoia A, Accardo C, Vannini F, et al. Outcomes in thread lift for facial rejuvenation: A study performed with happy lift revitalizing. Dermatol Ther (Heidelb). 2014;4:103-14.

Technique of Polycaprolactone Threads Placement

Local anesthesia was performed with 1-2% lidocaine, diluted epinephrine (1/200,000 cc) and the addition of diluted sodium hydrogen carbonate (NaHCO^3) (1/9 cc).

The free floating threads were introduced in flabby tissues of zygomatic area with a cannula needle (20/21 G caliber 9 6 9 1, 2 mm 9 15, 24 cm) and, subsequently, the cannula was removed, leaving the thread in its place. The thread, with bidirectional and convergent barbs towards the center, was inserted inside the needle carefully so that the barbs that had to maintain their efficiency were not damaged. The mechanical action exercised by the two halves of the thread had to be symmetrical and of the same entity; otherwise, the sliding of the thread in the insertion level and the "exiting" from one of the access holes was possible. The time necessary for the complete treatment required was an average of 35-55 min.[17]

Forehead, Mandibular Area, and the Neck Polycaprolactone Insertion Techniques[17]

- The double needle threads were utilized for these areas
- The protocol used for the revival of the eyebrow suggested the insertion of both straight needles at a point located in correspondence to the hairline
- One proceeds vertically downward until reaching the eyebrow where both needles protrude
- The course must be tangential to the bone surface and within the subcutaneous tissue
- The median needle reenters in the same exit hole and traces the eyebrow to exit the nasal edge. The needle placed more laterally undergoes the same path, symmetrically (Fig. 34).

Protocol for the Redefinition of the Mandibular Contour[17]

- It involves the use of a wire introduced through a straight needle in correspondence to the mandibular angle through two adjacent inlet holes
- The first needle goes along the ramus of the lower jaw to the temporal region and the second runs on the horizontal ramus of the mandible for 4-5 cm (Fig. 35)
- Finally, for the treatment of the neck, a wire double needle is introduced in correspondence to the aponeurosis of platysma with both needles, but in an alternating manner. It proceeds to the region of the sternum cleidomastoid drawing a "V" open towards the outside (Fig. 23C).

The time necessary for a complete treatment was, on average 20-40 min. The threads may displace themselves from their primal insertion position in the first 10 days following traumas and, therefore, loose the "gathering" established with the neighboring tissues.[23] The PCA threads demonstrate remarkable contouring results as seen in figure 36.

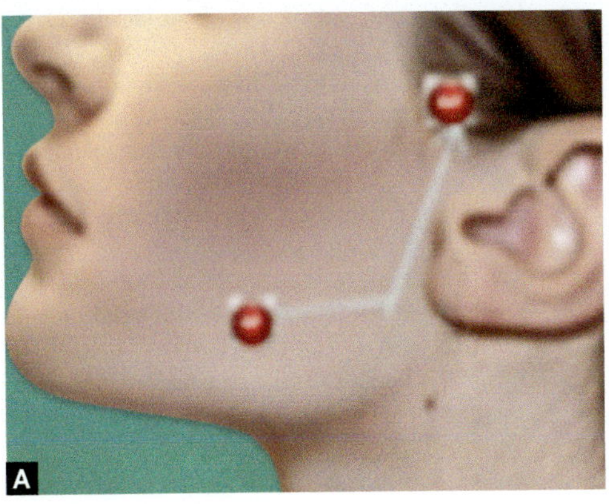

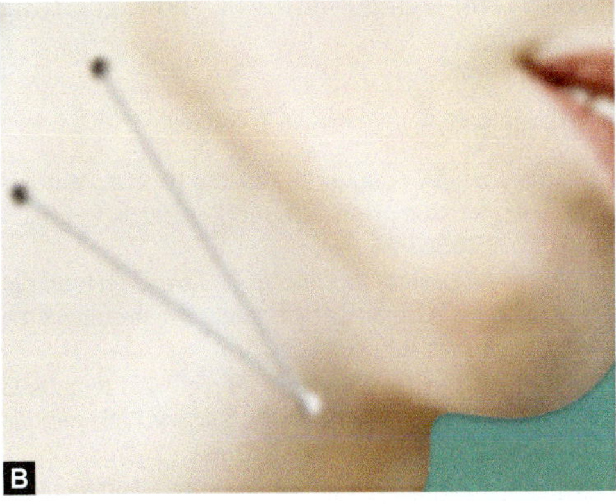

FIG. 35: A, Double needle for the redefinition of the mandibular contour; **B,** double needle for the treatment of the neck.

Source: Savoia A, Accardo C, Vannini F, et al. Outcomes in thread lift for facial rejuvenation: a study performed with happy lift revitalizing. Dermatol Ther (Heidelb). 2014;4:103-14.

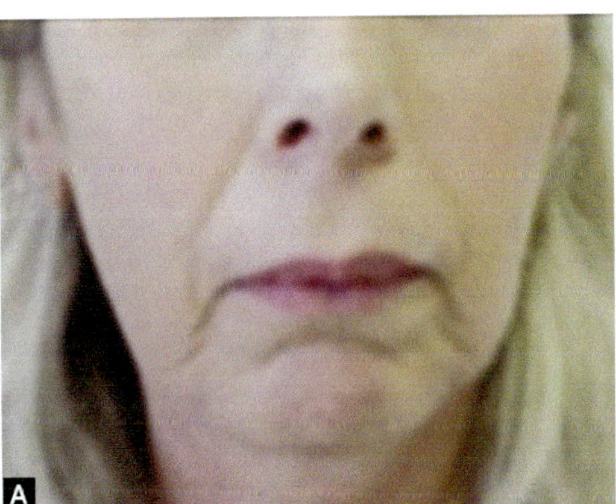

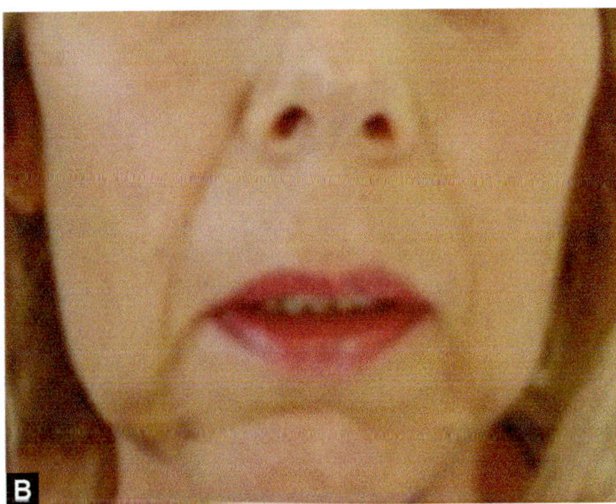

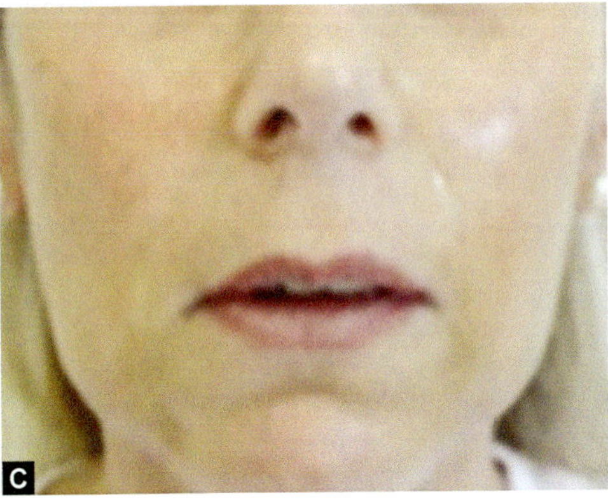

FIG. 36: Exemplificative case of facial rejuvenation. A patient treated for the redefinition of the mandibular contour. **A,** Before the treatment; **B,** immediately after the treatment; **C,** 6 months after the treatment.

Source: Savoia A, Accardo C, Vannini F, et al. Outcomes in thread lift for facial rejuvenation: A study performed with happy lift revitalizing. Dermatol Ther (Heidelb). 2014;4:103-14.

CONCLUSION

Thread lift is a minimally invasive, fast and easy procedure with no scarring. The new innovations, both in product and technique, make it a safe, satisfactory procedure with instant and long-lasting results. In recent times, Cogs PDO, PLLA, and PCA threads are the emerging, result oriented nonsurgical threads. The crucial tip for a successful thread lift is appropriate patient selection. A mild to moderate skin laxity and aging signs will show gratifying positive results.

REFERENCES

1. Sulamanidze MA, Fournier PF, Paikidze TG, et al. Removal of facial soft tissue ptosis with special threads. Dermatol Surg. 2002;28:367-71.
2. Abraham RF, DeFatta RJ, Williams EF. Thread-lift for facial rejuvenation: Assessment of long-term results. Arch Facial Plast Surg. 2009;11:178-83.
3. Sherrell J. Aston, Douglas S. Steinbrech, and Jennifer L. Walden, editors. Aesthetic Plastic Surgery. Philadelphia: Saunders, 2009. ISBN-10: 0702031682.
4. Abraham RF, DeFatta RJ, Williams EF. Thread-lift for facial rejuvenation: Assessment of long-term results. Arch Facial Plast Surg. 2009;11:178-83.
5. Sulamanidze M, Sulamanidze G, Vozdvizhensky I, et al. Avoiding complications with Aptos sutures. Aesthet Surg J. 2011;31:863-73.
6. Yongtrakul P, Sirithanabadeekul P, Siriphan P. Thread lift: Classification, technique, and how to approach to the patient. World Academy of Science, Engineering and Technology, International Journal of Medical, Health, Biomedical, Bioengineering and Pharmaceutical Engineering. 2016;10.12:535-43.
7. Bartholomew RS. PDS (polydioxanone suture): A new synthetic absorbable suture in cataract surgery. A preliminary study. Ophthalmologica. 1981;183(2):81-5.
8. Middleton JC, Tipton AJ. Synthetic Biodegradable Polymers as Medical Devices 1998. Biomaterials. 2000 Dec; 21(23):2335-46.
9. Boland ED, Coleman BD, Barnes CP, et al. Electrospinning polydioxanone for biomedical applications. Acta Biomater. 2005;1:115-23.
10. Gamboa GM, Vasconez LO. Suture suspension technique for midface and neck rejuvenation. Ann Plast Surg. 2009;62(5):478-81.
11. Kalra R. Use of barbed threads in facial rejuvenation. Indian J Plast Surg. 2008;41.
12. DeLorenzi CL. Barbed sutures: Rationale and technique. Aesthet Surg J. 2006;26(2):223- 9.
13. Rashid RM, Sartori M, White LE, et al. Breaking strength of barbed polypropylene sutures: rater-blinded, controlled comparison with nonbarbed sutures of various calibers. Arch Dermatol. 2007;143(7):869-72.
14. Suh DH, Jang HW, Lee SJ, et al. Outcomes of polydioxanone knotless thread lifting for facial rejuvenation. Dermatol Surg. 2015;41(6):720-5.
15. Horne DF, Kaminer MS. Reduction of face and neck laxity with anchored, barbed polypropylene sutures (Contour Threads). Skin Therapy Lett. 2006;11(1):5-7.
16. Wu WT. Nonsurgical facelifting with long barbed suture slings: The Woffleslift. J Asthet Chir. 2013;1:13-9.
17. Savoia A, Accardo C, Vannini F, et al. Outcomes in thread lift for facial rejuvenation: A study performed with happy lift revitalizing. Dermatol Ther (Heidelb). 2014;4:103-14.
18. Ruff G. Technique and uses for absorbable barbed sutures. Aesthet Surg J. 2006;26:620-8.
19. Athanasiou KA. Sterilization, toxicity, biocompatibilty and clinical applications of polylactic acid/polyglycolic acid copolymers. Biomaterials. 1996;17:93-102.
20. Gentile P. An overview of Poly (Lactic-co-glycolic) acid (PLGA)-based biomaterials for bone tissue engineering. Int J Mol Sci. 2014;15:3640-59.
21. Jamshidian M, et al. Poly-lactic acid: Production, applications, nanocomposites and release studies. Comprehensive Reviews in Food Science and Food Safety. 2010;9:552-71.
22. Council Directive 93/42/EEC of the European Parliament and of the Council of 14 June 1993. Available from: http://www.ce-mark.com/MDD.pdf. [Accessed 25 Nov 2013].
23. Villa MT, White LE, Alam M, et al. Barbed sutures: A review of the literature. Plast Reconstr Surg. 2008;121:102e-8e.

34

CHAPTER

Fractional Lasers

Venkatram Mysore, Anuj Pall, Elizabeth George

INTRODUCTION

The field of laser resurfacing for aesthetic enhancement has been improving since the 1980s. Fractional photothermolysis (FP) is a revolutionary change in this field. There are various machines and techniques available with a wide variety of applications. The various technologies developed include ablative, nonablative, and fractional lasers. They differ in their method of thermal damage, degrees of efficacy, downtime, and side effect profiles.[1] Fractional lasers provide better efficacy, decreased side effects with lesser recovery time. Ablative lasers have the superior most results with the disadvantage of increased side effects and an increased recovery time.[2]

PRINCIPLE

The concept of FP was introduced by Manstein and colleagues in 2004.[3] The first laser to incorporate FP utilized a wavelength targeting water (1,550 nm) in a nonablative fashion. While the laser thermally denatured dermal collagen and epidermal tissue, it was considered nonablative because the skin's barrier function was retained with the sparing of the stratum corneum. By pixelating the laser energy, small (<400 μm in diameter) columns of evenly spaced thermal damage were created, with depth of penetration proportional to energy per pixel. Each pixilated column of energy is referred to as a microscopic thermal zone (MTZ). By creating MTZ in only a fraction of the treatment area, the intervening, undamaged epidermis served as a reservoir of viable tissue for rapid repair of the coagulated MTZ in epidermal tissue, thus facilitating rapid and predictable epidermal healing.[3,4] The number, depth, and size of these vertical columns of MTZs are variable and depend on the type of machine, wavelength of the laser used, fluence, and the number of stacking or applications of laser. Each MTZ has a diameter ranging from 100 to 160 μ. The density of MTZs delivered at each treatment is 2,000 MTZs/cm^2.

Within the MTZ, coagulated material containing melanin, elastin, and other dermal contents has been histologically demonstrated to condense into a button-shaped conglomerate known as microepidermal necrotic debris (MEND).[2] Transepidermal elimination of the MEND correlates clinically with the bronzing of skin and mild exfoliation seen in the 1st week following treatment.[4] This is followed by reepithelialization and repair from the adjacent columns of intact tissue. Nonablative fractional lasers (NAFLs) have a similar mechanism of action except there is no epidermal ablation or extrusion of dermal contents which corresponds to rapid skin healing (Fig. 1). So, fractional lasers offer advantages of reduced edema and erythema, minimum downtime, reduced dyschromic changes, and suitability for darker skin types.[2]

INDICATIONS FOR FRACTIONAL LASER TREATMENT

Fractional lasers are currently approved by the Food and Drug Administration (FDA) for the treatment of pigmented lesions, periorbital rhytides, skin resurfacing, melasma and soft tissue coagulation, acne and surgical scars, and actinic keratosis. However, they are routinely used, for several off-label indications. Given here is a box 1 which lists out some important indications of fractional lasers.

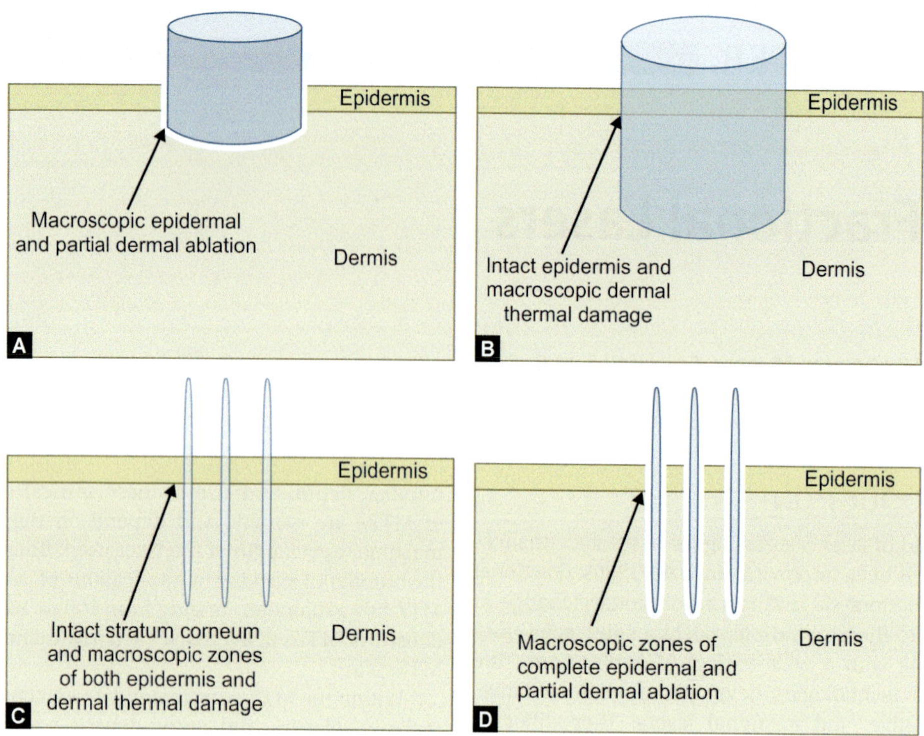

FIG. 1: Comparative zones of tissue damage for various laser systems. **A,** Conventional ablative lasers form macroscopic regions of complete epidermal vaporization and variable superficial dermal damage with accompanying risk of delayed healing and scarring; **B,** conventional nonablative lasers leave the epidermis completely intact and cause macroscopic regions of dermal thermal damage at varying depths, but the lack of epidermal damage is associated with modest clinical outcomes; **C,** fractional nonablative resurfacing leaves an intact stratum corneum and creates microscopic zones of epidermal and deep dermal thermal damage; and **D,** ablative fractional resurfacing creates microscopic zones of complete epidermal ablation as well as microscopic zones of deep dermal ablation.

BOX 1 Indications of fractional lasers

- Scars: Acne scar, traumatic scar, postburn scar, surgical scar, and stretch marks
- Aging changes: Photoaging on the face, neck, chest, hands; periorbital wrinkles
- Dyschromias: Melasma, postinflammatory pigmentation, minocycline pigmentation, poikiloderma of Civatte, and nevus of Ota
- Vascular lesions: Residual hemangiomas, telangiectatic matting
- Miscellaneous: Granuloma annulare, colloid milium, disseminated superficial actinic porokeratosis, lichen amyloidosis, mucinosis, shagreen patch, and morphea-related contracture

Aging and Photodamaged Skin

Aging, photodamaged skin is characterized by wrinkles, dark spots, and pigmentary changes. Mild-to-moderate facial wrinkles and periorbital wrinkles can be treated with both ablative and NAFLs.[5] Multiple treatments at intervals of 1 month are needed to achieve satisfactory improvement. Fractional lasers can also be used effectively for the treatment of photodamaged skin, rhytides, and fine lines.[6] Ablative fractional lasers (AFLs) produce greater textural improvement and dermal remodeling. Fractional ablative carbon dioxide (CO_2) laser is found to be effective in treating lower eyelid skin laxity and photoaging.[7] Ultrapulsed CO_2, short-pulse CO_2, and erbium-doped yttrium aluminum garnet (Erb:YAG) were found to be both effective and safe in treatment of neck laxity, rhytides, and texture.[8] Weiss et al. reported a comparative split-face trial study with half face treated with fractionated CO_2 laser and the contralateral half treated with a 1,550 nm nonablative fractional erbium laser. On blinded photographic analysis, significantly greater improvement (75% improvement) was observed in the fractionated CO_2 laser area than the 1,550 nm erbium laser (25% improvement) in periocular rhytides which suggest superior efficacy and patient satisfaction with fractional CO_2 laser resurfacing than 1,550 nm erbium laser.[9]

Study done by Friedmann et al. using newer 1,565 nm nonablative fractional erbium-doped fiber laser showed statistically significant decrease in Fitzpatrick-Goldman Wrinkle and Elastosis Score (FGWES) both at 3 months (-0.58 ± 0.23, $p = 0.02$) and 6 months (-0.66 ± 0.22, $p = 0.008$) after three treatment sessions in patient of facial photodamage and rhytides (Fig. 2). Lesser and discomfort (pain, erythema) and downtime (<2 days) are associated with better patient compliance.[10]

Post-acne Scars and Other Scars

Post-acne Scars

Post-acne scars can be of various types namely ice pick scars, box scars, rolling scars, keloidal, and hypertrophic scars. Treatment of acne scars depends on the type and severity of scarring. Fractional lasers have been used successfully and safely in the treatment of acne scars with good results in superficial and medium-depth scars (Fig. 3).[11] While macular, superficial, and medium-depth scars respond well, deep scars and ice pick scars may improve only marginally. In cases with severe scarring, combination with other approaches such as chemical peels, subcision, surgical dermabrasion, dermaroller, and trichloroacetic acid chemical reconstruction of skin scars (CROSS) technique may be needed.[12] There is 26–50% improvement in texture and atrophy, as well as overall improvement, in moderate-to-severe acne scarring with fractionated CO_2 laser. Although multiple treatments are required, the significant depth of penetration achieved with the NAFL has lead to improvements in scars similar

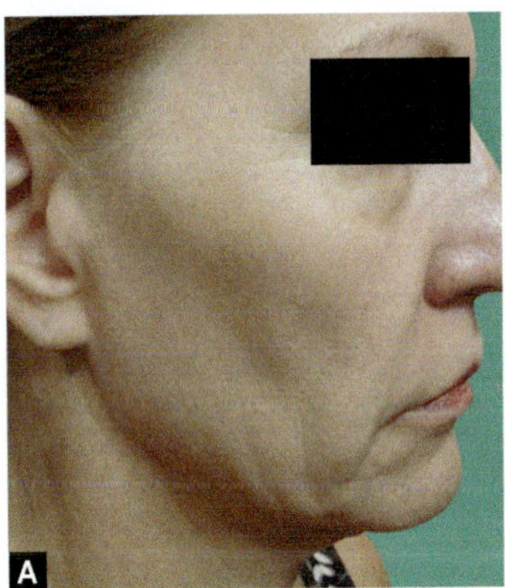

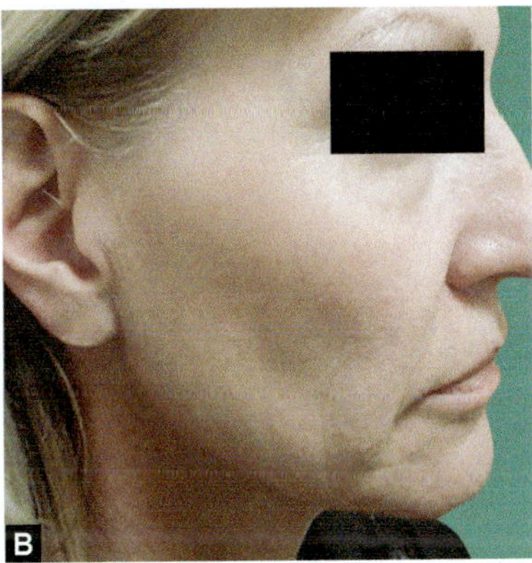

FIG. 2: Facial rejuvenation (before and 8 months after four sessions of 1,565 nm erbium fiber laser).

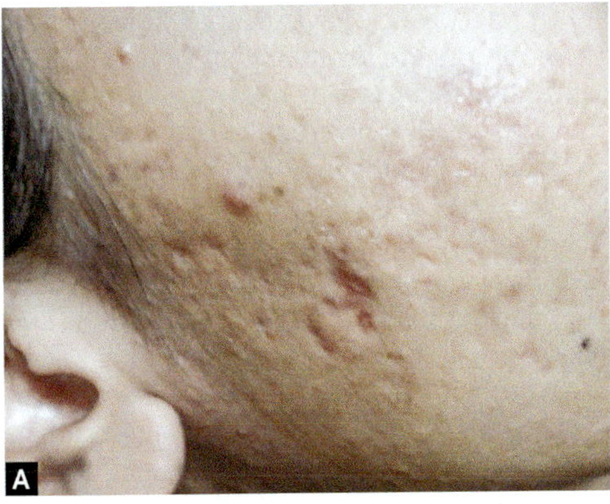

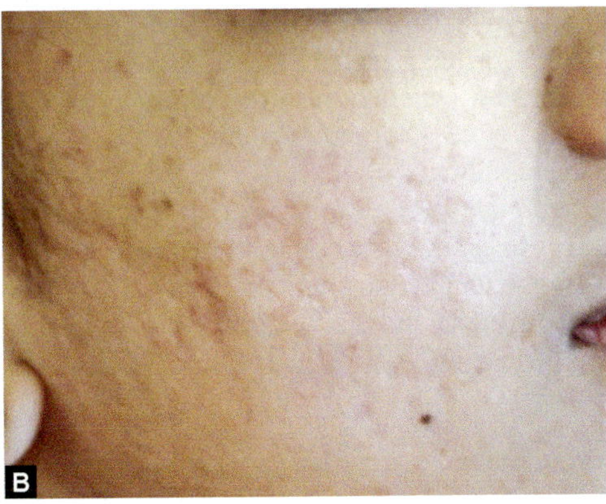

FIG. 3: A, Acne scars before treatment with fractional laser; and **B,** improvement in acne scars after treatment with fractional laser.

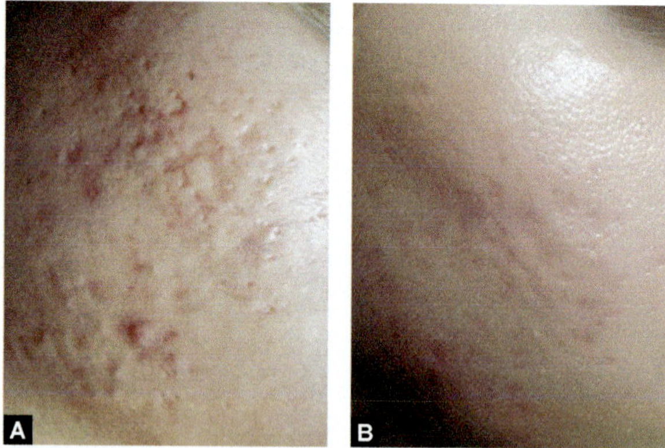

FIG. 4: A, Acne scar before treatment; and **B,** acne scars improvement 6 months after four sessions of 1,540 nm erbium glass laser.

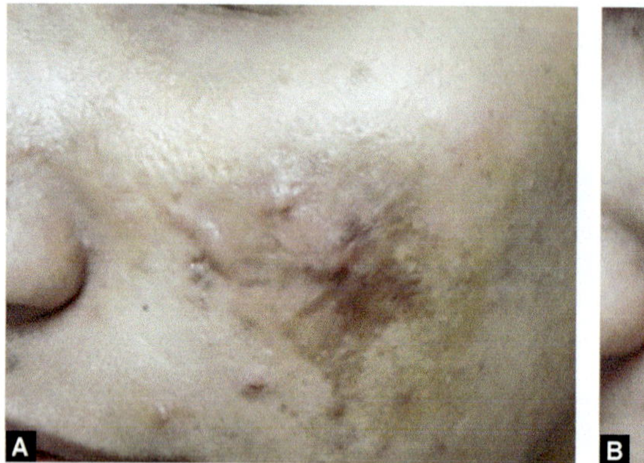

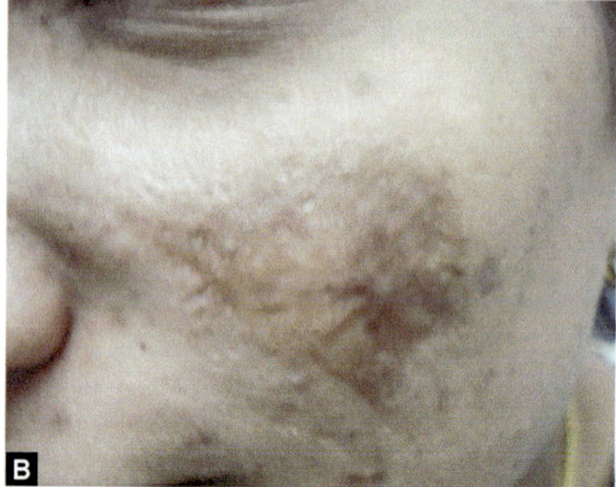

FIG. 5: A, Surgical scar before treatment; and **B,** surgical scar after treatment.

to those achieved with the ablative lasers. In a study of 87 patients, those patients with moderate acne scarring showed better improvement than those with severe scarring after six sessions of 1,540 nm NAFL (Fig. 4). Patients that undergo NAFL treatment for acne scarring experience 1–3 days of intense erythema that generally resolves within 1 week, a maximum of 26–50% improvement in scars, and a high tolerability.[11]

Fractional lasers carry a risk of transient erythema or edema, dryness, scabbing, milia or acne, hyperpigmentation or hypopigmentation, prolonged healing, or infection.[12] Hence proper counseling of patients and appropriate adjuvant medical treatment are essential.

Surgical Scars

Surgical, posttraumatic, and burn scars can also be treated with fractional lasers (Fig. 5).[13] Multiple treatments lead to improvement in texture, quality, and pigmentation of the scars in both atrophic and hypertrophic types. Atrophic and pigmented scars respond better than the hypertrophic scars.[14] Fractional lasers have demonstrated significant potential in the treatment of postsurgical, burn, and other traumatic scarring with minimal adverse effects, however, the optimal time to treat, treatment parameters, and appropriate follow-up have yet to be elucidated. Jung et al. treated 23 Korean females (Fitzpatrick skin type III–V) 2–3 weeks postthyroidectomy in an uncontrolled study using 10,600 nm ablative FP (AFP) (Lutronic Corporation, Goyang, Korea) and found statistical improvement in the Vancouver Scar Scale at 3-months follow-up ($p < 0.001$) when compared to pretreatment. Aesthetic improvement was accompanied by minimal adverse effects and high patient satisfaction (Fig. 6).[15]

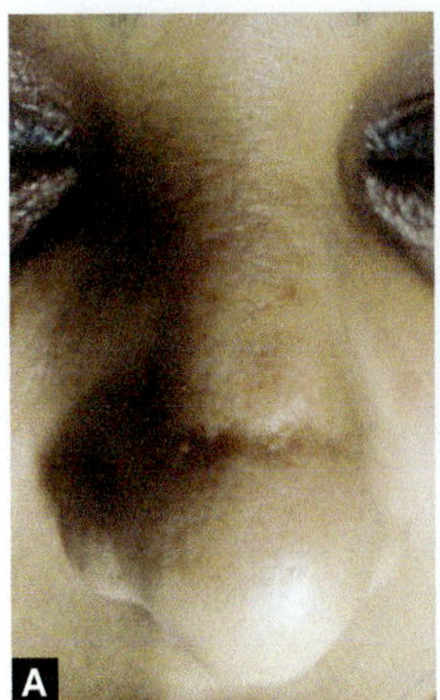

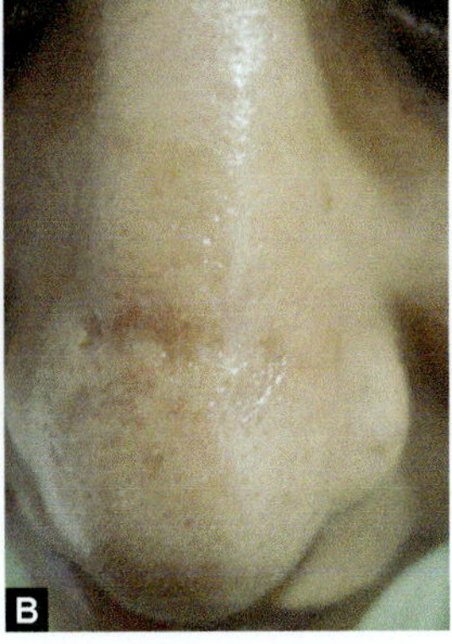

FIG. 6: A, Postsurgical scar before treatment; and **B,** postsurgical scar 4 months after five sessions of 1,540 nm erbium glass laser.

Burn Scars

Burn scars are unique because not only is there damage to tissue in the center of the injury as in a wound from a scalpel, but also the surrounding tissues have been altered structurally. Thus, most burn scars will go on to form a hypertrophic appearance. Hypertrophic scars are red, firm, and raised within the confines of the original wound. On a molecular level, hypertrophic scars result from imbalanced and excessive collagen deposition through aberrations in the fundamental wound healing phases of inflammation, proliferation, and remodeling.[16] Fractional lasers have a role in hypertrophic scars and improve surface irregularities, pigmentary abnormalities, hypertrophy, pruritus, and contraction.

Although no controlled trials have yet been conducted, case reports and series demonstrate a role for AFLs in the treatment of hypertrophic thermal burn scars.

Khandelwal A et al. did a retrospective chart review of adult and pediatric patients undergoing FP at a verified burn center examining treatment parameters as well as pre- and post-Vancouver Scar Scale scores. They found that FP is a safe and efficacious adjunct therapy for hypertrophic burn scars.[17]

Qu L et al. indicated that fractional CO_2 resulted in clinical improvement of mature burn scar. Alteration of types I and III procollagen, matrix metalloproteinase-1, transforming growth factor-β2, -β3, basic fibroblast growth factor, as well as miRNAs *miR-18a* and *miR-19a* expression may be responsible for the clinical improvement after treatment. They suggested that their finding may have implications for novel treatments and further the understanding of fractional CO_2 laser treatment.[18]

Waibel J et al. demonstrated significant improvement in 10 patients with second- and third-degree burn scars who underwent five sessions of 1,550 nm nonablative fractional erbium laser at 4-week intervals. 60% of patients showed moderate to excellent improvement. 90% of subjects had improved skin texture, 80% had improved dyschromia, and 80% had improved hypertrophy/atrophy.[19] Ozog et al. recently published a report of 10 burn scar patients who experienced similar benefit. Histological evaluation of treated areas suggested a reorganization of the type I and III collagen profile to that of unwounded skin may largely explain the observed benefit.[20]

Stretch Marks (Striae)

Stretch marks are a challenging condition to treat. Fractional photothermolysis is suggested to improve texture and pigmentation in striae.[21]

Histological sections from treatment areas revealed thickening of the epidermis and dermis, neocollagenesis, and increased elastin deposition. Improvement in striae with minimal adverse effects has also been demonstrated following treatment with 1,550 nm NAFL.[22]

Kim et al. reported a case series of patients with striae distensae who were treated with 1,550 nm FP showed satisfactory improvement in overall appearance, patient satisfaction, erythema index, melanin index, and skin elasticity. On histologic examination, a significant increase in epidermal thickness and new collagen and elastic fiber deposition were noted (Fig. 7).[23,24]

Pigmentary Disorders

Melasma

Fractional lasers have been used successfully in the management of melasma and postinflammatory pigmentation in a number of studies.[25,33] The possible mechanism for the efficacy of FP in melasma is by the elimination of melanocytes- and keratinocytes-containing melanin granules through a "melanin shuttle."[3] Histologic studies have shown melanin deprivation from the epidermal basal cell layer 1 day after FP NAFL at the 1,550 nm wavelength has been approved by the FDA since 2005 for the treatment of patients with melasma.

The limitations in treating melasma include variable response, recurrence of pigmentation, and postinflammatory pigmentation especially in patients with darker skin. For these reasons, lasers are not routinely recommended for treating melasma in Indian patients. Further studies need to be carried

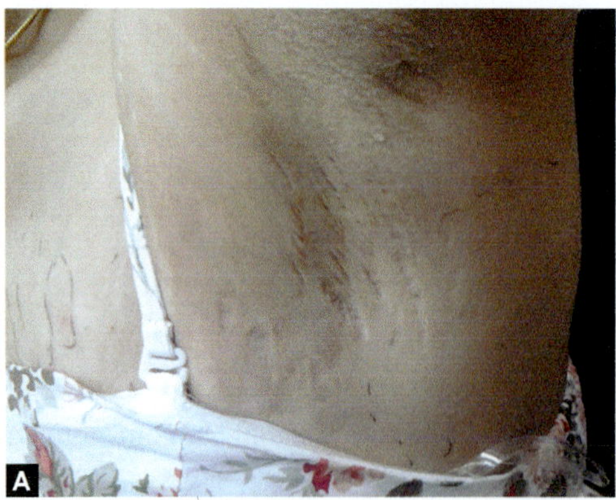
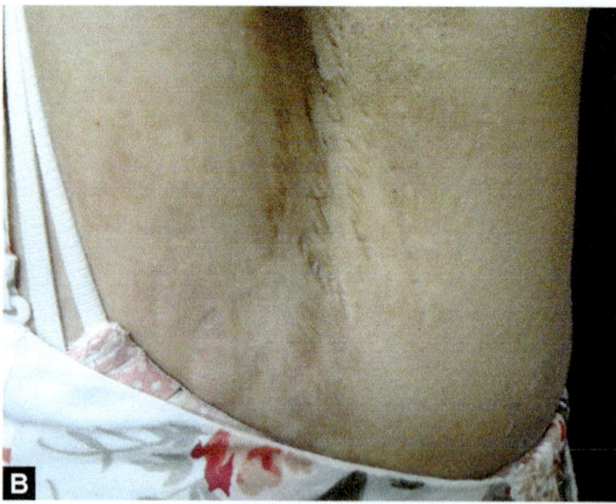

FIG. 7: A, Striae before treatment; and B, Striae 4 months after four sessions of 1565 mm erbium fiber laser.

out before fractional lasers can be recommended for routine treatment of melasma in darker skin types.

Other Pigmentary Disorders

Fractional photothermolysis has been used for the treatment of poikiloderma of Civatte (PC),[26] minocycline-induced pigmentation,[27] nevus of Ota,[28] and postinflammatory pigmentation.[29] Ablative fractional laser was found to be both safe and effective for the treatment of the vascular, pigmentary, and textural components of PC.[26]

Miscellaneous Indications

Fractional lasers have also been used for the treatment of residual hemangiomas,[30] telangiectatic matting,[31] granuloma annulare,[32] colloid milium,[33] and disseminated superficial actinic porokeratosis.[34] Blankenship et al. reported marked clinical improvement with 1,550 nm NAFL in case of residual hemangiomas.

There is a report of treating superficial lymphangioma with fractional ablative laser.[35] Fractional CO_2 laser was found to flatten fibrofatty residual tissue with improvement in color, texture, and overall appearance.[36] Silicone-induced foreign body reaction of face has been successfully treated with nonablative 1,550 nm erbium and ablative 10,600 nm CO_2 fractional laser.[37] There is evidence of use of fractional CO_2 in transfer of molecules through the skin and this, in turn, is used to optimize intracutaneous and transcutaneous delivery.[38] The author's experience fractional lasers have been found to be effective in treating lichen amyloidosis, shagreen patch, lentiginous hyperplasia, and port-wine stain with satisfactory results.

Port-wine Stain

The port-wine stain is described in figure 8.

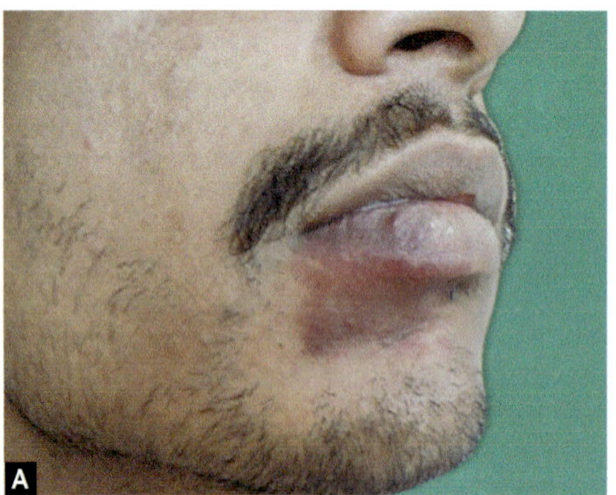
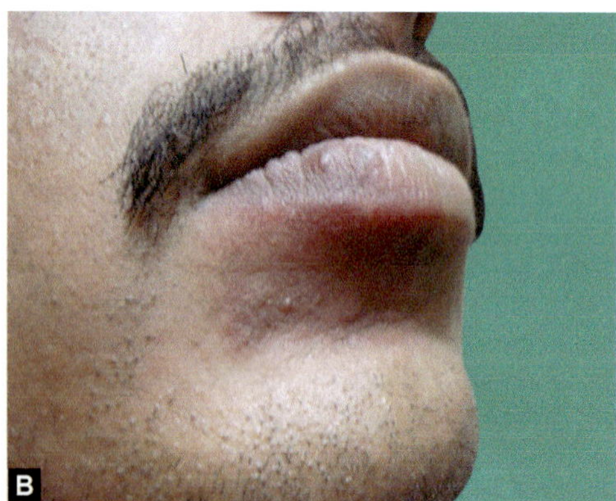

FIG. 8: A, Port-wine stain before treatment; and B, improvement in port-wine stain after treatment.

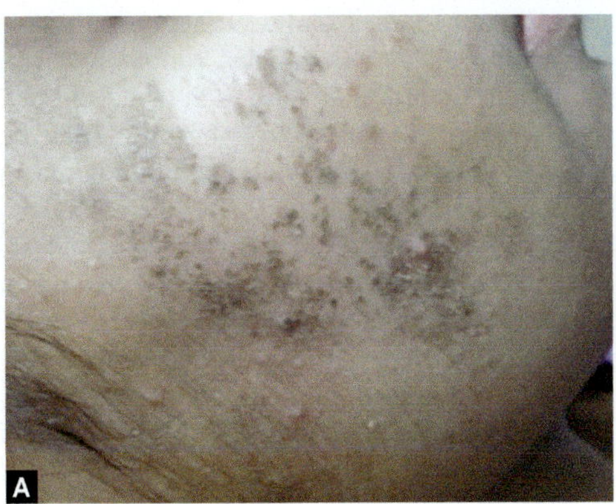

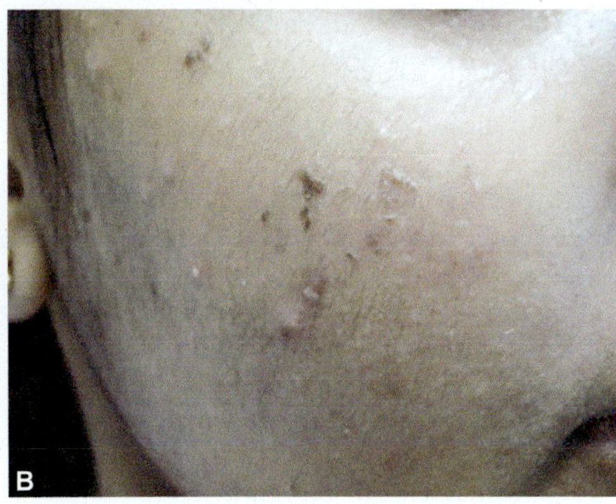

FIG. 9: A, Before treatment of disseminated actinic porokeratosis; and **A,** improvement after treatment.

Indications in Indian Skin

Of the earlier indications, the most common indications for fractional lasers include post-acne scarring, other types of scars, and dyschromias (Fig. 9). Their introduction has revolutionized the management of these conditions and also rendered the management of other difficult to treat dermatological conditions. Their safety also allows their usage in combination with other lasers such as Q-switched lasers in pigmentary conditions and tattoos.

FRACTIONAL LASERS AND PLATELET-RICH PLASMA

Platelet-rich plasma (PRP) combined with fractional laser has been shown to have a synergistic effect on facial rejuvenation, shortening duration of side effects, and promoting better therapeutic effect. In recent years, PRP has received extensive attention for various aesthetic indications. It is a small amount of plasma containing high concentration of platelets obtained from autologous whole blood after centrifugation. Platelet-rich plasma plays a vital role in the process of wound healing through secretion of a large number of growth factors. These can stimulate cellular migration, proliferation, and angiogenesis of PRP along with fractional laser therapy that may accelerate tissue repair and relieve pain. Combined application could not only effectively reduce facial wrinkles and texture, but also significantly relieve the coarse pores, pigmentation, and erythema caused by laser therapy.[39]

Lee JW et al. conducted a split face trial on 14 Korean participants with acne scars to evaluate the synergistic effects of autologous PRP with CO_2 fractional resurfacing for acne scars. They concluded that treatment with PRP after ablative CO_2 fractional resurfacing enhances recovery of laser damaged skin and synergistically improves the clinical appearance of acne scarring.[40]

In a study conducted by Shin MK et al., it was observed that PRP combined with fractional laser increased subject satisfaction and skin elasticity and decreased the erythema index. Platelet-rich plasma increased the length of the dermoepidermal junction, the amount of collagen, and the number of fibroblasts.[41]

Zhu JT et al., from their study, also concluded that PRP combined with erbium fractional laser therapy is an effective and safe approach for treating acne scars or acne, with minimal side effects, and it simultaneously enhanced the recovery of laser damaged skin.[42]

Tenna S et al. evaluated the efficacy of nanofat and PRP infiltration alone and combined with fractional CO_2 laser resurfacing to improve atrophic scars of the face and concluded that subcutaneous infiltration with nanofat and PRP seems to be effective to improve atrophic scars, either alone or combined with fractional CO_2 laser resurfacing. The FACE-Q module confirmed the impact of treatment of facial acne scars in social life and relationships.[43]

In another study by Abdelghani et al., 80 adult patients with nonsegmental vitiligo were treated with a combination of fractional CO_2 laser treatment and PRP for 2 months. More than 75% repigmentation was seen in 40% of the patients and more than 50% repigmentation was seen in 60% of the patients. Both fractional CO_2 laser and PRP injection gave poor results when done alone in patients of vitiligo.[44]

CONTRAINDICATIONS FOR FRACTIONAL LASERS

The contraindications for fractional lasers are listed as follows:

- History of immunocompromised status or active systemic disease that might interfere with wound healing
- Any active local or systemic infection
- Connective tissue disorders
- Pregnancy and lactation
- History of allergy to any medication necessary for treatment
- Active psoriasis or vitiligo, due to risk of koebnerization
- Unrealistic expectations
- Body dysmorphic disorder.

PATIENT SELECTION AND PREOPERATIVE MANAGEMENT

While fractional lasers are relatively safe, it is important to adhere to all standard precautions during their administration. Detailed informed consent should be obtained from all patients. Patients should be informed about the nature of treatment, precise procedural details, results expected, and the need for multiple sessions. Realistic expectation on the part of the patient should be stressed. Patients with dyspigmentation require two to three treatments, whereas those with rhytides require at least five or more treatments. Acne scars may need up to four to six sessions, depending on the depth, the type of scar, and also the machine used. Preprocedure photography is recommended in all patients before treatment and at each session.

Pretreatment History

Previous history of herpes labialis, keloid or hypertrophic scar, postinflammatory hyperpigmentation, isotretinoin intake, topical retinoid use, and lidocaine allergy should be noted.

Special Considerations

- Use in darker skin patients: All skin types can be treated with fractional lasers. However, it should be used with caution in patients with tendency for pigmentation and/or keloid formation. Proper counseling, priming with depigmenting agents and sunscreens, and initiation of treatment at lower fluences are advised in such patients
- All patients for facial resurfacing, with previous history of herpes labialis, should receive prophylactic oral antivirals such as acyclovir, famciclovir, or valacyclovir, starting 1 day before fractional resurfacing and continuing for 5 days postoperatively
- Oral antibiotics, such as cloxacillin or azithromycin, can be given to patients with a history of bacterial infections of the facial skin to reduce the chance of secondary bacterial infection
- While treating patients with melasma and postinflammatory pigmentation, prior priming with sunscreens and depigmenting agents for about 2–4 weeks is advised
- Pregnancy and lactation: Laser resurfacing is contraindicated in these cases
- Isotretinoin and fractional lasers: A 6-months waiting period following discontinuation of isotretinoin has been recommended before performing resurfacing procedures.[45] This is based on reports of keloid formation and atypical scar formation after use of dermabrasion and argon lasers, which are more invasive and ablative procedures.[46] However, several recent publications have documented the safety of fractional lasers in patients recently treated with isotretinoin.[47]

Kim HW et al. did one retrospective study to evaluate wound healing after ablative CO_2 fractional resurfacing for acne scarring which was conducted during and/or within 1–3 months of oral isotretinoin treatment. All patients showed normal reepithelialization and were satisfied with the results of the laser treatments and there were no report of hypertrophic scars or keloids.[48]

Ablation of a small test area may be a useful predictor of wound healing. Therefore, studies and published data on Indian skin are needed to make proper recommendations in this matter.

Anesthesia

This is patient and dosage specific. Lower fluences are tolerated well by most patients; but at higher fluence levels, topical anesthesia with mixture of lidocaine and prilocaine for 60 minutes prior to the procedure may be needed. Cold air or ice packs can also be used to decrease discomfort.[49]

Postoperative Care

Sunscreens and moisturizers are started soon after the procedure, and used daily. Mild topical steroid can be prescribed if erythema and edema persists.

Postoperative antibiotics are usually not necessary. Avoidance of rubbing and scratching is advised.

SIDE EFFECTS OF FRACTIONAL LASERS

The side effects of fractional lasers are minimal and transient. Mild erythema, edema, and peeling are common and can be managed by use of sunscreens and moisturizers. However, side effects do occur, particularly when aggressive doses/ multiple stackings are used, particularly in patients with darker skin.[47] Fractional ablative lasers are more likely to produce side effects than fractional nonablative lasers.[48]

- Erythema: There can be mild erythema for 2-3 days persisting up to a week. However, erythema persisting for 3-4 weeks has been noticed with higher fluences and multiple stackings[47,48]
- Posttreatment edema: This is mostly patient dependent. It can be seen for 2-3 days extending up to a week. The risk of edema increases with higher fluence levels
- Petechiae. Petechiae can be seen, especially in periorbital area, following use of higher fluences.[50] They usually develop after 3 days. This can be decreased by avoiding nonsteroidal anti-inflammatory drugs, aspirin, and other blood thinners in the immediate postoperative period
- Postinflammatory hypopigmentation and hyperpigmentation: The incidence of hyperpigmentation is considerably less when compared to ablative lasers, but it can still be seen in darker skin patients, especially patients with history of postinflammatory hyperpigmentation or melasma.[51] Higher fluences and multiple stackings should be used with caution in these patients. These patients should be pretreated with 2 weeks of depigmenting agents and a strict sun protection scheme. Hypopigmentation is rarely seen
- Bacterial infection: Bacterial infection is rare and seen in 0.1% of cases[52]
- Transient acneiform eruptions and milia can occur.[53] Flare-ups of acneiform eruptions can be prevented with antibiotics
- Cicatricial ectropion is a rare serious complication which has been reported with fractional CO_2 laser treatment[54]
- Another rare complication reported with fractional CO_2 laser used for neck rejuvenation is hypertrophic scarring.[55] Focal areas of erythema and induration, 2-4 weeks after treatment, are the first signs of potential scar formation. Neck is an area prone to such scarring. Postoperative wound infection, contact dermatitis, and tendency for keloidal scarring are other risk factors (Box 2).

BOX 2 Pearls to prevent complications and get better outcome[56]

- Careful patient selection
- Pre-treatment priming with sunscreens and skin lightening creams
- Post-procedure skin care such as using a broad spectrum sunscreen, instructions to avoid sun exposure, swimming and scrubs
- Keep treatment density low. Higher the treatment density (MTZ/cm^2), higher the risk of PIH
- Reduce the number of passes per treatment session
- Increasing treatment intervals if there is a history of PIH
- Provide additional cooling between passes to reduce bulk heating.

CONCLUSION

Fractional laser is an exciting technology to treat aging changes of skin, dyspigmentation, acne scars, and striae. Based on the wealth of studies noted earlier, it appears that NAFLs have less downtime and pain for most conditions. However, NAFLs may not be as effective per treatment compared to AFLs. Given that both ablative and nonablative fractional thermolysis are very effective and relatively safe, one could conclude that NAFL is a better approach due to decreased downtime and pain. Ablative fractional lasers certainly has the advantage in a new exciting area where one uses the ablative vertical channels to enhance drug and product delivery. As in all aesthetic treatments, proper training, judicious case selection, patient counseling about realistic expectations, and proper preoperative and postoperative care are important. Further, as in all new modalities, their use has to be done with caution, keeping the possible side effects in mind.

REFERENCES

1. Brightman LA, Brauer JA, Anolik R, et al. Ablative and fractional ablative lasers. Dermatol Clin. 2009;27(4):479-89.
2. Hantash BM, Mahmood MB. Fractional photothermolysis: a novel aesthetic laser surgery modality. Dermatol Surg. 2007;33(5):525-34.
3. Manstein D, Herron GS, Sink RK, et al. Fractional photothermolysis: a new concept for cutaneous remodeling

using microscopic patterns of thermal injury. Lasers Surg Med. 2004;34(5):426-38.
4. Walgrave S, Zelickson B, Childs J, et al. Pilot investigation of the correlation between histological and clinical effects of infrared fractional resurfacing lasers. Dermatol Surg. 2008;34(11):1443-53.
5. Rahman Z, Alam M, Dover JS. Fractional laser treatment for pigmentation and texture improvement. Skin Therapy Lett. 2006;11(9):7-11.
6. Chen KH, Tam KW, Chen IF, et al. A systematic review of comparative studies of CO_2 and erbium:YAG lasers in resurfacing facial rhytides (wrinkles). J Cosmet Laser Ther. 2017;19(4):199-204.
7. Mezzana P, Scarinci F, Costantino A, et al. Lower eyelid ablative fractional resurfacing: a new technique to treat skin laxity and photoaging. Acta Chir Plast. 2010;52(2-4):35-8.
8. Tierney EP, Hanke CW. Ablative fractionated CO_2, laser resurfacing for the neck: prospective study and review of the literature. J Drugs Dermatol. 2009;8(8):723-31.
9. Weiss R, Weiss M, Beasley K. Prospective split-face trial of a fixed spacing array computed scanned fractional CO_2 laser versus hand scanned 1550 nm fractional for rhytides. Am Soc Lasers Med Surg Confer. 2008.
10. Friedmann DP, Tzu JE, Kauvar AN, et al. Treatment of facial photodamage and rhytides using a novel 1,565 nm non-ablative fractional erbium-doped fiber laser. Lasers Surg Med. 2016;48(2):174-80.
11. Ong MW, Bashir SJ. Fractional laser resurfacing for acne scars: a review. Br J Dermatol. 2012;166(6):1160-9.
12. Rivera AE. Acne scarring: a review and current treatment modalities. J Am Acad Dermatol. 2008;59(4):659-76.
13. Lee Y. Combination treatment of surgical, post-traumatic and post-herpetic scars with ablative lasers followed by fractional laser and non-ablative laser in Asians. Lasers Surg Med. 2009;41(2):131-40.
14. Niwa AB, Mello AP, Torezan LA, et al. Fractional photothermolysis for the treatment of hypertrophic scars: clinical experience of eight cases. Dermatol Surg. 2009;35(5):773-7.
15. Jung JY, Jeong JJ, Roh HJ, et al. Early postoperative treatment of thyroidectomy scars using a fractional carbon dioxide laser. Dermatol Surg. 2011;37(2):217-23.
16. Gauglitz GG, Korting HC, Pavicic T, et al. Hypertrophic scarring and keloids: pathomechanisms and current and emerging treatment strategies. Mol Med. 2011;17(1-2):113-25.
17. Khandelwal A, Yelvington M, Tang X, et al. Ablative fractional photothermolysis for the treatment of hypertrophic burn scars in adult and pediatric patients: a single surgeon's experience. J Burn Care Res. 2014; 35(5):455-63.
18. Qu L, Liu A, Zhou L, et al. Clinical and molecular effects on mature burn scars after treatment with a fractional CO_2 laser. Lasers Surg Med. 2012;44(7):517-24.
19. Waibel J, Wulkan AJ, Lupo M, et al. Treatment of burn scars with the 1,550 nm nonablative fractional Erbium Laser. Lasers Surg Med. 2012;44(6):441-6.
20. Ozog DM, Liu A, Chaffins ML, et al. Evaluation of clinical results, histological architecture, and collagen expression following treatment of mature burn scars with a fractional carbon dioxide laser. JAMA Dermatol. 2013;149(1):50-7.
21. Clementoni MT, Lavagno R. A novel 1565 nm non-ablative fractional device for stretch marks: A preliminary report. J Cosmet Laser Ther. 2015;17(3):148-55.
22. de Angelis F, Kolesnikova L, Renato F, et al. Fractional nonablative 1540-nm laser treatment of striae distensae in Fitzpatrick skin types II to IV: clinical and histological results. Aesthet Surg J. 2011;31(4):411-9.
23. Kim BJ, Lee DH, Kim MN, et al. Fractional photothermolysis for the treatment of striae distensae in Asian skin. Am J Clin Dermatol. 2008;9(1):33-7.
24. Goldberg DJ, Berlin AL, Phelps R. Histologic and ultrastructural analysis of melasma after fractional resurfacing. Lasers Surg Med. 2008;40(2):134-8.
25. Neeley MR[h], Pearce FB, Collawn SS. Successful treatment of malar dermal melasma with a fractional ablative CO_2 laser in a patient with type V skin. J Cosmet Laser Ther. 2010;12(6):258-60.
26. Tierney EP, Hanke CW. Treatment of Poikiloderma of Civatte with ablative fractional laser resurfacing: prospective study and review of the literature. J Drugs Dermatol. 2009;8(6):527-34.
27. Izikson L, Anderson RR. Resolution of blue minocycline pigmentation of the face after fractional photothermolysis. Lasers Surg Med. 2008;40(6):399-401.
28. Kouba DJ, Fincher EF, Moy RL. Nevus of Ota successfully treated by fractional photothermolysis using a fractionated 1440-nm Nd:YAG laser. Arch Dermatol. 2008;144(2):156-8.
29. Rokhsar CK, Ciocon DH. Fractional photothermolysis for the treatment of postinflammatory hyperpigmentation after carbon dioxide laser resurfacing. Dermatol Surg. 2009;35(3):535-7.
30. Blankenship TM, Alster TS. Fractional photothermolysis of residual hemangioma. Dermatol Surg. 2008;34(8): 1112-4.
31. Glaich AS, Goldberg LH, Dai T, et al. Fractional photothermolysis for the treatment of telangiectatic matting: a case report. J Cosmet Laser Ther. 2007;9(2):101-3.
32. Karsai S, Hammes S, Rütten A, et al. Fractional photothermolysis for the treatment of granuloma annulare: a case report. Lasers Surg Med. 2008;40(5):319-22.
33. Marra DE, Pourrabbani S, Fincher EF, et al. Fractional photothermolysis for the treatment of adult colloid milium. Arch Dermatol. 2007;143(5):572-4.
34. Chrastil B, Glaich AS, Goldberg LH, et al. Fractional photothermolysis: a novel treatment for disseminated superficial actinic porokeratosis. Arch Dermatol. 2007;143(11):1450-2.
35. Tsilika K, Bahadoran P, Passeron T. Superficial lymphangioma treated with fractional ablative laser: a case report with clinical and reflectance confocal microscopy evaluation. Dermatol Surg. 2013;39(1 Pt 1):141-3.
36. Brightman LA, Brauer JA, Terushkin V, et al. Ablative Fractional Resurfacing for Involuted Hemangioma Residuum. Arch Dermatol. 2012;148(11):1294-8.

37. Cho S, Jung JY, Shin JU, et al. Silicone-induced foreign body reaction of the face successfully treated using nonablative 1,550-nm erbium-glass and ablative 10,600-nm carbon dioxide fractional lasers. Dermatol Surg. 2012;38(10):1744-6.
38. Haak CS, Bhayana B, Farinelli WA, et al. The impact of treatment density and molecular weight for fractional laser-assisted drug delivery. J Control Release. 2012;163(3):335-41.
39. Hui Q, Chang P, Guo B, et al. The Clinical Efficacy of Autologous Platelet-Rich Plasma Combined with Ultra-Pulsed Fractional CO_2 Laser Therapy for Facial Rejuvenation. Rejuvenation Res. 2017;20(1):25-31.
40. Lee JW, Kim BJ, Kim MN, et al. The efficacy of autologous platelet rich plasma combined with ablative carbon dioxide fractional resurfacing for acne scars: a simultaneous split-face trial. Dermatol Surg. 2011;37(7):931-8.
41. Shin MK, Lee JH, Lee SJ, et al. Platelet-rich plasma combined with fractional laser therapy for skin rejuvenation. Dermatol Surg. 2012;38(4):623-30.
42. Zhu JT, Xuan M, Zhang YN, et al. The efficacy of autologous platelet-rich plasma combined with erbium fractional laser therapy for facial acne scars or acne. Mol Med Rep. 2013;8(1):233-7.
43. Tenna S, Cogliandro A, Barone M, et al. Comparative Study Using Autologous Fat Grafts Plus Platelet-Rich Plasma With or Without Fractional CO_2 Laser Resurfacing in Treatment of Acne Scars: Analysis of Outcomes and Satisfaction with FACE-Q. Aesthetic Plast Surg. 2017;41(3):661-6.
44. Abdelghani R, Ahmed NA, Darwish HM. Combined treatment with fractional carbon dioxide laser, autologous platelet-rich plasma, and narrow band ultraviolet B for vitiligo in different body sites: A prospective, randomized comparative trial. J Cosmet Dermatol. 2017. [Epub ahead of print]
45. Dogan G. Possible isotretinoin-induced keloids in a patient with Behçet's disease. Clin Exp Dermatol. 2006; 31(4):535-7.
46. Rubenstein R, Roenigk HH, Stegman SJ, et al. Atypical keloids after dermabrasion of patients taking isotretinoin. J Am Acad Dermatol. 1986;15(2 Pt 1):280-5.
47. Leal H, Cantu P. Fractionated erbium laser during oral isotretinoin treatment. J Am Acad Dermatol. 2011;64(2 Suppl 1):AB18.
48. Kim HW, Chang SE, Kim JE, et al. The safe delivery of fractional ablative carbon dioxide laser treatment for acne scars in Asian patients receiving oral isotretinoin. Dermatol Surg. 2014;40(12):1361-6.
49. Fisher GH, Kim KH, Bernstein LJ, et al. Concurrent use of a handheld forced cold air device minimizes patient discomfort during fractional photothermolysis. Dermatol Surg. 2005;31(9 Pt 2):1242-3.
50. Fife DJ, Zachary CB. Delayed pinpoint purpura after fractionated carbon dioxide treatment in a patient taking ibuprofen in the postoperative period. Dermatol Surg. 2009;35(3):553.
51. Chan HH, Manstein D, Yu CS, et al. The prevalence and risk factors of post-inflammatory hyperpigmentation after fractional resurfacing in Asians. Lasers Surg Med. 2007;39(5):381-5.
52. Setyadi HG, Jacobs AA, Markus RF. Infectious complications after nonablative fractional resurfacing treatment. Dermatol Surg. 2008;34(11):1595-8.
53. Graber EM, Tanzi EL, Alster TS. Side effects and complications of fractional laser photothermolysis: experience with 961 treatments. Dermatol Surg. 2008;34(3): 301-5.
54. Fife DJ, Fitzpatrick RE, Zachary CB. Complications of fractional CO_2 laser resurfacing: four cases. Lasers Surg Med. 2009;41(3):179-84.
55. Avram MM, Tope WD, Yu T, et al. Hypertrophic scarring of the neck following ablative fractional carbon dioxide laser resurfacing. Lasers Surg Med. 2009;41(3): 185-8.
56. Kaushik SB, Alexis AF. Nonablative Fractional Laser Resurfacing in Skin of Color: Evidence-based Review. J Clin Aesthet Dermatol. 2017;10(6):51-67.

35

CHAPTER

Laser Hair Removal in Ethnic Skin

Keyvan Nouri, Anurag Tiwari

INTRODUCTION

Laser hair removal is one of the most commonly performed nonsurgical procedures and its popularity is growing rapidly in the field of cosmetic dermatology in India. Lasers for hair removal are currently approved for permanent hair reduction, meaning a complete (50–70%) but temporary loss of hair, after which, hair loss is partial, yet permanently reduced.[1] It is important, therefore, that patients are educated about laser capabilities and have realistic goals. With the advent of better laser technology, a greater understanding of selective photothermolysis, and appropriate safety precautions, lasers are safe and effective means of hair removal in all skin types.

MECHANISM OF ACTION

Lasers function on the principle of selective photothermolysis, a mechanism that permits the targeting of one particular structure over another by the selective wavelength absorption of different chromophores.[2] The skin contains many chromophores, some of which include melanin, hemoglobin, and water. In laser hair removal, lasers selectively target melanin in the hair bulge region while simultaneously protecting the outer, nontargeted tissue. By tailoring the laser's wavelength to the target chromophore, the chromophore's thermal relaxation time should be larger than the pulse duration, and the fluence must be large enough to destroy the chromophore.[3] Thus, when applying this theory to laser hair removal, particular chromophores in the skin can be targeted while protecting the adjacent tissue by changing parameters including fluence, pulse duration, and wavelength.[2]

The in-motion technology is said to cause photothermolysis of the bulge, the bulb, and the papillae of the hair follicle. Follicular stem cells in the bulge and dermal papillae are secondary targets. A hair conduction theory damaging the hair shafts thermally has also been proposed.

PATIENT SELECTION

Indications

Laser hair removal has been shown to be most efficacious in patients with fair skin and darkly pigmented hair; however, individuals from all demographics and varying skin phototypes can be treated with varying degrees of success.

Most commonly, hair removal is desired for cosmetic reasons. However, other conditions which require the laser hair reduction are (Figs 1–4):

- Hirsutism
- Hypertrichosis
- Pseudofolliculitis barbae
- Acne keloidalis nuchae
- Following skin grafting
- Pilonidal sinus.

Contraindications

- Active local infections: Patients with an active herpes simplex virus (HSV) outbreak should not be treated until the lesions have resolved. Antiviral prophylaxis for patients with history of HSV in treatment areas may be started 1 day prior to laser treatment, continuing for a total of 5–7 days[4]
- History of keloid and hypertrophic scarring: Possible problems with healing may occur if skin damage is sustained[5]
- Tattoos: Patients with tattoos in the area to be treated should be advised that changes in the

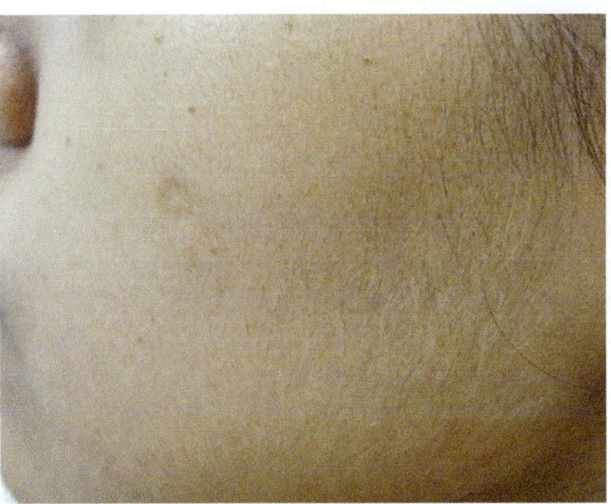

FIG. 1: Excessive vellus hair.
Courtesy: Dr Keyvan Nouri.

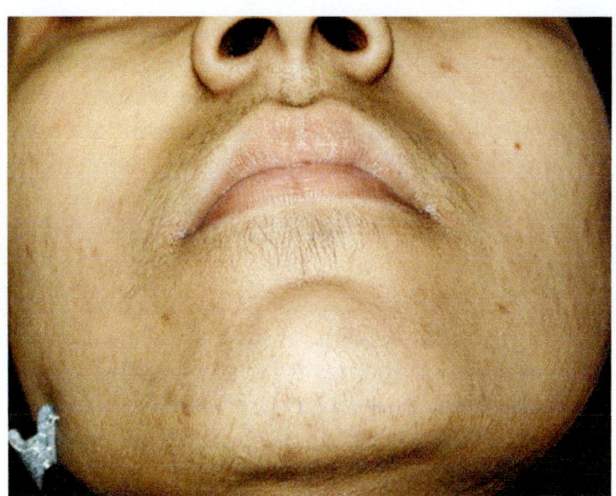

FIG. 2: Hirsutism.

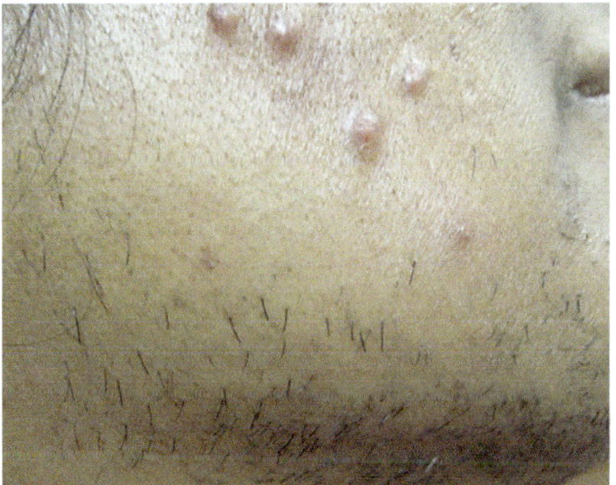

FIG. 3: Hirsutism.
Courtesy: Dr Keyvan Nouri.

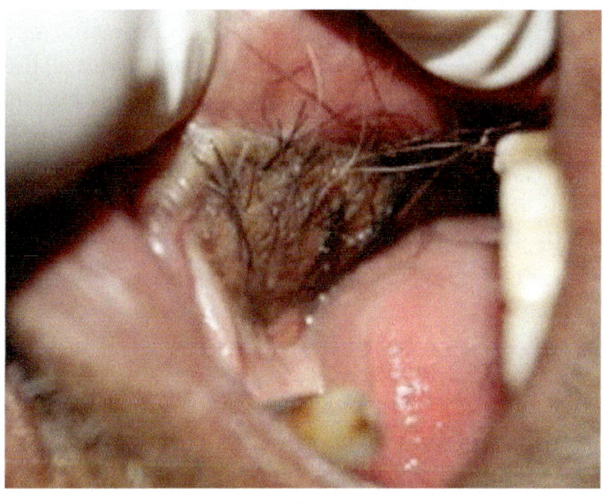

FIG. 4: Following skin grafting in oral mucosa.

tattoo color may occur. Treatment may lighten or darken certain pigments of the tattoo[6]

- Pregnancy: There is a paucity of studies investigating the safety of lasers for hair removal in pregnancy, it is recommended to avoid laser treatments because of the unknown effects on the fetus[6]
- Diseases that may be stimulated by light: Examples include porphyria, epilepsy, or lupus[4]
- Prior history of recent waxing, plucking, sugaring, electrolysis, or other methods of complete hair removal: Effective hair removal with laser-assisted devices requires the presence of a hair follicle for photothermolysis to commence.[4]

PREOPERATIVE MANAGEMENT

Laser Treatment Approach

As with any medical procedure, it is important to obtain a complete history and physical examination prior to treatment. This includes current medications, endocrine status, recent sun exposure, and history of other hair removal methods and their subsequent adverse reactions. Furthermore, it is important to examine for any infections in the treatment area as well as inquire about a history of scarring or postinflammatory hyperpigmentation from other procedures. Lastly, it is imperative to inquire about the patient's expectations as laser hair removal does not result in complete, permanent loss of all hair and many sessions may be required to achieve the desired effect. Patients should also be warned about the possibility of paradoxical hair growth following treatments. This effect may occur more frequently in those with a history of ovarian hyperandrogenism or polycystic ovarian syndrome (PCOS), as well as with darker phototypes.[7-9]

If the patient is considered a good candidate, preprocedure counseling is warranted. Patients who are scheduled to undergo laser hair removal should not pluck, wax, or use electrolysis for 2 weeks prior to treatment. Shaving is recommended. If the patient is of Fitzpatrick skin type IV, V, or VI, it may be beneficial to pretreat the area with hydroquinone/glycolic acid preparation as one study reported minimal adverse reactions with this regimen.[10]

If there is a history of severe or recurrent HSV, a 5–7 days regimen of antiviral prophylaxis may be initiated 2–3 days prior to treatment.[11] Protective eye shields must always be used when treating with all the types of lasers in all areas of the body.[12] While topical anesthetic may be applied before the procedure, the treatment area should be free of any makeup, deodorant, or topical agents before commencing. Lastly, test spotting in an inconspicuous, yet comparable region is recommended.

Appropriate Laser Parameters and Test Spots

Test spots should be chosen in an area with similar skin color, sun exposure, and hair density as the site to be treated. In general, 2–4 different fluence settings are recommended for testing and at least four, overlapping, spots should be administered for each fluence and pulse duration. By beginning with the safest parameters (longer pulse durations and lower fluences) and gradually progressing to shorter pulse durations and higher fluences, appropriate settings for every skin type may be achieved. For areas with higher hair density, such as the beard and upper back, the initial fluence must be even lower due to the increased risk of thermal damage that results from heat diffusion of closely adjacent hairs.[13] For patients with darker skin types, one should wait at least 2 days after performing test spots, as these patients may take 1–2 days to demonstrate side effects.

In all skin types, immediate effects classically include mild redness and perifollicular swelling that can last for a few minutes to a few hours. However, these responses are not always observed in darker skinned individuals due to the lower fluences that are typically used. In the setting of prolonged erythema or edema, however, fluence should be decreased. Blistering and crusting should be avoided, as these may result in discoloration and scarring. Severe or increased complaints of pain are additional indications for reducing fluence. Pain should be tolerable for most patients but topical anesthesia may be used for increased comfort.[13]

Techniques

Several different lasers and light sources have been successfully used in the treatment of unwanted or excessive hair; however, each hair removal device has its own inherent advantages and disadvantages. Certain lasers have been found to be safer and more efficacious in certain clinical scenarios; therefore, the clinician should be guided by both the laser's unique capabilities and limitations as well as the individual patient's potential for adverse outcomes.

Long-pulsed 694 nm Ruby Laser

The long-pulsed 694 nm ruby laser is the oldest laser used for hair removal. As it is primarily indicated for patients with fair skin and dark course hair, it is currently rarely used and not recommended for individuals with dark skin.

755 nm Alexandrite Laser

The wavelength can be produced by synthetic alexandrite crystal (conventional) or by diode crystal (newer machines).

They may be continuous or pulsed (both short and long), and typically have a larger spot size and higher repetition rate. While many studies have shown that the use of both short- and long-pulsed 755 nm alexandrite lasers are safe for use in ethnic skin, side effects such as erythema, edema, crusting, and transient hyper and hypopigmentation have still been documented.[10,14-17]

The short-pulsed 3 ms 755 nm alexandrite, along with a 10–18 mm spot size, has proven to be effective and appreciably safe in skin types I–VI. In darker skin types and tanned skin, the risk of epidermal damage increases due to laser targeting of epidermal melanosomes. In a study of skin types IV, V, and VI, Garcia et al. showed that three treatments at a fluence 18 J/cm^2 and 12 mm spot size resulted in a 2% incidence of side effects with no permanent scarring, albeit at just 40% effectiveness. The authors of this study, however, prescribed a pretreatment of hydroquinone/glycolic acid to the treatment area, directed patients to avoid sun exposure prior to and after each session, and applied topical betamethasone posttreatment. Therefore, it is unclear as to which factor played the greatest role in reducing side effects.

Longer pulses for the 755 nm alexandrite have been used as well. Lu et al. found that after five treatments with 20 ms pulse duration, 7–10 mm spot size, and 21–25 J/cm^2 fluence, hair quantity was reduced by 86–91%.[17] The alexandrite lasers were traditionally not used to treat dark skin due to lack of safety data, parameters, and high maintenance cost. However, after arrival of diode emitting alexandrite there is more acceptance of this wavelength. We now have stamping and in motion technology with contact cooling in these new machines.

Alexandrite is said to be more effective to treat fine hair. Initial results have been encouraging; however, long-term data needs to be looked at about its overall efficacy.

800 nm Pulsed Diode Laser

By producing light in the middle of the melanin absorption spectrum, the 800 nm diode laser is considered an effective system for melanin-targeted laser hair removal. When compared to the 1,064 nm neodymium-doped yttrium aluminum garnet (Nd:YAG), the shorter wavelength diode laser is more effective at hair removal due to its higher melanin absorption.[13] Furthermore, the 800 nm diode laser, like the 755 nm alexandrite laser, has a moderate depth of penetration and therefore is somewhat more selective in targeting dermal hair structures as opposed to epidermal melanin.

Diode laser has become very popular in our country. It is very effective and safe even in darker skin types when used with proper parameter's and care.

The initial fear has given way to bigger acceptance due to the efficacy, cost-benefit ratio, sturdiness, and less maintenance issues.

The in motion technology uses low energy with high repetition rate to progressively heat the epidermis. This is more suitable for body hair removal and is considered to be less painful than the stamping mode.

1,064 nm Long-pulsed Neodymium-doped Yttrium Aluminum Garnet Laser

Due to its longer wavelength, the 1,064 nm Nd:YAG laser has the deepest penetration and weakest absorption by melanin of all laser hair removal systems. By targeting hair structures approximately 5–7 mm below the skin's surface, the Nd:YAG may bypass the melanin-rich epidermis and result in less collateral damage in darker-skinned individuals despite the increased amounts of melanin present in ethnic skin. For this reason, the 1,064 nm Nd:YAG is considered safer for dark and tanned skin patients.[11,13,18,19]

Incidentally, the Nd:YAG laser may not be the most effective method of laser hair removal in fair-skinned individuals. A retrospective study of 805 consecutive laser-assisted hair removal treatments by means of either a long-pulsed Nd:YAG, a long-pulsed alexandrite, or a long-pulsed diode laser showed that the mean hair reduction was 42.4%, 65.6%, and 46.9% in Nd:YAG, alexandrite, and diode lasers, respectively. Although all were statistically significant changes, there was no mention if one method was statistically significant over the others. Incidence of side effects was the same for all lasers.[20]

Lasers with Multiple Wavelengths

Some machines have been developed to fire two or three wavelengths (diode ± alexandrite ± Nd:YAG) simultaneously. However, it is not yet clear if they have any advantage over the conventional single wavelength machines.

The possible logic behind combinations is to treat different kind of hair in the same sitting as each wavelength will travel to a different depth in the skin. The target chromophore (hair melanin) if deep would be hit by Nd:YAG and if in the upper layer then the diode/alexandrite will take care of it. The exact percentage of each wavelength in every shot is not known. We need to study these machines more before they can be considered safer and better.

Intense Pulsed Light (515–1,200 nm)

While not technically a laser, the intense pulsed light (IPL) system is indicated for nearly all conditions treatable by lasers, including hair removal. Intense pulsed light systems, like lasers, work on the principle of photothermolysis, and, therefore, target the endogenous chromophore melanin. Unlike lasers, however, IPL utilizes broadband flash lamps that emit incoherent light in the 515–1,200 nm spectrum, targeting additional chromophores such as water and hemoglobin. Optical filters are used to tailor the polychromatic light to specific needs and target one chromophore over others.[21]

There are several advantages to using IPL as opposed to other laser hair removal technologies.

The large spot size (120–450 mm^2) makes it easy to treat areas such as the back, chest, or legs, which would otherwise be time-consuming to treat with smaller spot-sized devices. Furthermore, IPL devices are usually less costly than monochromatic lasers. Due to their broad emission spectrum and selective filters, IPL systems also are easily tailored to treat a variety of conditions.

In terms of hair removal, effectiveness has been reported as high as 84% after four sessions.[22,23] A split-face comparison between IPL and the alexandrite 755 nm laser, however, proved that the alexandrite was more effective.[23] Moreover, disadvantages of IPL include decreased selectivity with inconsistent fluences, and thus a potentially increased risk of side effects. When compared to Nd:YAG (1,064 nm), IPL was shown to be less effective and resulted in significantly greater postinflammatory hyperpigmentation. Participants were of skin types IV, V, and VI.[24]

Radiofrequency

Radiofrequency devices have been used in combination with diode laser and IPL for hair removal. These combinations are safe in all skin types since radiofrequency energy is not absorbed by melanin in the epidermis.[25,26]

It is theorized that since IPL targets melanin within the hair shaft, heating the follicle from within, radiofrequency is a nonoptical energy source that works independently of melanin and heats the follicle from the outside. It is proposed that by combining these two mechanisms, destruction of nonpigmented hair may be obtained. However, practically the destruction of fine and nonpigmented hair is still beyond the capabilities of any available machine (Fig. 5).

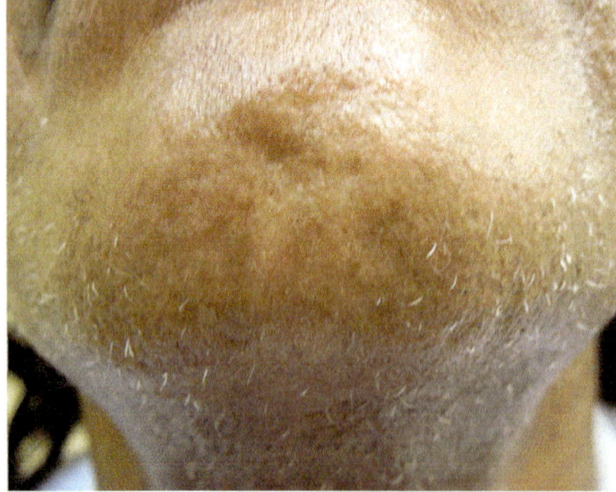

FIG. 5: Nonpigmented hair.
Courtesy: Dr Keyvan Nouri.

POSTOPERATIVE MANAGEMENT

After the procedure, ice packs may be placed over the treated area to minimize pain and edema. Analgesic medications are rarely necessary. To decrease posttreatment swelling and redness, mild topical steroid creams may be given. Topical antibiotics may be given for epidermal injury. Patients should avoid sun exposure and use sunblock.

Pediatric Population

Recently, hair removal lasers have been employed to treat a variety of pediatric conditions characterized by excessive or unwanted hair.

Often, the most concerning complication of hypertrichosis is the resultant cosmetic disfigurement; therefore, the decision to treat is dictated by both the extent of hypertrichosis and the degree of psychosocial impairment perceived by the patients and their families. While the safety and efficacy of lasers for hair removal has been extensively studied and is well established in adults, only a handful of studies have addressed these issues in children less than 16 years of age.

The pain and cost associated with treatments is also a major concern in the pediatric population. We need a more robust body for laser hair removal in children although it appears to be safe and efficacious.

SIDE EFFECTS AND COMPLICATIONS

Patient education must cover laser-induced side effects and a discussion with patients should be had before the procedure to address any expectations and concerns. Patients should be informed about possible discomfort during the procedure.

Side effects include scarring, pigmentary alterations, redness, bruising, swelling, blistering, erosions, crusting, superinfection, folliculitis, and superficial burns (Fig. 6).[27] Thermally-induced destruction of melanocytes contributes to hypopigmentation, while hyperpigmentation is the result of stimulated melanin production from melanocytes and is usually reversible (Fig. 7).[28] In a comparative evaluation of different lasers for hair removal in skin types IV, V, and VI, most of the side effects disappeared within 1–2 months.[29] There is also a greater risk of folliculitis in patients who swim or those with a predisposition for hyperhidrosis (Fig. 8).

Paradoxical Hypertrichosis

Paradoxical hypertrichosis has been defined as the development of a definite increase (when compared

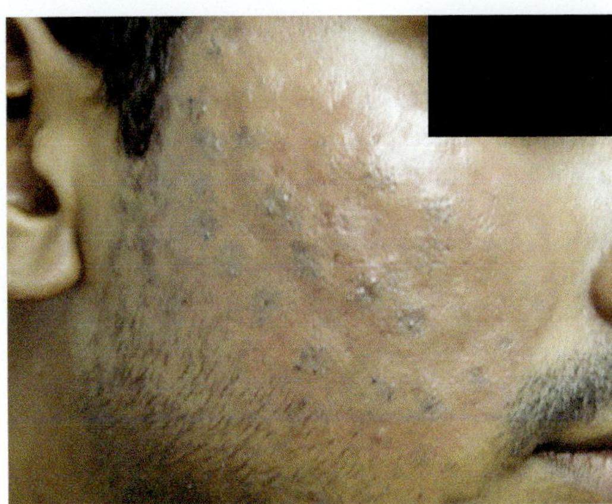

FIG. 6: Postlaser burns.

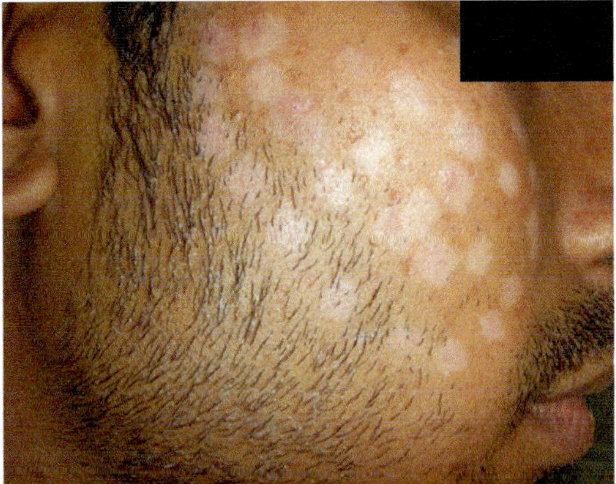

FIG. 7: Postinflammatory hypopigmentation.

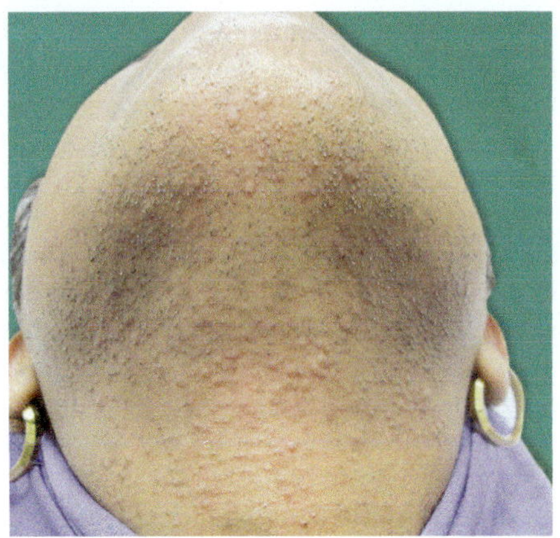

FIG. 8: Expected perifollicular erythema and edema immediately posttreatment.
Courtesy: Dr Keyvan Nouri.

to a patient's baseline) in hair density, color, coarseness, or a combination of these, at or around treated sites, in the absence of any other known cause of generalized hypertrichosis.[9] While the true incidence has yet to be established, estimates have been reported in the literature ranging anywhere from 0.06[9] to 4.5%[30] to as high as 10.2%.[7] Furthermore, the incidence of terminal hair induction likely varies depending on the laser or light source used.

Although usually associated with IPL, paradoxical hair induction has been reported with long-pulsed alexandrite, ruby, and diode lasers, and is most likely a potential side effect of all laser and light hair removal devices.[31-33]

The exact etiology of this adverse effect remains largely unknown. Bouzari et al. hypothesized that while the heat produced by the laser is insufficient to induce the thermal injury to the hair follicle required for miniaturization, the heat shock may be sufficient to induce follicular stem cell differentiation and growth by increasing the level of heat shock proteins.[34] Another proposed theory suggests that the process of laser depilation may serve to synchronize the cycling of hairs growing within the laser treatment sites. Theoretically, if all hairs were in the anagen phase for example, this would result in increased density compared to asynchronous growth.[33]

Paradoxical hair growth is most commonly observed in women on the face and neck, and on the back in men. Most cases occur several months (anywhere from 3 months to a year) after hair removal treatments and affected patients are reported to have undergone at least three treatments.[30]

Continuing hair removal treatments at the initial site and simply including the site of new hair growth have successfully treated most cases of paradoxical terminal hair differentiation. Due to the potential association with subtherapeutic fluences, it has been strongly encouraged to use higher fluence settings when possible to prevent this complication. Additionally, subsequent application of cold packs surrounding the treatment area during treatments and treating with two passes of the laser in the same session have been reported to effectively minimize the incidence of terminal hair growth.[31]

Tips While Treating Dark Skin (Types IV–VI)

- Wavelength: Opt for lasers with longer wavelengths in order to allow deeper penetration. This prevents the chances of epidermal melanin to compete as a target chromophore. It increases the ratio of the temperature of the hair bulb to the temperature of the epidermis allowing follicular destruction with relative sparing of the epidermis. This reduces the chances of PIH, burns, and scarring.

- Treatment parameters: Use conservative settings such as lower fluences and longer pulse durations to minimize the extent of epidermal and dermal injury and facilitate epidermal cooling, although these parameters may require a greater number of sessions.
- Pretreatment cooling with ice, cooling during treatment with inbuilt chill tip or external modalities, and post-treatment cooling with ice reduces chances of adverse effects.
- Pre- and post-treatment sun protection is mandatory.
- Use of exfoliants, scrubs, creams which cause exfoliation should be stopped a week before laser hair removal.
- Laser hair removal should not be done within two weeks of bleaching and chemical peels.
- Topical anesthetic preparations have a high potential of causing irritant reactions and subsequently burns with laser. Hence it is better to avoid topical anesthesia especially in dark or sensitive skin.
- Thin long hair which develop after a few treatment sessions need to be treated with a different wavelength such as 755 nm alexandrite laser or higher fluences with extensive cooling may be used.

FUTURE DIRECTIONS

Although lasers and IPL are considered as effective means of long-term hair removal, there is still much room for advancement. These can be made in exploring pretreatment regimens to help reduce the incidence of side effects, and in application of synthetic chromophores to aid in removal of nonpigmented hair. Optimization of these systems to produce the highest safety with lowest incidence of side effects to reduce side effects and increase effectiveness is always an aspiration.

CONCLUSION

Laser hair removal has become one of the most popular procedures in all of cosmetic dermatology. Excess hair is a condition that affects men and women of all ages. It is not only a cosmetic problem, but can also be associated with other conditions such as hypertrichosis, hirsutism, pseudofolliculitis barbae, and acne keloidalis nuchae. As with any medical procedure, it is important to obtain a complete history and do a physical examination prior to treatment. Laser and light technology offer a rapid, safe, and effective treatment for unwanted hair in patients of all skin types. The longer wavelength Nd:YAG laser is considered ideal for treating patients with darker skin, due to deeper penetration of laser light. The long-pulsed 755 nm alexandrite laser is also considered safe for use in ethnic skin. The use of longer pulse durations, conservative fluences, and multiple treatments increases the safety and efficacy of this procedure.

Prevention of unwanted side effects is especially important in darker skin tones, as there is a greater tendency to develop hypo- or hyperpigmentation. Despite many advances in this field, laser hair removal is largely limited to dark hairs. Further studies are needed to provide an effective treatment for patients with white, blond, or gray hairs.

REFERENCES

1. Dierickx C, Grossman MC. Laser hair removal. In: Dover JS, Alam M (Eds). Lasers and Lights. Philadelphia: Elsevier Saunders; 2005. pp. 61-76.
2. Anderson RR, Parrish JA. Selective photothermolysis: precise microsurgery by selective absorption of pulsed radiation. Science. 1983;220(4596):524-7.
3. Dierickx C, Alora MB, Dover JS. A clinical overview of hair removal using lasers and light sources. Dermatol Clin. 1999;17(2):357-66, ix.
4. Buddhadev RM, IADVL Dermatosurgery Task Force. Standard guidelines of care: laser and IPL hair reduction. Indian J Dermatol Venereol Leprol. 2008;74 Suppl:S68-74.
5. Kluger N, Hakimi S, Del Giudice P. Keloid occurring in a tattoo after laser hair removal. Acta Derm Venereol. 2009;89(3):334-5.
6. Kirman CN. (2015). Plastic Surgery for Laser Hair Removal Treatment and Management. [online] Available from: www.emedicine.medscape.com/article/1271154-treatment. [Accessed October, 2017].
7. Moreno-Arias GA, Castelo-Branco C, Ferrando J. Side-effects after IPL photodepilation. Dermatol Surg. 2002; 28(12):1131-4.
8. Navas E, Martín-Dávila P, Moreno L, et al. Paradoxical reactions of tuberculosis in patients with the acquired immunodeficiency syndrome who are treated with highly active antiretroviral therapy. Arch Intern Med. 2002;162(1):97-9.
9. Alajlan A, Shapiro J, Rivers JK, et al. Paradoxical hypertrichosis after laser epilation. J Am Acad Dermatol. 2005;53(1):85-8.

10. Garcia C, Alamoudi H, Nakib M, et al. Alexandrite laser hair removal is safe for Fitzpatrick skin types IV-VI. Dermatol Surg. 2000;26(2):130-4.
11. Battle EF. Advances in laser hair removal in skin of color. J Drugs Dermatol. 2011;10(11):1235-9.
12. Brilakis HS, Holland EJ. Diode-laser-induced cataract and iris atrophy as a complication of eyelid hair removal. Am J Ophthalmol. 2004;137(4):762-3.
13. Battle EF, Hobbs LM. Laser-assisted hair removal for darker skin types. Dermatol Ther. 2004;17(2):177-83.
14. Aldraibi MS, Touma DJ, Khachemoune A. Hair removal with the 3-msec alexandrite laser in patients with skin types IV-VI: efficacy, safety, and the role of topical corticosteroids in preventing side effects. J Drugs Dermatol. 2007;6(1):60-6.
15. Hussain M, Polnikorn N, Goldberg DJ. Laser-assisted hair removal in Asian skin: efficacy, complications, and the effect of single versus multiple treatments. Dermatol Surg. 2003;29(3):249-54.
16. Eremia S, Li CY, Umar SH, et al. Laser hair removal: long-term results with a 755 nm alexandrite laser. Dermatol Surg. 2001;27(11):920-4.
17. Lu SY, Lee CC, Wu YY. Hair removal by long-pulse alexandrite laser in oriental patients. Ann Plast Surg. 2001;47(4):404-11.
18. Battle EF. Cosmetic laser treatments for skin of color: A focus on safety and efficacy. J Drugs Dermatol. 2011;10(1):35-8.
19. Rao K, Sankar TK. Long-pulsed Nd:YAG laser-assisted hair removal in Fitzpatrick skin types IV-VI. Lasers Med Sci. 2011;26(5):623-6.
20. Bouzari N, Tabatabai H, Abbasi Z, et al. Laser hair removal: Comparison of long-pulsed Nd:YAG, long-pulsed alexandrite, and long-pulsed diode lasers. Dermatol Surg. 2004;30(4 Pt 1):498-502.
21. Babilas P, Schreml S, Szeimies RM, et al. Intense pulsed light (IPL): A review. Lasers Surg Med. 2010;42(2):93-104.
22. Feng Y, Zhao J, Gold MH. Skin rejuvenation in Asian skin: The analysis of clinical effects and basic mechanisms of intense pulsed light. J Drugs Dermatol. 2008;7(3):273-9.
23. McGill DJ, Hutchison C, McKenzie E, et al. A randomised, split-face comparison of facial hair removal with the alexandrite laser and intense pulsed light system. Lasers Surg Med. 2007;39(10):767-72.
24. Goh CL. Comparative study on a single treatment response to long pulse Nd:YAG lasers and intense pulse light therapy for hair removal on skin type IV to VI--is longer wavelengths lasers preferred over shorter wavelengths lights for assisted hair removal. J Dermatolog Treat. 2003;14(4):243-7.
25. Yaghmai D, Garden JM, Bakus AD, et al. Hair removal using a combination radio-frequency and intense pulsed light source. J Cosmet Laser Ther. 2004;6(4):201-7.
26. Karsai S, Schmitt L, Raulin C, et al. Combination of short- and long-pulsed mode of electro-optical synergy technology for photoepilation: a retrospective study with short- and long-term follow-up. J Eur Acad Dermatol Venereol. 2009;23(1):46-51.
27. Wanner M. Laser hair removal. Dermatol Ther. 2005; 18(3):209-16.
28. Lanigan SW. Incidence of side effects after laser hair removal. J Am Acad Dermatol. 2003;49(5):882-6.
29. Galadari I. Comparative evaluation of different hair removal lasers in skin types IV, V, and VI. Int J Dermatol. 2003;42(1):68-70.
30. Kontoes P, Vlachos S, Konstantinos M, et al. Hair induction after laser-assisted hair removal and its treatment. J Am Acad Dermatol. 2006;54(1):64-7.
31. Willey A, Torrontegui J, Azpiazu J, et al. Hair stimulation following laser and intense pulsed light photo-epilation: review of 543 cases and ways to manage it. Lasers Surg Med. 2007;39(4):297-301.
32. Hirsch RJ, Farinelli WA, Laughlin SA, et al. Hair growth induced by laser hair removal. Lasers Surg Med. 2003; 32(Suppl 15):63.
33. Radmanesh M. Paradoxical hypertrichosis and terminal hair change after intense pulsed light hair removal therapy. J Dermatolog Treat. 2009;20(1):52-4.
34. Bouzari N, Firooz AR. Lasers may induce terminal hair growth. Dermatol Surg. 2006;32(3):460.

36

CHAPTER

Lasers for Pigmentation

Anurag Tiwari

INTRODUCTION

Q-switched lasers (QSLs) are considered the gold standard for treating pigmented lesions and tattoos of the various types. Quality-switching (Q-switching) is actually creating very short pulses (5–100 ns) with extremely high peak powers. Of the various QSL available [Q-switched neodymium-doped yttrium aluminum garnet (Nd:YAG) (QSNY)] with its twin wavelength of 1,064 nm and frequency doubled 532 nm is the workhorse and most suited for treating darker skin types. Others which are available but better for skin type I–III are the QS alexandrite (755 nm), and the QS ruby (694 nm) due to increased chances of side effects like dyschromias, scarring, etc.

The longer wavelength of 1,064 nm of QSNY is useful for treating dermal lesions and blue-black tattoos. Whereas, the shorter wavelength of 532 nm is used for epidermal pigment and red color tattoos. Epidermal lesions need fewer sessions at shorter interval compared to dermal lesions.

BASICS AND MECHANISM OF ACTION

Melanin absorbs ultraviolet light up to 1,200 nm so there are many wavelengths and devices used to destroy it. Broadly, long wavelength and bigger spot size allow deeper penetration of the laser compared to shorter wavelengths. Various lasers like QS ruby 694 nm, QS alexandrite 755 nm, QSNY 1,064 nm, and frequency doubled 532 nm, intense pulsed light (IPL), etc. can be used.

Q-switched laser works on the principle of selective photothermolysis pioneered by Anderson and Parrish. According to this principle laser light targets a particular chromophore over another by preferential wavelength absorption of different structures. Few common chromophores in skin are water, melanin, and hemoglobin. To destroy the target chromophore the thermal relaxation time of target needs to be larger than the pulse duration, and the fluence of laser to be sufficiently high. The target chromophore here can be internal-melanin or external-tattoo particles. Apart from this, QSL also act by producing photoacoustic and photomechanical effects in the target by shock waves following irradiation with laser. These waves disrupt the melanosomes and the tattoo ink particles. These smaller particles are then phagocytosed and drained in the lymphatics for clearance from the body.

The 1,064 nm wavelength of QSNY laser penetrates 2–3 mm making it suitable for treating dermal pigmentation like nevus of Ota. When this beam is passed through potassium titanyl phosphate crystal, its frequency is doubled and wavelength is halved (532 nm). This new and short wavelength cannot penetrate deep, thus, making it useful to treat epidermal lesions like freckles.

Intense pulsed light systems use cutoff filters to block shorter wavelengths and to emit a broad band of light. These use wavelengths from 530 nm and above so can only be used to treat superficial conditions and not dermal lesions or for tattoo removal.[1-4]

INDICATIONS

Various lesions which can be treated by QSL:[5-7]

- Epidermal lesions: Freckles, lentigines, café-au-lait macule (CALM), solar lentigo, nevus spilus, etc.
- Dermal lesions: Nevus of Ota, blue nevus, and Hori's nevus (acquired bilateral nevus of Ota-like macules); tattoos—amateur, professional, cosmetic, traumatic, and fixed drug eruption
- Epidermal-dermal lesions: Postinflammation hyperpigmentation, nevus spilus, periorbital, perioral pigmentation, and melasma (Figs 1–3).

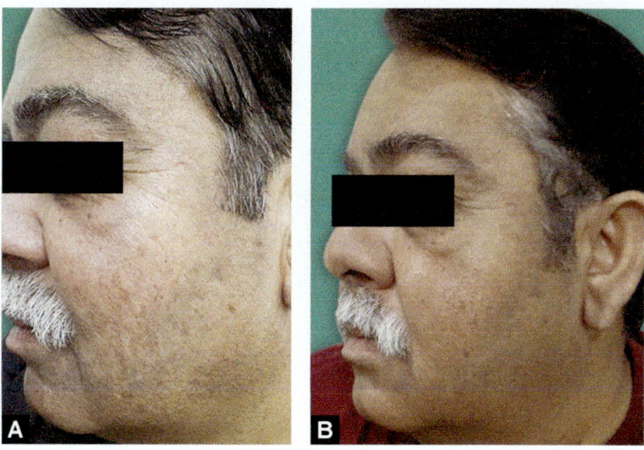

FIG. 1: A, Riehl's melanosis before treatment and **B,** Riehl's melanosis after treatment.
Courtesy: Dr Anuj Pall.

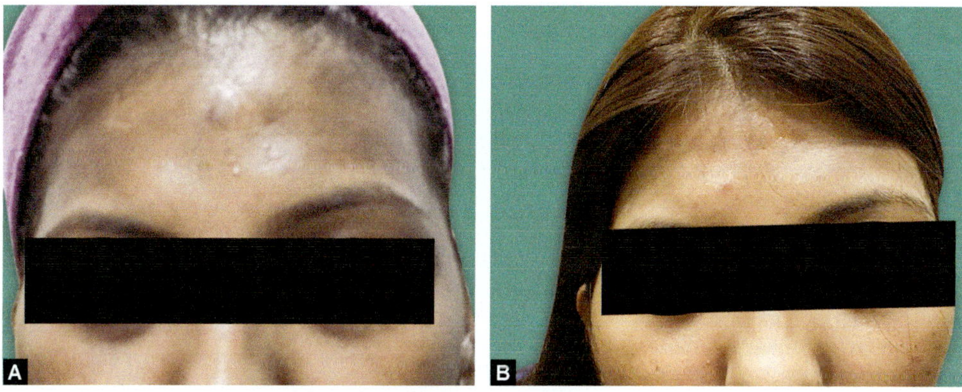

FIG. 2: A, Lichen planus pigmentosus before treatment and **B,** Lichen planus pigmentoses after treatment with 1064 nm Q switched Nd Yag laser. (Spectra XT).
Courtesy: Dr Abhay Talathi.

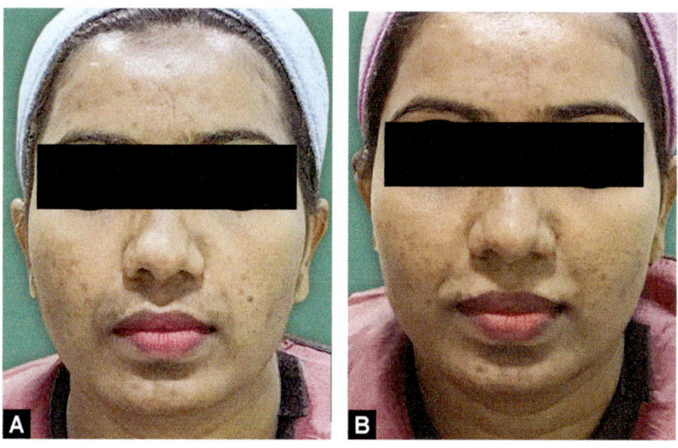

FIG. 3: A, Acne PIH before and **B,** Acne with PIH after treatment with 1064 nm Q switched Nd Yag laser. (Spectra XT).
Courtesy: Dr Abhay Talathi.

CONTRAINDICATIONS

Absolute

- Associated photoaggravated conditions like, systemic lupus erythematosus (SLE), etc.
- Treatment area having active infections, herpes labialis, staphylococcal infections, etc.
- Unstable vitiligo and psoriasis.
- Tattoo granuloma.
- Localized allergic reactions may result in urticaria and granulomatous reactions. During QS laser treatment, the ink particles are mobilized and travel all over, potentially triggering a systemic allergic response. These systemic reactions are more common in patients exhibiting a localized allergic response and pregnancy.
- Pregnancy.

Relative

In the following indications, laser has to be used cautiously, and after proper counseling of the patient; use of laser in these situations depends on individual situation and on treating dermatologist's judgment:

- Keloid and keloidal tendencies.
- Patient on isotretinoin.
- History of herpes simplex, the procedure should be performed after proper informed consent and only after starting oral acyclovir.
- Uncooperative patient and those with unrealistic expectation.

GENERAL GUIDELINES AND PATIENT SELECTION

Laser can be done as an outpatient procedure in the clinic/dedicated laser room/minor procedure room/operation theater, etc. The room should be devoid of mirrors and reflecting surfaces. Always have an assistant at the time of treatment with you, a female assistant is a must when the patient is a female. All persons in the room should have proper recommended eye protection while the lasing is going on. Try and indulge the patient in a monologue while doing the procedure particularly the first timers, it tends to take their mind off the laser sounds and relieves the apprehension. Soft music inside the room also gives a nice feel and comfort to the patient.

Prelaser Preparation

Take history regarding medical complaints, infections, allergies, and medicines being taken currently. Cause and outcome of previous surgeries with details about wound healing with reference to tendencies to develop scarring, keloid, postinflammatory hyper, or hypopigmentation should be inquired. Leading questions about allergies or irritation to topical anesthetic creams should be elicited.

Patient should undergo detailed counseling about the laser procedure. Incompletely informed patients generally have unrealistic expectations and create fuss that also brings disrepute. If possible, show pre and posttreatment photographs of patients who got average results rather than excellent results.

After clearly telling and counseling, take an informed written consent preferably in the language of understanding. In case of a minor, take the signature from parent/guardian. Good pretreatment photographs should be taken and then take them serially over successive visits.

Always put the patient on sunscreens and mild depigmenting creams. This prevents recurrence of epidermal lesions and also treats tanning, if present. Tanning alters the parameters to be used and it is advisable to either wait or remove the tan before laser procedure.

Test Patch

Beginners are advised to always do test patch preferably in a cosmetically unimportant area. This will help in determining the correct treatment parameters as they are individual specific. Parameters given in textbooks, and manuals acts as a reference point that needs to be adjusted. The response to test patch is seen after 6–8 weeks.

Test patch also acts as a confidence booster for patients and their family members.[6-11]

During Laser

Eye Protection

Q-switched laser can cause permanent retinal damage resulting in loss of vision.[8,12] It is absolutely essential that all the persons inside the laser room wear eye protective glasses. These are recommended and provided by the laser company as per the wavelength.

When treating eyelids, corneal shields must be used for the patient after putting topical anesthesia drops.

Selecting the Treatment Parameters

Fluence: Always use lowest fluence to produce an immediate whitening on the treated skin. If that does not happen then increase the fluence gradually. If there is significant debris or bleeding then lower the fluence.[6,7,11,13-16]

Spot size: For epidermal conditions choose a spot size just enough to cover the lesion. Larger spot will damage the normal skin and may lead to dyschromia. For conditions with dermal component use longer spot size which causes immediate whitening on the lasered area. As with all lasers, the larger the spot size deeper the penetration and lesser is the splatter.

Repetition rate: For small lesions and beginners a frequency of 1–2 Hz is recommended. For bigger lesions and when doing laser toning, it is better to treat with 5–10 Hz.

Endpoint: Immediate whitening (pseudo frosting) of the treated lesion is considered as the endpoint of the treatment.

Procedure

Once the appropriate laser parameters of correct spot size, fluence and frequency are selected, the treatment is completed keeping the handpiece perpendicular to the treatment area with up to 10% overlap. For larger lesions always start from one end and go across to avoid over treatment and skip areas. Immediate whitening is the desired outcome. Always tell the patient about the popping sound that occurs with each shot of laser becasuse they get startled with the strange loud noise and that may lead to an involuntary movement of the treated area. Never do stacking of pulses. Always cool the area to be treated with ice packs or air cooling devices before and after the laser.

Epidermal lesions may require one or two sittings, whereas dermal lesions may take five to seven sittings. As far as tattoos are concerned, it all depends on whether, it is an amateur, professional, or traumatic tattoo. Amateur tattoos respond most readily. Professional tattoos may require six to ten or more sessions to produce significant lightening. Traumatic tattoos clear with one or two treatments.

The treatment intervals range from 4 to 8 weeks. Dermal lesions like nevus of Ota are treated at intervals of 6–8 weeks and even longer intervals have been reported with good results. There is continued clearance of lesions in between the treatments due to removal of debris and particles by macrophages and lymphatics.[6,7,11,13-16]

Postlaser Care

Immediate postlaser the area is inflamed and sometimes tender with burning sensation, these are easily controlled by cooling with ice packs. This can be followed by application of topical antibiotic, if required and finally generous coating of sunscreen is applied before the patient leaves the clinic.

Oral antibiotics and anti-inflammatory drugs can be used as per the requirement and discretion of laser surgeon.

Strict instructions for avoidance of sun and regular applications of sunscreen are given. Patient is also instructed to report immediately, if any complications arise.[7,8]

COMPLICATIONS

- Postinflammatory hyperpigmentation: Most cases improve over a period of time. However, hydroquinone or other depigmenting creams along with sunscreens can be given for stubborn pigmentation
- Postinflammatory hypopigmentation: It can last for several weeks to months and is more dreaded by doctor and patient both. It is difficult to treat in few. Tacrolimus, narrowband ultraviolet-B (NBUVB), and targeted phototherapy have been used as a treatment modality
- Darkening of tattoo pigment, especially flesh-colored cosmetic tattoos. Red tattoos can turn black. If it occurs, it is difficult to treat
- Thermal injury and burns
- Localized allergic reactions can occur with almost any color of ink and can result in urticaria and granulomatous reactions. Red ink is the most common cause for allergic tattoo reactions. Other reactions which may occur are lichenoid and photoallergic reactions. After QSL treatment, the ink particles get further mobilized and trigger a severe systemic allergic response. For a patient having cutaneous reaction within a tattoo, QS should be used after treating the reaction with potent steroid creams. A test patch is always recommended. Patients with persistent allergic reactions in tattoos, may be treated with carbon dioxide (CO_2) or erbium-doped yttrium aluminum garnet (Er:YAG) laser ablation or dermabrasion
- Scarring: Happens rarely but could result from using very high fluence which may result in burn followed by secondary infection
- Infection: An antibiotic cream and a nonadherent dressing may be applied.[10,17-29]

TREATMENT PROTOCOL FOR VARIOUS INDICATIONS

Freckles

Respond very well in one or two treatments. They are notorious for recurrences and the patient should be told about maintenance sessions and sun protection.[30-32]

Lentigines

They can be removed completely in one or two sessions. Mucosal lesions also give good results.[30,32-38]

Café-au-lait Macules

Not easy to treat and require multiple sessions over a long period of time. However, recurrences occur in half of the patients. Also, there may be partial or incomplete clearance with pigmentary dyschromia (Fig. 4).[30,39,40]

Nevus Spilus

It does not respond uniformly to laser treatment due to the two components of pigmentation. The lighter base does not respond compared to the darker macular (junctional or compound nevus component) lesions which can be removed almost completely.[41-44]

Nevus of Ota

Laser treatment of nevus of Ota tends to give very good results. It requires six to ten sessions with 1,064 nm and a large spot size (6–8 mm) to achieve deeper penetration. The interval between two sessions varies from 6 weeks to 8 weeks. However, there are recommendations to do repetition after 6 months as well.[14,15,17,45-57]

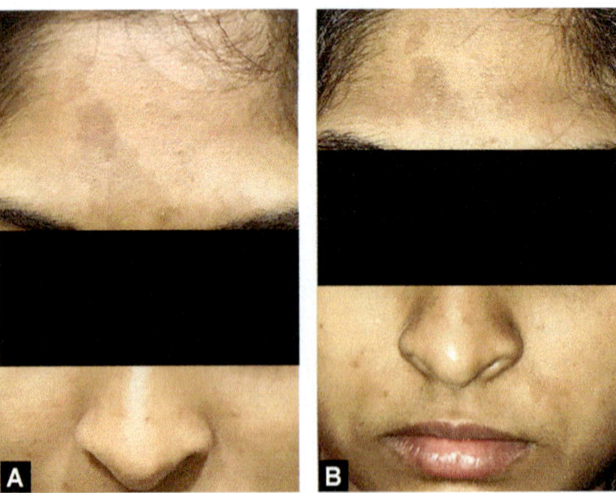

FIG. 4: A, CALM before treatment and **B,** CALM after treatment with 1064 nm Q switched Nd Yag laser. (Spectra XT). *Courtesy:* Dr Abhay Talathi.

Hori's Nevus

Hori's nevus mimics nevus of Ota closely but the late age of onset, bilateral and symmetrical occurrence, and also lack of mucosal involvement distinguishes it clinically. It responds well to long pulse 1,064 nm.[19,58-60]

Melasma

It is always better treated medically. Q-switched laser has been reported to be effective in treating melasma by many authors but overall the results have been varied. It can be used as an alternative treatment for stubborn melasma.

Chances of complication and recurrence are high. Hence, it is not recommended as a routine treatment. If the operator desires to treat, it should be done with utmost caution and preferably after doing a test patch on very low fluence.

Tattoos

Amateur Decorative Tattoos

They are blue or black in color due to the carbon-based ink which is superficially placed. They respond to treatment in 1–5 sessions.

Professional Tattoos

They are multicolored with deep and dense ink particles. Q-switched laser can remove black, and blue green colors (Fig. 5). Red color may darken on lasering, so test patches need to be done and use 532 nm wavelength. Green tattoos respond to 694 nm QS ruby laser. Some of these professional tattoos do not clear completely and leave a ghost image which may be treated with fractional devices. This needs multiple sessions or 8–10 or more at an interval of 6–8 weeks.

Traumatic Tattoos

It happens after road traffic accidents and responds very well in one or two treatments technique.

Advances in Tattoo Removal Techniques

R20 method: This involves multiple ablations in single session of laser.[61] During QSL, frosting is created which stops the penetration of laser into dermis. Frosting subsides in few minutes and the laser can penetrate again.

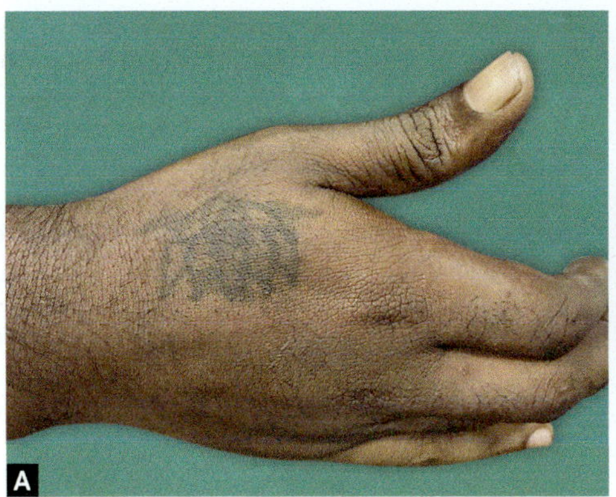

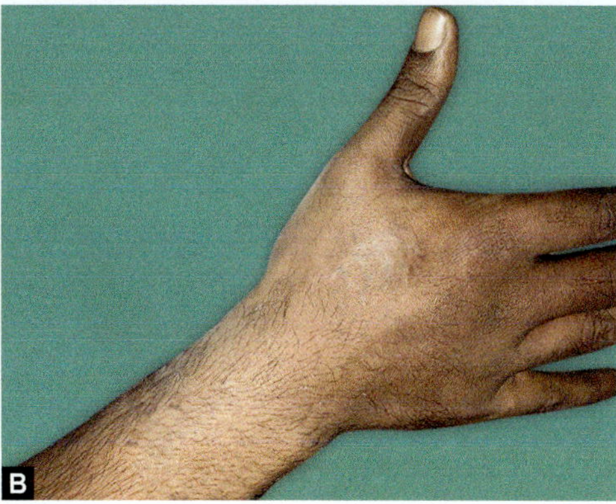

FIG. 5: A, Tattoo and **B,** Tattoo removed with 1064 nm Q switched Nd Yag laser.
Courtesy: Dr Abhay Talathi.

This principle is used for R20 method and four laser passes are done in single session after waiting for 20 minutes between each pass. The energy delivered remains the same for each pass. Higher rate of tattoo clearance has been observed compared to conventional method, however, the exact mechanism of action is not known. It is thought that the laser penetrates deeper following subsidence of frosting, thereby targeting more ink particles, also it fragments the ink into very small particles thereby getting easily phagocytized by macrophage and clearing it quickly.

R20 is more effective, number of treatment sessions required is reduced which increase the patient compliance. Particularly useful in army aspirants and patients who want quick results. However, it requires 3–4 hours to complete one session and may lead to increased chances of scarring, blistering, etc.

R0 method: The long waiting time in the clinic required for a session for R20 led to the development of this technique. First reported by Reddy et al., perfluorodecalin (PFD) is applied to reduce the frosting immediately and do the laser sessions quickly without waiting for 20 minutes.[62] Perfluorodecalin is a perfluorocarbon used by ophthalmologists for vitreous body replacement.

This compound absorbs the gas which is responsible for frosting during QSL and clears it in less than 5 seconds. Thereby, the next laser can be done immediately without waiting for 20 minutes and the treatment time reduces to approximately 5 minutes. Individuals have found comparable results from R20 and R0 methods.

Microencapsulated tattoo ink: Taking the research further, scientists have managed to make a permanent but easily removable ink in which the pigment is encapsulated in polymethylmethacrylate beads.[63] Unpublished data from Klitzman et al. shows 80% removal of tattoo in guinea pigs by a single laser session.

Laser toning: Laser toning is gradual removal of pigment by adjusting the total cumulative dose and interval of the treatment according to the response of each patient to the laser, beginning at the lowest fluence possible.[64]

PROPOSED MECHANISM OF ACTION

The use of peak powers and ultrashort pulse width of the 5 ns QSL with low fluence was demonstrated first in zebrafish and then in human melasma patients, whereby, the target melanin was selectively destroyed in the melanophores in the zebrafish and human keratinocytes, melanocytes, and dermal melanophores, but the cells containing the melanin were left alive. This was termed subcellular selective photothermolysis[65,66] and is the basis of laser toning.

The procedure is used by physicians to improve the quality, texture, and tone of skin. This technique involves using QSL with large spot size (>8 nm) with high frequency (8–10 Hz) with low fluence (1–1.5 J/cm^2). There are a number of protocols available for performing this ranging from once weekly to once a month. Laser session with 1–3 passes in each session.

Similar protocol is used in treating melasma. One should be cautious when starting this treatment as the speed at which the laser shoots (Hertz) is high so the hand movement should be well coordinated and equally fast else there are reports of depigmentation happening. The complications happen due to stacking of pulse or using higher energy.

PICOSECOND LASER

Q-switched laser has pulse duration in nanosecond range. In order to make it more effective the peak energy has to be higher which can be achieved if the pulse duration is shortened.

This shortening of pulse duration to picosecond has been achieved and the laser in the range of 50–100 picoseconds was introduced in the market. This machine heats up the pigment faster and creates finer fragmentation making it easier and faster for macrophages to remove these particles.

Brauer et al. demonstrated 75% removal of blue and green tattoos in 1–2 treatments.[67] Their safety in darker skin types needs to be evaluated and the cost is also a limiting factor.

COMBINATION OF LASERS

Monotherapy with lasers for pigmentation is effective. Combining QSL with fractional lasers both ablative and nonablative leads to quicker clearing and reducing the number of sessions and complications. This combination of lasers can be used for treating dermal pathologies like nevus of Ota, tattoos, etc. The combination can be in any order but doing fractional laser first followed by QSL reduces blister formation.[68]

The fractional laser (CO_2 or Er:YAG) drills microholes into the treated area and followed by QSL, these holes are said to protect the skin from higher fluence by allowing the gas to escape.

CONCLUSION

The search for an ideal laser for pigmented lesion is continuing. Q-switched laser is the gold standard for treating them today. However, we need safer quicker acting lasers which does away with need of multiple sessions.

Q-switched laser need a learning curve and like any other laser, needs to be treated and handled with respect and caution. Thorough knowledge of laser system and physics goes a long way in giving good results with the machine.

REFERENCES

1. Barlow RJ, Hruza GJ. Lasers and light tissue interactions. In: Goldberg DJ, Dover JS, Alam M (Eds). Procedures in Cosmetic Dermatology: Laser and Lights, 1st edition. Philadelphia: Elsevier; 2005. pp. 1-11.
2. OíShea DC, Callen WR, Rhodes WT. Introduction to lasers and their applications. Menlo Park: Addison-Wesley Publishing Co; 1978.
3. Anderson RR, Parrish JA. Selective photothermolysis: precise microsurgery by selective absorption of pulsed radiation. Science. 1983;220(4596):524-7.
4. Polla LL, Margolis RJ, Dover JS, et al. Melanosomes are a primary target of Q-switched ruby laser irradiation in guinea pig skin. J Invest Dermatol. 1987;89(3):281-6.
5. Kilmer SL. Laser eradication of pigmented lesions and tattoos. Dermatol Clin. 2002;20(1):37-53.
6. Goldberg DJ. Pigmented lesions, tattoos, and disorders of hypopigmentation. In: Goldberg DJ (Ed). Laser Dermatology: Pearls and Problems, 1st edition. Massachusetts: Blackwell publishing; 2008. pp. 71-114.
7. Kilmer SL, Garden JM. Laser treatment of pigmented lesions and tattoos. Semin Cutan Med Surg. 2000;19(4):232-44.
8. Schmults CD, Wheeland RG. Pigmented lesions and tattoos. In: Goldberg DJ, Dover JS, Alam M (Eds). Procedures in Cosmetic Dermatology: Laser and Lights, 1st edition. Philadelphia: Elsevier; 2005. pp. 41-66.
9. Kilmer SL. Laser treatment of tattoos. Dermatol Clin. 1997;15(3):409-17.
10. Grevelink JM, Duke D, van Leeuwen RL, et al. Laser treatment of tattoos in darkly pigmented patients: efficacy and side effects. J Am Acad Dermatol. 1996;34(4):653-6.
11. Adrian RM, Griffin L. Laser tattoo removal. Clin Plast Surg. 2000;27(2):181-92.
12. Russell SW, Dinehart SM, Davis I, et al. Efficacy of corneal eye shields in protecting patients' eyes from laser irradiation. Dermatol Surg. 1996;22(7):613-6.
13. Kilmer SL, Farinelli WF, Tearney G, et al. Use of a larger spot size for the treatment of tattoos increases clinical efficacy and decreases potential side effects. Lasers Surg Med. 1994;6:S51.
14. Chan HH, Lam LK, Wong DS, et al. Nevus of Ota: a new classification based on the response to laser treatment. Laser Surg Med. 2001;28(3):267-72.
15. Ueda S, Isoda M, Imayama S. Response of naevus of Ota to Q-switched ruby laser treatment according to lesion color. Br J Dermatol. 2000;142(1):77-83.
16. Kilmer SL, Lee MS, Grevelink JM, et al. The Q-switched Nd:YAG laser effectively treats tattoos. A controlled, dose-response study. Arch Dermatol. 1993;129(8):971-8.
17. Kono T, Nozaki M, Chan HH, et al. A retrospective study looking at the long-term complications of Q-switched ruby laser in the treatment of nevus of Ota. Lasers Surg Med. 2001;29(2):156-9.
18. Rheingold LM, Fater MC, Courtiss EH. Compartment syndrome of the upper extremity following cutaneous laser surgery. Plast Recontr Surg. 1997;99(5):1418-20.
19. Lam AY, Wong DS, Lam LK, et al. A retrospective study on the efficacy and complications of Q-switched

alexandrite laser in the treatment of acquired bilateral nevus of Ota-like macules. Dermatol Surg. 2001;27(11): 937-41.

20. Anderson RR, Geronemus R, Kilmer SL, et al. Cosmetic tattoo ink darkening. A complication of Q-switched and pulsed-laser treatment. Arch Dermatol. 1993;129(8): 1010-4.
21. Ross EV, Yashar S, Michaud N, et al. Tattoo darkening and nonresponse after laser treatment: a possible role for titanium dioxide. Arch Dermatol. 2001;137(1):33-7.
22. Fusade T, Toubel G, Grognard C, et al. Treatment of gunpowder traumatic tattoo by Q-switched Nd:YAG laser: an unusual adverse effect. Dermatol Surg. 2000;26(11):1057-9.
23. Jacob CI. Tattoo-associated dermatoses: a case report and review of the literature. Dermatol Surg. 2002;28(10):962-5.
24. Bhardwaj SS, Brodell RT, Taylor JS. Red tattoo reactions. Contact Dermatitis. 2003;48(4):236-7.
25. Ashinoff R, Levine VJ, Soter NA. Allergic reactions to tattoo pigment after laser treatment. Dermatol Surg. 1995;21(4):291-4.
26. England RW, Vogel P, Hagan L. Immediate cutaneous hypersensitivity after treatment of tattoo with Nd:YAG laser: a case report and review of the literature. Ann Allergy Asthma Immunol. 2002;89(2):215-7.
27. Kyanko ME, Pontasch MJ, Brodell RT. Red tattoo reactions: treatment with the carbon dioxide laser. J Dermatol Surg Oncol. 1989;15(6):652-6.
28. De Argila D, Chaves A, Moreno JC. Erbium:Yag laser therapy of lichenoid red tattoo reactions. J Eur Acad Dermatol Venereol. 2004;18(3):332-3.
29. Jimenez G, Weiss E, Spencer JM. Multiple color changes following laser therapy of cosmetic tattoos. Dermatol Surg. 2002;28(2):177-9.
30. Kilmer SL, Wheeland RJ, Goldberg DJ, et al. Treatment of epidermal pigmented lesions with the frequency-doubled Q-switched Nd:YAG laser. A controlled, single-impact, dose-response, multicenter trial. Arch Dermatol. 1994;130(12):1515-9.
31. Jang KA, Chung EC, Choi JH, et al. Successful removal of freckles in Asian skin with a Q-switched alexandrite laser. Dermatol Surg. 2000;26(3):231-4.
32. Wang CC, Sue YM, Yang CH, et al. A comparison of Q-switched alexandrite laser and intense pulsed light for the treatment of freckles and lentigines in Asian persons: a randomized, physician-blinded, split-face comparative trial. J Am Acad Dermatol. 2006;54(5):804-10.
33. Jiang SB, Levine V, Ashinoff R. The treatment of solar lentigines with the diode (Diolite 532 nm) and the Q-switched ruby laser: a comparative study. Laser Surg Med Suppl. 2000;12:55.
34. Todd MM, Rallis TM, Gerwels JW, et al. A comparison of 3 lasers and liquid nitrogen in the treatment of solar lentigines: a randomized, controlled, comparative trial. Arch Dermatol. 2000;136(7):841-6.
35. Li YT, Yang KC. Comparison of frequency-doubled Q-switched Nd:YAG laser and 35% trichloroacetic acid for the treatment of face lentigines. Dermatol Surg. 1999;25(3):202-4.
36. Bjerring P, Christiansen K. Intense pulsed light source for treatment of small melanocytic nevi and solar lentigines. J Cutan Laser Ther. 2000;2(4):177-81.
37. Kono T, Manstein D, Chan HH, et al. Q-switched ruby versus long-pulsed dye laser delivered with compression for treatment of facial lentigines in Asians. Laser Surg Med. 2006;38(2):94-7.
38. Chan HH, Fung WK, Ying SY, et al. An in vivo trial comparing the use of different types of 532 nm Nd:YAG lasers in the treatment of facial lentigines in Oriental patients. Dermatol Surg. 2000;26(8):743-9.
39. Levy JL, Mordon S, Pizzi-Anselme M. Treatment of individual cafè au lait macules with the Q-switched Nd:YAG: a clinicopathologic correlation. J Cutan Laser Ther. 1999;1(4):217-23.
40. Grossman MC, Anderson RR, Farinelli W, et al. Treatment of cafe au lait macules with lasers. A clinicopathologic correlation. Arch Dermatol. 1995;131(12):1416-20.
41. Grevelink JM, González S, Bonoan R, et al. Treatment of nevus spilus with the Q-switched ruby laser. Dermatol Surg. 1997;23(5):365-9.
42. Gold MH, Foster TD, Bell MW. Nevus spilus successfully treated with an intense pulsed light source. Dermatol Surg. 1999;25(3):254-5.
43. Moreno-Arias GA, Bulla F, Vilata-Corell JJ, et al. Treatment of widespread segmental nevus spilus by Q-switched alexandrite laser (755 nm, 100 nsec). Dermatol Surg. 2001;27(9):841-3.
44. Abecassis S, Spatz A, Cazeneuve C, et al. Melanoma within naevus spilus: 5 cases. Ann Dermatol Venereol. 2006;133(4):323-8.
45. Chan HH, Leung RS, Ying SY, et al. A retrospective analysis of complications in the treatment of nevus of Ota with the Q-switched alexandrite and Q-switched Nd:YAG lasers. Dermatol Surg. 2000;26(11):1000-6.
46. Chan HH, King WW, Chan ES, et al. In vivo trial comparing patients' tolerance of Q-switched Alexandrite (QS Alex) and Q-switched neodymium:yttrium-aluminum-garnet (QS Nd:YAG) lasers in the treatment of nevus of Ota. Lasers Surg Med. 1999;24(1):24-8.
47. Chan HH, Ying SY, Ho WS, et al. An in vivo trial comparing the clinical efficacy and complications of Q-switched 755 nm alexandrite and Q-switched 1064 nm Nd:YAG lasers in the treatment of nevus of Ota. Dermatol Surg. 2000;26(10):919-22.
48. Kilmer SL, Anderson RR. Clinical use of the Q-switched ruby and the Q-switched Nd:YAG (1064 nm and 532 nm) lasers for treatment of tattoos. J Dermatol Surg Oncol. 1993;19(4):330-8.
49. Goldberg DJ, Nychay SG. Q-switched ruby laser treatment of nevus of Ota. J Dermatol Surg Oncol. 1992;18(9):817-21.
50. Watanabe S, Takahashi H. Treatment of nevus of Ota with the Q-switched ruby laser. N Engl J Med. 1994;331(26):1745-50.
51. Geronemus RG. Q-switched ruby laser therapy of nevus of Ota. Arch Dermatol. 1992;128(12):1618-22.

52. Alster TS, Williams CM. Treatment of nevus of Ota by the Q-switched alexandrite laser. Dermatol Surg. 1995;21(7):592-6.
53. Turnbull JR, Assaf Ch, Zouboulis C, et al. Bilateral nevus of Ota: a rare manifestation in a Caucasian. J Eur Acad Dermatol Venereol. 2004;18(3):353-5.
54. Kopf AW, Bart RS. Malignant blue (otaís) nevus. J Dermatol Surg Oncol. 1982;8:442-5.
55. Patel BC, Egan CA, Lucius RW, et al. Cutaneous malignant melanoma and oculodermal melanocytosis (nevus of Ota): report of a case and review of the literature. J Am Acad Dermatol. 1998;38(5 Pt 2):862-5.
56. Lowe NJ, Wieder JM, Sawcer D, et al. Nevus of Ota: treatment with high energy fluences of the Q-switched ruby laser. J Am Acad Dermatol. 1993;29(6):997-1001.
57. Chan HH, Lam LK, Wong DS, et al. Role of skin cooling in improving patient tolerability of Q-switched alexandrite (QS Alex) laser in nevus of Ota treatment. Lasers Surg Med. 2003;32:148-51.
58. Kunachak S, Leelaudomlipi P. Q-switched Nd:YAG laser treatment for acquired bilateral nevus of ota-like maculae: a long-term follow-up. Laser Surg Med. 2000;26(4):376-9.
59. Polnikorn N, Tanrattanakorn S, Goldberg DJ. Treatment of Horís nevus with the Q-switched Nd:YAG laser. Dermatol Surg. 2000;26:477-80.
60. Lee B, Kim YC, Kang WH, et al. Comparison of characteristics of acquired bilateral nevus of Ota-like macules and nevus of Ota according to therapeutic outcome. J Korean Med Sci. 2004;19(4):554-9.
61. Kossida T, Rigopoulos D, Katsambas A, et al. Optimal tattoo removal in a single laser session based on the method of repeated exposures. J Am Acad Dermatol. 2012;66(2):271-7.
62. Zawar V, Sarda A, De A. Bindi tattoo on forehead: success with modified R-20 technique using low fluence q-switched nd yag laser: a case report. J Cutan Aesthet Surg. 2014;7(1):54-5.
63. Fox MA, Diven DG, Sra K, et al. Dermal scatter reduction in human skin: a method using controlled application of glycerol. Lasers Surg Med. 2009;41(4):251-5.
64. Kim HM. Effect of low fluence Q-switched 1,064 nm Nd:YAG laser therapy on melasma. Aesth Dermatol. 2010;20:343-7.
65. Mun JY, Jeong SY, Kim JH, et al. A low fluence Q-switched Nd:YAG laser modifies the 3D structure of melanocyte and ultrastructure of melanosome by subcellular-selective photothermolysis. J Electron Microsc (Tokyo). 2011;60(1):11-8.
66. Kim JH, Kim H, Park HC, et al. Subcellular selective photothermolysis of melanosomes in adult zebrafish skin following 1064-Nm Q-switched Nd:YAG laser irradiation. J Invest Dermatol. 2010;130(9):2333-5.
67. Brauer JA, Reddy KK, Anolik R, et al. Successful and rapid treatment of blue and green tattoo pigment with a novel picosecond laser. Arch Dermatol. 2012;148(7):820-3.
68. Marini L, Kozarev J, Grad L, et al. Fractional Er:YAG skin conditioning for enhanced efficacy for Nd:YAG Q-switched laser tattoo removal. J Laser Health Acad. 2012;1:35-40.

37 CHAPTER

Microneedling

Jaishree Sharad

INTRODUCTION

Microneedling is also known as skin needling therapy or percutaneous collagen induction therapy. It is an innovative, simple, and minimally invasive therapeutic technique which is used for the treatment of atrophic scars, stretch marks, alopecia, transdermal drug delivery, and skin rejuvenation. A handheld small rolling instrument with tiny protruding needles called as dermaroller is used to create multiple microinjuries in the skin, inducing new collagen synthesis. Microneedling can be used in combination with other techniques like chemical peels, lasers, platelet-rich plasma (PRP), and fillers for superior results.

Pioneered in 1995, Orentreich and Orentreich described subcision or dermal needling for scars.[1] This approach involves pricking or puncturing the skin and subcising the dermis with the needle to buildup connective tissue beneath the scars. Camirand and Doucet in 1997 used a tattoo gun to "needle abrade" scars.[2] Based on these principles, Fernandes developed a new technology, microneedling, to initiate the natural post-traumatic inflammatory cascade.[3]

INSTRUMENT

The Food and Drug Administration (FDA)-approved dermaroller is a handheld device equipped with medical-grade solid steel microneedles, projecting from a cylindrical roller. There are 24 circular arrays of eight needles each located on the roller (total 192 needles) and the needles vary in lengths ranging from 0.2 mm to 3 mm. The microneedles are synthesized by reactive ion etching techniques on silicon or medical-grade stainless steel. For adequate and uniform penetration, the needles are arranged at an angle of 15° to the center of the instrument. The most preferred needle length for dermatological use is 1.5 mm. The depth of penetration varies from 0.1 mm to 1.3 mm depending on the pressure and extent of skin stretching. The instrument is presterilized by gamma irradiation.[3]

PRINCIPLE

Microneedling involves the use of a handheld rolling instrument with tiny needles which create multiple superficial puncture wounds in the skin. Rolling a Dermaroller (192 needles, 200 μm length, and 70 μm diameter) over an area 15 times, results in approximately 250 holes/cm^2. Multiple superficial punctures are created that cause controlled injury by breaking down the collagen without any epidermal damage. The tiny microinjuries in the upper dermis release numerous growth factors, such as fibroblast growth factor, platelet-derived growth factor, and transforming growth factors (TGFs) α and β, which facilitate the production and propagation of intercellular matrix proteins.[4] The fibroblasts are laid down along the axis of the fibronectin matrix where they synthesize collagen and elastin. Collagen type III is the dominant form in the early wound-healing phase.[5,6]

Fibroblast synthesis causes tissue remodeling over the next few months. Collagen type III is gradually replaced by collagen type I over a period of 1 year or more.[4] Scar collagen synthesis due to thermal injury involves upregulation of TGF-β1 and β2, whereas natural collagen synthesis after microneedling is because of upregulation of TGF-β3.

Another hypothesis proposed is that when new wounds are formed with microneedling, the cells create a "demarcation current" which is further increased by the needles own electric potential.[7] This demarcation current (also called bioelectricity) triggers a cascade of growth factors that stimulate the healing phase. The generation of the demarcation current is based on the following principle: Under normal conditions, the interior of skin cells have a resting electrical potential of -70 mV.[8] The extracellular space as well as the skin surface is charged positively. If an epithelial injury occurs, the skin cells release potassium and proteins that in return change the conductivity of the interstitium. At the same time, the inner cellular current increases dramatically beyond -120 mV. This potential difference forces fibroblasts to migrate to the point of injury, to proliferate, and synthesize collagen fibers.[9]

During microneedling, the trauma to the skin results in a mild inflammatory response, which occurs due to bradykinins and histamine released from the mast cells.[10] The expression of matrix metalloproteinases induced by microneedling is speculated to help in the reduction of hyperpigmentation.[10] It has also been shown to cause significant widening of the follicular infundibulum by 47%, which may partly explain the increased penetration of the medication across the skin barrier. It also removes the scales and sebum residues in the neighborhood of the infundibulum.[11]

WOUND HEALING AFTER MICRONEEDLING

Inflammation

The inflammatory stage starts immediately after the procedure. Platelets release chemotactic factors and attract neutrophils, fibroblasts, and more platelets. In chronic wounds, progression toward healing often stalls in the inflammatory phase. At the wound edge, when reepithelialization is arrested, microneedling of the periwound skin may serve to induce a mild inflammatory response which may stimulate epithelial migration to occur.

Proliferation

The proliferation phase starts immediately after microneedling and may reach its peak after 2 months. Monocytes change to macrophages which, in turn, release several growth factors. This causes migration and proliferation of fibroblasts. Re-establishment of the basement membrane by the keratinocytes helps to build collagen.

Remodeling

New type III collagen fibers integrate into the existing skin matrix without any traces of fibrotic tissue. It gradually gets replaced by type I collagen over a period of 1 year resulting in tissue remodeling. Collagen type III is converted to type I by enzymes proteinases and collagenases. The new collagen formation is deposited from a depth of 0.6 mm upwards and towards the basal membrane, in most cases when needles with a length of 1.5 mm are used.[11]

HISTOPATHOLOGY

Various stains used to examine the changes are hematoxylin and eosin (H&E), picrosirius red, and Verhoeff-van Gieson (elastin stain). The picrosirius red stain shows the new collagen fibers as yellow to orange colored and the old fibers are stained red in color. In a study done by Fernandes and

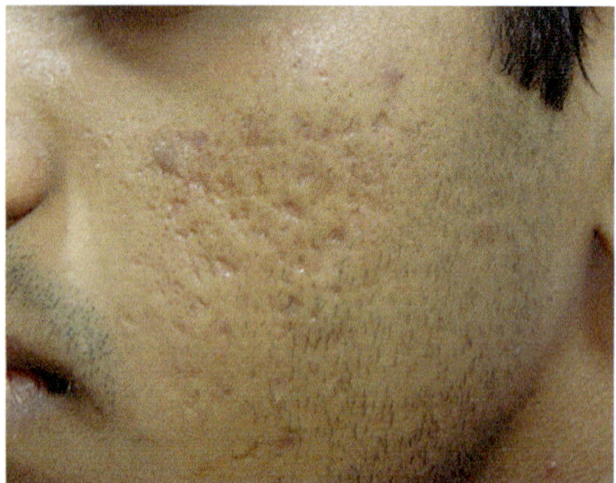

FIG. 1: Postacne scars before microneedling.

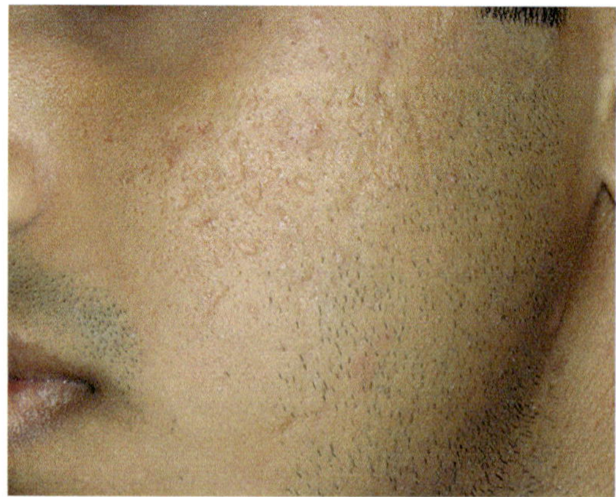

FIG. 2: Postacne scars after four sessions of microneedling.

Signorini, histological examination showed thicker skin, with greatly increased collagen type I and type III deposition and significantly more elastin, but otherwise, unremarkable from normal skin.[12] Type VII collagen which is the main component of anchoring fibrils also increases significantly. The collagen bundles are laid down in a normal lattice pattern rather than in parallel arrangement.

Aust et al. reported a considerable increase in collagen and elastin deposition at 6 months post procedure. The epidermis showed 40% thickening of the stratum spinosum and normal rete ridges at 1 year, postoperatively.[13]

INDICATIONS

- Post acne scars: Microneedling can be combined with various treatment modalities like subcision, chemical peels, and lasers. It is more effective in box and rolling scars. Fresh scars that have developed within last 1 year respond better to microneedling (Figs 1 and 2)[14]
- Drug delivery: Since, multiple microchannels are created in the skin, the transdermal penetration of drugs increases, facilitating higher drug concentrations in the dermis.[15] Thus, microneedling is being used as a tool for skin rejuvenation, skin lightening, melasma, and alopecia. Depending on the indication, products such as hyaluronic acid, growth factors, vitamin C, tranexamic acid, minoxidil, etc. are applied on to the skin immediately after microneedling.[16] It can also be synergistically combined with other procedures, such as iontophoresis, electroporation, and sonophoresis. It creates pores through the stratum corneum, and through delayed pore closure, allows for effective intradermal and transdermal drug delivery for a number of drugs including insulin and protein vaccines[17]
- Traumatic or surgical scars
- Skin rejuvenation
- Open pores
- Fine line and wrinkles
- Melasma: Microneedling in combination with tranexamic acid gives good results as it enhances the penetration of the drug
- Alopecia areata and androgenetic alopecia: Chandrashekar BS et al. treated resistant alopecia areata with microneedling combined with topical triamcinolone acetonide application and reported beneficial results.[18] Microneedling is believed to stimulate stem cells and induce growth factors, which are essential in the expression of hair growth-related genes[19]
- Actinic keratosis and photodamage: Microneedling can be combined with photodynamic therapy (PDT) for optimum results
- Microneedling is said to give fair results in cellulite and tightening of skin after liposuction.[20]

CONTRAINDICATIONS

- Patients with blood clotting disorders. It is advisable to stop the anticoagulants a week prior to the procedure
- Active infections like verrucae vulgaris, herpes labialis, and active acne[11]
- Keloids
- Uncontrolled diabetes, neuromuscular disease, and collagen vascular disease[12]
- Rosacea
- Chronic skin conditions like scleroderma, psoriasis, and eczema
- Pregnancy
- Skin malignancy, moles, and solar keratosis[21]
- Patients with unrealistic expectations.

PRECAUTIONS

- Any active infection or active acne should be treated before doing the microneedling procedure. Patient should be put on topical anti-acne creams about 2–3 weeks before doing the procedure if there is a history of acne flare ups. If there is a past history of recurrent herpes simplex, it is important to administer a prophylactic course of oral acyclovir or valacyclovir before starting the procedure
- Oral isotretinoin should be stopped at least 2 months before microneedling to prevent scarring. However, several experts believe that microneedling is safe in patients who are on low-dose isotretinoin
- Priming a patient before microneedling is very important. Topical bleaching agents such as hydroquinone, vitamin C, or kojic acid and peeling agents such as glycolic acid or vitamin A cream can be used for priming 2–3 weeks before the procedure. This enhances the efficacy and prevents post procedural pigmentation.[12,13]
- Patients should also be counseled about the importance of strict sun protection and should be advised to use a broad spectrum sunscreen regularly. Topical preparations containing hyaluronic acid help in faster healing.

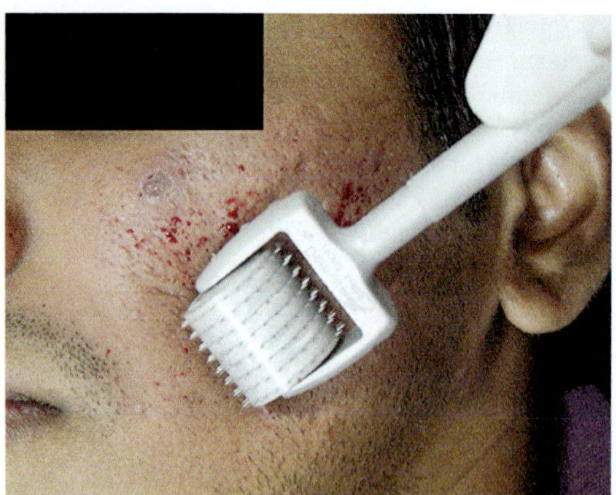

FIG. 3: Dermaroller rolled on affected part.

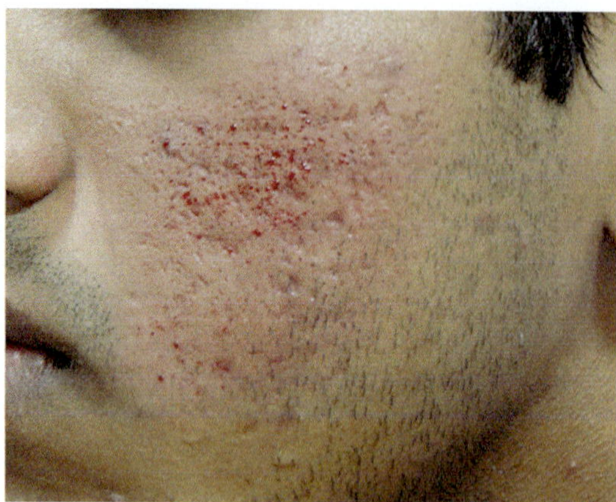

FIG. 4: Pinpoint bleeding immediately after procedure.

PRE-PROCEDURE PREPARATION

Written informed consent must be obtained before the procedure. Standardized digital photographs using identical patient positioning, lighting, and camera settings should be obtained. The patient must be explained about the procedure. The area to be treated should be thoroughly cleansed to remove makeup and dirt. Topical anesthesia in the form of a eutectic mixture of 2.5% lidocaine and 2.5% prilocaine is applied under occlusion. After an hour, the anesthetic cream is removed with acetone and the area is sterilized by cleansing with chlorhexidine, povidone-iodine and isopropyl alcohol solutions, and normal saline.

Technique

Counsel the patients prior to the procedure about the delayed response, multiple sittings, and downtime. With one hand, stretch the skin to be treated. With the other hand, grip the roller like a pen and roll it on the skin. The needles will penetrate at a greater depth if the skin is stretched. Roll the instrument to and fro 6–10 times in four directions; horizontally, vertically, and diagonally right and left, to cover an area of roughly 2 × 2 inches (Fig. 3). This ensures an even pricking pattern, resulting in about 250–300 pricks/cm^2. Pinpoint bleeding is considered as the clinical endpoint (Fig. 4). The movements have to be short and the pressure has to be moderate in order to assure a more uniform depth of penetration. The technique is operator-dependent and therefore, depth of penetration also depends on the pressure applied. Aggressive rolling or lateral pressure can lead to scarring and breakage of needles. Certain areas need special consideration. Lesser pressure is required over bony areas like the forehead and nose. When treating the orbital area, a needle length of 0.5 mm should be used to minimize the pain and also to prevent hematoma formation. The number of roller movements should also be less in the orbital region. While treating the skin around the lips, ask the patient to purse lips together so that the vermilion borders touch. Every needle initially penetrates at an angle and then goes deeper as the roller turns. Finally, the needle is extracted at a converse angle, therefore curving the tracts and redirecting the path of the needle as it rolls into and then out of the skin for about 1.5–2 mm into the dermis. Multiple microchannels are formed in the epidermis that closes within minutes of the treatment. If dermaroller with a needle size of less than 1.5 mm is used, there is only a flushed appearance on the skin and no serous ooze. Profuse bleeding is never seen. In case of deeper scars, rollers with 2 mm long needles are said to help in deeper penetration and thus, give better results. Also, longer needles result in better conductivity and lesser electrical resistance. The blood and the serous fluid is wiped using normal saline after the procedure. This is followed by local application of an antibacterial cream and sunscreen.

VARIATIONS IN DERMAROLLERS

Konstantinos has described five types of medical dermarollers that have been registered with the FDA:[21]

1. C-8 (cosmetic type), is the basic dermaroller as described above with a needle length of only 0.13 mm (130 µm) used for enhancing penetration of topical agents. It is completely painless
2. C-8HE (cosmetic type for hair-bearing surfaces, scalp) has a needle length of 0.2 mm (200 µm). Even this length is below the pain threshold

3. CIT-8 [collagen induction therapy (CIT), medical type] has a needle length of 0.5 mm (500 μm) and helps in collagen induction and skin remodeling
4. MF-8 type has a needle length of 1.5 mm (1,500 μm). This creates deeper microchannels on the entire epidermis and dermis and at the same time destroys scarred collagen bundles
5. MS-4 is the only dermaroller that has a smaller cylinder, 1 cm length, 2 cm diameter, and subsequently, four circular arrays of needles (total 96 needles) that have 1.5 mm length. It is used on areas where better precision and deeper penetration is required. It is mostly used on facial acne scars.

Devices similar to MS-4 are available with needle lengths of 0.5–0.75 mm, which are used for thin-skinned areas such as the periorbital and perioral regions.

POST-PROCEDURE CARE

There may be erythema, edema, and mild scabbing for 2–4 days posttreatment. The scabs usually fall after few days and patient should be instructed to avoid scratching. Patients should be advised broad-spectrum sunscreen and to avoid sun exposure for a week to prevent post-inflammatory hyperpigmentation. Antibacterial creams containing mupirocin should be used twice a day for 5–7 days. Moisturizers containing hyaluronic acid help in faster repair of the skin. A short course of oral anti biotic and oral nonsteroidal anti-inflammatory drug (NSAID) may be prescribed. The patient is advised to avoid any irritant substances like chloroxylenol, astringent, and abrasive scrubs. An interval of 6–8 weeks is preferred between two sessions.

COMPLICATIONS

The procedure is usually well tolerated. Erythema and swelling are observed few hours post procedure. The complications of microneedling include:

- Bruising
- Mild scabbing for a few days after the procedure
- Hematoma on the bony areas
- Secondary bacterial infection
- Milia formation
- Postinflammatory hyperpigmentation
- Tram track effect seen mainly on bony prominences
- Allergic and foreign body granulomatous reaction
- Reactivation of herpes simplex and activation of acne.

BOX 1 Tips to get better results

- Avoid lateral movement and aggressive downward pressure when rolling as this can cause scarring
- To increase the intensity, increase frequency of passes, not pressure
- Avoid abrasive substances such as scrubs and cleansing granules at least for a week posttreatment
- Patients are advised to not pick on the scabs
- Do not use one roller for more than one patient.
- There should be a minimum gap of 6 weeks between two sessions of microneedling to prevent scarring and to get optimum results

BENEFITS OF MICRONEEDLING

- Simple office procedure performed using topical anesthesia
- Less downtime
- Cost-effective treatment
- Does not damage the epidermal layer
- Acne scars with pigmented macular lesions and postinflammatory hyperpigmentation, can be treated by combining microneedling with glycolic acid peel alternately at 3 weekly intervals, each (Figs 5 and 6)[22]
- Downtime, postinflammatory hyperpigmentation, and scarring are less common as compared to other procedures like lasers
- It is safe in dark skin (skin types III–V) as there is neither any thermal damage nor is the epidermis injured
- Can be combined with other treatment modalities such as chemical peels, nonablative and fractional lasers, and fillers to enhance results.

DISADVANTAGES OF MICRONEEDLING

- It is a painful procedure, hence, topical anesthesia under occlusion must be used
- Microneedling requires multiple sessions as compared to ablative carbon dioxide (CO_2) laser because it a relatively milder procedure and less collagen is synthesized in a single sitting
- Scarring may be seen due to improper technique, excessive pressure, or aggressive needling
- Minimum improvement is seen when used for ice pick scars or grade 4 scars[23]
- The instrument cannot be used for multiple sittings as the needles become blunt in one sitting, especially when treating old fibrosed scars

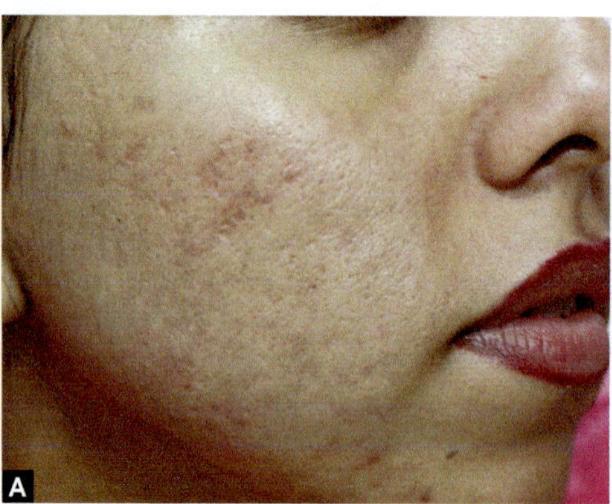

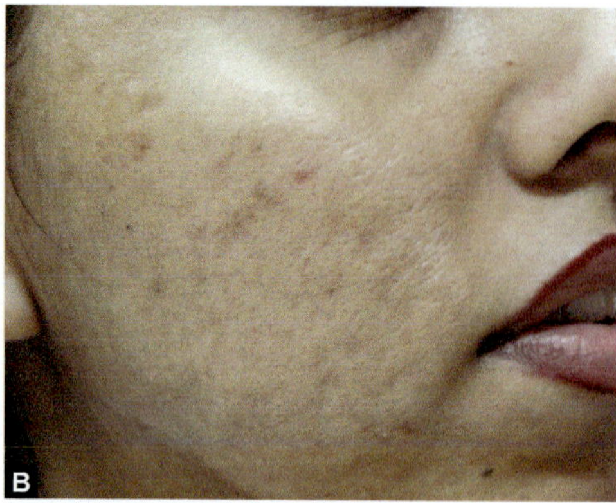

FIG. 5: **A,** Acne scars with postinflammatory hyperpigmentation before treatment; **B,** acne scars with postinflammatory hyperpigmentation after treatment—combination of microneedling and glycolic acid peels

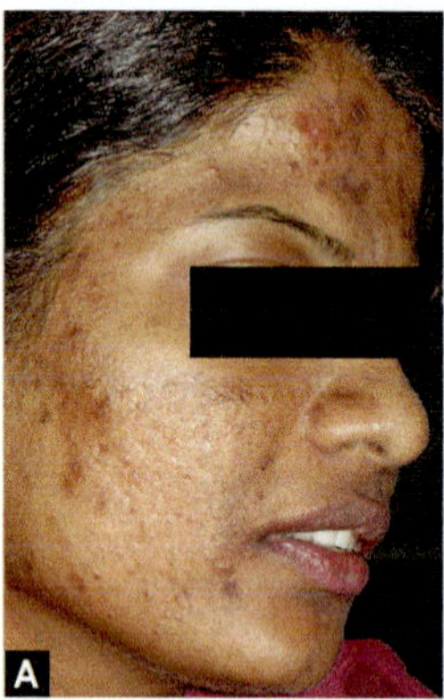

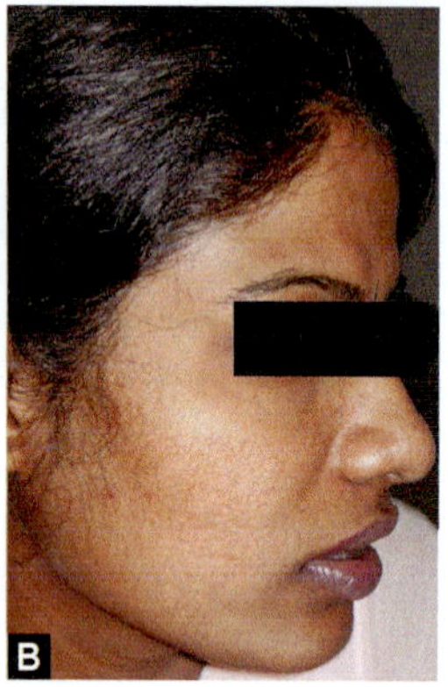

FIG. 6: **A,** Acne scars with postinflammatory hyperpigmentation before treatment; **B,** after treatment—combination of microneedling and 20% glycolic acid and 15% TCA peels done alternately every 3 weeks

- Proper aseptic precautions have to be taken to prevent any infection. Ice pick scars and grade 4 acne scars show less improvement, hence, it cannot be used to treat all types of scars.

TYPES OF MICRONEEDLING DEVICES

- The needles in dermarollers are mostly made of medical-grade stainless steel, but some instruments have needles made of titanium or gold coating that are believed to be less traumatic and safer than the uncoated needles. High ratio of tip length versus diameter of 13:1 is an important property of good needles[6,20]
- Automated rollers: Instruments with disposable heads and hence can be used for many patients. They are battery driven
- Instruments with a vibration mode to reduce pain
- Scalp rollers: They have titanium needles unlike stainless steel rollers and are used to treat thinning hair
- Instruments with a light-emitting diode (LED) photon light attached, mainly used for scarring and wrinkles. However, no published data is available regarding its efficacy. The various lights available are 405 nm blue, 633 nm red, 590 nm yellow, and 560 nm green
- Home care dermarollers: The needle size is less than 0.15 mm in length. They are used for the treatment of open pores, fine lines, cellulite, stretch marks, and to reduce sebum production, though with limited efficacy and no evidenced based results. They are also used for transdermal delivery of substances like lipopeptides and other antiaging products. They can be used twice a week for up to 100 times. After use, the rollers have to be cleaned in hot tap water and shaken dry[24]
- Dermastamp: They are the miniature versions of the Dermaroller with diameter of 0.12 mm and needle length varying from 0.2 mm to 3 mm. They are used for localized scars (e.g., varicella scars) and wrinkles. The procedure with the dermastamp can be performed in 2 minutes[24]
- Dermapen: It is an automated microneedling device which looks like a pen. This ergonomic device makes use of disposable needles and guides to adjust needle length for fractional mechanical resurfacing. It has 9–12 needles arranged in rows. It makes use of a rechargeable battery to operate in two modes, namely, (i) the high speed mode (700 cycles/min) and (ii) the low speed mode (412 cycles/min) in a vibrating

stamp-like manner. The needles are disposable and hence, the dermapen is reusable. It is safe as the needle tips are hidden inside the guide, and more convenient to treat narrow areas such as the nose, around the eyes, and lips without damaging the adjoining skin[25]

- DermaFrac: It is a newer modification of microneedling combining microdermabrasion, microneedling, simultaneous deep tissue serum infusion, and LED. It can be used for acne, uneven skin tone, fine lines and wrinkles, open pores, and photodamaged skin. It is noninvasive, and cost effective with less downtime with individualized selection of serums for infusion[26,27]
- Microneedle delivery systems: It is a painless method of transdermal drug administration, especially useful for vaccines.[28]
- Dermarollers with various types of microneedles:[28]
  - Hollow microneedles: For insertion into the skin and infusion of drug through the MN pore created
  - Coated microneedles: For deposition of active ingredient into the epidermis, followed by removal of the MN array
  - Solid microneedles: For skin pretreatment, followed by the application of an active-loaded reservoir
  - Dissolving microneedles: For delivery of active compound, incorporated into the matrix of the needles, into the skin
  - Swellable microneedles: For drug delivery through the hydrogel matrix from a drug-loaded reservoir.

CONCLUSION

Microneedling is a simple and affordable office procedure. It is most useful for the improvement of box and rolling acne scars. It is also an effective modality of treatment for open pores, facial rejuvenation, alopecia, transdermal drug delivery, and many more indications. It has gained popularity because of its simplicity, cost effectiveness, less downtime, and side effects as compared to other treatment modalities. It is considered safe in treating patients with Fitzpatrick's IV and V skin types because it overcomes the side effects of scarring and hyperpigmentation resulting from other procedures in which the epidermis is compromised. However, it is a lengthy procedure because multiple sittings are required to achieve adequate end results. Over-aggressive rolling or excessive pressure can cause scarring and tram tracking. It can be combined with other therapies like peels, lasers, and PRP for enhanced therapeutic effects.

REFERENCES

1. Orentreich DS, Orentreich N. Subcutaneous incisionless (subcision) surgery for the correction of depressed scars and wrinkles. Dermatol Surg. 1995;21(6):543-9.
2. Camirand A, Doucet J. Needle dermabrasion. Aesthetic Plast Surg. 1997;21(1):48-51.
3. Bhardwaj D. Collagen induction therapy with dermaroller. Community Based Med J. 2013;1:35-7.
4. Diegelmann RF, Evans MC. Wound healing: an overview of acute, fibrotic and delayed healing. Front Biosci. 2004;9:283-9.
5. Fabbrocini G, Fardella N, Monfrecola A, et al. Acne scarring treatment using skin needling. Clin Exp Dermatol. 2009;34(8):874-9.
6. Majid I, Sheikh G, September PI. Microneedling and its applications in dermatology. In Prime. 2014;4(7):44-9.
7. Kloth LC. Electrical stimulation for wound healing: A review of evidence from in vitro studies, animal experiments, and clinical trials. Int J Low Extrem Wounds. 2005;4:23-44.
8. Jaffe LF. Control of development by steady ionic currents. Fed Proc. 1981;40(2):125-7.
9. Sharad J, Yepuri V, Sitara GL. Microneedling. In: Mysore V (Ed). ACS(I) Textbook on Cutaneous and Aesthetic Surgery. New Delhi: Jaypee Brothers Medical Publishers (P) Ltd. 2016;85:885-91.
10. Liebl H, Kloth LC. Skin cell proliferation stimulated by microneedles. J Am Coll Clin Wound Spec. 2012;4(1):2-6.
11. Singh A, Yadav S. Microneedling: Advances and widening horizons. Indian Dermatol Online J. 2016;7(4):244-54.
12. Fernandes D, Signorini M. Combating photoaging with percutaneous collagen induction. Clin Dermatol. 2008;26(2):192-9.
13. Aust MC, Fernandes D, Kolokythas P, et al. Percutaneous collagen induction therapy: an alternative treatment for scars, wrinkles, and skin laxity. Plast Reconstr Surg. 2008;121(4):1421-9.
14. Sharad J. Microneedling. In: Khunger N (Ed). Step by Step Treatment of Acne Scars. New Delhi: Jaypee Brothers Medical Publishers (P) Ltd; 2014. pp. 102-13.
15. Escobar-Chávez JJ, Bonilla-Martínez D, Villegas-González MA, et al. Microneedles: a valuable physical enhancer to increase transdermal drug delivery. J Clin Pharmacol. 2011;51(7):964-77.
16. Vedamurthy M. Mesotherapy. Indian J Dermatol Venereol Leprol. 2007;73:60-2.
17. Hou A, Cohen B, Haimovic A, et al. Microneedling: A Comprehensive Review. Dermatol Surg. 2017;43(3):321-39.
18. Chandrashekar BS, Sriram R, Mysore R, et al. Evaluation of microneedling fractional radiofrequency device for treatment of acne scars. J Cutan Aesthet Surg. 2014;7(2):93-7.
19. Dhurat R, Sukesh M, Avhad G, et al. A randomized evaluator blinded study of effect of microneedling in

androgenetic alopecia: a pilot study. Int J Trichology. 2013;5(1):6-11.
20. Nair PA, Arora TH. Microneedling using dermaroller: A means of collagen induction therapy. GMJ. 2014;69:24-7.
21. Anastassakis K. (2016). The Dermaroller Series. [online] Available from: www.mtoimportadora.com.br/site_novo/wp.content/uploads/2014/04/Dr.-Anastassakis-Kostas.pdf. [Accessed October, 2017].
22. Sharad J. Combination of microneedling and glycolic acid peels for the treatment of acne scar in dark skin. J Cosmet Dermatol. 2011;10(4):317-23.
23. Majid I. Microneedling therapy in atrophic facial scars: an objective assessment. J Cutan Aesthet Surg. 2009; 2(1):26-30.
24. Doddaballapur S. Microneedling with dermaroller. J Cutan Aesthet Surg. 2009;2(2):110-1.
25. Arora S, Gupta BP. Automated microneedling device–A new tool in dermatologist's kit–A review. J Pak Med Assoc. 2012;22:354-7.
26. Lewis W. Is microneedling really the next big thing? Wendy Lewis explores the buzz surrounding skin needling. Plast Surg Pract. 2014;7:24-8.
27. Sahni K, Kassir M. Dermafrac™: an innovative new treatment for periorbital melanosis in a dark-skinned male patient. J Cutan Aesthet Surg. 2013;6(3):158-60.
28. McCrudden MT, McAlister E, Courtenay AJ, et al. Microneedle applications in improving skin appearance. Exp Dermatol. 2015;24(8):561-6.

38 CHAPTER

Microneedling Radiofrequency

Anuj Pall

INTRODUCTION

Fractional photothermolysis, as a concept, was introduced to overcome the drawbacks of ablative and nonablative resurfacing systems.[1] It induces homogeneous and fractional thermal injury at a particular level of the skin, followed by collagen remodeling process. This technique creates microscopic columns of thermal damage in the dermis, known as microscopic thermal zones or MTZ, around which are zones of normal tissue. Therefore, the re-epithelization process can occur faster with fewer side effects as compared to ablative skin resurfacing system.[2,3]

Ablative fractional lasers (AFLs) appear to lead to a more vigorous wound healing process and dermal fibrosis. This, in turn, causes more rapid and significant clinical effects that can be achieved with ablative than nonablative devices. However, AFLs cause longer downtime and an increased risk of postinflammatory hyperpigmentation (PIH), compared with that of nonablative fractional lasers (NAFLs).[3]

Nonablative fractional lasers (1,540 nm Erbium Glass) have the advantage of less downtime along with providing good efficacy. However, their clinical efficacy does not match that of the full ablative process, especially for moderate-to-severe rhytides and atrophic scars.

Fractional microneedling radiofrequency (MNRF) device is minimally invasive and may help overcome the disadvantages of fractional lasers. Microneedling radiofrequency system is one of the novel fractional resurfacing technique. In this, there are alternating rows of positive and negative electrode pins, between which the energy is conducted. Impedance is highest in the epidermis and is lesser in the dermis. There is a controlled thermal injury in the dermis which causes a wound healing response. This, in turn, initiates the collagen remodeling process by using heat production from tissue impedance and subsequently the thermal energy diffuses to the deeper tissues. An advantage of fractional radiofrequency is that it causes less epidermal disruption by only 5%, compared with 10–70% of that of fractional ablative laser systems.[4] The healing process is faster with minimal downtime. Therefore, this technique may be an alternative choice of facial rejuvenation and atrophic scars, especially in patients with darker skin complexion. This technique has shown to provide equivalent efficacy with less side effects, comparing with traditional ablative fractional resurfacing procedures.[5] Microneedling radiofrequency offers a great advantage over fractional lasers. The key differences of MNRF when compared to fractional lasers are:

- It can be used for all the skin types, with reduced risk of skin burns and PIH
- In insulated needles, radiofrequency (RF) energy which is delivered is particularly focused at the tip of the microneedle leading to very less injury to the epidermis. Thus, the down time and pain is reduced as compared to a conventional carbon dioxide fractional laser
- The depth of penetration of the microneedles can be adjusted from 0.5 to 4 mm depending upon the target areas. The maximum depth achieved safely with fractional lasers is 1 to 1.5 mm.

RADIOFREQUENCY ENERGY: BACKGROUND AND PRINCIPLES

High frequency (RF) electric energy has a history of over 70 years of practical clinical application in medicine. In this, the oscillation frequency of the current is about 3 kHz to 300 GHz, which is in the broadcasting band of the electromagnetic spectrum. Radiofrequency devices use electromagnetic radiation to generate electrical current.[2] Impedance, which is the resistance encountered on application to a tissue, is an inherent property of the particular tissue.[6,7] This transfer of energy from the electrical field to the charged particles in the target tissue generates heat energy. The energy output is calculated with the formula:

$$\text{Energy (J)} = I2 \times z \times t$$

Where I is current, z is impedance, and t is time in seconds,

Therefore, heat energy (J) is generated by impedance (z) to the motion of electrons, relative to the amount of current (I) and the time that current is transmitted to the tissue. Those parts of the body with more blood content have the lowest impedance, or highest electrical conductivity.[6] Bone, for example, has very high impedance and thus the electrical current cannot enter the bone tissue, so the current flows around it. Dry skin has high impedance, thus, to increase electrical current, hydration is required.[7,8]

Radiofrequency energy is not influenced by tissue diffraction and absorption of chromophore, which is in contrast to laser light that, can be scattered and absorbed before reaching the target tissue. Hence, the amount of RF energy is more controllable than laser light and it can be applied to any type of skin.[6]

Monopolar and Bipolar Radiofrequency

In monopolar RF, the current goes through the patient to complete the current cycle as the current is applied between a single electrode tip and the grounding plate. Whereas in bipolar RF, the current only goes through the tissue between the two electrodes of the instrument as the current is applied between two points on the tip of a probe. When same parameter is used, bipolar RF creates limited coagulative necrosis zone around the needle as compared to monopolar RF which causes wider denaturation zone.[7] The monopolar system has the advantage that it can achieve high penetration of emitted current and is considered to be ideal for skin tightening. The bipolar RF system provides more controlled distribution of energy at a certain depth but has its limitations on treating deeper skin area.[7-9] It makes bipolar RF more effective for treating acne scars, open pores, and surgical scars etc.

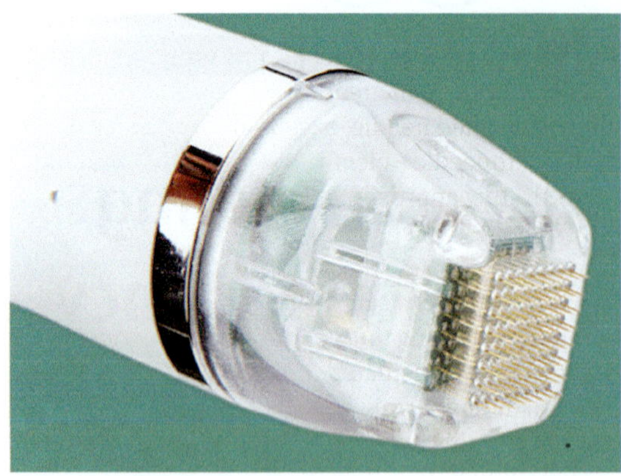

FIG. 1: Fractional microneedling radiofrequency probe.

FRACTIONAL MICRONEEDLING RADIOFREQUENCY DEVICE

The concept of "fractionating" the entire energy delivered by a device into multiple discrete points was seen in the early fractional nonablative lasers around 2005 for the first time. This concept of fractionating energy has spread from lasers to RF devices because of the obvious advantages such as fractional delivery, rapid wound healing, reduced discomfort and greater safety for the patient. By fractionating RF energy over multiple electrodes, the regions of controlled damage are surrounded by zones of normal tissue, reducing the pain, shortening the downtime, and accelerating the healing process. Fractional radiofrequency thermal zones (RFTZ) are created within the reticular dermis.[4] This is a minimally invasive nonablative system which delivers monopolar and bipolar RF energy in the form of an electrical current which causes generation of heat through the inherent electrical resistance of dermal and subcutaneous tissue.[9,10]

Most of the MNRF devices consist of a handheld applicator which has a disposable treatment tip for single-use, that contains 25–49 microneedle electrodes in an area of 1 cm^2 (Fig. 1). Needles are automatically inserted vertically into the skin, and after 0.2 seconds of insertion of the needles, RF is emitted to avoid epidermal damage. With varying energy levels, the amount of RF emission differs.

Microneedles

In noninsulated microneedles, an accurately controlled RF energy will directly be delivered into a particular depth of dermis through the entire length of minimally invasive microneedles (Fig. 2). The penetration length can be adjusted between 0.5 and 4 mm depth selectively depending on symptoms and the target treatment areas.

In insulated needle, except for the distal 0.3 mm, the microneedle electrodes are nonconductive (Fig. 3). The approximately 34 g surgical stainless steel needle, which is extremely sharp, is initially coated with gold for conductivity to the target tissue, followed by coating with a silicon insulating compound, leaving the 300 μm at the tip. As the shaft of the needle is insulated, there is no electrothermal injury at the epidermis, so skin cooling is not required. Thus, using this approach, it is possible to heat the deeper tissues to a reasonably high level, leading to greater collagen coagulation and remodeling, collagen contraction, and stimulation. Irrespective of insulation or noninsulation, the highest RF energy will be focused on the tip of microneedles. It is possible to treat whole length of scar by varying the depth of microneedles.

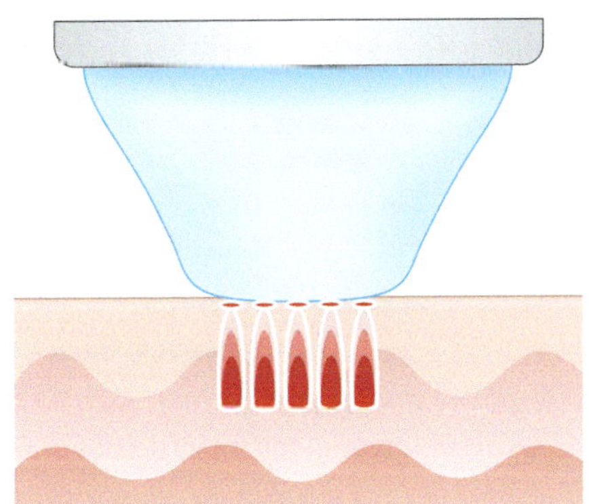

FIG. 2: Noninsulated needles.

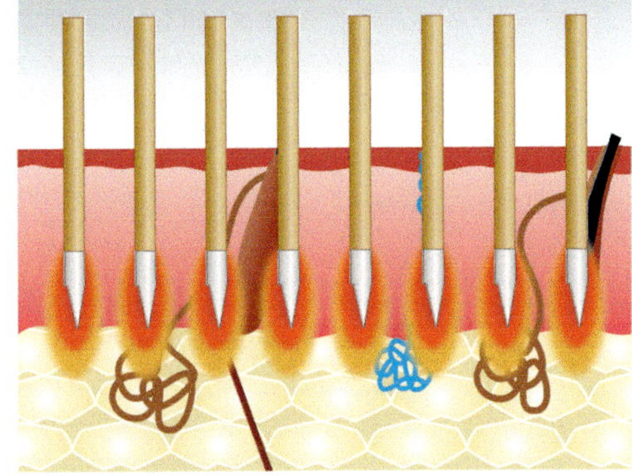

FIG. 3: Insulated needles.

Mechanism of Action

The RF energy is fractionally delivered leading to formation of RFTZ.[5] Fractional thermal injury of dermal collagen causes a strong wound healing process leading to inflammatory cascade. This leads to the formation of new collagen, elastin, and hyaluronic acid, eventually causing dermal remodeling.[5] Additionally, the actual penetration of the microneedles into the dermis has been shown to mechanically stimulate fibroblasts to produce collagen. It also stimulates the migration and proliferation of keratinocytes and fibroblasts by causing the release of several growth factors.[9] The untreated areas in between the treated areas serve as a reservoir of cells that promotes and expedite wound healing.

Histologic and Ultrastructural Changes

In a study conducted by Lim et al., pig skin was histologically evaluated up to 10 weeks after MNRF treatment using energies from 1.25 to 6.25 J/cm^2. They observed that thermally coagulated zone was localized in the reticular dermis without injuring the epidermis. After 10 weeks, new collagen was found to replace the coagulation necrosis zone (Fig. 4). The reverse transcription polymerase chain reaction studies indicated a rise in heat shock protein, matrix metalloproteinase and extracellular matrix protein. Raised collagen expressions posttreatment indicates that the thermal injury created by the RF device may trigger a wound healing response.[10]

Procedure

Before procedure, an informed consent and pre-treatment photographs are taken. Patients having

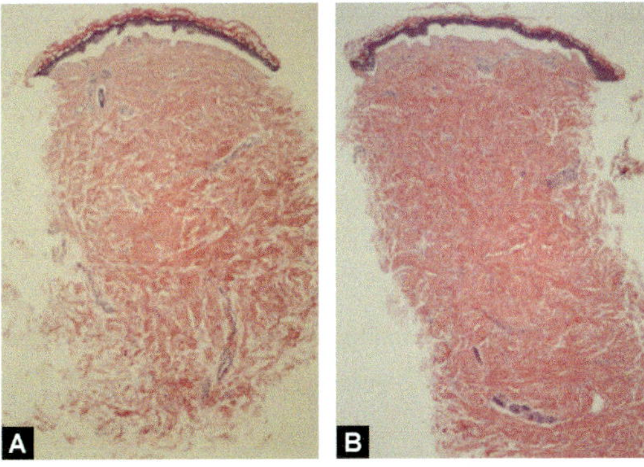

FIG. 4: A, Baseline (H&E x20) and B, after 2 months (H&E x20).

a history of herpes simplex may be advised to take oral valacyclovir on the day of treatment. Topical anesthetic cream under occlusion is applied an hour before the procedure. Prior to the treatment, the face should be cleansed with facial foam cleanser and alcohol swab. Depending on the clinical indication, desired depth of electrodes is selected and treatment is performed. Subsequent passes are made after reducing the depth and energy as the needle tips reach near the epidermis. There should be a proper contact of electrode to skin surface so as to reduce adverse events. Some vesiculation and superficial burn may occur after the treatment, although it is usually due to uneven electrode contact to skin. Lower RF energy and depth of the needle should be used in areas such as forehead and temple where underlying bones are in close proximity to the skin surface (Table 1).

Keep cleaning blood and fluid with sterile gauze during the treatment to avoid sliding of probe especially on the nose and bony prominences. There may be sunburn-like sensation and slight erythema for about 1-2 days. Patients can wash their face with a mild cleanser on the evening of treatment and can apply light makeup from the next day.

According to author's experience, fullface as well as neck treatment sessions take about 30 minutes. Each session is performed every 4 weeks for a maximum of 4–5 sessions. For the best results, 2–3 treatment sessions are required and it may take around 4–6 months posttreatment to visualize the maximum effect by which time the collagen remodeling is complete.

TABLE 1: Microneedling radiofrequency: Recommended guidelines

Condition	Needle depth	Radiofrequency mode	Passes	Interval	Comment
Face rejuvenation	2 mm 1.5 mm 0.8 mm	Monopolar Bipolar Bipolar	1 1 1	4–6 weeks	—
Forehead	0.8 mm	Bipolar	1-2	4–6 weeks	
Periorbital	0.5 mm 0.5 mm	Bipolar Monopolar	1 1	4–6 weeks	0.8 mm depth or more cause bruising
Perioral	0.5 mm 0.5 mm	Bipolar Monopolar	1 1	4–6 weeks	0.8 mm depth or more cause bruising
Telangiectasia	0.5 mm 0.8 mm	Bipolar Bipolar	1-3 1-3	6–8 weeks	—
Acne scars	1.5 mm 0.8 mm	Bipolar Bipolar	1-2 1-2	4 weeks	Combine with subcision, PRP or frational lasers
Traumatic scars	0.5–2 mm	Bipolar	2-3	4 weeks	Combine with intralesional steroids in case of hypertrophic scars
Active acne	1.5 mm 0.8 mm	Bipolar Bipolar	1-2 1	4–6 weeks	Avoid treating severe inflammatory acne
Chicken pox scars	2 mm 1.5 mm	Bipolar Bipolar	1-2 1-2	4 weeks	—
Strech marks	0.5–2 mm	Bipolar	2-3	4–6 weeks	Depth depends on type of stretch marks
Axillary hyperhidrosis	3 mm 2 mm 1.5 mm	Bipolar Bipolar Bipolar	2-3 2-3 2-3	4–6 weeks	—

PRP, plasma rich protein.

Posttreatment Care

For 2–3 days after treatment, the patient is advised to apply topical antibiotic. Prolonged direct sun exposure should be avoided and a sunscreen with sun protection factor (SPF30) or greater should be applied. Recently, light-emitting diode treatment has been performed immediately after MNRF treatment to reduce the intensity and duration of posttreatment erythema.

Indications

Microneedle fractional RF system is ideal for managing scars, skin rejuvenation, lifting, and tightening with minimally invasive microneedles (Box 1).

Skin Rejuvenation

Microneedling radiofrequency using monopolar radiofrequency may play a significant role in the cosmetic improvement of early skin laxity. It can, especially, be preferred by patients who want to avoid surgery due to associated risk of complications. According to a research, heating the dermis to a high enough temperature causes collagen coagulation that leads to immediate skin shrinkage that kick start the process of wound healing. This induces neocollagenesis and neoelastinogenesis eventually leading to skin tightening as the new collagen gradually replaces the old.[11] It can also be combined with other nonsurgical procedures such as botulinum toxin, fillers, protein rich plasma (PRP), high intensity focused ultrasound, and other nonablative laser treatments.

BOX 1 Indications of microneedling rediofrequency

- Nonsurgical face lifting
- Wrinkle reduction
- Skin tightening
- Skin rejuvenation
- Pore reduction
- Acne scars
- Traumatic scars
- Chicken pox scars
- Hyperhidrosis
- Stretch marks
- Spider veins

Acne Scars and Open Pores

Bipolar fractional microneedle RF has shown to be effective in improving acne scars. In various studies, 25 and 75% cosmetic improvement in affected skin can be expected with MNRF treatments. About 3–4 treatment sessions with 1–2 passes are required and it takes 3 months posttreatment for these results to be fully visible. This is the time required for optimal activation of fibroblasts and the stimulation of the collagen production which is needed to replace the dermal matrix. Side effects like transient pain, erythema, and scabbing are observed from MNRF treatments that resolve within 3–5 days. In comparison to fractional laser treatment, the pain is significantly less with RF. Along with the improvement in acne scars, patients may also observe aesthetic improvements in skin texture, skin tightening, fine lines, and wrinkles, and a reduction in pore size.[12] In a study of 30 patients with large facial pores and acne scars, there was improvement in more than 70% of all patients with respect to the grade of acne scars and Investigator Global Assessment of large pores. The dermal density, skin surface roughness and microscopic and composite images also showed improvement, whereas transepidermal waterloss and sebum measurement were unaltered.[9] Microneedling radiofrequency can be combined with subcision, PRP, amd fractional lasers to have more therapeutic effect on treating acne scars (Fig. 5).

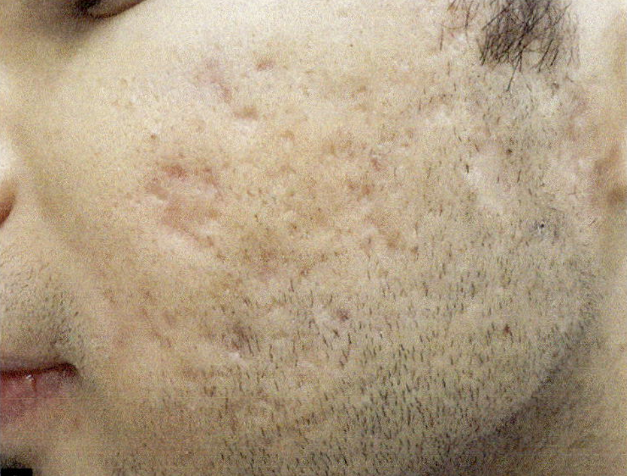

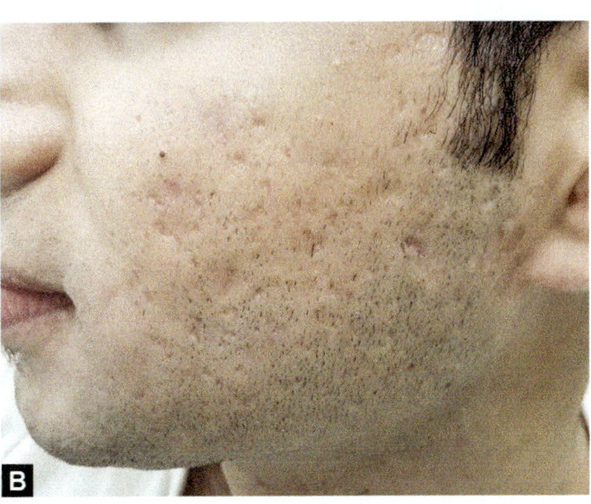

FIG. 5: A, Acne scars before treatment; and **B,** Acne scars after 4 sessions of subcision followed by MNRF. (Multiple passes, 1.5mm-2mm needle depth).

Acne Vulgaris

Microneedling radiofrequency devices can be used to treat acne vulgaris. In a study conducted on 20 patients with moderate inflammatory acne, significant clinical improvement was observed in reduction of lesion count and sebum secretion. Side effects noted were temporary redness, tingling, and burning sensation after treatment, which resolved in 2 days.[13]

Hyperhidrosis

Microneedling radiofrequency provides a good alternative to sweat gland suction curettage, and botulinum toxin treatment for axillary hyperhidrosis. The procedure is done every 4-6 weeks and is free from side effects. Overall, there was a high degree of satisfaction noted in all patients. Recently, a study conducted on 25 patients with severe primary axillary hyperhidrosis who were treated with 3 sessions of MNRF at 3-weeks interval, demonstrated significant improvement after treatment with a relapse rate of 45.9% after a year. It has been recommended to repeat the treatment after an year.[14]

Striae Distensae/Atrophic Scar

Striae distensae are atrophic dermal scars that have an overlying atrophy of the epidermis that may cause significant cosmetic concerns. Although various laser and light sources have been used for their treatment, to date there is no definite modality which is considered as a "gold standard".[15] In a study conducted on 30 female patients with moderate to severe striae distensae, optimal clinical results were seen with a few side effects (Fig. 6).[16]

According to author's experience, MNRF can be used as an effective modality to treat surgical scars, traumatic scars, chicken pox scars, and facial veins (Figs 7 to 9).

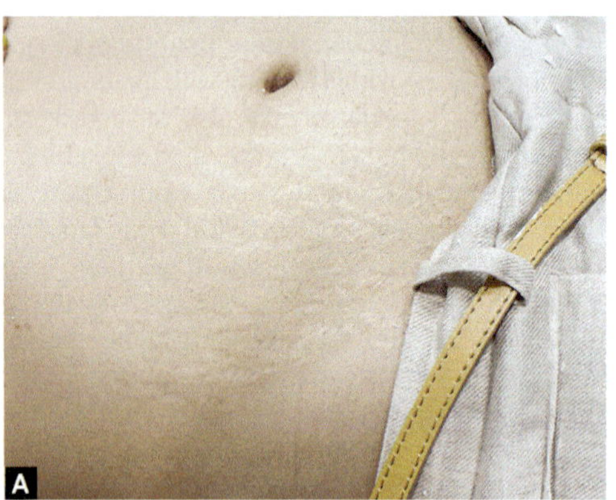
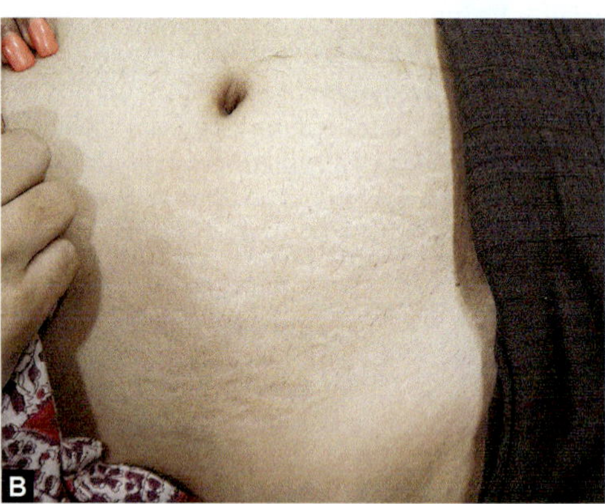

FIG. 6: A, Strech Marks before treatment; and **B,** Strech Marks after 5 sessions of MNRF, multiple passes, 0.8–2 mm needle depth.

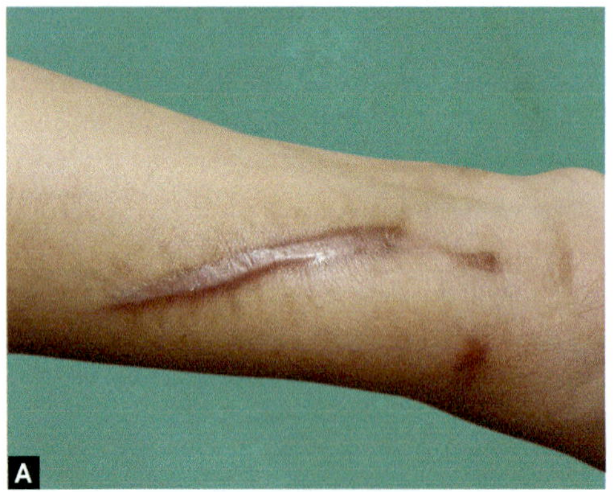
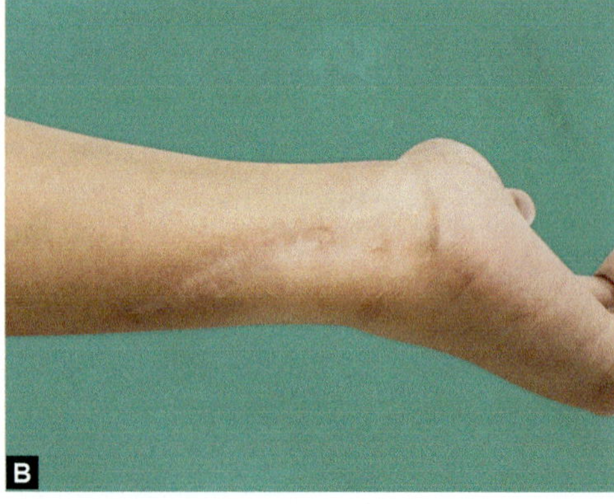

FIG. 7: A, Post surgical scar before treatment; **B,** post surgical scar after 4 sessions of MNRF. (Intralesional triamcinolone acetonide 10mg/ml in dilution followed by MNRF, multiple passes, 0.8–2 mm).

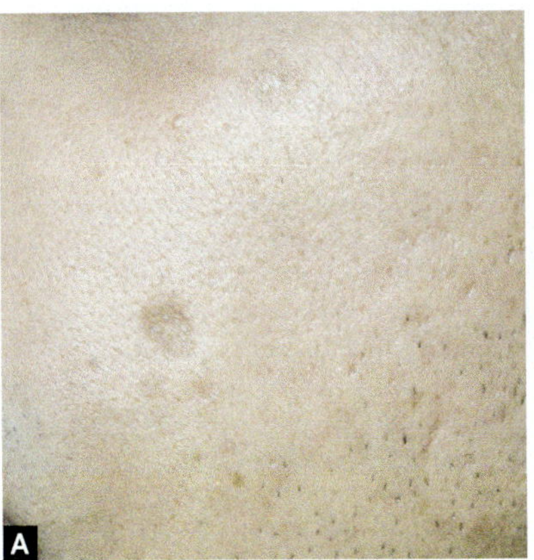
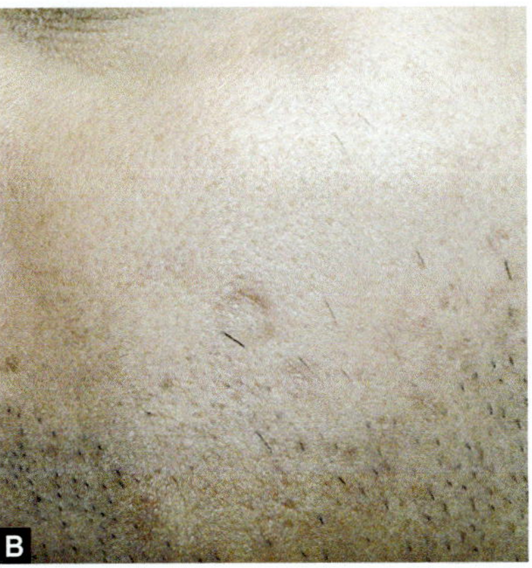

FIG. 8: A, Chicken Pox scar before treatment; **B,** chicken Pox scar after 4 sessions of subcision followed by MNRF, multiple passes, 0.8–2 mm.

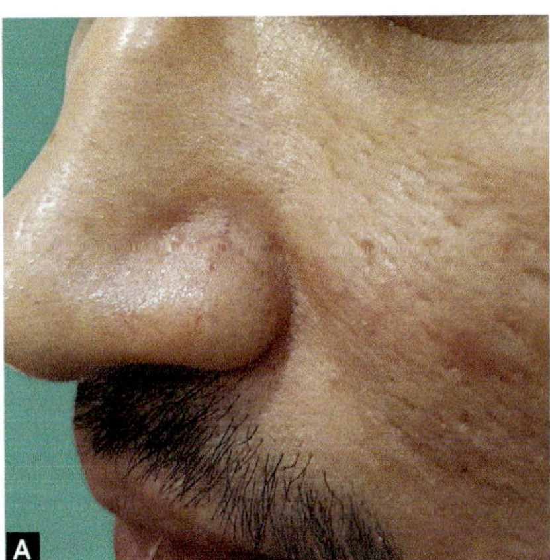
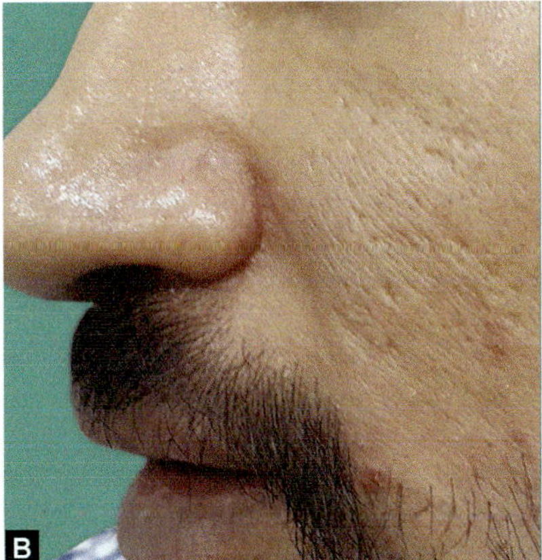

FIG. 9: A, Telangiectasias on the ala of nose before treatment; and **B,** after 2 sessions of MNRF, multiple passes, 0.8–1.5 mm.

Side Effects

Mild pain and temporary redness were common side effects seen during and post-procedure. In general, the incidence of side effects of MNRF treatment is lesser compared with conventional fractional lasers. Moreover, the risk of postinflammatory hyperpigmentation is minimal which also usually resolves within 4 weeks. The clinicians must use optimal treatment parameters according to the cosmetic units of the face, including energy level and needle depth. An uncommon side effect is persistence of shoe marks post MNRF treatment. They usually resolve after 3-6 months.

Cautions

- A probe once used should not be used again
- Some patients have skin allergy to topical anesthesia and develop erythematous rash after prolonged application
- Bruising may occur around the eyes even when using a needle length of 0.8 mm or more
- It is possible to have PIH if you overlap the treatment with high energy and same depth
- Put a little more pressure on the areas such as legs, stomach and thigh during treatment
- Treating vocal cords require special care. When performing such treatments, it is recommended not to use a needle length longer than 1.5 mm
- Patients who are taking drugs like isotretinoin and aspirin will have more bleeding than a normal person
- Avoid to have treatment on the area that had filler treatment or autologous fat injection

- In case of patients having dental prosthesis, put the gauze in their mouth between their teeth and lip in order to prevent flowing electric current.

Contraindications

- Skin infection
- Bleeding disorder
- Pregnancy
- Keloidal tendency
- Pacemaker, vascular stent, or metal implant
- Skin malignancy.

CONCLUSION

Radiofrequency offers a good treatment option for all types of scars in all skin types. Since it is a minimally invasive procedure with quick recovery time, the patients can return back to their daily routines immediately postprocedure. The author suggests that MNRF may be considered as the first choice for scar treatment as it has deeper treatment levels, reduced down time and a negligible risk of pigmentation in darker skin types as compared to certain fractional laser systems.

REFERENCES

1. Alexiades-Armenakas MR, Dover JS, Arndt KA. The spectrum of laser skin resurfacing: Nonablative, fractional, and ablative laser resurfacing. J Am Acad Dermatol. 2008;58(5):719-37.
2. Hantash BM, Bedi VP, Kapadia B, et al. In vivo histological evaluation of a novel ablative fractional resurfacing device. Lasers Surg Med. 2007;39(2):96-107.
3. Manuskiatti W, Triwongwaranat D, Varothai S, et al. Efficacy and safety of a carbondioxide ablative fractional resurfacing device for treatment of atrophic acne scars in Asians. J Am Acad Dermatol. 2010;63(2):274-83.
4. Hruza G, Taub AF, Collier SL, et al. Skin rejuvenation and wrinkle reduction using a fractional radiofrequency system. J Drugs Dermatol. 2009;8(3);259-65.
5. Vejjabhinanta V, Wanitphakdeedecha R, Limtanyakul P, et al. The efficacy in treatment of facial atrophic acne scars in Asians with a fractional radiofrequency microneedle system. J Eur Acad Dermatol Venereol. 2014;28(9):1219-25.
6. Lolis MS, Goldberg DJ. Radiofrequency in cosmetic dermatology: A review. Dermatol Surg. 2012;38(11):1765-76.
7. Alster TS, Lupton JR. Nonablative cutaneous remodeling using radiofrequency devices. Clin Dermatol. 2007; 25(5):487-91.
8. Elsaie ML. Cutaneous remodeling and photorejuvenation using radiofrequency devices. Indian J Dermatol. 2009;54(3):201-5.
9. Cho SI, Chung BY, Choi MG, et al. Evaluation of the clinical efficacy of fractional radiofrequency microneedle treatment in acne scars and large facial pores. Dermatol Surg. 2012;38(1):1017-24.
10. Lim SD, Yeo UC, Kim IH, et al. Surgical corner. Evaluation of the wound healing response after deep dermal heating by fractional micro-needle radiofrequency device. J Drugs Dermatol. 2013;12(9):1044-9.
11. Seo KY, Kim DH, Lee SE, et al. Skin rejuvenation by microneedle fractional radiofrequency and a human stem cell conditioned medium in Asian skin: A randomized controlled investigator blinded split-face study. J Cosmet Laser Ther. 2013;15(1):25-33.
12. Gold MH, Biron JA. Treatment of acne scars by fractional bipolar radiofrequency energy. J Cosmet Laser Ther. 2012;14(4):172-8.
13. Shin JU, Lee SH, Jung JY, et al. A split-face comparison of a fractional microneedle radiofrequency device and fractional carbon dioxide laser therapy in acne patients. J Cosmet Laser Ther. 2012;14(5):212-7.
14. Naeini BA, Pourazizi M, Naeini FF, et al. Treatment of primary axillary hyperhidrosis by fractional microneedle radiofrequency: Is it still effective after long-term follow-up? Indian J Dermatol. 2016;61(2):234.
15. Kim IS, Park KY, Kim BJ, et al. Efficacy of intradermal radiofrequency combined with autologous plateletrich plasma in striae distensae: A pilot study. Int J Dermatol. 2012;51(10):1253-8.
16. Naeini FF, Behfar S, Naeini BA, et al. Promising Option for treatment of striae alba: Fractionated microneedle radiofrequency in combination with fractional carbon dioxide Laser. Dermatol Res Pract. 2016;61-8.

39

CHAPTER

Body Contouring

Anuj Pall

INTRODUCTION

There is an increasing demand for body contouring procedures owing to the increasing number of obese patients, demand for aesthetical improvement devices, awareness and easy accessibility to such procedures, and emphasis on physical look. When there is an unsatisfactory improvement in body contour with diet and exercise, many invasive and noninvasive fat reduction options are available. Liposuction, an invasive procedure, can be applied for either localized or extensive fat removal. It is associated with a significant risk of complications and adverse effects such as postprocedural pain, prolonged recovery, infection, scarring, hematoma, bruising, or edema.[1] There can also be some long-term and potentially fatal complications like pulmonary embolism and deep vein thrombosis in addition to anesthesia-related complications.[2,3] Contour irregularity is another significant, although nonfatal complication, which may require surgical revision in 2–10% of cases.[1]

Noninvasive devices for body contouring are the emerging area of aesthetic medicine.[4] They are ideal for nonobese patients who are looking for safer, more affordable methods of modest reductions of stubborn localized fat deposits, and improved skin laxity without associated adverse effects or significant downtime that are usually seen with surgery. The surgical techniques are often combined with noninvasive methods so as to shorten the postoperative recovery, decrease bruising, and enhance to improve skin tightening of the treated areas.[5] At present, there are four leading noninvasive techniques for reduction of localized subcutaneous adipose tissue: cryolipolysis, high-intensity focused ultrasound (HIFU), low-level laser therapy (LLLT), and radiofrequency (RF) (Table 1). All of these techniques are believed to cause an efflux of triglycerides from adipocytes causing a decrease in size, necrosis, or apoptosis of targeted fat cells. The other methods include extracorporeal shockwave therapy, acoustic wave therapy, and topical creams. There are also various injectable treatments called as mesotherapy, which have been tried in attempts to decrease the subcutaneous fat tissue. However, their safety and efficacy is yet to be established.

CRYOLIPOLYSIS

Cryolipolysis is a noninvasive technology that leads to selective fat reduction, using controlled, localized cooling, thus causing an inflammatory reaction within adipose tissue and apoptosis of fat cells.[2] Cryolipolysis is performed via a vacuum applicator, which applies temperatures of –10°C (14°F) to the skin in cycles of 60 minutes each. Initially approved by the Food and Drug Administration (FDA) for treatment of flank adiposity in 2010, cryolipolysis has since been approved for treatment of the submental area, abdomen, thighs, flanks, fat around bra straps, on the back, and underneath the buttocks.[6] An advantage of cryolipolysis is that it does not require frequent treatment sessions for maximal efficacy (Fig. 1).

Krueger et al. have shown that precise application of cold temperatures elicits the death of adipocytes that are subsequently phagocytosed by macrophages. There are no noticeable changes in subcutaneous fat immediately posttreatment. Within 3 days of the treatment, an inflammatory response stimulated by apoptosis of adipocytes is seen as reflected by an influx of inflammatory cells. This process peaks at approximately 14 days, as the adipocytes get

TABLE 1: Non-invasive techniques for subcutaneous fat reduction

Technology	Devices
High-intensity focused ultrasound	Lipocel (body)
	Liposonix (body)
	Ultraformer (face)
	Doublo (face)
	Scizer (body)
	Ulthera (face)
	Ultrashape (body)
Cryolipolysis	CoolSculpting
	CoolTech
	Zimmer Cryo (OEM)
	CoolShaping
	Cymedics Cryo (OEM)
Radiofrequency (RF)	Venus Legacy (multipolar RF)
	Vanquish ME (operator independent selective RF)
	Exilis Elite (RF + ultrasound)
	Exilis (RF + ultrasound)
	Accent Ultra (RF + ultrasound)
	Reaction (vacuum and RF)
	Legend (TriLipo RF + DMA + TriFractional)
	Maximus (TriLipo RF + DMA + TriFractional)
	Thermage (monopolar RF 6.78 MHz 400 watt)
	Intragen (monopolar RF 6 MHz 200 watt)
Low-level laser therapy	Healite II

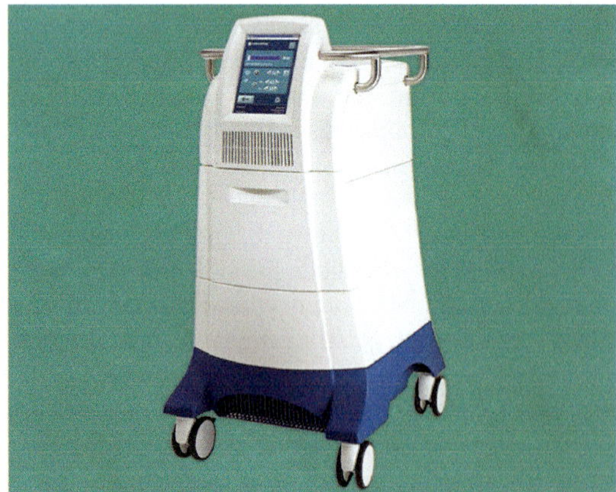

FIG. 1: CoolSculpting device.

surrounded by histiocytes, neutrophils, lymphocytes, and other mononuclear cells. After 14-30 days, macrophages and other phagocytes surround, and digest the lipid cells as a part of the body's natural reaction to injury. Thereafter, by 4 weeks, the inflammation decreases leading to reduction in adipocyte volume. After 2-3 months of treatment, the interlobular septa are significantly thickened and the inflammatory process further reduces. By this time, the fat volume in the treated area is apparently lesser and the septae form the majority of the tissue volume.[7]

Sasaki et al. have stated that the temperatures induced in cryolipolysis do not cause any permanent changes on the overlying dermis and epidermis. However, this cold ischemic injury may lead to cellular injury in adipose tissue via cellular edema, decreased Na^+/K^+-ATPase activity, decreased adenosine triphosphate, increased lactic acid levels, and release of mitochondrial free radicals. Another possible mechanism could be an initial insult of crystallization and cold ischemic injury induced by cryolipolysis, which is further compounded by ischemia-reperfusion injury. This leads to the generation of reactive oxygen species, increased cytosolic calcium levels, and stimulation of apoptotic pathways.[8]

Boey et al. suggested that manual massage improves clinical outcomes from cryolipolysis. Manual massage after cryolipolysis aid to lymphatic drainage and may also reduce discomfort, such as numbness, after the procedure.[9]

Cryolipolysis has been found to be safe and effective, with a satisfaction rate as high 73% after one treatment.[10] However, it has several limitations, such as a relatively long treatment duration (30-60 min for one application), discomfort during procedure, and limitations of the contour of an applicator. Side effects associated with cryolipolysis as seen in some studies, include temporary erythema, bruising, and numbness. These effects usually resolve within 2 weeks after treatment.[11] Cryolipolysis is considered safe for all skin types, even with repeated application and no reported pigmentary changes.[12]

HIGH-INTENSITY FOCUSED ULTRASOUND

High-intensity focused ultrasound was introduced in 1942 for therapeutic uses and is being used for treating kidney stones, uterine fibroids, and organ tumors for more than 50 years without using aggressive procedures.[13] However, recently HIFU has gained popularity as a noninvasive method for body contouring.[5] The currently available ultrasound technologies are nonselective, produce heat, and are thus liable to cause epidermal injury. Thus ideal ultrasound technology is needed, which will nonthermally and selectively disrupt/destroy adipocyte membrane integrity, without causing significant damage to the epidermis or to nearby cells in the adipose layer, such as blood vessels or nerves.

High-intensity focused ultrasound energy cuts off targeted adipose tissue with the help of an external transducer (Fig. 2) without having any effects on surrounding tissues. Due to elevated convergence of ultrasound energy at high frequencies, tissue damage is confined to a small focal point. Ultrasound energy causes molecular vibrations at the zone, which then stimulates a raised temperature at targeted tissue above 56°C and coagulative necrosis of adipocytes.[14]

High-intensity focused ultrasound can lyse fat cells through a mechanical compression wave (>20 kHz) and by formation of heat. Ultrasound

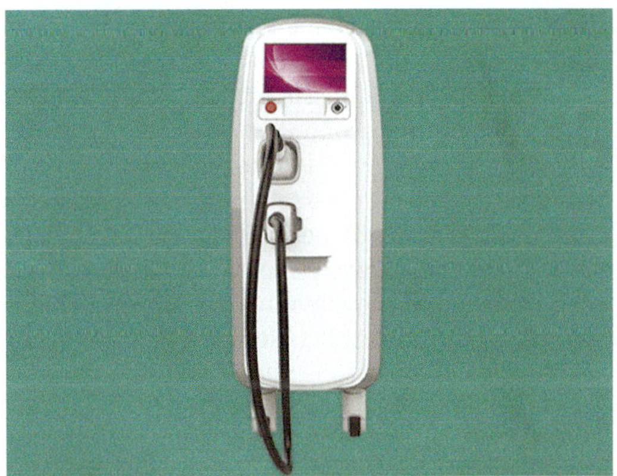

FIG. 2: Body high-intensity focused ultrasound.

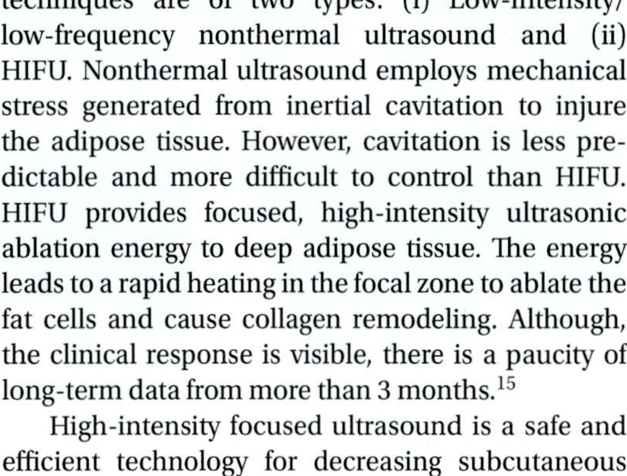

techniques are of two types: (i) Low-intensity/low-frequency nonthermal ultrasound and (ii) HIFU. Nonthermal ultrasound employs mechanical stress generated from inertial cavitation to injure the adipose tissue. However, cavitation is less predictable and more difficult to control than HIFU. HIFU provides focused, high-intensity ultrasonic ablation energy to deep adipose tissue. The energy leads to a rapid heating in the focal zone to ablate the fat cells and cause collagen remodeling. Although, the clinical response is visible, there is a paucity of long-term data from more than 3 months.[15]

High-intensity focused ultrasound is a safe and efficient technology for decreasing subcutaneous adipose tissue with minimal effects on blood lipid or inflammatory markers. Due to the availability of contact cooling in body HIFU devices, no local adverse effects such as epidermal burns or scarring are seen (Fig. 3). Studies have shown a self-reported patient's satisfaction of approximately 47–86% with the use of HIFU for body contouring. These results are not dependent on diet or physical activity. Moreover, it also has the advantage of minimal recovery time. There is no considerable reported effect on body mass index (BMI) or body weight.[16]

RADIOFREQUENCY

Although laser and light-based devices are able to reach up to deep dermal layers, light scattering and absorption of energy by chromophore melanin limit their thermal effects.[17] Radiofrequency is electromagnetic energy in frequency range of 3 kHz to 1 MHz. As the epidermal melanin does not scatter or absorb the radio waves, they are suitable for treating all skin types. Radiofrequency produces sufficient heat without causing a hazardous effect on epidermal integrity.[18]

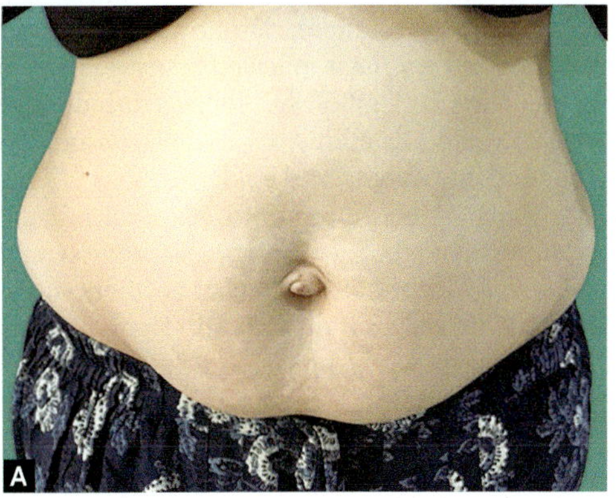

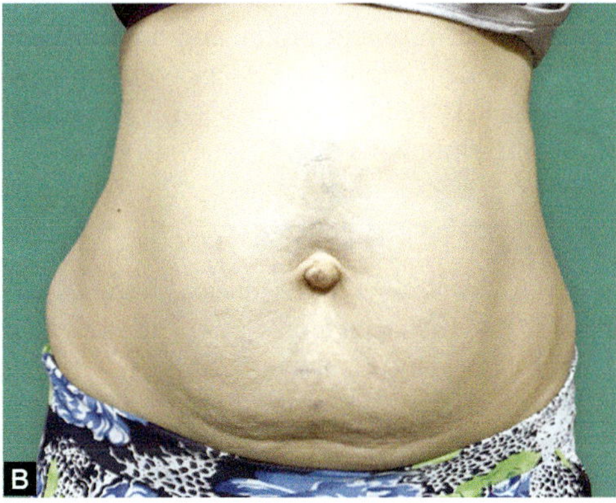

FIG. 3: Before and 3 months after three sessions of high-intensity focused ultrasound treatment.

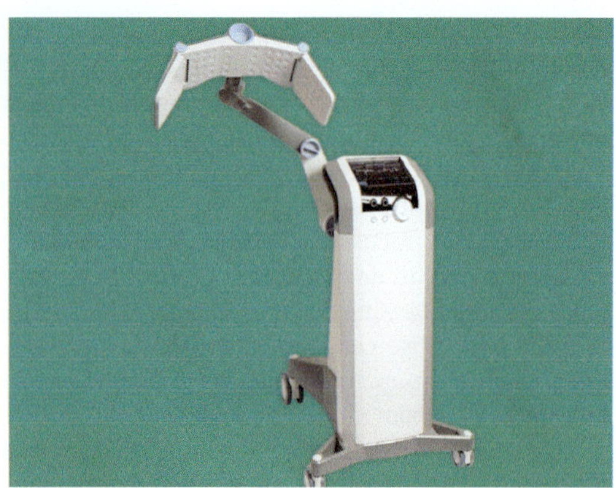

FIG. 4: Radiofrequency device for fat reduction.

Several RF devices have been developed since the year 2005, when the first RF device was approved by the FDA for cellulite. Radiofrequency devices generate thermal energy through the high tissue resistance of fat cells. Fat cells have relatively low heat transfer coefficients and thus transmit little heat to neighboring structures. This action mechanism leads to localized adipocyte thermolysis. In addition, RF heating has been shown to improve dermal collagen, elastin, and ground substances, causing skin tightening.[5]

Radiofrequency is used for skin tightening, and for fat or cellulite reduction. Radiofrequency can be employed in two ways with monopolar and bi/multipolar devices. In the former, energy passes from a single electrode to subcutaneous tissues through the skin and then to a return pad. The latter has two or more electrodes within the same handpiece where the energy passes in between the electrodes to generate heat. Thus, monopolar devices can enter deeper than bipolar devices.[19] Older RF devices caused skin tightening rather than fat destruction, with limitations in managing pain during the procedure and prolonging the transient effect.[20] Recently, various RF devices with reported effectiveness in fat reduction have been developed to overcome the limitations (Fig. 4).

LOW-LEVEL LASER THERAPY

External low-level laser is used as a noninvasive lipolysis technique, which has been approved in the United States and Canada. It works by forming pores in adipose cell membranes through which lipids are released. There is a concern that fat released from fat cells moves into the bloodstream, affecting the lipid profile. However, this issue is controversial.[21] Mark et al. suggested that the biochemical mechanism of action of LLLT appears to elevate cyclic adenosine monophosphate production via cytochrome C oxidase activation. C oxidase activation causes a breakdown of cell lipids in fat cells and form transitory pores in their cell membrane with subsequent cell collapse. Therefore, LLLT may be a safe and effective alternative for decreasing the subcutaneous tissue volume.[22] Recently, a new 1,060 nm diode laser with distinct affinity for adipose tissue was introduced, but clinical trial data are still pending.

Laser lipolysis approved by FDA in 2006 is now very well accepted and a commonly employed technique for removing unwanted fatty tissue. Studies have continued to corroborate early clinical findings of reduced adiposity, lesser recovery times, and improved skin tightening. Throughout the last 5 years, it has been observed that laser lipolysis liquefies fatty tissue, coagulates small blood vessels, stimulates collagenases with remodeling, and causing skin tightening. Low-level laser therapy has been shown to be an adequate adjunct therapy for various cosmetic procedures, including breast augmentation and lipoplasty.[23]

With respect to body contouring, a randomized, double-blind, sham-controlled study using a 635 nm LLLT device showed a circumferential reduction of the waist, hips, and thighs after six treatments done over a 2-week period.[24] While remaining noninvasive and relatively free of risk, this device has been observed to provide other significant benefits including reduction in cholesterol and leptin levels.[25]

MESOTHERAPY (INJECTION LIPOLYSIS)

Phosphatidylcholine and deoxycholate have independently been used in lipolysis. The first use of this class of drugs was done to dissolve the intramural accumulations of atherosclerotic plaques in systemic arteries and was later followed by usage to treat the pulmonary fat embolism. These compounds also demonstrated an affinity for adipose tissue, sparing the overlying dermis, and epidermis.

The FDA recently approved a formulation of sodium deoxycholate 10 mg/mL for subcutaneous injection with the indication of aesthetic improvement of excess submental fat. Deoxycholic acid (DCA) exists endogenously as a bile salt emulsifier and has been shown to cause dose-dependent adipocyte lysis, necrosis, disruption and dissolution of fat architecture, and inflammatory targeting of adipocytes by immune cells.[26] Thus, DCA causes targeted adipocytolysis and is a novel medical agent in the treatment of fat. Supplied in 2 mL vials, clinicians may inject 10 mL at each treatment for up to 6 treatments administered 1 month apart.

Overall, DCA demonstrated high rates of minor injection site AEs that resolved without sequelae and could be mitigated by comfort therapies (e.g., lidocaine, nonsteroidal anti-inflammatory drugs) as well as understanding the anatomy of the submental region. Adverse effects of particular interest included marginal mandibular nerve palsy, skin ulceration, and dysphagia.[27]

CONCLUSION

There are several body contouring technologies available in the market. However, it is important to choose the appropriate device, depending on the treatment area, and therapeutic aim. A novel body contouring device is one that is safe, efficacious, and can be used in treating small areas. According to the existing evidence, the noninvasive techniques such as cryolipolysis, RF, LLLT, and HIFU have shown statistically significant results on body contouring and in removing unwanted fat. The reported results of such devices were mild to moderate and the mentioned techniques have little or no effect on weight reduction and on total percentage of body fat. The circumference reduction after noninvasive methods was found to be around 2 cm. An important aspect of body contouring methods is patient satisfaction after treatment, which is not obvious in most cases because most of the patients expect outcomes at par to surgical procedures. Focusing on the reduction of subcutaneous fat as a sole defining method is too challenging. The best candidates for these treatments are those within their ideal weight range and those exercises regularly, eat a healthy diet, have visible fat bulges on the trunk, have realistic expectations, and are willing to maintain their results with a healthy and active lifestyle.

REFERENCES

1. Mordon S, Plot E. Laser lipolysis versus traditional liposuction for fat removal. Expert Rev Med Devices. 2009;6(6):677-88.
2. Garibyan L, Sipprell WH, Jalian HR, et al. Three-dimensional volumetric quantification of fat loss following cryolipolysis. Lasers Surg Med. 2014;46(2):75-80.
3. Alderman AK, Collins ED, Streu R, et al. Benchmarking outcomes in plastic surgery: National complication rates for abdominoplasty and breast augmentation. Plast Reconstr Surg. 2009;124(6):2127-33.
4. Body Shaping and Cellulite Reduction: Technology Proliferation Driven by Demand. Aliso Viejo: Medical Insight Inc.; 2009.
5. Mulholland RS, Paul MD, Chalfoun C. Noninvasive body contouring with radiofrequency, ultrasound, cryolipolysis, and low-level laser therapy. Clin Plast Surg. 2011;38(3):503-20.
6. Manstein D, Laubach H, Watanabe K, et al. Selective cryolysis: A novel method of non-invasive fat removal. Lasers Surg Med. 2008;40(9):595-604.
7. Krueger N, Mai SV, Luebberding S, et al. Cryolipolysis for noninvasive body contouring: Clinical efficacy and patient satisfaction. Clin Cosmet Investig Dermatol. 2014;7:201-5.
8. Sasaki GH, Abelev N, Tevez-Ortiz A. Noninvasive selective cryolipolysis and reperfusion recovery for localized natural fat reduction and contouring. Aesthet Surg J. 2014;34(3):420-31.
9. Boey GE, Wasilenchuk JL. Enhanced clinical outcome with manual massage following cryolipolysis treatment: A 4-month study of safety and efficacy. Lasers Surg Med. 2014;46(1):20-6.
10. Dierickx CC, Mazer JM, Sand M, et al. Safety, tolerance, and patient satisfaction with noninvasive cryolipolysis. Dermatol Surg. 2013;39(8):1209-16.
11. Coleman SR, Sachdeva K, Egbert BM, et al. Clinical efficacy of noninvasive cryolipolysis and its effects on peripheral nerves. Aesthetic Plast Surg. 2009;33(4):482-8.
12. Stevens WG, Pietrzak LK, Spring MA. Broad overview of a clinical and commercial experience with CoolSculpting. Aesthet Surg J. 2013;33(6):835-46.
13. Wu F, Wang ZB, Chen WZ, et al. Extracorporeal high intensity focused ultrasound ablation in the treatment of 1038 patients with solid carcinomas in China: An overview. Ultrason Sonochem. 2004;11(3-4):149-54.
14. Shek SY, Yeung CK, Chan JC, et al. Efficacy of high-intensity focused ultrasonography for noninvasive body sculpting in Chinese patients. Lasers Surg Med. 2014;46(4):263-9.
15. Fatemi A, Kane MA. High-intensity focused ultrasound effectively reduces waist circumference by ablating adipose tissue from the abdomen and flanks: A retrospective case series. Aesthetic Plast Surg. 2010; 34(5):577-82.
16. Gadsden E, Aguilar MT, Smoller BR, et al. Evaluation of a novel high-intensity focused ultrasound device for ablating subcutaneous adipose tissue for noninvasive body contouring: safety studies in human volunteers. Aesthet Surg J. 2011;31(4):401-10.
17. Nassab R. The evidence behind noninvasive body contouring devices. Aesthet Surg J. 2015;35(3):279-93.
18. Brightman L, Weiss E, Chapas AM, et al. Improvement in arm and post-partum abdominal and flank subcutaneous fat deposits and skin laxity using a bipolar radiofrequency, infrared, vacuum and mechanical massage device. Lasers Surg Med. 2009;41(10):791-8.
19. Goldberg DJ, Fazeli A, Berlin AL. Clinical, laboratory, and MRI analysis of cellulite treatment with a unipolar

radiofrequency device. Dermatol Surg. 2008;34(2): 204-9.

20. Manuskiatti W, Wachirakaphan C, Lektrakul N, et al. Circumference reduction and cellulite treatment with a TriPollar radiofrequency device: a pilot study. J Eur Acad Dermatol Venereol. 2009;23(7):820-7.
21. Jewell ML, Solish NJ, Desilets CS. Noninvasive body sculpting technologies with an emphasis on high-intensity focused ultrasound. Aesthetic Plast Surg. 2011;35(5):901-12.
22. Nestor MS, Zarraga MB, Park H. Effect of 635nm Low-Level Laser Therapy on Upper Arm Circumference Reduction: A Double-blind, Randomized, Sham-controlled Trial. J Clin Aesthet Dermatol. 2012;5(2):42-8.
23. McBean JC, Katz BE. Laser lipolysis: An update. J Clin Aesthet Dermatol. 2011;4(7):25-34.
24. Neira R, Ortiz-Neiraq C. Low-level laser-assisted liposculpture: clinical report of 700 second cases. Aesthetic Surg J. 2002;22(1):451-5.
25. Maloney R, Shanks S, Jenney E. The reduction in cholesterol and triglyceride serum levels following low-level laser irradiation: a non-controlled, non-randomized pilot study. Laser Surg Med. 2009;21:66.
26. Yagima Odo ME, Cucé LC, Odo LM, et al. Action of sodium deoxycholate on subcutaneous human tissue: local and systemic effects. Dermatol Surg. 2007;33(2):178-88.
27. Fagien S, McChesney P, Subramanian M, et al. Prevention and Management of Injection-Related Adverse Effects in Facial Aesthetics: Considerations for ATX-101 (Deoxycholic Acid Injection) Treatment. Dermatol Surg. 2016 Nov;42 Suppl 1:S300-S304.

Index

Page numbers followed by *b* refer to box, *f* refer to figure, *fc* refer to flowchart, and *t* refer to table.

B

C

D

E

O

P

W

X

Y

Z